Craig's
RESTORATIVE
DENTAL
MATERIALS

Craig's
RESTORATIVE DENTAL MATERIALS

THIRTEENTH EDITION

EDITED BY

Ronald L. Sakaguchi, DDS, MS, PhD, MBA
Associate Dean for Research and Innovation
Professor
Division of Biomaterials and Biomechanics
Department of Restorative Dentistry
School of Dentistry
Oregon Health and Science University
Portland, Oregon

John M. Powers, PhD
Editor
The Dental Advisor
Dental Consultants, Inc
Ann Arbor, Michigan

Professor of Oral Biomaterials
Department of Restorative Dentistry and Biomaterials
UTHealth School of Dentistry
The University of Texas Health Science Center at Houston
Houston, Texas

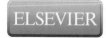

MOSBY

1600 John F. Kennedy Blvd.
Ste 1800
Philadelphia, PA 19103-2899

CRAIG'S RESTORATIVE DENTAL MATERIALS ISBN: **978-0-3230-8108-5**

Copyright © 2012, 2006, 2002, 1997, 1993, 1989, 1985, 1980, 1975, 1971, 1968, 1964, 1960 by Mosby, Inc.,
an affiliate of Elsevier Inc.

Library of Congress Cataloging-in-Publication Data

Craig's restorative dental materials / edited by Ronald L. Sakaguchi, John M. Powers. -- 13th ed.
 p. ; cm.
 Restorative dental materials
 Order of editors reversed on prev. ed.
Includes bibliographical references and index.
 ISBN 978-0-323-08108-5 (pbk. : alk. paper) 1. Dental materials. I. Sakaguchi, Ronald L.
II. Powers, John M., 1946- III. Title: Restorative dental materials.
 [DNLM: 1. Dental Materials. 2. Dental Atraumatic Restorative Treatment. WU 190]
 RK652.5.P47 2012
 617.6'95--dc23

                  2011015522

Vice President and Publishing Director: Linda Duncan
Executive Editor: John J. Dolan
Developmental Editor: Brian S. Loehr
Publishing Services Manager: Catherine Jackson/Hemamalini Rajendrababu
Project Manager: Sara Alsup/Divya Krish
Designer: Amy Buxton

Printed in United States
Last digit is the print number: 9 8 7 6 5 4 3 2 1

To the many mentors and colleagues
with whom we have collaborated.

Contributors

Roberto R. Braga, DDS, MS, PhD
Professor
Department of Dental Materials
School of Dentistry
University of São Paulo
São Paulo, SP, Brazil
Chapter 5: Testing of Dental Materials and Biomechanics
Chapter 13: Materials for Adhesion and Luting

Isabelle L. Denry, DDS, PhD
Professor
Department of Prosthodontics and Dows Institute
for Dental Research
College of Dentistry
The University of Iowa
Iowa City, Iowa
Chapter 11: Restorative Materials—Ceramics

Jack L. Ferracane, PhD
Professor and Chair
Department of Restorative Dentistry
Division Director, Biomaterials and Biomechanics
School of Dentistry
Oregon Health & Science University
Portland, Oregon
Chapter 6: Biocompatibility and Tissue Reaction to
*   Biomaterials*

Sharukh S. Khajotia, BDS, MS, PhD
Professor and Chair
Department of Restorative Dentistry
College of Dentistry
University of Oklahoma Health Sciences Center
Oklahoma City, Oklahoma
Chapter 2: The Oral Environment

David B. Mahler, PhD
Professor Emeritus
Division of Biomaterials and Biomechanics
Department of Restorative Dentistry
School of Dentistry
Oregon Health and Science University
Portland, Oregon
Chapter 10: Restorative Materials—Metals

Grayson W. Marshall, DDS, MPH, PhD
Distinguished Professor and Chair
Division of Biomaterials and Bioengineering
Vice-Chair, Department of Preventive and
Restorative Dental Sciences
School of Dentistry
University of California San Francisco
San Francisco, California
Chapter 2: The Oral Environment

Sally J. Marshall, PhD
Vice Provost, Academic Affairs
Director of the Office of Faculty Development and
Advancement
Distinguished Professor Division of Biomaterials
and Bioengineering
Department of Preventive and Restorative Dental
Sciences
School of Dentistry
University of California San Francisco
San Francisco, California
Chapter 2: The Oral Environment

John C. Mitchell, PhD
Associate Professor
Division of Biomaterials and Biomechanics
Department of Restorative Dentistry
School of Dentistry
Oregon Health and Science University
Portland, Oregon
Chapter 6: Biocompatibility and Tissue Reaction to
*   Biomaterials*
Chapter 15: Dental and Orofacial Implants
Chapter 16: Tissue Engineering

Sumita B. Mitra, PhD
Partner
Mitra Chemical Consulting, LLC
West St. Paul, Minnesota
Chapter 9: Restorative Materials—Polymers
Chapter 13: Materials for Adhesion and Luting

Kiersten L. Muenchinger, AB, MS
Program Director and Associate Professor
Product Design
School of Architecture and Allied Arts
University of Oregon
Eugene, Oregon
Chapter 3: Design Criteria for Restorative Dental Materials

Carmem S. Pfeifer, DDS, PhD
Research Assistant Professor
Department of Craniofacial Biology
School of Dental Medicine
University of Colorado
Aurora, Colorado
Chapter 4: Fundamentals of Materials Science
Chapter 5: Testing of Dental Materials and Biomechanics

John M. Powers, PhD
Editor
The Dental Advisor
Dental Consultants, Inc.
Ann Arbor, Michigan

Professor of Oral Biomaterials
Department of Restorative Dentistry
and Biomaterials
UTHealth School of Dentistry
The University of Texas Health Science Center
at Houston
Houston, Texas
Chapter 12: Replicating Materials—Impression and Casting
*Chapter 14: Digital Imaging and Processing for
  Restorations*

Ronald L. Sakaguchi, DDS, MS, PhD, MBA
Associate Dean for Research and Innovation
Professor
Division of Biomaterials and Biomechanics
Department of Restorative Dentistry
School of Dentistry
Oregon Health and Science University
Portland, Oregon
*Chapter 1: Role and Significance of Restorative Dental
  Materials*
Chapter 3: Design Criteria for Restorative Dental Materials
Chapter 4: Fundamentals of Materials Science
Chapter 5: Testing of Dental Materials and Biomechanics
Chapter 7: General Classes of Biomaterials
Chapter 8: Preventive and Intermediary Materials
Chapter 9: Restorative Materials—Composites and Polymers
Chapter 10: Restorative Materials—Metals
*Chapter 14: Digital Imaging and Processing for
  Restorations*
Chapter 15: Dental and Orofacial Implants

Preface

The thirteenth edition of this classic textbook has been extensively rewritten to include the many recent developments in dental biomaterials science and new materials for clinical use. One of our goals for this edition is to include more clinical applications and examples, with the hope that the book will be more useful to practicing clinicians. The book continues to be designed for predoctoral dental students and also provides an excellent update of dental biomaterials science and clinical applications of restorative materials for students in graduate programs and residencies.

Dr. Ronald L. Sakaguchi is the new lead editor of the thirteenth edition. Dr. Sakaguchi earned a BS in cybernetics from University of California Los Angeles (UCLA), a DDS from Northwestern University, an MS in prosthodontics from the University of Minnesota, and a PhD in biomaterials and biomechanics from Thames Polytechnic (London, England; now the University of Greenwich). He is currently Associate Dean for Research & Innovation and a professor in the Division of Biomaterials & Biomechanics in the Department of Restorative Dentistry at Oregon Health & Science University (OHSU) in Portland, Oregon.

Dr. John M. Powers is the new co-editor of the thirteenth edition. He served as the lead editor of the twelfth edition and contributed to the previous eight editions. Dr. Powers earned a BS in chemistry and a PhD in mechanical engineering and dental materials at the University of Michigan, was a faculty member at the School of Dentistry at the University of Michigan for a number of years, and is currently a professor of oral biomaterials in the Department of Restorative Dentistry and Biomaterials at the UTHealth School of Dentistry, The University of Texas Health Science Center at Houston. He was formerly Director of the Houston Biomaterials Research Center. Dr. Powers is also senior vice president of Dental Consultants, Inc., and is co-editor of *The Dental Advisor*.

The team of editors and authors for the thirteenth edition spans three generations of dental researchers and educators. Dr. Sakaguchi received his first exposure to dental biomaterials science as a first-year dental student at Northwestern University Dental School. Drs. Bill and Sally Marshall were the instructors for those courses. After many years of mentoring received from Drs. Bill Douglas and Ralph DeLong, and Ms. Maria Pintado at the University of Minnesota, Dr. Sakaguchi joined the biomaterials research team in the School of Dentistry at OHSU with

Drs. David Mahler, Jack Mitchem and Jack Ferracane. The OHSU laboratory benefited from the contributions of many visiting professors, post-doctoral fellows, and graduate students, including Dr. Carmem Pfeifer who conducted her PhD research in our laboratory. Thanks to the many mentors who generously contributed directly and indirectly to this edition of the book.

We welcome the following new contributors to the thirteenth edition and thank them for their effort and expertise: Drs. Bill and Sally Marshall of University of California San Francisco (UCSF); Dr. Sumita Mitra of Mitra Chemical Consulting, LLC, and many years at 3M ESPE; Dr. Jack Ferracane of OHSU; Dr. Roberto Braga of the University of São Paulo; Dr. Sharukh Khajotia of the University of Oklahoma; Dr. Carmem Pfeifer of the University of Colorado, and Professor Kiersten Muenchinger of the University of Oregon. We also thank the following returning authors for their valuable contributions and refinements of content in the thirteenth edition: Dr. David Mahler of OHSU, Dr. John Mitchell of OHSU, and Dr. Isabelle Denry of the University of Iowa, previously at The Ohio State University.

The organization of the thirteenth edition has been modified extensively to reflect the sequence of content presented to predoctoral dental students at OHSU. Chapters are organized by major clinical procedures. Chapter 2 presents new content on enamel, dentin, the dentinoenamel junction, and biofilms. Chapter 3, another new chapter, describes the concepts of product design and their applications in restorative material selection and treatment design. Fundamentals of materials science, including the presentation of physical and mechanical properties, the concepts of biomechanics, surface chemistry, and optical properties, are consolidated in Chapter 4. Materials testing is discussed in extensively revised Chapter 5, which has a greater emphasis on contemporary testing methods and standards. Chapter 14, new to this edition, is devoted to digital imaging and processing techniques and the materials for those methods. All other chapters are reorganized and updated with the most recent science and applications.

A website accompanies this textbook. Included is the majority of the procedural, or materials handling, content that was in the twelfth edition. The website can be found at http://evolve.elsevier.com/Sakaguchi/restorative/, where you will also find mindmaps of each chapter and extensive text and graphics to supplement the print version of the book.

Acknowledgments

We are deeply grateful to John Dolan, Executive Editor at Elsevier, for his guidance in the initial planning and approval of the project; to Brian Loehr, Senior Developmental Editor at Elsevier, for his many suggestions and support and prodding throughout the design process and writing of the manuscript. Jodie Bernard and her team at Lightbox Visuals were amazing in their ability to create new four-color images from the original black and white figures. We thank Sara Alsup, Associate Project Manager at Elsevier, and her team of copyeditors for greatly improving the style, consistency, and readability of the text. Thanks also to many others at Elsevier for their behind-the-scenes work and contributions to the book.

Lastly, we thank our colleagues in our respective institutions for the many informal chats and suggestions offered and our families who put up with us being at our computers late in the evenings and on many weekends. It truly does take a community to create a work like this textbook and we thank you all.

Ronald L. Sakaguchi
John M. Powers

Contents

1

Role and Significance of Restorative Dental Materials

Developments in materials science, robotics, and biomechanics have dramatically changed the way we look at the replacement of components of the human anatomy. In the historical record, we find many approaches to replacing missing tooth structure and whole teeth. The replacement of tooth structure lost to disease and injury continues to be a large part of general dental practice. Restorative dental materials are the foundation for the replacement of tooth structure.

Form and function are important considerations in the replacement of lost tooth structure. Although tooth form and appearance are aspects most easily recognized, function of the teeth and supporting tissues contributes greatly to the quality of life. The links between oral and general health are widely accepted. Proper function of the elements of the oral cavity, including the teeth and soft tissues, is needed for eating, speaking, swallowing, and proper breathing.

Restorative dental materials make the reconstruction of the dental hard tissues possible. In many areas, the development of dental materials has progressed more rapidly than for other anatomical prostheses. Because of their long-term success, patients often expect dental prostheses to outperform the natural materials they replace. The application of materials science is unique in dentistry because of the complexity of the oral cavity, which includes bacteria, high forces, ever changing pH, and a warm, fluid environment. The oral cavity is considered to be the harshest environment for a material in the body. In addition, when dental materials are placed directly into tooth cavities as restorative materials, there are very specific requirements for manipulation of the material. Knowledge of materials science and biomechanics is very important when choosing materials for specific dental applications and when designing the best solution for restoration of tooth structure and replacement of teeth.

SCOPE OF MATERIALS COVERED IN RESTORATIVE DENTISTRY

Restorative dental materials include representatives from the broad classes of materials: metals, polymers, ceramics, and composites. Dental materials include such items as resin composites, cements, glass ionomers, ceramics, noble and base metals, amalgam alloys, gypsum materials, casting investments, dental waxes, impression materials, denture base resins, and other materials used in restorative procedures. The demands for material characteristics and performance range from high flexibility required by impression materials to high stiffness required in crowns and fixed dental prostheses. Materials for dental implants require integration with bone.

Some materials are cast to achieve excellent adaptation to existing tooth structure, whereas others are machined to produce very reproducible dimensions and structured geometries. When describing these materials, physical and chemical characteristics are often used as criteria for comparison. To understand how a material works, we study its chemical structure, its physical and mechanical characteristics, and how it should be manipulated to produce the best performance.

Most restorative materials are characterized by physical, chemical, and mechanical parameters that are derived from test data. Improvements in these characteristics might be attractive in laboratory studies, but the real test is the material's performance in the mouth and the ability of the material to be manipulated properly by the dental team. In many cases, manipulative errors can negate the technological advances for the material. It is therefore very important for the dental team to understand fundamental materials science and biomechanics to select and manipulate dental materials appropriately.

BASIC SCIENCES APPLIED TO RESTORATIVE MATERIALS

The practice of clinical dentistry depends not only on a complete understanding of the various clinical techniques but also on an appreciation of the fundamental biological, chemical, and physical principles that support the clinical applications. It is important to understand the 'how' and 'why' associated with the function of natural and synthetic dental materials.

A systems approach to assessing the chemical, physical, and engineering aspects of dental materials and oral function along with the physiological, pathological, and other biological studies of the tissues that support the restorative structures provides the best patient outcomes. This integrative approach, when combined with the best available scientific evidence, clinician experience, patient preferences, and patient modifiers results in the best patient-centered care.

APPLICATION OF VARIOUS SCIENCES

In the chapters that follow, fundamental characteristics of materials are presented along with numerous practical examples of how the basic principles relate to clinical applications. Test procedures and techniques of manipulation are discussed briefly but not emphasized. Many of the details of manipulation have been moved to the book's website at http://evolve.elsevier.com/sakaguchi/restorative ⊖

A more complete understanding of fundamental principles of materials and mechanics is important for the clinician to design and provide a prognosis for restorations. For example, the prognosis of long-span fixed dental prostheses, or bridges, is dependent on the stiffness and elasticity of the materials. When considering esthetics, the hardness of the material is an important property because it influences the ability to polish the material. Some materials release fluoride when exposed to water, which might be beneficial in high-caries-risk patients. When selecting a ceramic for in-office fabrication of an all-ceramic crown, the machining characteristic of ceramics is important. Implants have a range of bone and soft tissue adaptation that are dependent on surface texture, coatings, and implant geometry. These are just a few examples of the many interactions between the clinical performance of dental materials and fundamental scientific principles.

The toxicity of and tissue reactions to dental materials are receiving more attention as a wider variety of materials are being used and as federal agencies demonstrate more concern in this area. A further indication of the importance of the interaction of materials and tissues is the development of recommended standard practices and tests for the biological interaction of materials through the auspices of the American Dental Association (ADA).

After many centuries of dental practice, we continue to be confronted with the problem of replacing tooth tissue lost by either accident or disease. In an effort to constantly improve our restorative capabilities, the dental profession will continue to draw from materials science, product design, engineering, biology, chemistry, and the arts to further develop an integrated practice of dentistry.

FUTURE DEVELOPMENTS IN BIOMATERIALS

In the United States over 60% of adults aged 35 to 44 have lost at least one permanent tooth to an accident, gum disease, a failed root canal, or tooth decay. In the 64- to 65-year-old category, 25% of adults have lost all of their natural teeth. For children aged 6 to 8, 26% have untreated dental caries, and 50% have been treated for dental decay. The demand for restorative care is tremendous. Advances in endodontology and periodontology enable people to retain teeth longer, shifting restorative care from replacement of teeth to long-term restoration and maintenance. Development of successful implant therapies has encouraged patients to replace individual teeth with fixed, single tooth restorations rather than with fixed or removable dental prostheses. For those patients with good access to dental care, single tooth replacements with

implants are becoming a more popular option because they do not involve the preparation of adjacent teeth as for a fixed, multi-unit restoration. Research into implant coatings, surface textures, graded properties, alternative materials, and new geometries will continue to grow. For those with less adequate access, removable prostheses will continue to be used.

An emphasis on esthetics continues to be popular among consumers, and this will continue to drive the development of tooth whitening systems and esthetic restorations. There appears to be an emerging trend for a more natural looking appearance with some individuality as opposed to the uniform, sparkling white dentition that was previously requested by many patients. This will encourage manufacturers to develop materials that mimic natural dentition even more closely by providing the same depth of color and optical characteristics of natural teeth.

With the aging of the population, restorations for exposed root surfaces and worn dentitions will become more common. These materials will need to function in an environment with reduced salivary flow and atypical salivary pH and chemistry. Adhesion to these surfaces will be more challenging. This segment of the population will be managing multiple chronic diseases with many medications and will have difficulty maintaining an adequate regimen of oral home care. Restorative materials will be challenged in this difficult environment.

The interaction between the fields of biomaterials and molecular biology is growing rapidly. Advances in tissue regeneration will accelerate. The developments in nanotechnology will soon have a major impact on materials science. The properties we currently understand at the macro and micro levels will be very different at the nano level. Biofabrication and bioprinting methods are creating new structures and materials. This is a very exciting time for materials research and clinicians will have much to look forward to in the near future as this body of research develops new materials for clinical applications.

Bibliography

American Association of Oral and Maxillofacial Surgeons: *Dental implants*. http://www.aaoms.org/dental_implants.php. Accessed August 28, 2011.

Centers for Disease Control and Prevention: *National Health and Nutrition Examination Study*. http://www.cdc.gov/nchs/nhanes/nhanes2005-2006/nhanes05_06.htm. Accessed August 28, 2011.

Choi CK, Breckenridge MT, Chen CS: Engineered materials and the cellular microenvironment: a strengthening interface between cell biology and bioengineering, *Trends Cell Biol* 20(12):705, 2010.

Horowitz RA, Coelho PG: Endosseus implant: the journey and the future, *Compend Contin Educ Dent* 31(7):545, 2010.

Jones JR, Boccaccini AR: Editorial: a forecast of the future for biomaterials, *J Mater Sci: Mater Med* 17:963, 2006.

Kohn DH: Current and future research trends in dental biomaterials, *Biomat Forum* 19(1):23, 1997.

Nakamura M, Iwanaga S, Henmi C, et al: Biomatrices and biomaterials for future developments of bioprinting and biofabrication, *Biofabrication* 2(1):014110, 2010 Mar 10. Epub.

National Center for Chronic Disease Prevention and Health Promotion (CDC): Oral health, preventing cavities, gum disease, tooth loss, and oral cancers, at a glance, 2010.

National Institute of Dental Research: National Institutes of Health (NIH): *International state-of-the-art conference on restorative dental materials*, Bethesda, MD, Sept 8-10, 1986, NIH.

National Institute of Dental and Craniofacial Research: *A plan to eliminate craniofacial, oral, and dental health disparities*, 2002. http://www.nidcr.nih.gov/NR/rdonlyres/54B65018-D3FE-4459-86DD-AAA0AD51C82B/0/hdplan.pdf.

Oregon Department of Human Services, Public Health Division: The burden of oral disease in Oregon, Nov, 2006.

U.S. Department of Health and Human Services: *Oral health in America: a report of the Surgeon General—executive summary*, Rockville, MD, 2000, U.S. Department of Health and Human Services, National Institute of Dental and Craniofacial Research, National Institutes of Health.

The Oral Environment

The tooth contains three specialized calcified tissues: enamel, dentin, and cementum (Figure 2-1). Enamel is unique in that it is the most highly calcified tissue in the body and contains the least organic content of any of these tissues. Enamel provides the hard outer covering of the crown that allows efficient mastication. Dentin and cementum, like bone, are vital, hydrated, biological composite structures formed mainly from a collagen type I matrix reinforced with the calcium phosphate mineral called *apatite*. Dentin forms the bulk of the tooth and is joined to the enamel at the dentin-enamel junction (DEJ). The dentin of the tooth root is covered by cementum that provides connection of the tooth to the alveolar bone via the periodontal ligament. Although the structure of these tissues is often described in dental texts, the properties are often discussed only superficially. However, these properties are important in regard to the interrelationships of the factors that contribute to the performance necessary for the optimum function of these tissues.

In restorative dentistry we are interested in providing preventive treatments that will maintain tissue integrity and replace damaged tissues with materials that ideally will mimic the natural appearance and performance of those tissues when necessary. Thus knowledge of the structure and properties of these tissues is desirable both as a yardstick to measure the properties and performance of restorative materials and as a guide to the development of materials that will mimic their structure and function. In addition, many applications, such as dental bonding, require us to attach synthetic materials to the calcified tissues, and these procedures rely on detailed knowledge of the structure and properties of the adhesive tissue substrates.

ENAMEL

Figure 2-1 shows a schematic diagram of a posterior tooth sectioned to reveal the enamel and dentin components. Enamel forms the hard outer shell of the crown and as the most highly calcified tissue is well suited to resisting wear due to mastication.

Enamel is formed by ameloblasts starting at the dentin-enamel junction (DEJ) and proceeding outward to the tooth surface. The ameloblasts exchange signals with odontoblasts located on the other side of the DEJ at the start of the enamel and dentin formation, and the odontoblasts move inward from the DEJ as the ameloblasts forming enamel move outward to form the enamel of the crown. Most of the enamel organic matrix composed of amelogenins and enamelins is resorbed during tooth maturation to leave a calcified tissue that is largely composed of mineral and a sparse organic matrix. The structural arrangement of enamel forms keyhole-shaped structures known as *enamel prisms* or *rods* that are about 5 μm across as seen in Figure 2-2.

The overall composition is about 96% mineral by weight, with 1% lipid and protein and the remainder being water. The organic portion and water probably play important roles in tooth function and pathology, and it is often more useful to describe the composition on a volume basis. On that basis we see the organic components make up about 3% and water 12% of the structure. The mineral is formed and grows into very long crystals of hexagonal shape about 40 nm across; these have not been synthetically duplicated. There is some evidence that the crystals may span the whole enamel thickness, but this is difficult to prove because most preparation procedures lead to fracture of the individual crystallites. It appears that they are at least thousands of nanometers long. If this is true, then enamel crystals provide an extraordinary "aspect" ratio (length to width ratio) for a nanoscale material, and they are very different from the much smaller dentin crystals. The crystals are packed into enamel prisms or rods that are about 5 μm across as shown in Figure 2-2. These prisms are revealed easily by acid etching and extend in a closely packed array from the DEJ to the enamel surface and lie roughly perpendicular to the DEJ, except in cuspal areas where the rods twist and cross, known as *decussation*, which may increase fracture resistance. About 100 crystals of the mineral are needed to span the diameter of a prism, and the long axes of the crystals tend to align themselves along the prism axes, as seen in Figure 2-2.

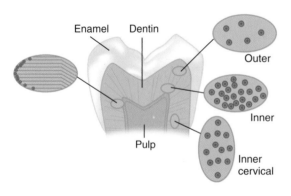

FIGURE 2.1 **Schematic diagram of a tooth cut longitudinally to expose the enamel, dentin, and the pulp chamber.** On the right side are illustrations of dentin tubules as viewed from the top, which shows the variation in the tubule number with location. At the left is an illustration of the change in direction of the primary dentin tubules as secondary dentin is formed. *(From Marshall SJ, et al: Acta. Mater. 46, 2529-2539, 1998.)*

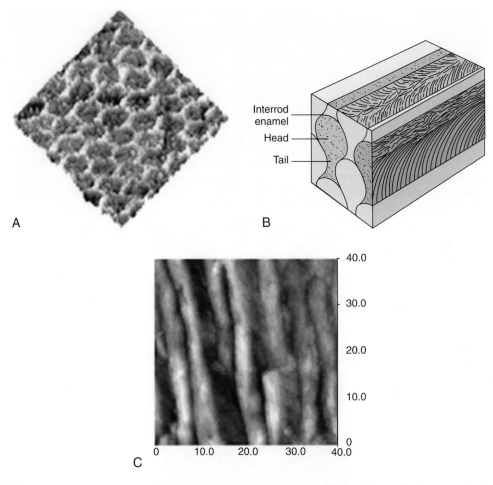

FIGURE 2.2 Enamel microstructure showing a schematic diagram of keyhole-shaped enamel prisms or rods about 5 μm in diameter (**B**). Atomic force microscopy (AFM) images showing prism cross sections in **A** and along axes of the prisms in **C**. Crystallite orientation deviates in the inter-rod and tail area, and the organic content increases in the inter-rod area. *(Modified from Habelitz S, et al: Arch. Oral Biol. 46, 173-183, 2001.)*

The crystals near the periphery of each prism deviate somewhat from the long axis toward the interface between prisms. The deviation in the tail of the prism is even greater. The individual crystals within a prism are also coated with a thin layer of lipid and/or protein that plays important roles in mineralization, although much still remains to be learned about the details. Recent work suggests that this protein coat may lead to increased toughness of the enamel. The interfaces between prisms, or inter-rod enamel, contain the main organic components of the structure and act as passageways for water and ionic movement. These areas are also known as *prism sheaths*. These regions are of vital importance in etching processes associated with bonding and other demineralization processes, such as caries.

Etching of enamel with acids such as phosphoric acid, commonly used in enamel bonding, eliminates smear layers associated with cavity preparation, dissolves persisting layers of prismless enamel in deciduous teeth, and differentially dissolves enamel crystals in each prism. The pattern of etched enamel is categorized as type 1 (preferential prism core etching, Figure 2-2, A); type 2 (preferential prism periphery etching, Figure 2-3, C), and type 3 (mixed or uniform). Sometimes these patterns appear side by side on the same tooth surface (Figure 2-3, E). No differences in micromechanical bond strength of the different etching patterns have been established. In a standard cavity preparation for a composite, the orientation of the enamel surfaces being etched could be perpendicular to enamel prisms (perimeter of the cavity outline), oblique cross section of the prisms (beveled occlusal or proximal margins), and axial walls of the prisms (cavity preparation walls). During the early stages of etching, when only a small amount of enamel crystal dissolution occurs, it may be difficult or impossible to detect the extent of the

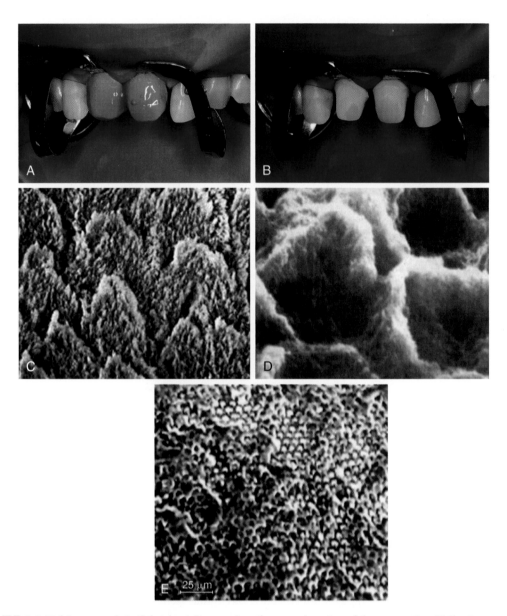

FIGURE 2.3 Etching enamel. A, Gel etchant dispensed on the enamel portion of the preparation. **B,** Frosty appearance after etching, rinsing and drying. **C,** Magnified view of etch pattern with preferential prism periphery etch (type 1). **D,** Bonding agent revealed after dissolving enamel. **E,** Mixed etch patterns showing type 1 (light prisms with dark periphery) and type 2 (dark cores with light periphery) etching on same surface after Marshall et al, 1975 JDR. Marshall GW, Olson LM, Lee CV: SEM Investigation of the variability of enamel surfaces after simulated clinical acid etching for pit and fissure sealants, J Dent Res 54:1222–1231, 1975. Part C from Marshall, Olson and Lee, JDR 1975 (same as above) and Part E from Marshall, Marshall and Bayne, 1988: Marshall GW, Marshall SJ, Bayne SC: Restorative dental materials: scanning electron microscopy and x-ray microanalysis, Scanning Microsc 2:2007–2028, 1988.

process. However, as the etching pattern begins to develop, the surface etched with phosphoric acid develops a frosty appearance (Figure 2-3, *B*), which has been used as the traditional clinical indicator for sufficient etching. This roughened surface provides the substrate for infiltration of bonding agents that can be polymerized after penetration of the etched enamel structure so that they form micromechanical bonds to the enamel when polymerized. With self-etching bonding agents, this frosty appearance cannot be detected.

There are two other important structural variations of enamel. Near the DEJ the enamel prism structure is not as well developed in the very first

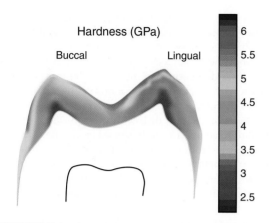

Hardness (GPa)

Buccal   Lingual

6
5.5
5
4.5
4
3.5
3
2.5

FIGURE 2.4 **Nanoindentation mapping of the mechanical properties of human molar tooth enamel.** *(From Cuy JL, et al: Arch. Oral Biol. 47(4), 281-291, 2002.)*

enamel formed, so that the enamel very close to the DEJ may appear aprismatic or without the prism like structure. Similarly, on the outer surface of the enamel, at completion of the enamel surface, the ameloblasts degenerate and leave a featureless layer, called *prismless enamel*, on the outer surface of the crown. This layer is more often observed in deciduous teeth and is often worn off in permanent teeth. However, if present, this causes some difficulty in getting an effective etching pattern and may require roughening of the surface or additional etching treatments. The outer surface of the enamel is of great clinical significance because it is the surface subjected to daily wear and undergoes repeated cycles of demineralization and remineralization. As a result of these cycles, the composition of the enamel crystals may change, for example, as a result of exposure to fluoride. Thus the properties of the enamel might be expected to vary from the external to the internal surface. Such variations, including a thin surface veneer of fluoride-rich apatite crystals, create differences in the enamel properties within the enamel. Enamel is usually harder at the occlusal and cuspal areas and less hard nearer the DEJ. Figure 2-4 shows an example of the difference in hardness.

THE MINERAL

The mineral of all calcified tissues is a highly defective relative of the mineral hydroxyapatite, or HA. The biological apatites of calcified tissues are different than the ideal HA structure in that the defects and chemical substitutions generally make it weaker and more soluble in acids. Hydroxyapatite has the simple formula $Ca_{10}(PO_4)_6(OH)_2$, with an ideal molar ratio of calcium to phosphorus (Ca/P) of 1.67 and a hexagonal crystal structure. The apatite of

enamel and dentin has a much more variable composition that depends on its formative history and other chemical exposures during maturity. Thus the mineral in enamel and dentin is a calcium-deficient, carbonate-rich, and highly substituted form related to HA. Metal ions such as magnesium (Mg) and sodium (Na) may substitute for calcium, whereas carbonate substitutes for the phosphate and hydroxyl groups. These substitutions distort the structure and make it more soluble. Perhaps the most beneficial substitution is the fluorine (F) ion, which substitutes for the hydroxyl group (OH) in the formula and makes the structure stronger and less soluble. Complete substitution of F for (OH) in hydroxyapatite yields fluoroapatite mineral, $Ca_{10}(PO_4)_6(F)_2$, that is much less soluble than HA or the defective apatite of calcified tissues. It is worth noting that HA has attracted considerable attention as an implantable calcified tissue replacement. It has the advantage of being a purified and stronger form of the natural mineral and releases no harmful agents during biological degradation. Its major shortcoming is that it is extremely brittle and sensitive to porosity or defects and therefore fractures easily in load-bearing applications.

The approximate carbonate contents of the enamel and dentin apatites are significantly different, about 3% and 5% carbonate, respectively. All other factors being equal, this would make the dentin apatite more soluble in acids than enamel apatite. Things are not equal, however, and the dentin apatite crystals are much smaller than the enamel crystals. This means that the dentin crystals present a higher surface area to attacking acids and contain many more defects per unit volume and thus exhibit considerably higher solubility. Finally, as discussed further below, the dentin mineral occupies only about 50% of the dentin structure, so there is not as much apatite in the dentin as there is in enamel. All of these factors multiply the susceptibility of dentin to acid attack and provide insight into the rapid spread of caries when it penetrates the DEJ.

DENTIN

Dentin is a complex hydrated biological composite structure that forms the bulk of the tooth. Furthermore, dentin is modified by physiological, aging, and disease processes that result in different forms of dentin. These altered forms of dentin may be the precise forms that are most important in restorative dentistry. Some of the recognized variations include primary, secondary, reparative or tertiary, sclerotic, transparent, carious, demineralized, remineralized, and hypermineralized. These terms reflect alterations in the fundamental components of the structure as defined by changes in their arrangement, interrelationships, or chemistry. A number of these may have important implications for our ability to develop long-lasting adhesion or bonds to dentin.

Primary dentin is formed during tooth development. Its volume and conformation, reflecting tooth form, vary with the size and shape of the tooth. Dentin is composed of about 50 volume percent (vol%) carbonate-rich, calcium-deficient apatite; 30 vol% organic matter, which is largely type I collagen; and about 20 vol% fluid, which is similar to plasma. Other noncollagenous proteins are thought to be involved in dentin mineralization and other functions such as

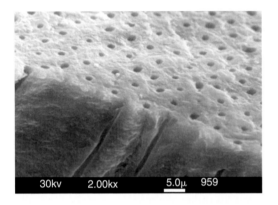

FIGURE 2.5 **Scanning electron microscopy (SEM) image of normal dentin showing its unique structure as seen from two directions.** At the top is a view of the tubules, each of which is surrounded by peritubular dentin. Tubules lie between the dentin-enamel junction (DEJ) and converge on the pulp chamber. The perpendicular surface at the bottom shows a fracture surface revealing some of the tubules as they form tunnel-like pathways toward the pulp. The tubule lumen normally contains fluid and processes of the odontoblastic cells. *(From Marshall GW: Quintessence Int. 24, 606-617, 1993.)*

controlling crystallite size and orientation; however, these functions are not discussed further in this text. The major components are distributed into distinctive morphological features to form a vital and complex hydrated composite in which the morphology varies with location and undergoes alterations with age or disease.

The tubules, one distinct and important feature of dentin, represent the tracks taken by the odontoblastic cells from the DEJ or cementum at the root to the pulp chamber and appear as tunnels piercing the dentin structure (Figure 2-5). The tubules converge on the pulp chamber, and therefore tubule density and orientation vary from location to location (see Figure 2-1). Tubule number density is lowest at the DEJ and highest at the predentin surface at the junction to the pulp chamber, where the odontoblastic cell bodies lie in nearly a close-packed array. Lower tubule densities are found in the root. The contents of the tubules include odontoblast processes, for all or part of their course, and fluid. The extent of the odontoblast process is still uncertain, but evidence is mounting that it extends to the DEJ. For most of its course, the tubule lumen is lined by a highly mineralized cuff of peritubular dentin roughly 0.5 to 1 µm thick (Figure 2-6). Because the peritubular dentin forms after the tubule lumen has been formed, some argue that it may be more properly termed *intratubular dentin* and contains mostly apatite crystals with little organic matrix. A number of studies have concluded that the peritubular dentin does not contain collagen, and therefore might be considered a separate calcified tissue. The tubules are separated by intertubular dentin composed of a matrix of type I collagen reinforced by apatite (see Figures 2-5 and 2-6). This arrangement means that the amount of intertubular dentin varies with location. The apatite

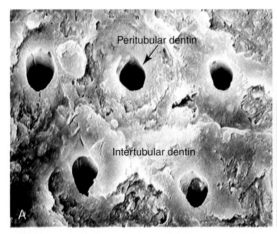
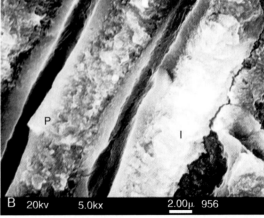

FIGURE 2.6 **Fracture surface of the dentin viewed from the occlusal in A and longitudinally in B.** Peritubular (*P*) (also called *intratubular*) dentin forms a cuff or lining around each tubule. The tubules are separated from one another by intertubular dentin (*I*). *(Courtesy of G. W. Marshall.)*

crystals are much smaller (approximately 5 × 30 × 100 nm) than the apatite found in enamel and contain 4% to 5% carbonate. The small crystallite size, defect structure, and higher carbonate content lead to the greater dissolution susceptibility described above.

Estimates of the size of tubules, the thickness of the peritubular region, and the amount of intertubular dentin have been made in a number of studies. Calculations for occlusal dentin as a function of position from these data show the percent tubule area and diameter vary from about 22% and 2.5 μm near the pulp to 1% and 0.8 μm at the DEJ. Intertubular matrix area varies from 12% at the predentin to 96% near the DEJ, whereas peritubular dentin ranges from over 60% down to 3% at the DEJ. Tubule densities are compared in Table 2-1 based on work by various investigators. It is clear that the structural components will vary considerably over their course, and necessarily result in location-dependent variations in morphology, distribution of the structural elements, and important properties such as permeability, moisture content, and available surface area for bonding and may also affect bond strength, hardness, and other properties.

Because the odontoblasts come to rest just inside the dentin and line the walls of the pulp chamber after tooth formation, the dentin-pulp complex can be considered a vital tissue. This is different than mature enamel. Over time secondary dentin forms and the pulp chamber gradually becomes smaller. The border between primary and secondary dentin is usually marked by a change in orientation of the dentin tubules. Furthermore, the odontoblasts react to form tertiary dentin in response to insults such as caries or tooth preparation, and this form of dentin is often less well organized than the primary or secondary dentin.

Early enamel carious lesions may be reversed by remineralization treatments. However, effective remineralization treatments are not yet available for dentin and therefore the current standard of care dictates surgical intervention to remove highly damaged tissue and then restoration as needed. Thus it is

important to understand altered forms of dentin and the effects of such clinical interventions.

When dentin is cut or abraded by dental instruments, a smear layer develops and covers the surface and obscures the underlying structure (Figure 2-7). The bur cutting marks are shown in Figure 2-7, A, and at higher magnification in Figure 2-7, B. Figure 2-7, C, shows the smear layer thickness from the side and the development of smear plugs as the cut dentin debris is pushed into the dentin tubule lumen. The advantages and disadvantages of the smear layer have been extensively discussed for several decades. It reduces permeability and therefore aids in maintaining a drier field and reduces infiltration of noxious agents into the tubules and perhaps the pulp. However, it is now generally accepted that it is a hindrance to dentin bonding procedures and, therefore, is normally removed or modified by some form of acid conditioning.

Acid etching or conditioning allows for removal of the smear layer and alteration of the superficial dentin, opening channels for infiltration by bonding agents. Figure 2-8 shows what happens in such an etching treatment. The tubule lumens widen as the peritubular dentin is preferentially removed because it is mostly mineral with sparse protein. The widened lumens form a funnel shape that is not very retentive.

Figure 2-9 shows these effects in a slightly different way. Unetched dentin in Figure 2-9, A, has small tubules and peritubular dentin, which is removed in the treated dentin at the exposed surface after etching (*bottom*). The two-dimensional network of collagen type I fibers is shown after treatment in Figure 2-9, A. Figure 2-9, B, shows progressive demineralization of a dentin collagen fibril in which the external mineral and proteins are slowly removed to reveal the typical banded pattern of type I collagen. In Figure 2-9, C, this pattern is seen at high magnification of the treated dentin in Figure 2-9, A.

If the demineralized dentin is dried, the remaining dentin matrix shrinks and the collagen fibrils become matted and difficult to penetrate by bonding agents. This is shown in Figure 2-10, which compares demineralized and dried dentin with demineralized and hydrated dentin.

Most restorative procedures involve dentin that has been altered in some way. Common alterations include formation of carious lesions that form various zones and include transparent dentin that forms under the caries infected dentin layer. Transparent dentin results when the dentin tubules become filled with mineral, which changes the refractive index of the tubules and produces a translucent or transparent zone.

Figure 2-11 shows a section through a tooth with a carious lesion, which has been stained to reveal its zones. The gray zone under the stained and severely

TABLE 2.1 Comparison of Mean Numerical Density of Tubules in Occlusal Dentin[*]

Outer Dentin	Middle Dentin	Inner Dentin
15,000/mm^2	35,000/mm^2	65,000/mm^2
20,000/mm^2	35,000/mm^2	43,000/mm^2
24,500/mm^2	40,400/mm^2	51,100/mm^2
18,000/mm^2	39,000/mm^2	52,000/mm^2

*From data reported in the literature (Marshall GW: Quintessence Int. 24, 606-617, 1993.)

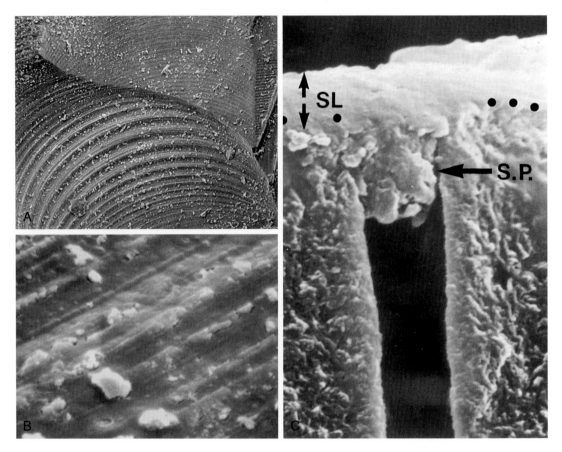

FIGURE 2.7 **Smear layer formation.** **A**, Bur marks on dentin preparation **B**, Higher magnification showing smear layer surface and cutting debris. **C**, Section showing smear layer (*SL*) and smear plugs (S.P.). *(A and B from Marshall GW, et al: Scanning Microsc. 2, 2007-2028, 1988; C from Pashley DH, et al: Arch. Oral Biol. 33, 265-270, 1988.)*

demineralized dentin is the transparent layer (Figure 2-11, *A*). Figure 2-11, *B*, shows the transparent dentin in which most of the tubule lumens are filled with mineral. After etching, as shown in Figure 2-11, *C* the peritubular dentin is etched away, but the tubules retain plugs of the precipitated mineral, which is more resistant to etching. This resistance to etching makes bonding more difficult.

Several other forms of transparent dentin are formed as a result of different processes. A second form of transparent dentin results from bruxism. An additional form of transparent dentin results from aging as the root dentin gradually becomes transparent. In addition noncarious cervical lesions (NCCLs), often called *abfraction* or *notch* lesions, form at the enamel-cementum or enamel-dentin junction, usually on facial or buccal surfaces. Their etiology is not clear at this point; their formation has been attributed to abrasion, tooth flexure, and erosion or some combination of these processes. Nonetheless these lesions occur with increasing frequency with age, and the exposed dentin becomes transparent as the tubules are filled. Figure 2-12 shows examples of

transparent dentin in which the tubule lumens are completely filled.

The properties of the transparent dentin may differ from one to another depending on the processes that lead to deposit of the mineral in the tubules. Several studies have shown that elastic properties of the intertubular dentin are not altered by aging, although the structure may become more susceptible to fracture. Similarly, arrested caries will contain transparent dentin and this has often been called *sclerotic dentin*, a term that implies it may be harder than normal dentin. However, other studies have shown that the elastic properties of the intertubular dentin may actually be unaltered or lower than normal dentin.

Physical and Mechanical Properties

The marked variations in the structural elements of dentin when located within the tooth imply that the properties of dentin will vary considerably with location. That is, variable structure leads to variable properties.

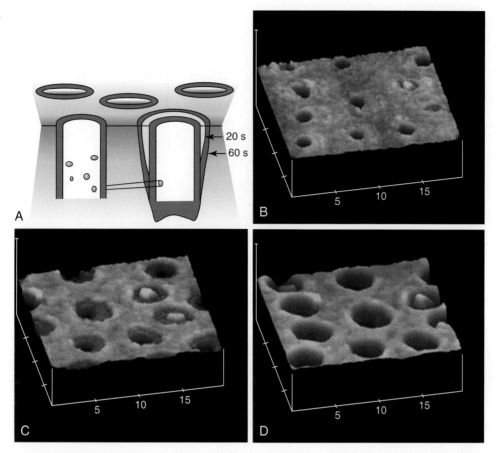

FIGURE 2.8 **Stages of dentin demineralization. A**, Schematic showing progressive stages of dentin demineralization. **B** to **D**, Atomic force microscopy (AFM) images showing stages of etching. The etching leads to wider lumens as peritubular dentin is dissolved and funnel-shaped openings are formed. *(AFM images from Marshall GW: Quintessence Int. 24, 606-617, 1993.)*

Because one major function of tooth structure is to resist deformation without fracture, it is useful to have knowledge of the forces that are experienced by teeth during mastication. Measurements have given values on cusp tips of about 77 kg distributed over the cusp tip area of 0.039 cm^2, suggesting a stress of about 200 MPa.

Difficulties in Testing

In Table 2-2, values are presented for some important properties of enamel and dentin. The wide spread of values reported in the literature is remarkable. Some of the reasons for these discrepancies should be appreciated and considered in practice or when reading the literature.

First, human teeth are small, and therefore it is difficult to get large specimens and hold them in such a way that you can measure properties. This makes the use of standard mechanical testing such as tensile, compressive, or shear tests difficult. When testing bonded teeth, the problem is even more complicated,

and special tests have been developed to obtain insights into these properties. From the previous discussion of structural variations, it is also clear that testing such small inhomogeneous specimens means that the properties will not be uniform.

Another problem is the great variation in structure in both tissues. Enamel prisms are aligned generally perpendicular to the DEJ, whereas dentin tubules change their number density with depth as they course toward the pulp chamber. Preparing a uniform sample with the structures running all in one direction for testing is challenging. In addition, properties generally vary with direction and location and the material is not isotropic; therefore, the best a single value can tell you is some average value for the material.

Storage and time elapsed since extraction are also important considerations. Properties that exist in a natural situation or *in situ* or *in vivo* are of greatest interest. Clearly this condition is almost impossible to achieve in most routine testing, so changes that

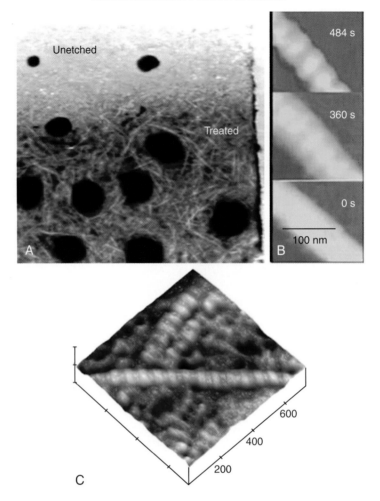

FIGURE 2.9 **Etching of dentin removes mineral from the intertubular dentin matrix leaving a collagen-rich layer and widening the dentin tubule orifices. A,** After etching the tubule lumens are enlarged and the collagen network surrounding the tubules can be seen after further treatment. **B,** Isolated dentin collagen fiber is slowly demineralized revealing the typical 67 nm repeat pattern of type I collagen. **C,** High magnification view of collagen fibers in **A**. *(A and C from Marshall GW, et al: Surface Science. 491, 444-455, 2001; B modified from Balooch M, et al: J. Struct. Biol. 162, 404-410, 2008.)*

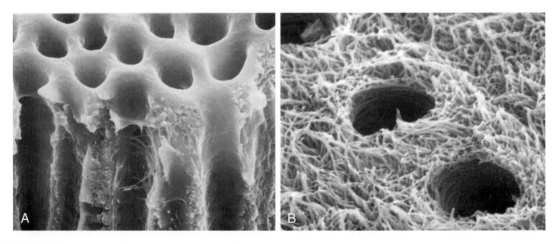

FIGURE 2.10 **Demineralized dentin is sensitive to moisture and shrinks on drying. A,** Demineralized dentin undergoes shrinkage when air dried forming a collapsed layer of collagen that is difficult to infiltrate with resin bonding agents. **B,** When kept moist, the collagen network is open and can be penetrated by bonding agents. *(From Marshall GW, et al: J. Dent. 25, 441-458, 1997.)*

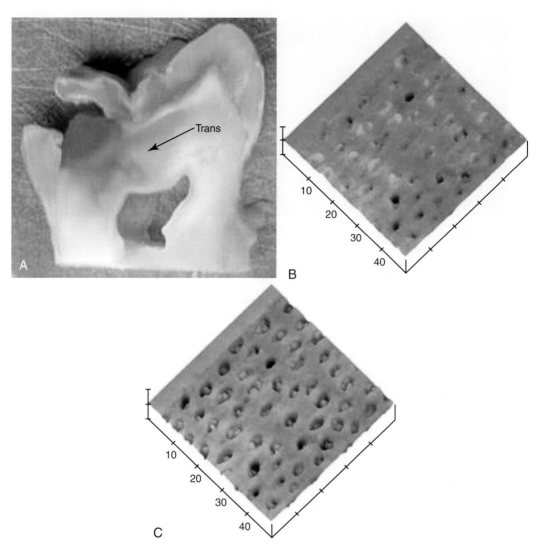

FIGURE 2.11 **Transparent dentin associated with carious lesions. A,** Carious lesion showing dentin carious zones revealed by staining, including the grayish transparent zone. **B,** Atomic force microscopy (AFM) of carious transparent dentin before etching. **C,** After etching the tubule lumens remain filled even as the peritubular dentin is etched away. *(A from Zheng L, et al: Eur. J. Oral Sci. 111, 243-252, 2003; **B** and **C** from Marshall GW, et al: Dent. Mater. 17, 45-52, 2001b.)*

have occurred as a result of storage conditions prior to testing must be considered. It is also important to consider biological hazards because extracted teeth must be treated as potentially infective. How do you sterilize the teeth without altering their properties? Autoclaving undoubtedly alters the properties of proteins, and is therefore not appropriate for dentin, and might also affect enamel.

Finally, the fluid content of these tissues must be considered. Moisture is a vital component of both tissues and *in vivo* conditions cannot be replicated if the tissues have been desiccated (see Figure 2-10). This becomes a critically important consideration in bonding to these tissues, as is discussed further in Chapter 13. In contrast to the importance of this issue

is the issue of convenience. It is much more difficult to test the tissues in a fully hydrated condition than in a dry condition. All of these factors and a number of others, such as temperature of testing, will influence the results and contribute to a spread in the values reported for the properties.

Despite these limitations, some generalizations about the properties of these tissues are useful (see Table 2-1). Root dentin is generally weaker and softer than coronal dentin. Enamel also appears to vary in its properties, with cuspal enamel being stronger and harder than other areas, presumably as an adaption to masticatory forces. Dentin is less stiff than enamel (i.e., has a lower elastic modulus), and has a higher fracture toughness. This may be counterintuitive but

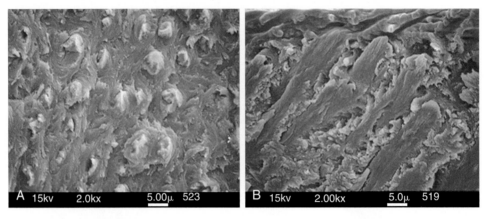

FIGURE 2.12 **Transparent dentin.** As seen from the facial, **A,** and longitudinal, **B,** directions. The transparent dentin results from filling of the tubules with mineral deposits that alter the optical properties of the tooth. *(Courtesy of Marshall GW.)*

TABLE 2.2   Properties of Enamel and Dentin

Property	Enamel	Dentin
Density	2.96 g/cm^3	2.1 g/cm^3
Compressive		
Modulus of elasticity	60-120 GPa	18-24 GPa
Proportional limit	70-353 MPa	100-190 MPa
Strength	94-450 MPa	230-370 MPa
Tensile		
Modulus of elasticity		11-19 GPa
Strength	8-35 MPa	30-65 MPa
Shear strength	90 MPa	138 MPa
Flexural strength	60-90 MPa	245-280 MPa
Hardness	3-6 GPa	0.13-.51 GPa

will become clearer when we define these terms in Chapter 4. In addition, dentin is viscoelastic, which means that its mechanical deformation characteristics are time dependent, and elastic recovery is not instantaneous. Thus dentin may be sensitive to how rapidly it is strained, a phenomenon called *strain rate sensitivity*. Strain rate sensitivity is characteristic of polymeric materials; the collagen matrix imparts this property to tissues such as dentin. Under normal circumstances, enamel and other ceramic materials do not show this characteristic in their mechanical properties.

The Dentin-Enamel Junction

The dentin-enamel junction (DEJ) is much more than the boundary between enamel and dentin. Because enamel is very hard and dentin is much softer and tougher, they need to be joined together to provide a biomechanically compatible system. Joining such dissimilar materials is a challenge, and it is not completely clear how nature has accomplished this. However, the DEJ not only joins these two tissues but also appears to resist cracks in the enamel from penetrating into dentin and leading to tooth fracture as shown in Figure 2-13, *A*. Many such cracks exist in the enamel but do not seem to propagate into the dentin. If the DEJ is intact, it is unusual to have tooth fracture except in the face of severe trauma. In Figure 2-13, *B*, microhardness indentations have been placed to drive cracks toward the DEJ (*orange*). The crack stops at or just past the interface. This image also shows that the DEJ is scalloped with its concavity directed toward the enamel. This means that most cracks approach the DEJ at an angle, and this may lead to arrest of many of the cracks. The scalloped structure actually has three levels: scallops, microscallops within the scallops, and a finer structure. Figures 2-13, *C*, and 2-13, *D*, show images of larger scallops in molars (~24 µm across) and smaller scallops (~15 µm across) in anterior teeth after the removal of the enamel. Finite element models suggest that the scallops reduce stress concentrations at the interface, but it is not known whether the larger scallop size in posterior teeth is an adaption to higher masticatory loads or a developmental variation. In Figure 2-13, *E*, the crystals of dentin are almost in contact with those of the enamel, so that the anatomical DEJ is said to be optically thin. However, measurements of property variations across the DEJ show that this is a graded interface with properties varying from those of the enamel to the adjacent mantle dentin over a considerable distance. This gradient, which is due in part to the scalloped nature of the DEJ, makes the functional width of the DEJ much larger than its anatomical appearance and further

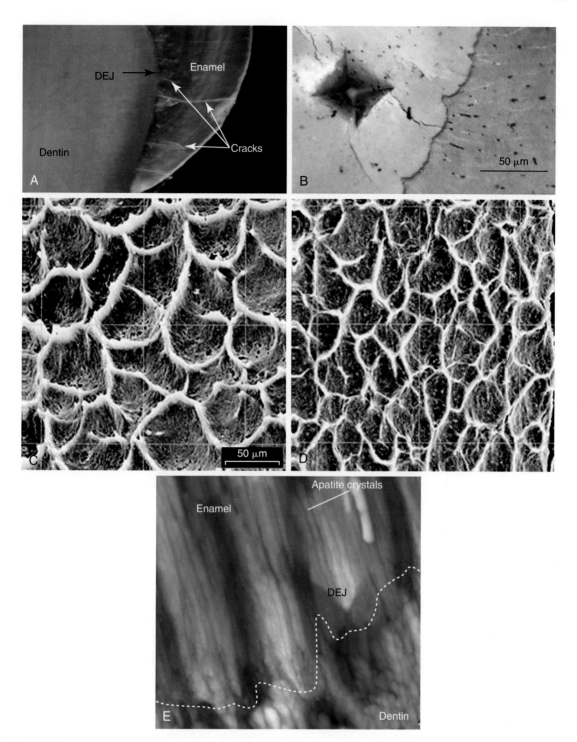

FIGURE 2.13 **Cracks in enamel appear to stop at the dentin-enamel junction (DEJ). A,** Low-magnification view of cracks in enamel. **B,** Indentation-generated cracks stop near or at the scalloped DEJ (*orange*). **C,** Large scallops in molars. **D,** Smaller scallops in anterior teeth. **E,** Crystals of the enamel are nearly in contact with dentin crystals at the DEJ forming an optically thin but functionally wide union. (*A, C-E from Marshall SJ, et al: J. European Ceram. Soc. 23, 2897-2904, 2003; **B** from Imbeni V, et al: Nature Mater. 4, 229-232, 2005.*)

reduces stresses. In addition, although collagen is absent from enamel, collagen fibers cross the DEJ from dentin into enamel to further integrate the two tissues. At this point, no unique components, such as proteins, have been identified that could serve as a special adhesive that bonds the enamel to the dentin.

ORAL BIOFILMS AND RESTORATIVE DENTAL MATERIALS

Biofilms are complex, surface-adherent, spatially organized polymicrobial communities containing bacteria surrounded by a polysaccharide matrix. Oral biofilms that form on the surfaces of teeth and biomaterials in the oral cavity are also known as *dental plaque*. When the human diet is rich in fermentable carbohydrates, the most prevalent organisms shown to be present in dental plaque are adherent acidogenic and aciduric bacteria such as streptococci and lactobacilli that are primarily responsible for dental caries. Other consequences of long-term oral biofilm accumulation can also include periodontal diseases and peri-implantitis (inflammation of the soft and hard tissues surrounding an implant), depending on the location of attachment of the biofilm.

Biofilm formation on hard surfaces in the oral cavity is a sequential process. A conditioning film from saliva (known as *pellicle*) containing adsorbed macromolecules such as phosphoproteins and glycoproteins is deposited on tooth structure and biomaterials within minutes after a thorough cleaning. This stage is followed by the attachment of planktonic (free-floating) bacteria to the pellicle. Division of the attached initial colonizing bacterial species produces microcolonies, and subsequent attachment of later colonizing species results in the formation of matrix-embedded multispecies biofilms. These biofilms can mature over time if they are not detached by mechanical removal or intrinsic factors.

Biofilm formation occurs via complicated physical and cellular interactions between the substrate, pellicle, and bacteria. These interactions occur at several levels and can include physical proximity, metabolic exchange, signal molecule-mediated communication, exchange of genetic material, production of inhibitory factors, and co-aggregation ("specific cell-to-cell recognition between genetically distinct cell types," as defined by Kolenbrander et al., 2006).

The pellicle contains a variety of receptor molecules that are recognized primarily by streptococci (Figure 2-14). This is evident in healthy individuals, who typically have biofilms containing a thin layer of adherent gram-positive cocci. The ability to bind to nonshedding surfaces such as enamel gives streptococci a tremendous advantage and is consistent with the observation that streptococci constitute

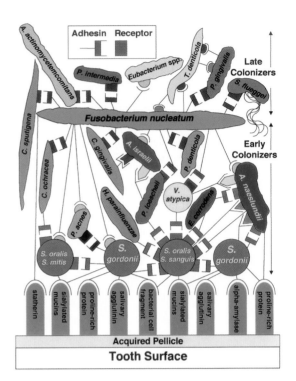

FIGURE 2.14 Spatiotemporal model of oral bacterial colonization, showing recognition of salivary pellicle receptors by early colonizing bacteria and co-aggregations between early colonizers, fusobacteria, and late colonizers of the tooth surface. Starting at the bottom, primary colonizers bind via adhesins (*round-tipped black line symbols*) to complementary salivary receptors (*blue-green vertical round-topped columns*) in the acquired pellicle coating the tooth surface. Secondary colonizers bind to previously bound bacteria. Sequential binding results in the appearance of nascent surfaces that bridge with the next co-aggregating partner cell. The bacterial strains shown are *Actinobacillus actinomycetemcomitans, Actinomyces israelii, Actinomyces naeslundii, Capnocytophaga gingivalis, Capnocytophaga ochracea, Capnocytophaga sputigena, Eikenella corrodens, Eubacterium* spp., *Fusobacterium nucleatum, Haemophilus parainfluenzae, Porphyromonas gingivalis, Prevotella denticola, Prevotella intermedia, Prevotella loescheii, Propionibacterium acnes, Selenomonas flueggei, Streptococcus gordonii, Streptococcus mitis, Streptococcus oralis, Streptococcus sanguis, Treponema* spp., and *Veillonella atypica.* (*From Kolenbrander PE, et al: Microbiol. Mol. Biol. Rev. 66, 486-505, 2002.*)

60% to 90% of the initial bacterial flora on enamel in situ. Furthermore, the streptococci are less sensitive to exposure to air than most oral bacteria because they are facultatively anaerobic and can participate in modifying the biofilm environment to a more reduced state, a condition often considered to favor an ecological shift towards gram-negative anaerobes.

Interactions among human oral bacteria are pivotal to the development of oral biofilms (see Figure 2-14). In the first 4 hours of biofilm formation, gram-positive cocci appear to predominate, particularly mitis group streptococci. After 8 hours of growth, the majority of the bacterial population continues to be largely coccoid, but rod-shaped organisms are also observed. By 24 to 48 hours, thick deposits of cells with various morphologies can be detected, including coccoid, coccobacilliary, rod-shaped, and filamentous bacteria. Within 4 days of biofilm growth, an increase in the numbers of gram-negative anaerobes is observed, and particularly of *Fusobacterium nucleatum*. The latter organism has the unique ability to co-aggregate with a wide variety of bacteria and is believed to play a pivotal role in the maturation of biofilm because it forms co-aggregation bridges with both early and late colonizers. As the biofilm matures, a shift is observed toward a composition of largely gram-negative morphotypes, including rods, filamentous organisms, vibrios, and spirochetes. These shifts in the microbial composition of biofilm are important because they correlate with the development of gingivitis (inflammation of gingival tissues).

Even though biofilms accumulate on restorative, orthodontic, endodontic, and implant biomaterials, the remainder of this section focuses on biofilms that accumulate on the surfaces of restorative and implant materials only. The precise mechanisms of bacterial adhesion and biofilm formation on the surfaces of dental materials have not yet been identified in spite of decades of research effort but are accepted to be complex processes that depend on a large number of factors. In vitro studies have shown that the adhesion of salivary proteins and bacteria at small distances (5-100 nm) from the surfaces of biomaterials is influenced by a combination of Lifshitz-van der Waals forces, electrostatic interactions, and acid-base bonding. Other properties such as substrate hydrophobicity, surface free energy, surface charge, and surface roughness have commonly been investigated in vitro for correlation with the number of adhering bacteria. Many of the above-mentioned surface properties are described in later chapters.

The role of surface roughness in biofilm formation has been widely investigated. Smooth surfaces have been shown to attract less biofilm in vivo than rough surfaces. It has also been observed that hydrophobic surfaces that are located supragingivally attract less biofilm in vivo than more hydrophilic surfaces over a 9-day period. An increase in the mean surface roughness parameter (R_a) above a threshold value of 0.2 μm or an increase in surface free energy were both found to result in more biofilm accumulation on dental materials. When both of those surface properties interact with each other, surface roughness was observed to have a greater effect on biofilm accumulation. The creation of a rough restoration surface caused by abrasion, erosion, air polishing or ultrasonic instrumentation, or a lack of polishing after the

fabrication of a restoration, has also been associated with biofilm formation.

Bacterial adhesion in vivo is considerably reduced by the formation of a pellicle, regardless of the composition of the underlying substrate. Pellicle formation has also been shown to have a masking effect on specific surface characteristics of biomaterials to a certain extent. Surfaces having a low surface energy were observed to retain the smallest amount of adherent biofilm due to the lower binding forces between bacteria and substrata even after several days of exposure in the human oral cavity. Reciprocally, the higher surface energy of many restorative materials compared with that of the tooth surface could result in a greater tendency for the surface and margins of the restoration to accumulate debris, saliva, and bacteria. This may in part account for the relatively high incidence of secondary (recurrent) carious lesions seen in enamel at the margins of resin composite and amalgam restorations.

Investigations of oral biofilms on restorative materials can generally be divided into in vivo, in situ, and in vitro studies, with the latter comprising monospecies or multispecies investigations. Biofilms that are formed on restorative materials can vary in thickness and viability. In vivo and in situ studies of biofilm formation on dental materials have produced inconsistent results, and a trend for accumulation on materials has not been determined so far.

Levels of cariogenic organisms (capable of producing or promoting caries) such as *Streptococcus mutans* have been shown to be higher in biofilms adjacent to posterior resin restorations than in biofilms adjacent to amalgam or glass ionomer restorations. The formation of oral biofilms has been associated with an increase in the surface roughness of resin composites, degradation of the material due to acid production by cariogenic organisms, hydrolysis of the resin matrix, and a decrease in microhardness of the restoration's surface. Additionally, it has been theorized that planktonic bacteria can enter the adhesive interface between the restorative material and the tooth, leading to secondary caries and pulp pathology. On the other hand, trace amounts of unpolymerized resin, resin monomers, and the products of resin biodegradation have been shown to modulate the growth of oral bacteria in the vicinity of resin restorations. All of these factors create a cycle of bacteria-surface interaction that further increases surface roughness and encourages bacterial attachment to the surface, thereby placing the adjacent enamel at greater risk for secondary caries.

Bacterial adhesion to casting alloys and dental amalgams has received limited attention in recent times. Biofilms on gold-based casting alloys are reported to be of low viability, possibly due to the bacteriostatic effect of gold. Biofilms on amalgam are also reported to have low viability, which could be attributed to the presence of the Hg(II) form of mercury in dental amalgam. Interestingly, amalgam restorations have been shown to promote the levels of mercury (Hg)-resistant bacteria in vitro and in vivo. Resistance to antibiotics, and specifically tetracycline, was observed to be concurrent with Hg-resistance in oral bacteria. However, it is worth noting that Hg-resistant bacteria were also found in children without amalgam fillings or previous exposure to amalgam.

Information regarding the morphology of biofilms on ceramic restorations is limited, although it is generally accepted that ceramic crowns accumulate less biofilm than adjacent tooth structure. The recent demonstration of increased surface roughness of zirconia surfaces in vitro after the use of hand and ultrasonic scaling instruments could be theorized to produce greater biofilm accumulation on zirconia restorations subsequent to dental prophylaxis procedures.

Biofilms that adhere to denture base resins predominantly contain the *Candida* species of yeast. However, initial adhesion of bacteria such as streptococci to the denture base may have to occur before *Candida* species can form biofilms. This is attributed to the observation of bacteria on dentures within hours and *Candida* species after days, and to the ability of *Candida* species to bind to the cell wall receptors in streptococci. Biofilms on dentures have commonly been associated with denture stomatitis (chronic inflammation of the oral mucosa) in elderly and immunocompromised patients. Removal of biofilms from dentures typically requires mechanical and/or chemical means and is a significant clinical problem because of biofilm adherence to the denture base resins.

The accumulation of biofilms on titanium and titanium alloys that are used in dental implants has received much attention because biofilms play a significant role in determining the success of an implant. The sequence of microbial colonization and biofilm formation on dental implants has been shown to be similar to that on teeth, but differs in early colonization patterns. Several in vivo studies have confirmed that a reduction in mean surface roughness (R_a) of implant materials below the threshold value of 0.2 μm has no major effect on adhesion, colonization, or microbial composition. Compared to polished titanium surfaces, titanium implant surfaces that were modified with titanium nitride (TiN) showed significantly less bacterial adhesion and biofilm formation in vivo, thereby potentially minimizing biofilm accumulation and subsequent peri-implantitis. Other contributing factors such as the hydrophobicity, surface chemistry, and surface free energy of the implant material have been found to play vital roles in bacterial adhesion to dental implant materials. In addition, the surface characteristics of the bacteria, the design of the implant and the abutment, and the micro-gap between the implant and abutment have also been shown to influence microbial colonization on dental implants.

The most common reason for the replacement of dental restorations is secondary caries at the gingival tooth-restoration margin. It is estimated that 50% to 80% of resin restorations are replaced annually in the United States alone. The cost of replacing restorations is estimated to be in the billions of dollars worldwide, and the number and cost of replacing restorations is increasing annually. Although bacteriological studies of secondary caries indicate that its etiology is similar to that of primary caries, the mechanisms by which secondary caries occur are a focus of ongoing investigations.

The removal of tenaciously adherent oral biofilms from hard surfaces is crucial to caries control and is most effectively accomplished by mechanical brushing with toothpaste, especially in interproximal regions and posterior teeth along with the use of adjunctive chemical agents. Although tooth brushing has been associated with increased surface roughness of restorations over time due to the process of wear, which could permit additional bacterial attachment on the surface, mechanical removal has been shown to be more effective than chemical intervention. This is because bacteria in biofilms are typically well protected from the host immune response, antibiotics, and antibacterials when embedded within a complex biofilm matrix. Furthermore, most antimicrobial agents have commonly been tested against planktonic bacteria, which are killed by much lower concentrations of antimicrobials than biofilm bacteria. Chemical control of biofilms has also been limited by concerns regarding the development of resistant microorganisms resulting from the prolonged use of antimicrobials, and acceptance of the hypothesis that the microflora should not be eliminated but should instead be prevented from shifting from a favorable ecology to an ecology favoring oral disease.

The accumulation of biofilms on glass ionomer and resin-modified glass ionomer biomaterials is a factor that has been associated with an increase in the surface roughness of those biomaterials. Fluoride-releasing materials, and glass-ionomers and compomers in particular, can neutralize acids produced by bacteria in biofilms. Fluoride can provide cariostatic benefits and may affect bacterial metabolism under simulated cariogenic conditions in vitro. Although the large volume of saliva normally present in the oral cavity is hypothesized to result in fluoride concentrations that are too low for cavity-wide antibacterial protection, the amount of fluoride released could theoretically be sufficient to minimize demineralization in the tooth structure adjacent to glass ionomer and resin-modified glass ionomer restorations. In addition, glass ionomer materials can be recharged by daily exposure to fluoride-containing dentifrices, thereby compensating for the significant decrease in fluoride release that occurs over time. Interestingly, clinical studies have not clearly demonstrated that fluoride-releasing restorative materials significantly reduce the incidence of secondary caries as compared to non-fluoride-releasing biomaterials. More studies are therefore needed to determine the impact of fluoride-releasing restorations on the development and progression of secondary caries.

SELECTED PROBLEMS

PROBLEM 1

The enamel microstructure is unique among the dental calcified tissues in that it is the hardest tissue in the body. Explain why its unique structure is important to its function and how this has been used in restorative treatments to provide reliable bonding.

Solution

Enamel has the highest mineral content of the calcified tissues providing high hardness and wear resistance needed for mastication. The small amount of organic substances coats each crystallite and increases toughness in comparison to pure apatite. The very long crystals are packed into keyhole–shaped enamel rods that are separated by regions of higher organic content. This structure etches differently when exposed to acids, such as phosphoric acid, leading to a clean, high-energy surface with varying roughness within and between the rods.

When infiltrated with resins and subsequently polymerized, the resins form a tight and reliable bond between the enamel structure and the resin.

PROBLEM 2

Apatite is the mineral component of both enamel and dentin, but there are important differences between these critical forms of apatite. What are the critical differences and how do these differences affect restorative dentistry?

Solution

Enamel and dentin mineral contain calcium-deficient carbonate-rich hydroxyapatite. However, the crystallite size is different, with enamel having much larger crystals that comprise 85 vol% of the structure, compared to about 50 vol% in dentin. The larger surface area of the dentin apatite increases its dissolution susceptibility when exposed to acids. This susceptibility is further increased because of the higher carbonate content of the dentin mineral. Thus the dentin mineral is dissolved more rapidly than the enamel mineral, and because there is less total mineral in dentin than in enamel, the acid attack proceeds more quickly in dentin. The dentin tubules also provide pathways for this dissolution. Therefore caries proceed more quickly once into dentin and generally require surgical intervention and restoration. In contrast, early enamel caries can be treated and the enamel remineralized.

PROBLEM 3

Dentin tubules are an important structural feature of dentin and are the pathways taken by odontoblasts during formation, starting from the DEJ and proceeding to the pulp chamber. Why does this result in a different number of tubules per unit area and difference in moisture level with distance from the pulp?

Solution

Each odontoblast forms one tubule during dentinogenesis. Because the DEJ surface is larger than the surface of the pulp chamber, the tubules are more concentrated at deeper levels, resulting in an increased number of tubules per unit area. Because tubules are filled with fluid and there is a positive pressure from the pulp, the higher number of (and somewhat larger diameter) tubules in deeper dentin results in more moisture when deep dentin is cut than when superficial dentin is cut. Thus deep dentin is inherently wetter than superficial dentin. This has important implications for bonding because moisture may interfere with bonding procedures and there is less solid dentin in deeper dentin available for bonding.

PROBLEM 4

Cavity preparations in the crown nearly always involve both enamel and dentin, and often at least some portions of the dentin may have been affected by caries. What difficulties does this situation present for restorative dental treatments?

Solution

These difficulties are particularly important in bonding to such mixed substrates and are less important for amalgam or crown preparations. In bonding applications we seek to make micromechanical bonds to the enamel and dentin substrates. This is generally easier for enamel than dentin, and the enamel portions of most preparations are in sound enamel. Furthermore, enamel is not as sensitive to moisture content, and the enamel can be thoroughly dried if necessary to promote bonding. Dentin is inherently wet with moisture level increasing with depth in the crown. In dentin demineralized by etching or caries, drying causes collapse of the exposed matrix, which makes it difficult to penetrate by bonding agents. In addition, cutting dentin results in smear layer formation, which may interfere with bonding. This may be of less concern with some self-etching systems that incorporate smear layer or its remnants in the bonding layer. In addition, the dentin substrate may have been altered by caries. Such alterations may include loss of mineral, making it more susceptible to etchants, or the formation of a transparent layer that blocks the tubule orifices and may restrict bonding. Most research has suggested that bond strengths to caries-altered dentin are lower than to normal dentin.

PROBLEM 5

The dentin-enamel junction (DEJ) is the starting surface (starting line) for dentinogenesis. After tooth formation, the DEJ joins enamel and dentin and is an important crack-arresting interface. It is also an important landmark for restorative procedures. What are the current concepts concerning this junction and how it assists tooth function, minimizes tooth fracture, and defines an important landmark to determine treatment?

Solution

Enamel tends to be brittle and less tough than dentin. The dentin is needed to support and distribute stresses. The DEJ joins these two different calcified tissues and helps provide an integrated structure that resists crack propagation from enamel to dentin. It appears to function this way by providing a complex geometrical surface that helps deflect cracks and provides the tooth structure with a more gradual transition in properties from enamel to dentin. Both the geometrical complexity and the graduated properties enhance bonding between the tissues and prevent abrupt transitions in mechanical properties. Such abrupt changes would lead to higher stresses at the interface that otherwise would favor separation of the enamel from the dentin. In addition, the DEJ is a key diagnostic marker in current practice because caries that progress past this junction are treated restoratively, but lesions restricted to the enamel may be treated by remineralization. In restorative treatments that require removal of tooth structure beyond the DEJ, the restored tooth is likely to be weaker and more prone to fracture.

PROBLEM 6

List some of the factors that contribute to the increased accumulation of oral biofilms on resin composite restorations.

Solution

Bacterial adhesion and biofilm formation on the surfaces of dental biomaterials are complex processes that depend on a large number of factors. An increase in the surface roughness of a restoration due to abrasion or erosion and factors affecting the degradation of the resin restoration, such as acid production by cariogenic organisms and hydrolysis of the resin matrix by saliva, are all capable of influencing biofilm accumulation on a resin restoration. Insufficient polishing of a resin restoration has also been associated with biofilm formation. Additionally, the release of trace amounts of unpolymerized resin and the products of resin biodegradation can affect the growth of oral bacteria in the vicinity of resin composite restorations.

PROBLEM 7

You have a patient who has a large number of cervical restorations made of resin-modified glass ionomer. The patient's restorations and teeth were recently cleaned with an ultrasonic scaler. What should you be concerned about?

Solution

The creation of a rough restoration surface by abrasion, erosion, air polishing, or ultrasonic instrumentation has been associated with increased biofilm formation. The restorations could be repolished or coated with a surface sealant (liquid polish) to rectify the roughening of the surfaces. The restorations should be monitored periodically because clinical studies have not clearly demonstrated that fluoride-releasing dental biomaterials significantly reduce the incidence of secondary caries, and because secondary caries most commonly occur at the gingival margin of restorations.

Bibliography

Arola D, Bajaj D, Ivancik J, et al: Fatigue of biomaterials: hard tissues, *Int J Fatigue* 32(9):1400–1412, 2010.

Bajaj D, Arola D: Role of prism decussation on fatigue crack growth and fracture of human enamel, *Acta Biomater* 5(8):3045, 2009.

Balooch M, Habelitz S, Kinney JH, et al: Mechanical properties of mineralized collagen fibrils as influenced by demineralization, *J Struct Biol* 162:404–410, 2008.

Brauer D, Marshall GW, Marshall SJ: Variation in DEJ scallop size with tooth type, *J Dent* 38:597–601, 2010.

Cuy JL, Mann AB, Livi KJ, et al: Nanoindentation mapping of the mechanical properties of human molar tooth enamel, *Arch Oral Biol* 47(4):281–291, 2002 Apr.

Fosse G, Saele PK, Eide R: Numerical density and distributional pattern of dentin tubules, *Acta Odontologica Scand* 50:201–210, 1992.

Garberoglio R, Brannstrom M: Scanning electron microscopic investigation of human dentinal tubules, *Arch Oral Biol* 21:355–362, 1976.

Habelitz S, Marshall SJ, Marshall GW, et al: Mechanical properties of human dental enamel on the nanometer scale, *Arch Oral Biol* 46:173–183, 2001.

Habelitz S, Rodriguez BJ, Marshall SJ, et al: Peritubular dentin lacks piezoelectricity, *J Dent Res* 86:908–911, 2007.

Imbeni V, Kruzic JJ, Marshall GW, et al: The dentin-enamel junction and the fracture of human teeth, *Nature Mater* 4:229–232, 2005.

Marshall GW, Olson LM, Lee CV: SEM Investigation of the variability of enamel surfaces after simulated clinical acid etching for pit and fissure sealants, *J Dent Res* 54:1222–1231, 1975.

Marshall GW, Marshall SJ, Bayne SC: Restorative dental materials: scanning electron microscopy and x-ray microanalysis, *Scanning Microsc* 2:2007–2028, 1988.

Marshall GW: Dentin: microstructure and characterization, *Quintessence Int* 24:606–617, 1993.

Marshall GW, Marshall SJ, Kinney JH, et al: The dentin substrate: structure and properties related to bonding, *J Dent* 25:441–458, 1997.

Marshall GW, Chang JY, Gansky SA, et al: Demineralization of caries-affected transparent dentin by citric acid: an atomic force microscopy study, *Dent Mater* 17:45–52, 2001b.

Marshall GW, Habelitz S, Gallagher R, et al: Nanomechanical properties of hydrated carious human dentin, *J Dent Res* 80:1768–1771, 2001a.

Marshall GW, Yucel N, Balooch M, et al: Sodium hypochlorite alterations of dentin and dentin collagen, *Surface Science* 491:444–455, 2001.

Marshall SJ, Balooch M, Breunig T, et al: Human dentin and the dentin-resin adhesive interface, *Acta Mater* 46:2529–2539, 1998.

Marshall SJ, Balooch M, Habelitz S, et al: The dentin-enamel junction—a natural, multilevel interface, *J European Ceram Soc* 23:2897–2904, 2003.

Nazari A, Bajaj D, Zhang D, et al: Aging and the reduction in fracture toughness of human dentin, *J Mech Behav Biomed Mater* 2(5):550–559, 2009.

Olsson S, Olio G, Adamczak E: The structure of dentin surfaces exposed for bond strength measurements, *Scand J Dent Res* 101:180–184, 1993.

Pashley DH: Dentin: a dynamic substrate—a review, *Scanning Microscopy* 3:161–176, 1989.

Pashley DH, Tao L, Boyd L, et al: Scanning electron microscopy of the substructure of smear layers in human dentine, *Arch Oral Biol* 33(4):265–270, 1988.

Shimizu D, Macho GA: Functional significance of the microstructural detail of the primate dentino-enamel junction: a possible example of exaptation, *J Hum Evol* 52(1):103–111, 2007 Jan.

Zheng L, Hilton JF, Habelitz S, et al: Dentin caries activity status related to hardness and elasticity, *Eur J Oral Sci* 111(3):243–252, 2003.

Oral Biofilms

Bernardo M, Luis H, Martin MD, et al: Survival and reasons for failure of amalgam versus composite posterior restorations placed in a randomized clinical trial, *J Am Dent Assoc* 138(6):775–783, 2007.

Bollen CM, Lambrechts P, Quirynen M: Comparison of surface roughness of oral hard materials to the threshold surface roughness for bacterial plaque retention: a review of the literature, *Dent Mater* 13(4):258–269, 1997.

Busscher HJ, Rinastiti M, Siswomihardjo W, et al: Biofilm formation on dental restorative and implant materials, *J Dent Res* 89(7):657–665, 2010.

Drummond J: Degradation, fatigue, and failure of resin dental composite materials, *J Dent Res* 87(8):710–719, 2008.

Hannig C, Hannig M: The oral cavity—a key system to understand substratum-dependent bioadhesion on solid surfaces in man, *Clin Oral Investig* 13(2):123–139, 2009.

Khalichi P, Singh J, Cvitkovitch DG, et al: The influence of triethylene glycol derived from dental composite resins on the regulation of Streptococcus mutans gene expression, *Biomaterials* 30(4):452–459, 2009.

Kolenbrander PE, Andersen RN, Blehert DS, et al: Communication among oral bacteria, *Microbiol Mol Biol Rev* 66(3):486–505, 2002.

Kolenbrander PE, Palmer RJ Jr, Rickard AH, et al: Bacterial interactions and successions during plaque development, *Periodontol 2000* 42:47–79, 2006.

Mjor IA, et al: Clinical diagnosis of recurrent caries, *J Am Dent Assoc* 136(10):1426–1433, 2005.

Quirynen M, Bollen CM, Papaioannou W, et al: The influence of titanium abutment surface roughness on plaque accumulation and gingivitis: short-term observations, *Int J Oral Maxillofacial Implants* 11(2):169–178, 1996.

Ready D, Qureshi F, Bedi R, et al: Oral bacteria resistant to mercury and to antibiotics are present in children with no previous exposure to amalgam restorative materials, *FEMS Microbiology Letters* 223(1):107–111, 2003.

Subramani K, Jung RE, Molenberg A, et al: Biofilm on dental implants: a review of the literature, *Int J Oral Maxillofac Implants* 24(4):616–626, 2009.

Teughels W, Van Assche N, Sliepen I, et al: Effect of material characteristics and/or surface topography on biofilm development, *Clin Oral Implants Res* 17(Suppl 2):68–81, 2006.

von Fraunhofer JA, Loewy ZG: Factors involved in microbial colonization of oral prostheses, *Gen Dent* 57(2):136–143, 2009:quiz 44–5.

Wiegand A, Buchalla W, Attin T: Review on fluoride-releasing restorative materials–fluoride release and uptake characteristics, antibacterial activity and influence on caries formation, *Dent Mater* 23(3):343–362, 2007.

Design Criteria for Restorative Dental Materials

As discussed in Chapter 2, restorative materials are exposed to chemical, thermal, and mechanical challenges in the oral environment. The combination of forces, displacements, bacteria, biofilm, fluids, thermal fluctuations, and changing pH contribute to the degradation of natural and synthetic biomaterials. Each patient has a unique combination of these factors. When considering a new or replacement restoration for a patient, the performance history of the patient's existing restorations can provide insight into the prognosis of the new restoration. The performance of materials in controlled conditions, in vitro and in vivo, is also useful when selecting materials and predicting their service life. Making the final materials choices involves a complex decision-making process that can be informed by principles of product design.

DESIGN CYCLE

Considering many factors and integrating many specifications into one final product is a requirement of any object that requires fabrication. In product design, a cyclical approach of analyzing and then testing problems is used to determine the best design for the final production piece. Three categories of problem-solving are used in the design cycle: observe, plan, and build. Then the steps are repeated as the time, number of problems, and difficulty of problems allow (Figure 3-1).

To illustrate how this process can be applied to the design of a materials-sensitive product for dental hygiene, we use the simple example of dental floss. The job this product needs to accomplish is removal of interproximal plaque and debris. All interproximal regions and surfaces are not the same. Some interproximal contacts are tight, others are open, and some regions might have proximal restorations with varying degrees of marginal adaptation. The development of a new dental floss product might start with the problem of a potential customer who has a two-surface posterior restoration with an overhang. Current floss products on the market shred or tear when flossing in such a region. This main *observation* is analyzed and deemed significant, because many people with this problem and similar problems could be helped by a design change to this dental floss. Multiple and varied ideas are generated to address the problem: (1) the dental floss cross section could be a ribbon rather than a rope to ease the floss over the overhang; (2) the floss could be a single strand rather than a braid of multiple strands to reduce the number of surfaces on the floss that could catch; or (3) the floss could be made of a different material or a slippery coating could be added to reduce friction. (Note that all of these designs have been presented to consumers at one time or another.)

Based on these possible design changes, a *plan* is made that incorporates a method or combination of methods that appear to be most promising in regard to addressing the observed problem. All of the possibilities could have merit, but by selecting those that address the *observed problem* most directly, one can test the solutions most directly. In this example, we will say that the floss will be formed as a ribbon cross section and a change of material will be made to reduce friction. The new floss is *built* and tested in simulated and actual environments.

One cycle of our design process for a new dental floss has been completed. We hope to find in our testing that we solved the observed problem. That would be an effective solution. What we may observe through testing our built product, however, is that the material is too slippery to remove plaque effectively, or the ribbon is too wide to stay flat when drawn through the interproximal contact and into the gingival sulcus. Based on these observations, a new plan is made, a new product version is created, and we find that we have completed another design cycle. We repeat this process creating more refined versions of the product that provide more exacting solutions to the observed problems. We also observe use of the product in as broad a range of consumer groups as possible to ensure the product addresses the needs of the target market.

The design cycle for developing new products can be used in the planning of restorations as well. When selecting materials for a restoration, one observes the patient's oral and medical condition and prioritizes the observed problems. The observation data are integrated with valid materials performance data to create a plan of treatment. A restoration is built and tested for occlusion, compatibility, esthetics, feel, and so forth. Adjustments are made in recurring observe,

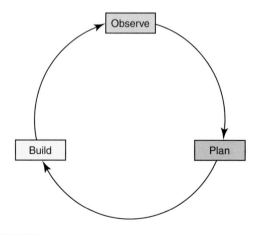

FIGURE 3.1 **The design cycle: Observe, Plan, Build, ...** **Repeat.**

plan, build steps, refining the restoration to satisfy both patient and clinician.

EVIDENCE USED IN PRODUCT DESIGN

The entire design cycle is based on evidence. Observation provides evidence about the history of performance of existing materials and solutions and identifies the job that new solutions must perform. The thoroughness of the observation phase depends on the skills and experience of the designer. In the plan phase, material properties and characteristics and test data for performance of materials in controlled conditions are added to the observation data. The build phase integrates knowledge of the job or problem with the skill and experience of the designer and considers variations in the operating conditions and properties and known performance of the materials. Without this systematic and integrative approach, the design process would be haphazard and wasteful. The evidence-based design cycle just described is analogous to evidence-based decision making in health care and evidence-based dentistry.

EVIDENCE-BASED DENTISTRY

The American Dental Association (ADA) defines *evidence-based dentistry* as an approach to oral health care that requires the judicious integration of systematic assessments of clinically relevant scientific evidence relating to the patient's oral and medical condition and history, along with the dentist's clinical expertise and the patient's treatment needs and preferences (http://ebd.ada.org). This approach is patient centered and tailored to the patient's needs and preferences. Our goal is to practice at the intersection of the three circles (Figure 3-2).

Patient Evidence

Patient needs, conditions, and preferences are considered throughout the diagnostic and treatment planning process. *Observation* of patient needs and medical/dental history occurs first. In this phase, performance of prior and existing restorations, in terms of success or failure, should be noted. This is often a good indicator of conditions in the oral environment and the prognosis of success of similar materials in this environment. The patient's facial profile and orofacial musculature is a good indicator of potential occlusal forces. Wear patterns on occlusal surfaces are indicators of bruxing, clenching, occlusal forces, and mandibular movements. Cervical

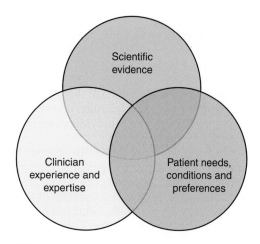

FIGURE 3.2 **The elements of evidence-based dentistry.**

abfractions may indicate heavy occlusal contact accompanied by bruxing or occlusal interferences. Erosion on anterior teeth suggests elevated levels of dietary acids, and generalized wear without occlusal trauma could involve a systemic disorder such as gastroesophageal reflux disease (GERD). Any of these conditions would compromise the longevity of restorative therapy. Unusually harsh environments require careful restoration design and selection of materials, sometimes different from the norm.

The options for material to be selected then need to be considered in accord with the problems and needs exhibited by the patient. These data are found in the scientific literature. The integration of patient data and materials data helps make a more fully considered plan for treatment.

Laboratory (In Vitro) Evidence

When searching for scientific evidence, the best available evidence, usually compiled from a review of the scientific literature, provides scientific evidence to inform the clinician and patient. The highest level of validity is chosen to minimize bias. These studies are typically meta-analyses of randomized controlled trials (RCTs), systematic reviews, or individual RCTs. Lower levels of evidence are found in case studies, cohort studies, and case reports. Laboratory studies are listed as "other evidence" because a clinical correlation can be made only as an extrapolation of the laboratory data. The listing of bench or laboratory research as "other evidence" should not be construed as meaning that bench research is not valid. The hierarchy of evidence as presented for evidence-based data (EBD) is based on human clinical data, for which bench data can only be a surrogate.

When searching for scientific evidence, the best available, or most valid, data should be chosen. New material developments that are enhancements to existing products are not required to undergo clinical testing by the Food and Drug Administration (FDA). Published laboratory or in vitro studies are often the only forms of scientific evidence available for materials. This does not mean that no evidence is available. It is simply an indication that laboratory studies should be admitted into evidence for making the clinical decision (Table 3-1).

Researchers in dental materials science have sought to correlate one or two physical or mechanical properties of materials with clinical performance. Although it is possible to use laboratory tests to rank the performance of different formulations of the same class of material, the perfect clinical predictor remains elusive. Often the comparison of laboratory-based materials studies is difficult because of an incomplete description of methods and materials. Researchers in dental materials are encouraged to provide a complete set of experimental conditions in their publications to enable the comparison of data among studies. This process will facilitate systematic reviews of laboratory studies that can be used as a source of scientific evidence when clinical studies are not available.

Every patient is unique, including the patient's oral environment and general physiology. This provides a unique set of circumstances and challenges for implementing successful materials choices in a treatment plan. The elements of EBD and material properties should be considered as a system to provide the best patient-centered care. The observed evidence in an assessment of the patient, the analyzed evidence of the laboratory data, the experience of the clinician, and the needs and wants of the patient are all related and all impact the prognosis of the restoration. Although it might be tempting to categorize a patient's needs by age, gender, or general clinical presentation, careful data gathering, planning, and analysis provides the best solution. This assessment is the basis for the complex process of oral rehabilitation (Figure 3-3).

CREATING THE PLAN

The *plan phase* integrates elements of evidence-based decision making and a consideration of material properties and performance. The process of treatment planning is familiar to clinicians, but the practice of designing restorations with material properties in mind might not be done routinely. To begin, performance requirements are analyzed. The environment in which the restoration will serve is used as a modifier to the performance requirements. For example, when treatment planning a three-unit

TABLE 3.1   Assessing the Quality of Evidence

Study Quality	Diagnosis	Treatment/Prevention/ Screening	Prognosis
Level 1: good-quality, patient-oriented evidence	Validated clinical decision rule SR/meta-analysis of high-quality studies High-quality diagnostic cohort study*	SR/meta-analysis or RCTs with consistent findings High-quality individual RCT[†] All-or-none study[‡]	SR/meta-analysis of good-quality cohort studies Prospective cohort study with good follow-up
Level 2: limited-quality patient-oriented evidence	Unvalidated clinical decision rule SR/meta-analysis of lower quality studies or studies with inconsistent findings Lower quality diagnostic cohort study or diagnostic case-control study	SR/meta-analysis of lower quality clinical trials or of studies with inconsistent findings Lower quality clinical trial Cohort study Case-control study	SR/meta-analysis of lower quality cohort studies or with inconsistent results Retrospective cohort study or prospective cohort study with poor follow-up Case-control study Case series
Level 3: other evidence	Consensus guidelines, extrapolations from bench research, usual practice, opinion, disease-oriented evidence (intermediate or physiologic outcomes only), or case series for studies of diagnosis, treatment, prevention, or screening		

From Newman MG, Weyant R, Hujoel P: J. Evid. Based Dent. Pract. 7, 147-150, 2007.
*High-quality diagnostic cohort study: cohort design, adequate size, adequate spectrum of patients, blinding, and a consistent, well-defined reference standard.
†High-quality RCT: allocation concealed, blinding if possible, intention-to-treat analysis, adequate statistical power, adequate follow-up (greater than 80%).
‡In an all-or-none study, the treatment causes a dramatic change in outcomes, such as antibiotics for meningitis or surgery for appendicitis, which precludes study in a controlled trial.
SR, Systematic review; RCT, randomized controlled trial.

posterior fixed dental prosthesis, the usual considerations will include the length of the span, location, condition of the abutments, opposing occlusion, periodontal support of the abutments, parafunctional habits, oral hygiene, existing restorations in the abutment teeth, shape of the edentulous area, and esthetic concerns. Other elements for the integrative plan and design are the three-dimensional geometry of the edentulous area, potential occlusal force that can be generated, history of other restorations in the region, the cause of tooth loss, and potential materials and their properties. Tooth preparation occurs after the restoration is conceptually designed because the design of the restoration will determine the amount and shape of the tooth reduction.

When creating a plan, the goal is to be succinct, which is difficult to do considering a goal of the observe phase is to be comprehensive in the gathering of data. Some pieces of information will be extraneous to the treatment problem and can conceal the best plan of treatment. There will be synergistic and contradictory materials solutions for the possible plans of action. There will be features and constraints presented by each possible materials choice. Prioritization of this information will guide the clinician toward the solutions that will be most effective.

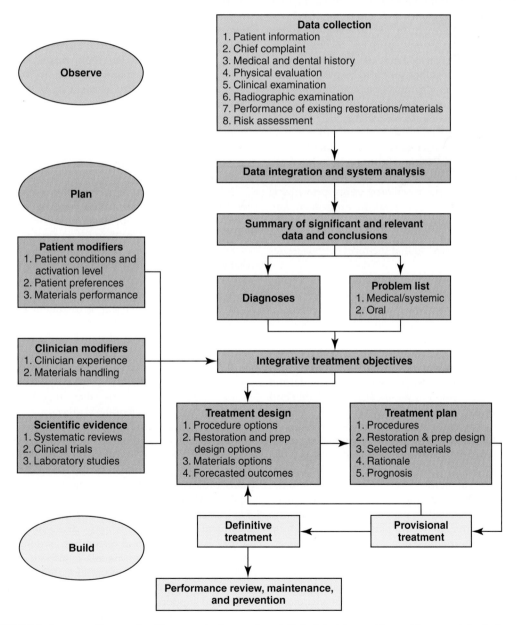

FIGURE 3.3 A process diagram that illustrates the integration of clinical decision making, evidence, and the design cycle.

Some diagnoses of a clinical situation may have a strong basis in the care that was previously provided. A patient may have an upper posterior tooth that is exhibiting an excessive amount of wear. A lower posterior crown with a porcelain occlusal surface could be the culprit. Porcelain was chosen for esthetic reasons. However, the hard porcelain occlusal surface is abrading the upper tooth, resulting in severe occlusal wear of the enamel surface. This prognosis could be addressed by restoring the upper tooth, and/or by changing the restoration on the lower tooth to a softer material or less abrasive material. Because the preservation of natural tooth material is a high priority, replacement of the lower crown with a material that is more harmonious with the occlusal scheme would provide the best service for the patient. The importance of a systems approach to observation and planning is illustrated here, where all factors are to be considered together, followed by prioritization.

Prioritization is also an opportunity to provide education and to enhance the patient's level of activation. It is not uncommon for patients to be unaware of serious oral problems. For example, interproximal caries or oral lesions might not be evident to the patient, whereas a single discolored anterior tooth can be very noticeable. Although the patient's desire for care could be the discolored tooth, prioritizing the care and first acting to treat the immediate danger of infection and disease progression helps the patent's overall oral health. The priorities and expectations can be altered so that the most serious issues are addressed first.

The patient may arrive with a materials-specific treatment in mind, such as a ceramic veneer on the discolored tooth mentioned earlier. If the tooth is in malocclusion or potentially abutting an opposing natural enamel surface, a ceramic material could be an unwise choice because of the potential for chipping or wear of the opposing tooth. In this case, composite is a better choice for longevity of the natural dentition. Discussion of the materials available and the potential plans of action can shift the patient's understanding of the problem to include the unique nature of the case, the desire for a long-lasting, naturally colored restoration, and the materials that are best suited for the case to meet the patient's initial goal. The planning then shifts away from the predetermined material specification of a ceramic veneer. Including the patient in prioritizing his or her care provides an immediate and personal feedback loop that can be incorporated into the planning phase.

The materials used are both features and constraints of a restoration. Composites, ceramics, and metals offer features and constraints that allow their applications to vary slightly in different treatments. The *observe, plan, build…repeat* cycle is a process that aids the identification and analysis of features and constraints. Each step of the cycle offers opportunities to prioritize the features and constraints of materials for the case and select those that best fit the occlusal scheme. In every design cycle, the solution and problem become more convergent and the quality of the final product or service increases.

BUILDING THE RESTORATION

Building is the next phase. The building required for the restoration may be directly applied to the tooth or may require several iterative steps to create the final product, including a laboratory procedure. In many intracoronal restorations and some veneers, the restoration is applied directly to the tooth and typically completed in one visit. These are referred to as *direct procedures*. For these procedures, final material decisions are made prior to any "building" procedures. The plan of treatment must include all materials selections. Fine adjustments are made by adding and/or removing material based on assessment of the occlusion, questioning the patient about tactile feel, and evaluating the esthetics and harmony of the restoration with the rest of the dentition and oral environment.

Some restorative materials are more sensitive to technique variations than others. For example, placement of resin composite restorations in posterior teeth requires more steps than for an amalgam. Each of these steps require a specified level of precision, that when totaled, equate to a more complex process. An error in any step could affect the success of the restoration. *Clinical expertise* therefore is an important factor when developing a treatment plan and selecting restorative materials, particularly when the restoration is a direct application to the tooth. The handling properties of a material are an important consideration that is often difficult to measure and describe.

In indirect restorations that require several appointments and a laboratory procedure, *prototyping* occurs before building. Prototyping can also be done with direct restorations, for example, by simulating the shape and color of a composite veneer without curing the material. For indirect restorations, prototyping is done routinely. Creating models of the final restoration is helpful because that allows the clinician and patient to discuss and agree on treatment outcomes. This early discussion reduces surprises when the final restoration is delivered to the patient. The use of models is also an excellent aid for designing tooth preparations that optimally transfer occlusal force through the restoration to the tooth and supporting tissues.

The concept of *prototyping* is also useful in the fabrication of provisional or transitional restorations for indirect restorations. When the provisional restoration accurately simulates the final design in form and appearance, the patient and clinician can discuss design outcomes, expectations, and required modifications. Esthetics is particularly important to simulate as accurately as possible because of its subjectivity. Color, shape, size, and position are all important factors to evaluate to ensure the patient's satisfaction with the restoration. Provisional restorations also act as important diagnostic aids for studying occlusion, occlusal forces, parafunctional habits, oral hygiene, and soft tissue response. Analysis of the performance of carefully fabricated transitional restorations can provide many clues for optimal design and fabrication of the permanent restoration. The transitional restoration is the place for *testing* and making *iterative modifications* to design concepts before the permanent restoration is fabricated. Observations of occlusal wear facets, cracks, dislodgements, discoloration, and discomfort from the provisional restoration are all indicators of conditions that might be beyond the usual design limits. Studying the cause of these events can help specify material properties for the dental laboratory.

Material selection is best made during planning and design rather than after tooth preparation. Material options for a particular restorative scenario will differ in their mechanical and physical properties. For example, casting alloys for a fixed dental prosthesis differ in their stiffness, hardness, malleability, and corrosion resistance. Higher stiffness alloys will transfer more occlusal stress to the abutments, whereas lower stiffness alloys will deform and cause the prosthesis to deflect. Corrosion resistance is important when patients have diets high in acids and consume foods and fluids with high staining potential. In another example, ceramics might satisfy the esthetic requirements of the restoration, but might not be suitable for the high occlusal loads of patients who brux and clench.

The concepts of the design process—*observe, plan, build…repeat*—integrate well with evidence-based decision making and materials selection. When all of these elements are considered together, an integrative treatment plan and design can be achieved that provides the optimal outcome for the patient. The iterative cycle of design also provides many opportunities for discussion between the clinician and patient to facilitate agreement on expectations well ahead of the delivery of the final restoration.

Chapter 4 presents concepts of material science, including the physical and mechanical properties of materials. A good understanding of the fundamental properties of materials enables the clinician to design treatment and prepare oral tissues to best distribute forces in the oral environment.

Bibliography

American Dental Association: *ADA Center for Evidence-Based Dentistry.* http://ebd.ada.org/. Accessed August 28, 2011.

Ashby MF: *Materials Selection and Process in Mechanical Design.* 1999, Butterworth Heinemann, Oxford.

Ashby MF, Johnson K: *Materials and Design, the Art and Science of Materials Selection in Product Design,* 2002, Butterworth Heinemann, Oxford.

Bader JD: Stumbling into the age of evidence, *Dent Clin North Am* 53(1):15, 2009.

Brown T: Design thinking, *Harv Bus Rev* 86(6):84, 2008.

Forrest JL: Introduction to the basics of evidence-based dentistry: concepts and skills, *J Evid Based Dent Pract* 9(3):108, 2009.

Forrest JL, Miller SA: Translating evidence-based decision making into practice: EBDM concepts and finding the evidence, *J Evid Based Dent Pract* 9(2):59, 2009.

Martin R: How successful leaders think, *Harv Bus Rev* 85(6):60, 2007.

Miller SA, Forrest JL: Translating evidence-based decision making into practice: appraising and applying the evidence, *J Evid Based Dent Pract* 9(4):164, 2009.

Newman MG, Weyant R, Hujoel P: JEBDP improves grading system and adopts strength of recommendation taxonomy grading (SORT) for guidelines and systematic reviews, *J Evid Based Dent Pract* 7:147–150, 2007.

Sakaguchi RL: Evidence-Based Dentistry: Achieving a Balance, *J Am Dent Assoc* 141(5):496–497, 2010.

Vossoughi S: Designing the 'care' into health care, Business Week Nov 21, 2007.

Fundamentals of Materials Science

Restorative dental materials are subjected to a very hostile environment, in which pH, salivary flow, and mechanical loading fluctuate constantly and often rapidly. These challenges have required substantial research and development to provide products for the clinician. Much of this is possible through the application of fundamental concepts of materials science. The understanding of properties of polymers, ceramics, and metals is crucial to their selection and design of dental restorations.

No single property defines the quality of a material. Often several properties, determined from standardized laboratory and clinical tests, are used to describe quality. Laboratory tests, although they are only surrogates for clinical studies, provide standardized measures for comparing materials and guiding the interpretation of clinical trials.

Standardization of laboratory tests is essential, however, to control quality and permit comparison of results between investigators. When possible, test specimens should mimic the size and shape of the structure in the clinical setting, with mixing and manipulating procedures being equivalent to routine clinical conditions.

Although it is important to know the comparative values of properties of different restorative materials, it is also essential to know the quality of the supporting and investing hard and soft tissues. Many restorations fail clinically because of fracture or deformation. This is a material property issue. Some well-constructed restorations become unserviceable because the supporting tissue fails. This is an interface or substrate failure. Consequently, when designing restorations and interpreting test results, it is important to remember that the success of a restoration depends not only on its physical qualities but also on the biophysical or physiological qualities of the supporting tissues.

The physical properties described in this chapter include mechanical properties, thermal properties, electrical and electromechanical properties, color, and optical properties.

MECHANICAL PROPERTIES

In the oral environment, restorative materials are exposed to chemical, thermal, and mechanical challenges. These challenges can cause deformation of the material. The science that studies how biological materials interact and deform is called *biomechanics*. This section introduces concepts of elastic, plastic, and viscoelastic deformation and mechanical quantities including force, stress, strain, strength, toughness, hardness, friction, and wear in terms of performance of materials in the oral environment.

Force

One body interacting with another generates force. Forces may be applied through actual contact of the bodies or at a distance (e.g., gravity). The result of an applied force on a body is translation or deformation of the body depending on whether the body is rigid or deformable and whether the body is constrained. If the body is constrained (i.e., does not move or translate), the force causes the body to deform or change its shape. If the body is free of constraints, an applied force results in movement or translation.

A force is defined by three characteristics: point of application, magnitude, and direction of application. The direction of a force is characteristic of the type of force. The International System of Units (SI) unit of force is the Newton (N). One pound-force (lb-f) equals 4.4 Newtons (N).

Occlusal Forces

Maximum occlusal forces range from 200 to 3500 N. Occlusal forces between adult teeth are highest in the posterior region closest to the mandibular hinge axis and decrease from the molar region to the incisors. Forces on the first and second molars vary from 400 to 800 N. The average force on the bicuspids, cuspids, and incisors is about 300, 200, and 150 N, respectively. A somewhat nonlinear but definite increase in force from 235 to 494 N occurs in growing children, with an average yearly increase of about 22 N.

Forces on Restorations

Occlusal forces with dental prosthetic devices are generally lower than with natural dentition. Patients with removable partial dentures generate occlusal forces in the range of 65 to 235 N. For patients with complete dentures, the average force on the molars and bicuspids is about 100 N; the forces on the incisors averages 40 N. Age and gender variations in the patient populations contribute to the large variation in force values. In general, the occlusal force produced by women is about 90 N less than that applied by men. Facial form and muscle definition are good predictors of occlusal force capacity. Patients with high mandibular angles generally exhibit lower occlusal forces than patients with low angles and square mandibular form.

Maximum occlusal force and the response of underlying tissues change with anatomic location, age, occlusal scheme, and placement of a dental prosthesis. When designing restorations and selecting materials, it is important to consider the location, opposing dentition, and force-generating capacity of the patient. These factors can often be estimated by the success or failure of other restorations in the patient's mouth. A material or design sufficient to withstand the forces of occlusion in the anterior segment may not be sufficient for the posterior segment.

Stress

When a force acts on a constrained body, the force is resisted by the body. This internal reaction is equal in magnitude and opposite in direction to the applied external force, and is called *stress,* typically denoted as S or σ. Both the applied force and the internal resistance (stress) are distributed over an area of the body, so the stress in an object is defined as the *force per area,* or stress = force/area. Stress is difficult to measure directly, so the force and the area to which the force is applied are measured, and stress is calculated from the ratio of force per area. The unit of stress therefore is the unit of force (N) divided by a unit of area, and is commonly expressed in SI units as Pascal ($1 \text{ Pa} = 1 \text{ N/m}^2 = 1 \text{ MN/mm}^2$). It is common to report stress in units of megaPascals (MPa) or millions of Pascals, $1 \text{ MPa} = 10^6 \text{ Pa}$.

Because the stress in a structure varies directly with the force and inversely with area, the area over which the force acts is an important consideration. This is particularly true in dental restorations in which the areas over which the forces are applied often are extremely small. For example, cusp areas of contact may have cross-sectional areas of only 0.16 to 0.016 cm^2.

As a numerical example, a 20-gauge orthodontic wire has a diameter of 0.8 mm and a cross-sectional area of 0.5 mm^2. If a 220-N force is applied to a wire of this diameter, the stress developed is equivalent to 220 N/0.5 mm^2, or 440 N/mm^2 (MPa).

Stress is always normalized to a 1 m^2 area, but a dental restoration such as a small occlusal pit restoration may have no more than 4 mm^2 of surface area, if the restoration is 2 mm on a side. If an occlusal force of 440 N is concentrated on this area, the stress developed would be 100 MPa. Therefore, stresses equivalent to several hundred MPa occur in many types of restorations. Stresses can be produced in the range of thousands of MPa when the contact area of a cusp or dental explorer is used to apply the force. This is one reason that premature contacts, in which small surface areas are supporting large occlusal forces, are so damaging. When equilibrating the occlusion, multiple simultaneous occlusal contacts are desirable. Distributing occlusal forces over larger surface areas reduces the local occlusal stress.

Types of Stress

A force can be applied from any angle or direction, and often several forces combine to develop complex stresses in a structure. It is rare for forces and stresses to be isolated to a single axis. Individually applied forces can be defined as axial, shear, bending, or torsional. These directional forces are illustrated in a simplified manner in Figure 4-1. All stresses, however, can be resolved into combinations of two basic types—axial and shear.

Tension results from two sets of forces directed away from each other in the same straight line or when one end is constrained and the other end is subjected to a force directed away from the constraint. *Compression* results from two sets of forces directed toward each other in the same straight line or when one surface is constrained and the other is subjected to a force directed toward the constraint. *Shear* occurs from two sets of forces directed parallel to each other, but not along the same straight line. *Torsion* results from the twisting of a body, and *bending* or *flexure* results from an applied bending moment. When tension is applied, the molecules making up the body resist being pulled apart. When compression is applied, they resist being forced more closely together. As a result of a shear stress application, one portion of the body must resist sliding past another. These resistances of a material to deformation represent the basic qualities of elasticity of solid bodies.

An example of the complexity and varying direction and magnitude of stresses in the oral cavity is shown in Figure 4-2, in which a finite element model of a dental implant is loaded in compression. Figure 4-2, *A*, shows the stresses on the shoulder of the implant resulting from occlusal forces. Figure 4-2, *B*, shows the distribution of stresses in the implant abutment.

Strain

Each type of stress is capable of producing a corresponding deformation in a body (see Figure 4-1). The deformation from a tensile force is an elongation

FORCE	DEFORMATION	
Axial, tension	Elongation	
Axial, compression	Compression	
Shear	Shear	
Twisting moment	Torsion	
Bending moment	Bending	

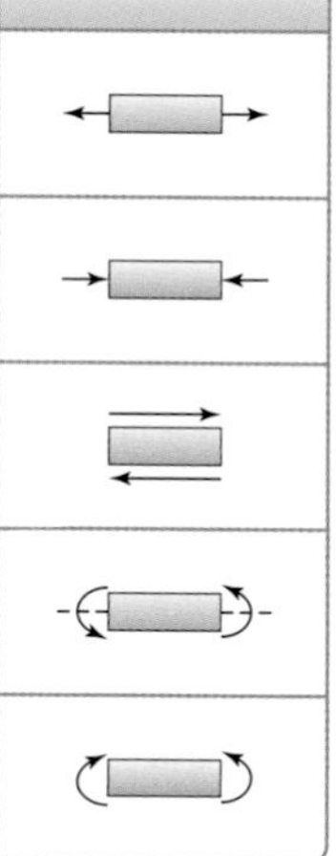

FIGURE 4.1 **Schematic of the different types of stresses and their corresponding deformations.**

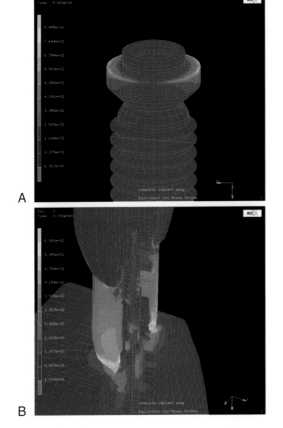

FIGURE 4.2 **Stress distribution in an implant supported restoration. A,** Stresses on the shoulder of the implant body from an oblique occlusal load. **B,** Stresses within the implant abutment and alveolar bone. *(Courtesy of Dr. Svenn Borgersen, Eagan, MN and Dr. Ronald Sakaguchi.)*

in the axis of applied force, whereas a compressive force causes compression or shortening of the body in the axis of loading. Strain, ε, is described as the change in length ($\Delta L = L - L_o$) per original length (L_o) of the body when it is subjected to a load. The units of measurement (length/length) cancel in the calculation of strain.

$$\text{Strain } (\varepsilon) = \text{Deformation / Original length}$$
$$= (L - L_o) / L_o = \Delta L / L_o$$

If a load is applied to a wire with an original length of 2 mm resulting in a new length of 2.02 mm, it has deformed 0.02 mm and the strain is 0.02/2 = 0.01, or 1%. Strain is often reported as a percentage. Although the length units cancel in the calculation of strain, it is best to report the units with the final result to specify the scale of the measurement (m/m; mm/mm; μm/μm). The amount of strain will differ with each type of material and with the magnitude of the load applied. Note that regardless of the composition or nature of the material, and regardless of

the magnitude and type of load applied to the material, deformation and strain result with each stress application. Strain is an important consideration in dental restorative materials, such as orthodontic wires or implant screws, in which a large amount of strain can occur before failure. Wires can be bent and adjusted without fracturing. Strain is also important in impression materials, where the material needs to recover without permanent distortion when removing it from hard tissue undercuts.

Stress-Strain Curves

If a bar of material is subjected to an applied force, *F*, the magnitude of the force and the resulting deformation (δ) can be measured. In another bar of the same material, but different dimensions, the same applied force produces different force-deformation characteristics (Figure 4-3, *A*). However, if the applied force is normalized by the cross-sectional area *A* of the bar (stress), and the deformation is normalized by the original length of the bar (strain), the resulting stress-strain curve is independent of the geometry of the bar (Figure 4-3, *B*). It is therefore preferred that the stress-strain relations of an object be reported rather than the force-deformation characteristics. The stress-strain relationship of a dental material can be studied by measuring the load and deformation and then calculating the corresponding stress and strain.

When testing materials, loads should be applied at a uniform rate, and deformation should occur at a uniform rate. A typical universal testing machine can analyze materials in tension, compression, or shear. In the scheme illustrated in Figure 4-4, a rod is clamped between two jaws and a tensile force is applied. The load is measured with a force transducer and the deformation is measured with an extensometer clamped over a specified length of the specimen. A plot of load versus deformation is produced, which can be converted to a plot of stress versus strain (Figure 4-5) by the simple calculations described previously. By convention, strain is plotted on the x-axis as an independent variable because most tests are operated in strain control, where a constant strain is applied to the specimen and the resulting force is measured as the dependent, or y-axis, variable.

In the calculation of stress, it is assumed that the cross-sectional area of the specimen remains constant during the test. Using this assumption, the stress-strain curve is called an *engineering stress-strain curve*, and stresses are calculated using the original cross-sectional area. When large loads are applied, or the object is tested in tension, the cross-sectional area might change dramatically during testing. In that case, the true stress, calculated with the actual cross-sectional area in the denominator, is very

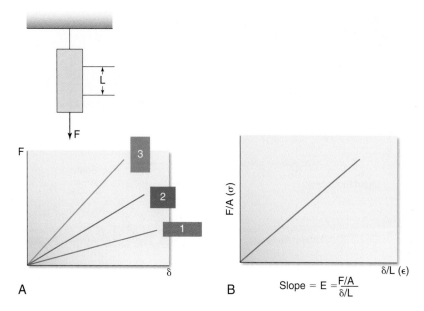

FIGURE 4.3 Force-deformation characteristics. A, Force-deformation characteristics for the same material but having different dimensions. **B,** Stress-strain characteristics of the same group of bars. The stress-strain curve is independent of the geometry of the bar.

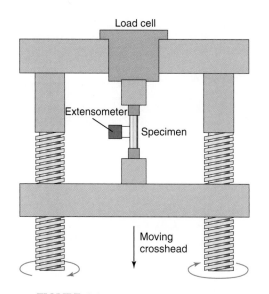

FIGURE 4.4 Universal testing machine.

different than the engineering stress, calculated with the original cross-sectional area. If the cross-sectional area decreases during the test, the true stress will be higher than the engineering stress because the denominator is smaller. In most mechanical tests, particularly those of small specimen dimensions, the original cross-sectional area is used for calculating stress because it is often very difficult to measure the cross-sectional area as it changes throughout the experiment. Engineering stress is used in the presentation of stress-strain curves obtained in tension in this chapter.

Proportional and Elastic Limits

A stress-strain curve for a hypothetical material subjected to increasing tensile stress until failure is shown in Figure 4-5. As the stress is increased, the strain is increased. In the initial portion of the curve, from 0 to A, the stress is linearly proportional to the strain. As the strain is doubled, the stress is also doubled. After point A, the stress is no longer linearly proportional to the strain. Hence the value of the stress at A is known as the *proportional limit (S_{PL} or σ_{PL})*, defined as the highest stress at which the stress-strain curve is a straight line, that is, stress is linearly proportional to strain. Below the proportional limit, no permanent deformation occurs in a structure. When the force is removed, the object will return to its original dimensions. Below the proportional limit, the material is elastic in nature.

The region of the stress-strain curve before the proportional limit is called the *elastic region*. When an object experiences a stress greater than the proportional limit, permanent or irreversible strain occurs. The region of the stress-strain curve beyond the proportional limit is called the *plastic region*. This characterization refers to linearly elastic materials such as many metals in which the relation between stress and strain is linear up to the proportional limit, and nonlinear thereafter. There are exceptions to this general rule, however. Materials described as *super-elastic* exhibit nonlinear elastic behavior; that is, their

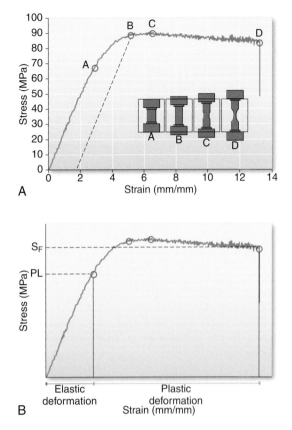

A

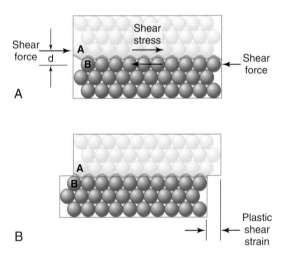

B

FIGURE 4.5 **Plotting stress-strain curves. A,** Stress-strain curve for a material subjected to tensile stress. Specimens illustrate amount of deformation at each point (*A-D*). **B,** Elastic deformation is exhibited up to the proportional limit (*PL*) and plastic deformation is exhibited from *PL* to the failure point (FP).

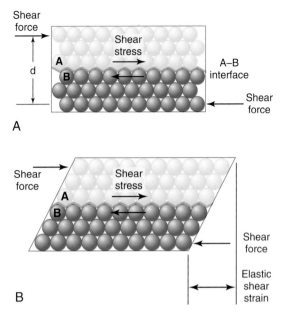

FIGURE 4.6 Sketch of an atomic model showing atoms in **A,** original position, and **B,** after elastic deformation. (*Modified from Anusavice KJ: Phillips' Science of Dental Materials, ed 11, Saunders, St. Louis, p. 79, 2003.*)

FIGURE 4.7 Sketch of an atomic model showing atoms in **A,** original position, and **B,** after plastic deformation. (*Modified from Anusavice KJ: Phillips' Science of Dental Materials, ed 11, Saunders, St. Louis, p. 79, 2003.*)

relationship between stress and strain in the elastic region does not follow a straight line, but removal of the load results in a return to zero strain.

The *elastic limit* (S_{EL} or σ_{EL}) is defined as the maximum stress that a material will withstand without permanent deformation. For linearly elastic materials, the proportional limit and elastic limit represent the same stress within the structure, and the terms are often used interchangeably in referring to the stress involved. An exception is when superelastic materials are considered. It is important to remember, however, that the two terms differ in fundamental concept; one deals with the proportionality of strain to stress in the structure, whereas the other describes the elastic behavior of the material. For the same material, values for proportional or elastic limit obtained in tension versus compression will differ.

The concepts of elastic and plastic behavior can be illustrated with a simple schematic model of the deformation of atoms in a solid under stress (Figures 4-6 and 4-7). The atoms are shown in

Figure 4-6, *A,* without stress, and in Figure 4-6, *B,* with a resulting stress that is below the value of the proportional limit. When the stress shown in *B* is removed, the atoms return to their positions shown in *A,* indicating that the deformation was reversible. When the stress is greater than the proportional limit, the atoms move to a position as shown in Figure 4-7, *B,* and on removal of the stress, the atoms remain in this new position, indicating an irreversible, permanent deformation. When the stress is less than the proportional or elastic limit, the strain is reversible, whereas when the stress is greater than the proportional or elastic limit, there is an irreversible or permanent strain in the object.

Yield Strength

It is often difficult to explicitly measure the proportional and elastic limits because the precise point of deviation of the stress-strain curve from linearity is difficult to determine. The *yield strength* or *yield stress* or *yield point (YS* or σ_Y) of a material is a property that can be determined readily and is often used to describe the stress at which the material begins to function in a plastic manner. At this point, a small, defined amount of permanent strain has occurred in the material. The yield strength is defined as the stress at which a material deforms plastically and there is a defined amount of permanent strain. The amount of permanent strain is arbitrarily selected for the material being examined and may be indicated as 0.1%, 0.2%, or 0.5% (0.001, 0.002, 0.005) permanent strain. The amount of permanent strain is referred to as the *percent offset*. Many specifications use 0.2% as a convention, but this depends on the plastic behavior of the material tested. For stiff materials with small elongation, the calculation of yield stress will include greater offsets than those materials with larger elongation or deformation.

The yield stress is determined by selecting the desired offset or strain on the x-axis and drawing a line parallel to the linear region of the stress-strain curve. The point at which the parallel line intersects the stress-strain curve is the yield stress. On the stress-strain curve shown in Figure 4-5, for example, the yield strength is represented by the value *B*. This represents a stress of about 360 MPa at a 0.25% offset. This yield stress is slightly higher than that for the proportional limit because it includes a specified amount of permanent deformation. Note that when a structure is permanently deformed, even to a small degree (such as the amount of deformation at the yield strength), it does not return completely to its original dimensions when the stress is removed. For this reason, the elastic limit and yield strength of a material are among its most important properties because they define the transition from elastic to plastic behavior.

Any dental restoration that is permanently deformed through the forces of mastication is usually a functional failure to some degree. For example, a fixed partial denture that is permanently deformed by excessive occlusal forces would exhibit altered occlusal contacts. The restoration is permanently deformed because a stress equal to or greater than the yield strength was generated. Recall also that malocclusion changes the stresses placed on a restoration; a deformed restoration may therefore be subjected to greater stresses than originally intended because the occlusion that was distributed over a larger number of occlusal contacts may now be concentrated on a smaller number of contacts. Under these conditions, fracture does not occur if the material is able to plastically deform. Permanent deformation results, which represents a destructive example of deformation. Permanent deformation and stresses in excess of the elastic limit are desirable when shaping an orthodontic arch wire or adjusting a clasp on a removable partial denture. In these examples, the stress must exceed the yield strength to permanently bend or adapt the wire or clasp. Elastic deformation occurs as the wire or clasp engages and disengages a retentive undercut in the cervical area of the tooth. Retention is achieved through small-scale elastic deformation. This elastic or reversible deformation describes the function of elastic bands, clasps, o-rings, and implant screws.

Ultimate Strength

In Figure 4-5, the test specimen exhibits a maximum stress at point C. The *ultimate tensile strength* or *stress (UTS)* is defined as the maximum stress that a material can withstand before failure in tension, whereas the *ultimate compressive strength* or *stress (UCS)* is the maximum stress a material can withstand in compression. The ultimate engineering stress is determined by dividing the maximum load in tension (or compression) by the original cross-sectional area of the test specimen. The ultimate tensile strength of the material in Figure 4-5 is about 380 MPa.

The ultimate strength of an alloy as used in dentistry specifies the maximum load and minimum cross-sectional area when designing a restoration. Note that an alloy that has been stressed to near the ultimate strength will be permanently deformed, so a restoration receiving that amount of stress during function would be useless. A safety margin should be incorporated into the design of the restoration and choice of material to ensure that the ultimate strength is not approached in normal function. The yield strength is often of greater importance than ultimate strength in design and material selection because it is an estimate of when a material will start to deform permanently.

Fracture Strength

In Figure 4-5 the test specimen fractured at point D. The stress at which a brittle material fractures is called the *fracture strength* or *fracture stress (S_F* or σ_F). Note that a material does not necessarily fracture at the point at which the maximum stress occurs. After a maximum tensile force is applied to some materials, the specimen begins to elongate excessively, resulting in "necking" or a reduction of cross-sectional area (see Figure 4-5). The stress calculated from the force and the original cross-sectional area may drop before final fracture occurs because of the reduction in cross-sectional area. Accordingly, the stress at the end of the curve is less than at some intermediate point on the curve. Therefore, in materials that exhibit necking, the ultimate and fracture strengths are different. However, for the specific cases of many dental alloys and ceramics subjected to tension, the ultimate and fracture strengths are similar, as is shown later in this chapter. Note that the reduction in stress that is observed after the ultimate stress in materials that show necking is an artifact of using the original cross-sectional area in the calculation of stress. If the true cross-sectional area is used, the stress would increase.

Elongation

The deformation that results from the application of a tensile force is *elongation*. Elongation is extremely important because it gives an indication of the possible manipulation of an alloy. As may be observed from Figure 4-5, the elongation of a material during a tensile test can be divided conveniently into two parts: (1) the increase in length of the specimen below the proportional limit (from 0 to *A*), which is not permanent and is proportional to the stress; and (2) the elongation beyond the proportional limit and up to the fracture strength (from *A* to *D*), which is permanent. The permanent deformation may be measured with an extensometer while the material is being tested and calculated from the stress-strain curve. Total elongation is commonly expressed as a percentage. The percent elongation is calculated as follows:

$$\% \text{ Elongation} = (\text{Increase in length} / \text{Original length}) \times 100\%$$

The total percent elongation includes both the elastic elongation and the plastic elongation. The plastic elongation is usually the greatest of the two, except in materials that are quite brittle or those with very low stiffness. A material that exhibits a 20% total elongation at the time of fracture has increased in length by one fifth of its original length. Such a material, as in many dental gold alloys, has a high value for plastic or permanent elongation and, in general, is a ductile type of alloy, whereas a material with only 1% elongation would possess little permanent elongation and be considered brittle.

An alloy that has a high value for total elongation can be bent permanently without danger of fracture. Clasps can be adjusted, orthodontic wires can be adapted, and crowns or inlays can be burnished if alloys with high values for elongation are used.

Elongation and yield strength are generally related in many materials, including dental gold alloys, where, generally, the higher the yield strength, the lower the elongation.

Elastic Modulus

The measure of elasticity of a material is described by the term *elastic modulus,* also referred to as *modulus of elasticity* or *Young's modulus,* and denoted by the variable *E*. The word *modulus* means ratio. The elastic modulus represents the stiffness of a material within the elastic range. The elastic modulus can be determined from a stress-strain curve (see Figure 4-5) by calculating the ratio of stress to strain or the slope of the linear region of the curve. The modulus is calculated from the following equation:

$$\text{Elastic modulus} = \text{Stress} / \text{Strain}$$

or

$$E = \sigma / \varepsilon$$

This equation is also known as Hooke's law. Because strain is unitless, the modulus has the same units as stress and is usually reported in MPa or GPa (1 GPa = 1000 MPa).

The elastic qualities of a material represent a fundamental property of the material. The interatomic or intermolecular forces of the material are responsible for the property of elasticity (see Figure 4-6). The stronger the basic attraction forces, the greater the values of the elastic modulus and the more rigid or stiff the material. Because this property is related to the attraction forces within the material, it is usually the same when the material is subjected to either tension or compression. The property is generally independent of any heat treatment or mechanical treatment that a metal or alloy has received, but is quite dependent on the composition of the material.

The elastic modulus is determined by the slope of the elastic portion of the stress-strain curve, which is calculated by choosing any two stress and strain coordinates in the elastic or linear range. As an example, for the curve in Figure 4-5, the slope can be calculated by choosing the following two coordinates:

$$\sigma_1 = 150 \text{ MPa}, \ \varepsilon_1 = 0.005$$

and

$$\sigma_2 = 300 \text{ MPa}, \ \varepsilon_2 = 0.010$$

The slope is therefore:

$$(\sigma_2 - \sigma_1) / (\varepsilon_2 - \varepsilon_1) = (300 - 150) / (0.010 - 0.005)$$
$$= 30,000 \text{ MPa} = 30 \text{ GPa}$$

Stress-strain curves for two hypothetical materials, *A* and *B,* of different composition are shown in Figure 4-8. Inspection of the curves shows that for a given stress, *A* is elastically deformed less than *B,*

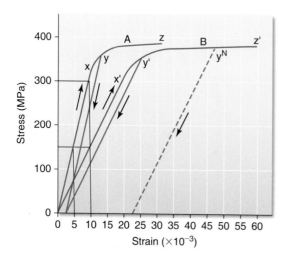

FIGURE 4.8 **Stress-strain curves of two hypothetical materials subjected to tensile stress.**

TABLE 4.1 Elastic Modulus (GPa) of Selected Dental Materials

Material	Elastic Modulus (GPa)
Enamel	84
Dentin	17
Gold (type IV) alloy	90-95
Amalgam	28-59
Cobalt-chromium partial denture alloy	218-224
Feldspathic porcelain	69-70
Resin composite with hybrid filler	17-21
Poly (methyl methacrylate)	2.4
Silicone elastomer for maxillofacial prosthesis	0.002-0.003

with the result that the elastic modulus for *A* is greater than for *B*. This difference can be demonstrated numerically, by calculating the elastic moduli for the two materials subjected to the same stress of 300 MPa. At a stress of 300 MPa, material *A* is strained to 0.01 (1%) and the elastic modulus is as follows:

$$E = 300 \text{ MPa} / 0.010 = 30{,}000 \text{ MPa} = 30 \text{ GPa}$$

On the other hand, material *B* is strained to 0.02 (2%), or twice as much as material *A* for the same stress application. The equation for the elastic modulus for *B* is

$$E = 300 \text{ MPa} / 0.020 = 15{,}000 \text{ MPa} = 15 \text{ GPa}$$

The fact that material *A* has a steeper slope in the elastic range than material *B* means that a larger force is required to deform material *A* to a given amount than is required for material *B*. From the curves shown in Figure 4-8, it can be seen that a stress of 300 MPa is required to deform *A* to the same amount elastically to which *B* is deformed by a stress of 150 MPa. Therefore, *A* is stiffer or more rigid than *B*. Conversely, *B* is more flexible than *A*. Materials such as elastomers and other polymers have low values for elastic modulus, whereas many metals and ceramics have much higher values, as shown in Table 4-1.

Poisson's Ratio

During axial loading in tension or compression there is a simultaneous strain in the axial and transverse, or lateral, directions. Under tensile loading, as a material elongates in the direction of load, there is a reduction in cross section, known as *necking*. Under compressive loading, there is an increase in the cross section. Within the elastic range, the ratio of the lateral to the axial strain is called *Poisson's ratio* (v). In

tensile loading, the Poisson's ratio indicates that the reduction in cross section is proportional to the elongation during the elastic deformation. The reduction in cross section continues until the material is fractured. Poisson's ratio is a unitless value because it is the ratio of two strains.

Most rigid materials, such as enamel, dentin, amalgam, and dental composite, exhibit a Poisson's ratio of about 0.3. Brittle substances such as hard gold alloys and dental amalgam show little permanent reduction in cross section during a tensile test. More ductile materials such as soft gold alloys, which are high in gold content, show a higher degree of reduction in cross-sectional area and higher Poisson's ratios.

Ductility and Malleability

Two significant properties of metals and alloys are ductility and malleability. The *ductility* of a material represents its ability to be drawn and shaped into wire by means of tension. When tensile forces are applied, the wire is formed by permanent deformation. The *malleability* of a substance represents its ability to be hammered or rolled into thin sheets without fracturing. Malleability comes from the Latin *malleus*, or hammer.

A high degree of elongation indicates good malleability and ductility, although some metals show some exception to this rule. The reduction in area in a specimen, together with the elongation at the breaking point, is, however, a good indication of the relative ductility of a metal or alloy.

Ductility is a property that has been related to the workability of a material in the mouth (e.g., burnishability of the margins of a casting). Although ductility is important, the amount of force necessary to cause permanent deformation during the burnishing operation also must be considered. A burnishing index has been used to rank the ease of burnishing alloys and is equal to the ductility (elongation) divided by the yield strength.

Gold and silver, used extensively in dentistry, are the most malleable and ductile of the metals, but other metals do not follow the same order for both malleability and ductility. In general, metals tend to be ductile, whereas ceramics tend to be brittle.

Resilience

Resilience is the resistance of a material to permanent deformation. It indicates the amount of energy necessary to deform the material to the proportional limit. Resilience is therefore measured by the area under the elastic portion of the stress-strain curve, as illustrated in Figure 4-9, *A.*

Resilience has particular importance in the evaluation of orthodontic wires. An example is the amount of work expected from a particular spring to move a tooth. The amount of stress and strain at the proportional limit is also of interest because these factors determine the magnitude of the force that can be applied to the tooth and how far the tooth can move before the spring is no longer effective. For example, Figure 4-10 illustrates the load-deflection curve for a nickel-titanium (Ni-Ti) orthodontic wire. Note that the loading (activation) portion of the curve is different from the unloading (deactivation) portion. This difference is called *hysteresis.* The units of resilience are mMN/m^3 or mMPa/m.

Toughness

Toughness, which is the resistance of a material to fracture, is an indication of the amount of energy necessary to cause fracture. The area under the *elastic* and *plastic* portions of a stress-strain curve, as shown in Figure 4-9, *B,* represents the toughness of a material. The units of toughness are the same as the units of resilience—mMN/m^3 or mMPa/m. Toughness represents the energy required to stress the material to the point of fracture. Note that a material can be tough by having a combination of high yield and ultimate strength and moderately high strain at rupture, or by having moderately high yield and ultimate strength and a large strain at rupture. Brittle materials tend to have low toughness because little plastic deformation occurs before failure, thus the area under the elastic and plastic regions of the curve is not significantly different from the area under the elastic region alone.

Fracture Toughness

Recently the concepts of fracture mechanics have been applied to a number of problems in dental materials. Fracture mechanics characterizes the behavior

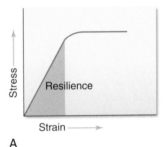

A

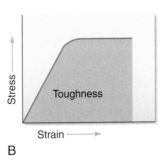

B

FIGURE 4.9 Stress-strain curves showing **A,** the area indicating the resilience, and **B,** the area representing the toughness of a material.

of materials with cracks or flaws. Flaws or cracks may arise naturally in a material or nucleate after a time in service. In either case, any defect generally weakens a material, and as a result, sudden fractures can arise at stresses below the yield stress. Sudden, catastrophic fractures typically occur in brittle materials that do not have the ability to plastically deform and redistribute stresses. The field of fracture mechanics analyzes the material behavior during these types of failures.

Two simple examples illustrate the significance of defects on the fracture of materials. Plates of glass or ceramic tiles are often scribed with a diamond or carbide instrument. The purpose of the scribe is to create a defect that propagates when additional stresses are introduced. Both are difficult to break without a scribed line or defect. If the same experiment is performed on a ductile material, the small surface notch has no effect on the force required to break the plate, and the ductile plate can be bent without fracturing (Figure 4-11). For a brittle material such as glass, no local plastic deformation is associated with fracture, whereas for a ductile material, plastic deformation, such as the ability to bend, occurs without fracture. The ability to be plastically deformed without fracture, or the amount of energy required for fracture, is the *fracture toughness.*

In general, the larger a flaw, the lower the stress needed to cause fracture. This is because the stresses, which would normally be supported by material, are

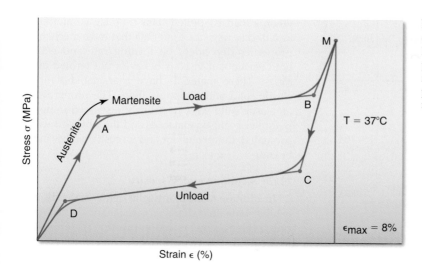

FIGURE 4.10 **Load-deflection curve for Ni-Ti orthodontic wire.** Note that the loading (activation) portion of the curve is different from the unloading (deactivation) portion, indicating hysteresis in the material. *Ni-Ti,* Nickel-titanium.

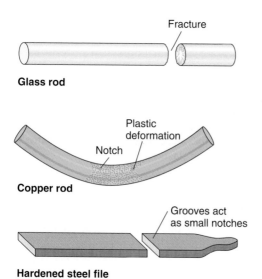

FIGURE 4.11 **Schematic of different types of deformation in brittle (glass, steel file) and ductile (copper) materials of the same diameter and having a notch of the same dimensions.** *(From Flinn RA, Trojan PK: Engineering Materials and Their Applications. Houghton Mifflin, Boston, p. 535, 1981.)*

TABLE 4.2   Fracture Toughness (K_{IC}) of Selected Dental Materials

Material	K_{IC} (MN m$^{-3/2}$)
Enamel	0.7-1.3
Dentin	3.1
Amalgam	1.3-1.6
Ceramic	1.2-3.0
Resin composite	1.4-2.3
Porcelain	0.9-1.0

toughening are presumed to be matrix-filler interactions, but these have not yet been established. Similarly, the addition of up to 50% by weight of zirconia to ceramic increases fracture toughness. As with other mechanical properties, aging or storage in a simulated oral environment or at elevated temperatures can decrease fracture toughness, but there is no uniform agreement on this in the literature. Attempts to correlate fracture toughness with wear resistance have had mixed results. Fracture toughness is not a reliable predictor of the wear of restorative materials.

Properties and Stress-Strain Curves

The shape of a stress-strain curve and the magnitudes of the stress and strain allow classification of materials with respect to their general properties. The idealized stress-strain curves in Figure 4-12 represent materials with various combinations of physical properties. For example, materials 1 to 4 have high stiffness, materials 1, 2, 5, and 6 have high strength, and materials 1, 3, 5, and 7 have high ductility. If the only requirement for an application is stiffness, materials 1 to 4 are all satisfactory. However,

now concentrated at the tip of the flaw. The ability of a flaw to cause fracture depends on the fracture toughness of the material. Fracture toughness is a material property and is proportional to the energy consumed in plastic deformation.

Fracture toughness (K_{Ic}) has been measured for a number of important restorative materials, including amalgam, acrylic denture base materials, composites, ceramics, orthodontic brackets, cements, and human enamel and dentin. Typical values for composites, ceramics, enamel, and dentin are listed in Table 4-2.

The presence of fillers in polymers substantially increases fracture toughness. The mechanisms of

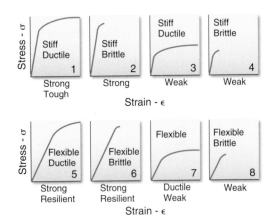

FIGURE 4.12 Stress-strain curves for materials with various combinations of properties.

if the requirements are both stiffness and strength, only materials 1 and 2 are acceptable. If the requirements are to also include ductility, the choice would be limited to material 1. It is clear that the properties of stiffness, strength, and ductility are independent, and materials may exhibit various combinations of these three properties.

Tensile Properties of Brittle Materials

Many restorative materials, including dental amalgam, cements, ceramics, plaster, and stone, are much weaker in tension than in compression. Tests traditionally used for ductile materials can be adapted to brittle materials such as the ones listed previously, but brittle materials must be tested with caution, because any stress concentrations at the grips or anywhere else in the specimen can lead to premature fracture. As a result, there is large variability in tensile data on brittle materials. Although special grips have been used to provide axial tensile loading with a minimum of localized stress, obtaining uniform results is still difficult, and such testing is relatively slow and time consuming.

Viscoelasticity

The mechanical properties of many dental materials, such as alginate, elastomeric impression materials, waxes, amalgam, polymers, bone, dentin, oral mucosa, and periodontal ligaments, depend on how fast they are loaded. For these materials, increasing the loading (strain) rate produces a different stress-strain curve with higher rates giving higher values for the elastic modulus, proportional limit, and ultimate strength. Materials that have mechanical properties independent of loading rate are termed *elastic*. In these materials, strain occurs when the load is applied. Other materials exhibit a lag in response

when a load is applied. This time lag is referred to as a *viscous response*. Materials that have mechanical properties dependent on loading rate and exhibit both elastic and viscous behavior are termed *viscoelastic*. These materials have characteristics of an elastic solid and a viscous fluid. The properties of an elastic solid were previously discussed in detail. Before viscoelastic materials and their properties are presented, fluid behavior and viscosity are reviewed below.

Fluid Behavior and Viscosity

In addition to the many solid dental materials that exhibit some fluid characteristics, many dental materials, such as cements and impression materials, are in the fluid state when formed. Therefore fluid (viscous) phenomena are important. Viscosity (η) is the resistance of a fluid to flow and is equal to the shear stress divided by the shear strain rate, or:

$$\eta = \tau / [d\varepsilon/dt]$$

When a cement or impression material sets, the viscosity increases, making it less viscous and more solid-like. The units of viscosity are poise, p (1 p = 0.1 Pa s = 0.1 N s/m^2), but often data are reported in centipoise, cp (100 cp = 1 p).

Rearranging the equation for viscosity, we see that fluid behavior can be described in terms of stress and strain, just like elastic solids.

$$\tau = \eta [d\varepsilon/dt]$$

In the case of an elastic solid, stress (σ) is proportional to strain (ε), with the constant of proportionality being the modulus of elasticity (E). The equation above indicates a similar situation for a viscous fluid, where the stress (shear) is proportional to the strain rate and the constant of proportionality is the viscosity. The stress is therefore time dependent because it is a function of the strain rate, or rate of loading. To better comprehend the concept of strain rate dependence, consider two limiting cases—rapid and slow deformation. A material pulled extremely fast ($dt \rightarrow 0$) results in an infinitely high stress, whereas a material pulled infinitesimally slow results in a stress of zero. This concept will be important in understanding stress relaxation and delayed gelation phenomena, explored later in this chapter. The behavior of elastic solids and viscous fluids can be understood from studying simple mechanical models. An elastic solid can be viewed as a spring (Figure 4-13). When the spring is stretched by a force, F, it displaces a distance, x. The applied force and resultant displacement are proportional, and the constant of proportionality is the spring constant, k. Therefore, according to Hooke's law:

$$F = kx$$

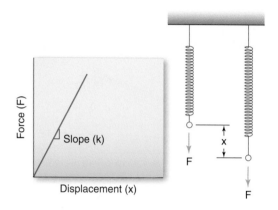

FIGURE 4.13 **Force versus displacement of a spring, which can be used to model the elastic response of a solid.** *(From Park JB: Biomaterials Science and Engineering. Plenum Press, New York, p. 26, 1984.)*

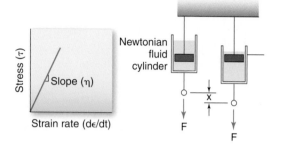

FIGURE 4.14 **Stress versus strain rate for a dashpot, which can be used to model the response of a viscous fluid.** *(From Park JB: Biomaterials Science and Engineering. Plenum Press, New York, p. 26, 1984.)*

Note that this relation is equivalent to the equation presented in the stress × strain section of this chapter.

$$\sigma = E\varepsilon$$

Also note that the model of an elastic element does not involve time. The spring acts instantaneously when stretched. In other words, an elastic solid is independent of loading rate.

A viscous fluid can be viewed as a dashpot, or a piston moving through a viscous fluid (Figure 4-14). When the fluid-filled cylinder is pulled, the rate of strain ($d\varepsilon/dt$) is proportional to the stress (τ) and the constant of proportionality is the viscosity of the fluid (π).

Although the viscosity of a fluid is proportional to the shear rate, the proportionality differs for different fluids. Fluids may be classified as Newtonian, pseudoplastic, or dilatant depending on how their viscosity varies with shear rate, as shown in Figure 4-15. The viscosity of a Newtonian fluid is constant and independent of shear rate. Some dental cements and impression materials are Newtonian. The viscosity of a pseudoplastic fluid decreases with increasing shear rate. Monophase elastomeric impression materials are pseudoplastic. When subjected to low shear rates during spatulation or while an impression is positioned in a tray in preparation of placing it into the mouth, these impression materials have a high viscosity and stay in place without flowing. These materials, however, can also be used in a syringe, because at the higher shear rates encountered as they pass through the syringe tip, the viscosity decreases by as much as tenfold. This characteristic is sometimes referred to as *thixotropy*, although that term actually describes the change in viscosity of a material with time. Ketchup is also pseudoplastic, which makes it difficult to remove from a bottle. Shaking the bottle

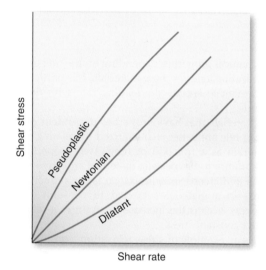

FIGURE 4.15 **Shear diagrams of Newtonian, pseudoplastic, and dilatant liquids.** The viscosity is shown by the slope of the curve at a given shear rate.

or rapping the side of the bottle increases its shear rate, decreases its viscosity, and improves its pourability. The viscosity of a dilatant fluid increases with increasing shear rate. Examples of dilatant fluids in dentistry include the fluid denture base resins.

Viscoelastic Materials

For viscoelastic materials, the strain rate can alter the stress-strain properties. The tear strength of alginate impression material, for example, is increased about four times when the rate of loading is increased from 2.5 to 25 cm/min. Alginate impressions should therefore be removed from the mouth quickly to improve its tear resistance. Another example of strain-rate dependence is the elastic modulus of dental amalgam, which is 21 GPa at slow rates of loading and 62 GPa at high rates of loading. A viscoelastic material therefore may have widely different

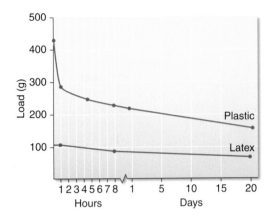

FIGURE 4.16 **Decrease in load of latex rubber and plastic bands as a function of time at a constant extension of 95 mm.** *(From Craig RG (Ed.): Dental Materials: A Problem-oriented Approach. Mosby–Year Book, St. Louis, 1978.)*

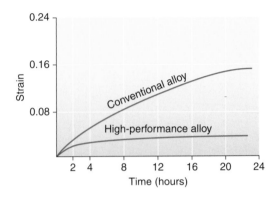

FIGURE 4.17 **Creep curves for conventional (low-copper) and high-performance (high-copper) amalgams.** *(From O'Brien WJ: Dental Materials: Properties and Selection. Quintessence, Chicago, p. 25, 1989.)*

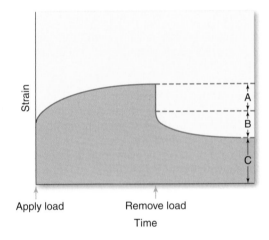

FIGURE 4.18 **Creep recovery curve, showing, *A*, elastic, *B*, anelastic, and, *C*, viscous strain.**

mechanical properties depending on the rate of load application, and for these materials, it is particularly important to specify the loading rate with the test results.

Materials that have properties dependent on the strain rate are better characterized by relating stress or strain as a function of time. Two properties of importance to viscoelastic materials are stress relaxation and creep. *Stress relaxation* is the reduction in stress in a material subjected to constant strain, whereas *creep* is the increase in strain in a material under constant stress.

As an example of stress relaxation, consider how the load-time curves at constant deformation are important in the evaluation of orthodontic elastic bands. The decrease in load (or force) with time for latex and plastic bands of the same size at a constant extension of 95 mm is shown in Figure 4-16. The initial force was much greater with the plastic band, but the decrease in force with time was much less for the latex band. Therefore, plastic bands are useful for applying high forces, although the force decreases rapidly with time, whereas latex bands apply lower forces, but the force decreases slowly with time in the mouth; latex bands are therefore useful for applying more sustained loads.

The importance of creep can be seen by interpretation of the data in Figure 4-17, which shows creep curves for low- and high-copper amalgam. For a given load at a given time, the low-copper amalgam has a greater strain. The implications and clinical importance of this are that the greater creep in the low-copper amalgam makes it more susceptible to strain accumulation and fracture, and also marginal breakdown, which can lead to secondary decay. The high creep behavior of low-copper amalgam contributed to its decline in popularity.

Creep Compliance

A creep curve yields insight into the relative elastic, viscous, and inelastic response of a viscoelastic material; such curves can be interpreted in terms of the molecular structure of the associated materials, which have structures that function as elastic, viscous, and inelastic elements. Creep recovery curves are produced from data collected during removal of a load (Figure 4-18). In such a curve, after the load is removed, there is an instantaneous drop in strain and slower strain decay to some steady-state strain value, which may be nonzero. The instantaneous drop in strain represents the recovery of elastic strain. The slower recovery represents the inelastic strain, and the remaining, permanent strain represents the viscous strain. A family of creep curves can be determined by using different loads. A more useful way of presenting these data is by calculating the

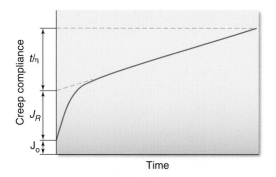

FIGURE 4.19 Creep compliance versus time for a viscoelastic material. *(Modified from Duran RL, Powers JM, Craig RG: J. Dent. Res. 58, 1801, 1979.)*

creep compliance. *Creep compliance* (J_t) is defined as strain divided by stress at a given time. Once a creep curve is obtained, a corresponding creep compliance curve can be calculated. The creep compliance curve shown in Figure 4-19 is characterized by the following equation:

$$J_t = J_0 + J_R + (t / \eta)$$

where J_0 is the instantaneous elastic compliance, J_R is the retarded elastic (inelastic) compliance, and t/η represents the viscous response at time t for a viscosity η. The strain associated with J_0 and J_R is completely recoverable after the load is removed; however, the strain associated with J_R is not recovered immediately but requires some finite time. The strain associated with t/η is not recovered and represents a permanent deformation. If a single creep compliance curve is calculated from a family of creep curves determined at different loads, the material is said to be linearly viscoelastic. In this case, the viscoelastic qualities can be described concisely by a single curve.

The creep compliance curve therefore permits an estimate of the relative amount of elastic, inelastic, and viscous behavior of a material. J_0 indicates the flexibility and initial recovery after deformation, J_R the amount of delayed recovery that can be expected, and t/η the magnitude of permanent deformation to be expected. Creep compliance curves for elastomeric impression materials are shown in Chapter 12, Figure 12-17.

Dynamic Mechanical Properties

Although static properties can often be related to the function of a material under dynamic conditions, there are limitations to using static properties to estimate the properties of materials subjected to dynamic loading. *Static testing* refers to continuous application of force at slow rates of loading, whereas

dynamic testing involves cyclic loading or loading at high rates (*impact*). Dynamic methods, including a forced oscillation technique used to determine dynamic modulus and a torsion pendulum used for impact testing, have been used to study viscoelastic materials such as dental polymers. Ultrasonic techniques have been used to determine elastic constants of viscoelastic materials such as dental amalgam and dentin. Impact testing has been applied primarily to brittle dental materials.

Dynamic Modulus

The *dynamic modulus* (E_D) is defined as the ratio of stress to strain for small cyclical deformations at a given frequency and at a particular point on the stress-strain curve. When measured in a dynamic oscillation instrument, the dynamic modulus is computed by:

$$E_D = mqp^2$$

where m is the mass of the loading element, q is the height divided by twice the area of the cylindrical specimen, and p is the angular frequency of the vibrations.

In general, elastic modulus calculated from dynamic testing is higher than when calculated by static testing. For ideal elastic materials subjected to an oscillatory strain, the sinusoidal wave of the resultant stress matches perfectly the strain wave; it is said then that stress and strain are "in phase" (Figure 4-20, A and B), or that there is no energy lost to the environment because all the energy is used to provide a deformation. For Newtonian fluids (ideal liquids), the strain response lags in time, and the phase lag equals the greatest possible angle ($\delta = 90$ degrees) between stress and strain waves, for any given cycle (see Figure 4-20, A). As discussed earlier, from the stress-strain curves, a complex modulus (E^*) can be calculated. The complex modulus, therefore, is the ratio of the stress amplitude to the strain amplitude and represents the stiffness of the material.

Most real materials subjected to oscillatory strain behave somewhere in between a perfectly elastic and a perfectly plastic material, and in those cases, by resolving the complex modulus (E^*) into an "in phase" elastic component (called *storage modulus*, or E') and an "out of phase" viscous component (called *loss modulus*, or E''), it is possible to gain insight into the elastic and viscous components, respectively (see Figure 4-20, B). They correlate according to the mathematical relationship shown in Figure 4-20, C, where $E' = E^* \sin \delta$ and $E'' = E^* \cos \delta$. One useful concept that arises is the loss factor tan δ (calculated as tan $\delta = E'/E''$). This relationship allows us to determine whether a material presents a predominantly elastic or viscous response when subjected to load while in service.

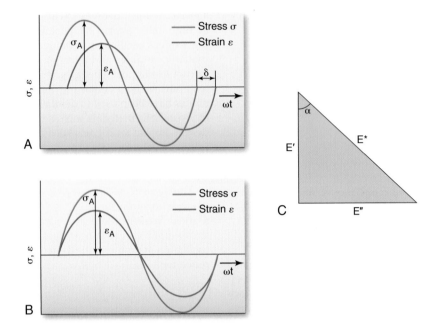

FIGURE 4.20 Sinusoidal oscillation and response of **(A)** an ideal liquid and **(B)** a purely elastic material; δ = phase angle. **(C)** Mathematical correlation of complex (E^*), storage (E') and loss (E'') moduli.

In conjunction with the dynamic modulus, values of internal friction and dynamic resilience can be determined. For example, cyclical stretching or compression of an elastomer results in irreversibly lost energy that is exhibited as heat. The internal friction of an elastomer is comparable with the viscosity of a liquid. The value of internal friction is necessary to calculate the *dynamic resilience*, which is the ratio of energy lost to energy expended.

The dynamic modulus and dynamic resilience of some dental elastomers are listed in Table 4-3. These properties are affected by temperature (−15 to 37° C) for some maxillofacial elastomers, such as plasticized polyvinylchloride and polyurethane, but less so in silicones. As shown in Table 4-3, the dynamic modulus decreases and the dynamic resilience increases as the temperature increases. As a tangible example, the dynamic resilience of a polymer used for an athletic mouth protector is a measure of the ability of the material to absorb energy from a blow and thereby protect the oral structures.

Surface Mechanical Properties

In our discussion so far, we have introduced and discussed mechanical properties that are mainly dependent on the bulk characteristics of a material. In this section, mechanical properties that are more a function of the surface condition of a material are presented. In particular, the concepts of hardness, friction, and wear are summarized.

TABLE 4.3   Values of Dynamic Modulus and Dynamic Resilience as a Function of Temperature for Some Dental Elastomers

Material	Temperature (° C)	Dynamic Modulus (MPa)	Dynamic Resilience (%)
MAXILLOFACIAL MATERIALS			
Polyurethane	−15	5.98	15.0
	37	3.06	19.9
Polyvinylchloride	−15	12.2	6.0
	37	2.51	19.6
Silicone elastomer	−15	2.84	16.0
	37	2.36	23.2
POLYVINYLACETATE-POLYETHYLENE MOUTH PROTECTOR			
New	37	9.39	23.4
Worn	37	7.23	20.2

Hardness

Hardness may be broadly defined as the resistance to permanent surface indentation or penetration. Formulating a more rigorous definition of hardness is difficult because any test method will, at a microscopic level, involve complex surface morphologies and stresses in the test material, thereby involving

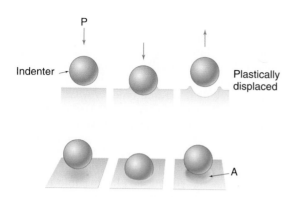

P

Indenter

Plastically
displaced

A

FIGURE 4.21 **Schematic representation of a hardness test.** *A*, Area of plastic deformation; *P*, normal load. *(From Park JB: Biomaterials Science and Engineering. Plenum Press, New York, p. 18, 1984).*

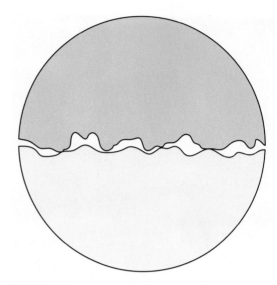

FIGURE 4.22 **Microscopic area of contact between two objects.** The frictional force, which resists motion, is proportional to the normal force and the coefficient of friction.

a variety of qualities in any single hardness test. Despite this condition, the most common concept of hard and soft substances is their relative resistance to indentation. Hardness is therefore a measure of the resistance to plastic deformation and is measured as a force per unit area of indentation (Figure 4-21).

Based on this definition of hardness, it is clear why this property is so important to dentistry. Hardness influences ease of cutting, finishing, and polishing an object and its resistance to in-service scratching. Finishing or polishing a structure is important for esthetic purposes and, as discussed previously, scratches can compromise fatigue strength and lead to premature failure.

Some of the most common methods of testing the hardness of restorative materials are the Brinell, Knoop, Vickers, Rockwell, Barcol, and Shore A hardness tests. Each of these tests differs slightly in the indenter used and in the calculation of hardness. Each presents certain advantages and disadvantages, described in detail in Chapter 5. They have a common quality, however, in that each depends on the penetration of some small, symmetrically shaped indenter into the surface of the material being tested. The choice of a hardness test depends on the material of interest, the expected hardness range, and the desired degree of localization.

Friction

Friction is the resistance between contacting bodies when one moves relative to another (Figure 4-22). A restraining force that resists movement is the (static) frictional force and results from the molecules of the two objects bonding where their surfaces are in close contact. The frictional force, F_s, is proportional to the normal force (F_N) between the surfaces and the (static) coefficient of friction (μ_s):

$$F_S = \mu_S F_N$$

The coefficient of friction varies between 0 and 1 and is a function of the two materials in contact, their composition, surface finish, and lubrication. Similar materials in contact have a greater coefficient of friction, and if a lubricating medium exists at the interface, the coefficient of friction is reduced.

Motion is possible when the applied force is greater than F_s. Once motion occurs, molecular bonds are made and broken, and microscopic pieces break off from the surfaces. With motion, a sliding or kinetic friction is produced, and the force of kinetic friction opposes the motion:

$$F_k = \mu_k F_N$$

Frictional behavior therefore arises from surfaces that, because of microroughness, have a small real contact area (see Figure 4-22). These small surface areas result in high contact stresses, which lead to local yielding, or permanent deformation. The resistance to shear failure of the junctions results in the frictional force. When static friction is overcome and relative motion takes place, it is accompanied by the modification of the interface through kinetic friction and wear.

An example of the importance of friction in dentistry lies in the concept of sliding mechanics used in orthodontics. A known and controlled frictional force is required when an orthodontic wire is slid through a bracket. Combinations of different materials result in different frictional forces. Friction is also an important consideration when dissimilar restorative materials contact and slide against each other in the oral cavity such as in protrusive or working movements of the mandible.

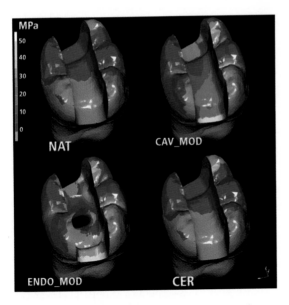

FIGURE 4.23 **Stress distribution in a finite element model of a molar with a 100 N occlusal load.** *(Magne P: Dent. Mater. 23(5), 539-548, 2007.)*

Wear

Wear is a loss of material resulting from removal and relocation of materials through the contact of two or more materials. When two solid materials are in contact, they touch only at the tips of their most protruding asperities (Figure 4-23). Wear is usually undesirable, but under controlled conditions during finishing and polishing, controlled wear can be very useful.

Several factors make wear of biomaterials unique. Most important, wear can produce particles that can elicit an inflammatory response. The wear process can also produce shape changes in the object that can affect function. For example, wear of teeth and restorative materials is characterized by the loss of the original anatomical form of the material. Wear may result from mechanical, physiological, or pathological conditions. Normal mastication may cause attrition of tooth structure or materials, particularly in populations that consume unprocessed foods. Bruxism is an example of a pathological form of wear in which clenching and grinding of teeth produces occlusal and incisal wear. Abrasive wear occurs when excessively abrasive toothpastes and hard toothbrush bristles are used when brushing teeth.

Wear is a function of a number of material and environmental factors, including the characteristics of wearing surfaces (i.e., inhomogeneity, crystal orientation, phases, and inclusions present); the microscopic contact; interaction between sliding surfaces (i.e., elevated stress, temperature, and flow at contact points, leading to localized yielding, melting, and hardening); lubrication; and different material combinations. In general, wear is a function of opposing materials and the interface between them. The presence of a lubricating film, such as saliva, separates surfaces during relative motion and reduces frictional forces and wear.

In general, there are four types of wear: (1) adhesive wear; (2) corrosive wear; (3) surface fatigue wear; and (4) abrasive wear. Adhesive wear is characterized by the formation and disruption of microjunctions. Microregions are pulled from one object and transferred to the other. Abrasive wear involves a harder material cutting or plowing into a softer material. There can be two types of abrasive wear: two- and three-body abrasive wear. This type of wear can be minimized if surfaces are smooth and hard and if third party particles are kept off the surfaces. Corrosive wear is secondary to physical removal of a protective layer and is therefore related to the chemical activity of the wear surfaces. The sliding action of the surfaces accelerates corrosion. In surface fatigue wear, asperities or free particles with small areas of contact contribute to high localized stresses and produce surface or subsurface cracks. Particles break off under cyclic loading and sliding.

In general, metals are susceptible to adhesive, corrosive and three-body wear, whereas polymers are susceptible to abrasive and fatigue wear.

The Colloidal State

Colloids were first described by Thomas Graham (1861) as a result of his studies of diffusion in solutions. He observed that substances such as starch, albumin, and other gelatinous materials did not behave in the same manner as acids, bases, and salts. The term *colloid* now is used to describe a *state* of matter rather than a *kind* of matter. The main characteristic of colloidal materials is their high degree of microsegmentation. These fine particles also have certain physical properties, such as electrical charges and surface energies that control the characteristics of the colloids. Particle size alone does not adequately define colloids.

Nature of Colloids

Substances are called *colloids* when they consist of two or more phases, with the units of at least one of the phases having a dimension slightly greater than simple molecular size. Although the range of size is somewhat arbitrary, it is usually recognized as being approximately 1 to 500 nm in maximum dimension. Thus colloidal systems can be fine dispersions, gels, films, emulsions, or foams. In other words, the colloidal state represents a highly dispersed system of fine particles of one phase in another, and a characteristic property of the dispersed phase is an enormous surface area. This is true whether a dispersed phase of oil droplets in an emulsion or a finely divided solid suspended in a liquid is considered. This increase in surface area gives rise to a corresponding increase in surface energy and surface reactions. Not only is the surface energy important, but the interface between the two phases also imparts important and characteristic properties to the system.

Except for a dispersion of a gas in a gas, which is a true solution, each of the three forms of matter—gas, liquid, and solid—may be dispersed as colloidal particles in the other and in itself as well. The dispersed phase, which may be in the form of a gas, liquid, or solid, may also exist in a variety of conditions. Some examples of these dispersed phases are (1) colloidal silica as a filler in resin composites, (2) colloidal silica in water to be mixed with high-strength dental stone to improve abrasion resistance, (3) droplets of oil in water used during steam sterilization to prevent rusting of dental instruments, (4) fillers used in elastomeric impression materials to control such properties as viscosity, and (5) agglomerates of detergent molecules in water that serve as wetting agents for wax patterns.

Typical Colloid Systems

A few colloid systems are more important than others in relation to restorative materials. For example, the distinction between a sol and a gel is important because several of each are found in dental applications. A sol resembles a solution, but it is made up of colloidal particles dispersed in a liquid. When a sol is chilled or caused to react by the addition of suitable chemicals, it may be transformed into a gel. In the gel form the system takes on a semisolid, or jellylike, quality.

The liquid phase of either a sol or a gel is usually water, but may be some organic liquid such as alcohol. Systems having water as one component are described as *hydrosols* or *hydrogels.* A more general term might be *hydrocolloid,* which is often used in dentistry to describe the alginate gels used as flexible impression materials. A general term to describe a system having an organic liquid as one component would be *organosol* or *organogel.*

Two examples of materials that involve gel structures are the agar and alginate hydrocolloid impression materials. Gels possess an entangled framework of solid colloidal particles in which liquid is trapped in the interstices and held by capillarity. Such a gel has some degree of rigidity, depending on the extent of the structural solids present.

Gels that are formed with water are hydrophilic (water loving) in character and tend to imbibe large quantities of water if allowed to stand submerged. The imbibition is accompanied by swelling and a change in physical dimensions. In dry air, the gel loses water to the atmosphere, with an accompanying shrinkage. Such changes may be observed readily in alginate gels.

Diffusion Through Membranes and Osmotic Pressure

Osmotic pressure is the pressure developed by diffusion of a liquid or solvent through a membrane. The solvent passes from the dilute to the more concentrated solution through the membrane separating the two solutions. The presence of dissolved material in a solvent lowers the escaping tendency of the solvent molecules; the greater the concentration, the more the escaping tendency is lowered. Accordingly, the solvent will diffuse or pass through a membrane to a region of greater concentration, thus diluting the concentration of the solution.

Osmotic pressure is a concept that has been used to explain the hypersensitivity of dentin. The change in pressure in carious, exposed dentin from contact with saliva or concentrated solutions causes diffusion throughout the structure that increases or decreases the pressure on the sensory system.

Just as diffusion through membranes is important, so also is the diffusion from a substance of a given concentration to that of another concentration important in many materials in dentistry. Salts and dyes diffuse through human dentin. Stains and discoloring agents diffuse through polymeric restorative materials. Diffusion of salts and acids through some cavity liners is a potential problem.

Adsorption, Absorption, and Sorption

In the adsorption process, a liquid or gas adheres to the surface of the solid or liquid firmly by the attachment of molecules, thus reducing their surface free energy. In a physical sense, if the two substances are alike, as, for example, two pieces of the same metal in the solid state pressed closely together, the mass is said to *cohere.* When a dissimilar substance, such as a gas or liquid, is in intimate contact with the surface of the solid, it is said to *adhere* to the surface. The process of adsorption or adhesion to the surface of a substance is important in the wetting process, in which the substance is coated or wetted with a foreign substance such as a liquid. The degree to which saliva, for example, will wet or adhere to the enamel surface of a tooth depends on the tendency for surface adsorption. A substance that is readily wetted on the surface by water, as is glass or porcelain or tooth enamel, is considered to have adsorbed on its surface a layer of water molecules. When a wet, human enamel surface is desiccated, the first water to evaporate is bulk water, leaving physically and chemically adsorbed water. Considerable heat is required to remove physically adsorbed water, and even higher temperatures are needed to remove chemically adsorbed water. Thus any attempt to bond a restorative material to enamel must consider that adhesion will be to adsorbed water and not hydroxyapatite. High-energy surfaces such as metals will adsorb molecules more readily than low-energy surfaces such as waxes; oxides have intermediate surface energies.

The process of adsorption differs somewhat from the process of absorption. In the process of absorption, the substance absorbed diffuses into the solid material by a diffusion process, and the process is characterized by concentration of molecules at the surface.

In instances in which both adsorption and absorption are known to exist and it is not clear which process predominates, the whole process is known as *sorption*. In measurement of the moisture content of dental resins, the process is described as one of sorption of moisture by the resin.

Numerous examples of these processes are found in the use of various restorative dental materials. The process of absorption of water by alginate impression materials is particularly important to its stability. When the quantity of liquid absorbed into a substance is relatively large, there is likely to be an accompanying swelling of the absorbent.

Surface Tension and Wetting

Surface tension is measured in terms of force (dynes) per centimeter of the surface of liquid. In the case of water at 20° C, the value is 72.8 dynes/cm. At the same temperature, benzene has a value of 29 dynes/cm; alcohol, 22 dynes/cm; and ether, 17 dynes/cm. By contrast, mercury at 20° C has a surface tension of 465 dynes/cm. The values for each of these substances are influenced by factors such as temperature and purity. In general, there is a reduction in surface tension of all liquids as the temperature is increased. For example, the surface tension of water (in dynes/cm) is 76 at 0° C, 72 at 25° C, 68 at 50° C, and 59 at 100° C.

The surface tension of liquids is also reduced by the presence of impurities, some of which are exceedingly effective. Detergents, such as sodium lauryl sulfate, or the ingredients of soaps, including sodium stearate or sodium oleate, which have long hydrocarbon chains attached to hydrophilic groups (such as COONa), are particularly effective in reducing the surface tension of water.

These surface-active agents affect the surface tension by concentrating at the liquid-air interface or other interfaces or surfaces. As these molecules occupy surface positions in the water-air surface, they displace surface water molecules, thus reducing the cohesive force between water molecules over the surface area, because the cohesion between water

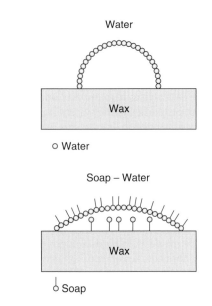

FIGURE 4.24 **Spreading of pure water (top) and water containing soap molecules on wax (bottom).**

and surface-active agent is less than that between water and water. This effect is demonstrated in Figure 4-24, which represents two drops placed on wax, one of which is water and the other water with detergent. The presence of the surface-active agent molecules in the surface layer reduces the pull on the surface molecules toward the liquid mass. This reduces the surface tension to increase wetting. The soap molecules are oriented so that the hydrophilic end is in the water and the hydrophobic (hydrocarbon) end is oriented toward the wax or air.

The increased wettability of solids with liquids of reduced surface tension is important in numerous dental applications. The wetting power of a liquid is represented by its tendency to spread on the surface of the solid. In restorative dental laboratory procedures, wax patterns are formed that are to be wetted by water or water suspensions of a casting investment. Wax is not well wetted by water, so a dilute solution of some wetting agent (such as 0.01% aerosol) is first painted on the wax in small quantities to aid in the spreading of the casting investment. Without adequate wetting, the investment could not flow over the surface of the wax and replicate fine detail.

Much can be learned about the spreading of liquids on solids, or the tendency for wetting surfaces, by measuring the angle of contact between the liquid and the solid surface. The angles of contact for different liquid droplets on a plane glass surface are illustrated in Figure 4-25. The contact angle results from a balance of surface and interfacial energies. The greater the tendency to wet the surface, the lower the contact angle, until complete wetting occurs at an angle equal to zero.

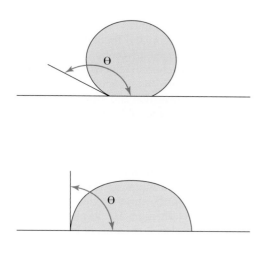

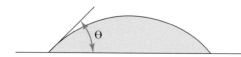

FIGURE 4.25 **Relation of contact angle to the spreading or wetting of a liquid on a solid.**

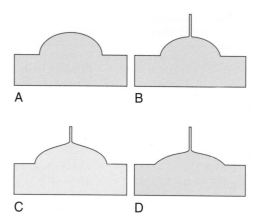

FIGURE 4.26 **Diagrams show the contact angle formed by a drop of water or saliva on wax and acrylic plastic. A,** Water on wax. **B,** Water on plastic. **C,** Fresh saliva on plastic. **D,** Saliva after remaining in contact with plastic.

TABLE 4.4   Contact Angles of Water on Solids at 27° C

Solid	Advancing Angle (degrees)
Acrylic polymer	74
Teflon	110
Glass	14
Amalgam	77
Acrylic filling material	38
Composite filling material	51

Modified from O'Brien WJ: Capillary Penetration of Liquids Between Dissimilar Solids, doctoral thesis, University of Michigan, Ann Arbor, p. 40, 1967.

Contact angles of water and saliva in dental materials: The determination of contact angle is important in a number of clinically relevant situations. For example, the contact angle of water and saliva on complete denture plastics relates to the retention of the denture. The contact angle and the tendency of a drop of water to spread on paraffin wax and methyl methacrylate are shown for comparison in Figure 4-26. The contact angle of saliva freshly applied to an acrylic surface is similar to the one formed by water. This angle drops if saliva is allowed to stand overnight in contact with the plastic material, which indicates that the surface wetting is somewhat improved. Table 4-4 gives contact angle values for water on selected materials.

Contact angles can also provide important information regarding the wettability of dental elastomeric materials, defining the ease of pouring a mix of dental stone and water to produce a model. The contact angles of water on various dental elastomeric impression materials are listed in Table 4-5, along with the castability of an impression of a very critical comb-like model. Surfactants can be added to the surface to artificially decrease the contact angle.

Contact angles between metals during casting, soldering and amalgamation: The surface tension of metals is relatively high in comparison with that of other liquids, because of the greater cohesive forces between the liquid metal atoms in the liquid-air surface compared to water. The surface tension of most metals, except mercury, cannot be measured at room temperature because of their high melting points. Typical values of a few metals are included in Table 4-6. This is important because it defines the ease of spreading of the molten metal or alloy on the investment material surface during casting, and determines the accuracy and reproduction of detail in the final restoration. The same applies to the spreading of molten flux on hot metal during melting or soldering operations. If the contact angle of the solder is too great, it will not penetrate into the fine detail of the structures to be joined.

Adhesion

Surface Considerations

Atoms or molecules at the surfaces of solids or liquids differ greatly from those in the bulk of the solid or liquid, and neighboring atoms may be arranged anisotropically. Also, some atoms or molecules may

TABLE 4.5   Wettability and Castability of Stone Models in Flexible Impression Materials

	Advancing Contact Angle of Water (degrees)	Castability of Water Mixes of High Strength Stone (%)
Condensation silicone	98	30
Addition silicone-hydrophobic	98	30
Polysulfide	82	44
Polyether	49	70
Addition silicone-hydrophobic	53	72

TABLE 4.6   Surface Tension of Metals

Metal	Temperature (° C)	Surface Tension (dynes/cm)
Lead	327	452
Mercury	20	465
Zinc	419	758
Copper	1131	1103
Gold	1120	1128

accumulate at the surface and thus cause unusual physical and chemical properties. These solid surfaces have atoms of higher energy than bulk atoms because of the absence of some neighboring atoms and thus readily adsorb ambient atoms or molecules. To produce a clean solid surface, one with less than 1% of an adsorbed monolayer, a vacuum of 10^{-9} Torr or 1.33×10^{-7} Pa is required to keep a surface clean for about an hour. At a vacuum of about 3×10^{-6} Torr, a newly cleaned surface would be coated with ambient atoms or molecules in only a few seconds. Therefore, all dental materials and dental surfaces would be covered with a layer of ambient atoms or molecules and thus adhesives would be bonding to these adsorbed monolayers.

The energy involved in the adsorption of atoms or molecules onto the substrate may be at the level of a chemical reaction, or chemisorption, or may be at the level of van der Waals reaction, or physiosorption. The former is irreversible, whereas the latter is reversible.

Thus an important concept in surface chemistry is that critically important properties of a material may be more related to the chemistry of the surface layer and its composition than to the bulk properties.

Such surface effects dominate the surface mechanical properties of adhesion and friction, the optical surface phenomena of the perception of color and texture, the tissue reaction to materials, the attachment of cells to materials, the wettability and capillarity of surfaces, the nucleation and growth of solids, and many other areas of crucial interest in biomaterials.

Dental applications of surface chemistry can be seen in the elements chosen in metal alloys. Stainless steel used mainly in orthodontics is 72% to 74% iron, but has acceptable corrosion resistance in the mouth because the 18% chromium content forms an adherent oxide layer on the surface, which provides corrosion resistance. Titanium and its alloys, and noble alloys containing small amounts of indium and tin, have excellent biocompatibility properties as a result of oxides of titanium, indium, and tin on the surface.

Penetration Coefficient

The rate of penetration of a liquid into a crevice is an important aspect of capillary phenomena. An example is the penetration of a liquid prepolymer sealant into a fissure and the fine microscopic spaces created by etching of an enamel surface. The properties of the liquid affecting the rate of penetration may be related to the penetration coefficient (PC) where γ is the surface tension, η is the viscosity, and θ is the contact angle of the sealant on the enamel:

$$PC = \gamma \cos / 2\eta$$

The penetration coefficients for sealants have been shown to vary from 0.6 to 12 cm/sec. Narrow occlusal fissures can be filled almost completely if the penetration coefficient value is at least 1.30 cm/s, provided that no air bubbles trapped in the fissure are present. The same analysis applies to the penetration of liquid sealants into the etched surface of enamel to form tags, as shown in Figure 4-27.

Optical Properties
Color

The perception of color is the result of a physiological response to a physical stimulus. The sensation is a subjective experience, whereas the beam of light, which is the physical stimulus that produces the sensation, is entirely objective. The perceived color response results from either a reflected or a transmitted beam of white light or a portion of that beam. According to one of Grassmann's laws, the eye can distinguish differences in only three parameters of color. These parameters are dominant wavelength, luminous reflectance, and excitation purity.

The dominant wavelength (λ) of a color is the wavelength of a monochromatic light that, when mixed in suitable proportions with an achromatic color (gray), will match the color perceived. Light having short

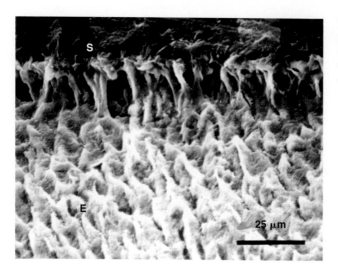

FIGURE 4.27 Scanning electron micrograph of the interface of sealant *(S)* and enamel *(E)* showing sealant tags that had penetrated into the etched enamel surface. *(From O'Brien WJ, Fan PL, Apostolidis A: Oper. Dent. 3, 53, 1978.)*

wavelengths (400 nm) is violet in color, and light having long wavelengths (700 nm) is red. Between these two wavelengths are those corresponding to blue, green, yellow, and orange light. This attribute of color perception is also known as *hue.*

Of all the visible colors and shades, there are only three primary colors: red, green, and blue (or violet). Any other color may be produced by the proper combination of these colors. For example, yellow light is a mixture of green and red lights.

The luminous reflectance of a color classifies an object as equivalent to a member of a series of achromatic, grayscale objects ranging from black to white for light-diffusing objects and from black to perfectly clear and colorless for transmitting objects. A black standard is assigned a luminous reflectance of 0, whereas a white standard is assigned 100. This attribute of color perception is described as *value* in one visual system of color measurement.

The excitation purity or saturation of a color describes the degree of its difference from the achromatic color perception most resembling it. Numbers representing excitation purity range from 0 to 1. This attribute of color perception is also known as *chroma.*

Measurement of Color

The color of dental restorative materials is most commonly measured in reflected light using a color measuring instrument or a visual method.

COLOR MEASURING INSTRUMENT

Curves of spectral reflectance versus wavelength can be obtained over the visible range (405 to 700 nm) with a recording spectrophotometer and integrating sphere. Typical curves for a resin composite before and after 300 hours of accelerated aging in a weathering chamber are shown in Figure 4-28. From the reflectance values and tabulated color-matching

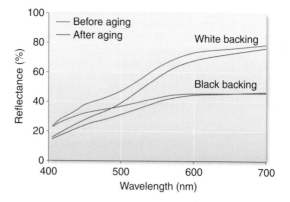

FIGURE 4.28 **Curves of spectral reflectance versus wavelength for a resin composite before and after exposure to conditions of accelerated aging.** The specimen was exposed continuously for 300 hours to the radiation of a 2500-watt xenon lamp and intermittently sprayed with water. The aging chamber was held at 43° C and 90% relative humidity. Spectral reflectance curves for translucent specimens often are obtained with both black and white backings.

functions, the tristimulus values *(X, Y, Z)* can be computed relative to a particular light source. These tristimulus values are related to the amounts of the three primary colors required to give, by additive mixture, a match with the color being considered. Typically, the tristimulus values are computed relative to the Commission Internationale de l'Eclairage (CIE) (International Commission on Illumination) source D55, D65, or C. The ratios of each tristimulus value of a color to their sum are called the *chromaticity coordinates (x, y, z).* Dominant wavelength and excitation purity of a color can be determined by referring its chromaticity coordinates to a chromaticity diagram such as the one shown in Figure 4-29. The luminous

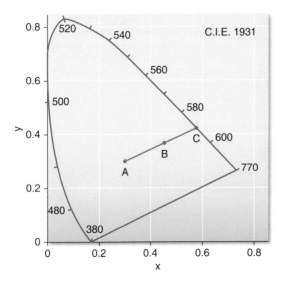

FIGURE 4.29 Chromaticity diagram (x, y) according to the 1931 CIE Standard Observer and coordinate system. Values of dominant wavelength determine the spectrum locus. The excitation purity is the ratio of two lengths (AB/AC) on the chromaticity diagram, where A refers to the standard light source and B refers to the color being considered. The point C, the intersection of line AB with the spectrum locus, is the dominant wavelength.

reflectance is equal to the value of the second (Y) of the three tristimulus values.

A diagram of the CIE $L^*a^*b^*$ color space is shown in Figure 4-30. The $L^*a^*b^*$ color space is characterized by uniform chromaticities. Value (black to white) is denoted as L^*, whereas chroma (a^*b^*) is denoted as red $(+a^*)$, green $(-a^*)$, yellow $(+b^*)$, and blue $(-b^*)$. Ranges of CIE $L^*a^*b^*$ values for bleaching shades of resin composites are listed in Table 4-7.

Differences between two colors can be determined from a color difference formula. One such formula has the following form:

$$\Delta E_{ab}^* (L^* a^* b^*) = [(\Delta L^*)^2 + (\Delta a^*)^2 + (\Delta b^*)^2]^{1/2}$$

where L^*, a^*, and b^* depend on the tristimulus values of the specimen and of a perfectly white object. A value of ΔE^* of 1 can be observed visually by half of the observers under standardized conditions. A value of ΔE^* of 3.3 is considered perceptible clinically.

VISUAL METHOD

A popular system for the visual determination of color is the Munsell color system, the parameters of which are represented in three dimensions, as shown in Figure 4-31. A large set of color tabs is used to determine the color. Value (lightness) is determined first by the selection of a tab that most nearly corresponds with the lightness or darkness of the color.

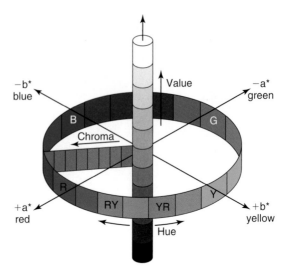

FIGURE 4.30 CIE $L^*a^*b^*$ color arrangement. *(From Seghi RR, Johnston WM, O'Brien WJ: J. Prosthet. Dent. 56, 35, 1986.)*

TABLE 4.7   Ranges of CIE $L^*a^*b^*$ (D55, 10°, CIE 1964) Values for Bleaching Shades of Resin Composites

Material	L^*	a^*	b^*
Microhybrid composites	56.3 to 82.4	−0.4 to −3.8	−4.1 to 3.3
Microfilled composites	62.1 to 77.8	−1.9 to −2.8	−2.9 to 1.7
Control shade 1M1	62.9	−0.8	2.9
Control shade B1	58.2	−0.8	1.5

Modified from Paravina RD, Ontiveros JC, Powers JM: J. Esthet. Restor. Dent., 16, 117, 2004.

Value ranges from white (10/) to black (0/). Chroma is determined next with tabs that are close to the measured value but are of increasing saturation of color. Chroma ranges from achromatic or gray (/0) to a highly saturated color (/18). The hue of the color is determined last by matching with color tabs of the value and chroma already determined. Hue is measured on a scale from 2.5 to 10 in increments of 2.5 for each of the 10 color families (red, R; yellow-red, YR; yellow, Y; green-yellow, GY; green, G; blue-green, BG; blue, B; purple-blue, PB; purple, P; red-purple, RP). For example, the color of the attached gingiva of a healthy patient has been measured as 5R 6/4 to indicate a hue of 5R, a value of 6, and a chroma of 4.

Two similar colors also can be compared in the Munsell color system by a color difference formula such as one derived by Nickerson:

$$I = (C/5)(2 \Delta H) + 6 \Delta V + 3 \Delta C$$

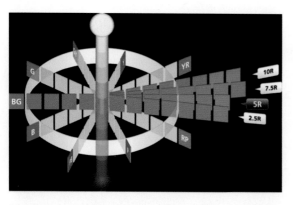

FIGURE 4.31 Munsell scales of hue, value, and chroma in color space. *(Image courtesy of Munsell Color, Grand Rapids, MI.)*

where *C* is the average chroma and ΔH, ΔV, and ΔC are differences in hue, value, and chroma of the two colors. For example, if the color of attached gingiva of a patient with periodontal disease was 2.5R 5/6, the color difference, *I*, between the diseased tissue and the aforementioned healthy tissue (5R 6/4) would be as follows:

$$I = (5/5)(2)(2.5) + (6)(1) + (3)(2) = 17$$

A trained observer can detect a color difference, *I*, equal to 5.

SURFACE FINISH AND THICKNESS

When white light shines on a solid, some of the light is directly reflected from the surface and remains white light. This light mixes with the light reflected from the body of the material and dilutes the color. As a result, an extremely rough surface appears lighter than a smooth surface of the same material. This problem is associated with unpolished or worn glass ionomer and resin composite restorations. For example, as the resin matrix of a composite wears away, the restoration appears lighter and less chromatic (grayer).

The thickness of a restoration can affect its appearance. For example, as the thickness of a composite restoration placed against a white background increases, the lightness and the excitation purity decrease. This is observed as an increase in opacity as the thickness increases.

Pigmentation

Esthetic effects are sometimes produced in a restoration by incorporating colored pigments in nonmetallic materials such as resin composites, denture acrylics, silicone maxillofacial materials, and dental ceramics. The perceived color results from the absorption of specific wavelengths of light by the pigments and the reflection of other wavelengths.

Mercuric sulfide, or vermilion, is red because it absorbs all colors except red and it reflects red. The mixing of pigments therefore involves the process of subtracting colors. For example, a green color may be obtained by mixing a pigment such as cadmium sulfide, which absorbs blue and violet, with ultramarine, which absorbs red, orange, and yellow. The only color reflected from such a mixture of pigments is green, which is the color observed.

Inorganic pigments are often preferred to organic dyes because the pigments are more permanent and durable in their color qualities. When colors are combined with the proper translucency, restorative materials can be made to closely match the surrounding tooth structure or soft tissue. To match tooth tissue, various shades of yellow and gray are blended into the white base material, and occasionally some blue or green pigments are added. To match the pink gingival tissues, various blends of red and white are used, with occasional additions of blue, brown, and black in small quantities. The color and translucency of gingival tissues vary widely from patient to patient and from one area of the mouth to another.

Metamerism

Metameric colors are color stimuli of identical tristimulus values under a particular light source but with different spectral energy distributions. The spectral reflectance curves of two such pairs would be complicated, with perhaps three or more crossing points. Under some lights the pairs would appear to match, but under other lights they would be different (Figure 4-32).

The quality and intensity of light are factors that must be controlled when matching colors in dental restorations. Because the light spectrum of incandescent lamps, fluorescent lamps, and the sun differ from each other, a color match between a restorative material and tooth structure in one lighting condition might not match in another. Whenever possible, shade matching should be done in conditions where most of the patient's activities will occur.

Fluorescence

Fluorescence is the emission of luminous energy by a material when a beam of light is shone on it. The wavelength of the emitted light usually is longer than that of the exciting radiation. Typically, blue or ultraviolet light produces fluorescent light that is in the visible range. Light from most fluorescent substances is emitted in a single, broad, well-shaped curve, the width and peak depending on the fluorescing substance.

Sound human teeth emit fluorescent light when excited by ultraviolet radiation (365 nm), the

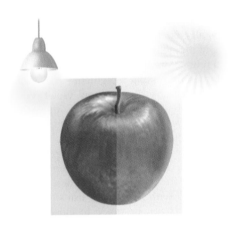

FIGURE 4.32 **Example of metamerism: the apple changes color depending on the light source used to illuminate it.**

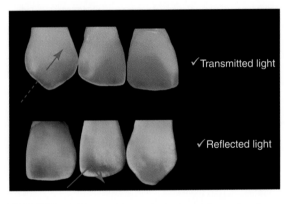

FIGURE 4.33 **Demonstration of opalescence in a ceramic restoration.** The tooth appears brown under transmitted light and blue under reflected light.

fluorescence being polychromatic with the greatest intensity in the blue region (450 nm) of the spectrum. Some anterior restorative materials and dental porcelains are formulated with fluorescing agents to reproduce the natural appearance of tooth structure.

Opacity, Translucency, Transparency, and Opalescence

The color of an object is modified not only by the intensity and shade of the pigment or coloring agent but also by the translucency or opacity of the object. Hard and soft tissues vary in their degree of opacity. Most exhibit some translucency. This is especially true of tooth enamel and the surrounding gingival tissues.

Opacity is a property of materials that prevents the passage of light. When all of the colors of the spectrum from a white light source such as sunlight are reflected from an object with the same intensity as received, the object appears white. When all the spectrum colors are absorbed equally, the object appears black. An opaque material may absorb some of the light and reflect the remainder. If, for example, red, orange, yellow, blue, and violet are absorbed, the material appears green in reflected white light.

Translucency is a property of substances that permits the passage of light but disperses the light, so objects cannot be seen through the material. Some translucent materials used in dentistry are ceramics, resin composites, and acrylics.

Transparent materials allow the passage of light so little distortion takes place and objects may be clearly seen through them. Transparent substances such as glass may be colored if they absorb certain wavelengths and transmit others. For example, if a piece of glass absorbed all wavelengths except red, it would appear red by transmitted light. If a light

beam containing no red wavelengths were shone on the glass, it would appear opaque, because the remaining wavelengths would be absorbed.

Opalescent materials, such as dental enamel, are able to scatter shorter wavelengths of light. Under transmitted light, they appear brown/yellow, whereas shades of blue are perceptible under reflected light (Figure 4-33). To produce highly esthetic restorations that truly mimic the natural appearance of the tooth, materials with opalescent properties should be used. This has popularized the use of porcelain veneering materials, as well as direct restorative composites.

Index of Refraction

The index of refraction (n) for any substance is the ratio of the velocity of light in a vacuum (or air) to its velocity in the medium. When light enters a medium, it slows from its speed in air (300,000 km/sec) and may change direction. For example, when a beam of light traveling in air strikes the surface of water at an oblique angle, the light rays are bent toward the normal. The *normal* is a line drawn perpendicular to the water surface at the point where the light contacts the water surface. If the light is traveling through water and contacts a water-air surface at an oblique angle, the beam of light is bent or refracted away from the normal. The index of refraction is a characteristic property of the substance (Table 4-8) and is used extensively for identification. One of the most important applications of refraction is the control of the refractive index of the dispersed and matrix phases in materials such as resin composites and dental ceramics, designed to have the translucent appearance of tooth tissue. A perfect match in the refractive indices results in a transparent solid, whereas large differences result in opaque materials.

TABLE 4.8 Index of Refraction (n) of Various Materials

Material	Index of Refraction
Feldspathic porcelain	1.504
Quartz	1.544
Synthetic hydroxyapatite	1.649
Tooth structure, enamel	1.655
Water	1.333

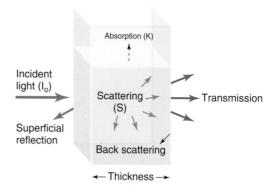

FIGURE 4.34 **Schematic of the possible interactions of light with a solid.**

Optical Constants

As light interacts with an object, several phenomena can be observed. Incident light can be reflected, absorbed, scattered (or backscattered) or transmitted. These parameters can all be calculated to more objectively characterize the optical properties of the material (Figure 4-34). Esthetic dental materials such as ceramics, resin composites, and tooth structure are turbid, or intensely light-scattering, materials. In a turbid material the intensity of incident light is diminished considerably when light passes through the specimen. These considerations are important not only for shade matching but also in situations where the restorative material is used to conceal imperfections in the tooth being restored, such as stains or other flaws. The optical properties of restorative materials are described by the Kubelka-Munk equations, which develop relations for monochromatic light between the reflection of an infinitely thick layer of a material and its absorption and scattering coefficients. These equations can be solved algebraically by hyperbolic functions derived by Kubelka.

Secondary optical constants (a and b) can be calculated as follows:

$$a = [R(B) - R(W) - R_B + R_W - R(B)R(W)R_B \\ + R(B)R(W)R_W + R(B)R_BR_W - R(W)R_BR_W \\ - R(W)R_BR_W] / \{2[R(B)R_W - R(W)RB]\}$$

and

$$b = (a^2 - 1)^{\frac{1}{2}}$$

where R_B is the reflectance of a dark backing (the black standard), R_W is reflectance of a light backing (the white standard), $R(B)$ is the light reflectance of a specimen with the dark backing, and $R(W)$ is the light reflectance of the specimen with the light backing.

These equations are used under the assumptions that (1) the material is turbid, dull, and of constant finite thickness; (2) edges are neglected; (3) optical inhomogeneities are much smaller than the thickness of the specimen and are distributed uniformly; and (4) illumination is homogeneous and diffused.

SCATTERING COEFFICIENT

The scattering coefficient is the fraction of incident light flux lost by reversal of direction in an elementary layer. The scattering coefficient, S, for a unit thickness of a material is defined as follows:

$$S = (1/bX) \, Ar \, ctgh \, [1 - a(R + R_g) + RR_g/b \\ (R - R_g)], \, mm^{-1}$$

where X is the actual thickness of the specimen, $Ar \, ctgh$ is an inverse hyperbolic cotangent, and R is the light reflectance of the specimen with the backing of reflectance, R_g.

The scattering coefficient varies with the wavelength of the incident light and the nature of the colorant layer, as shown in Figure 4-35 for several shades of a resin composite. Composites with larger values of the scattering coefficient are more opaque.

ABSORPTION COEFFICIENT

The absorption coefficient is the fraction of incident light flux lost by absorption in an elementary layer. The absorption coefficient, K, for a unit thickness of a material is defined as follows:

$$K = S(a - 1), \, mm^{-1}$$

The absorption coefficient also varies with the wavelength of the incident light and the nature of the colorant layer, as shown in Figure 4-36 for several shades of a resin composite. Composites with larger values of the absorption coefficient are more opaque and more intensely colored.

LIGHT REFLECTIVITY

The light reflectivity, RI, is the light reflectance of a material of infinite thickness, and is defined as follows:

$$RI = a - b$$

This property also varies with the wavelength of the incident light and the nature of the colorant layer.

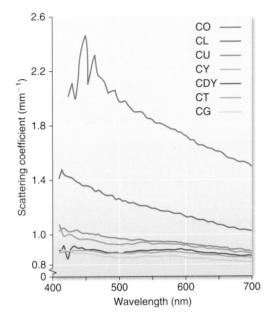

FIGURE 4.35 **Scattering coefficient versus wavelength for shades of a composite, *C.*** Shades are *O,* opaque; *L,* light; *U,* universal; *Y,* yellow; *DY,* dark yellow; *T,* translucent; and *G,* gray. *(From Yeh CL, Miyagawa Y, Powers JM: J. Dent. Res. 61, 797, 1982.)*

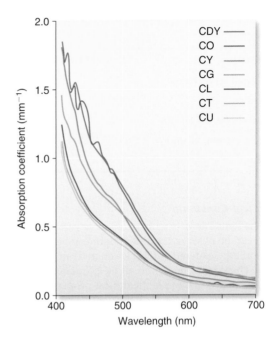

FIGURE 4.36 **Absorption coefficient versus wavelength for shades of a composite, *C.*** Shades are *DY,* dark yellow; *O,* opaque; *Y,* yellow; *G,* gray; *L,* light; *T,* translucent; and *U,* universal. *(From Yeh CL, Miyagawa Y, Powers JM: J. Dent. Res. 61, 797, 1982.)*

The light reflectivity can be used to calculate a thickness, XI, at which the reflectance of a material with an ideal black background would attain 99.9% of its light reflectivity. The infinite optical thickness, XI, is defined for monochromatic light as follows:

$$XI = (1/bS)\ Ar\ \mathrm{ctgh}\ [(1 - 0.999aRI)/0.999bRI],\mathrm{mm}$$

The variation of XI with wavelength is shown in Figure 4-37 for a resin composite. It is interesting that composites are more opaque to blue than to red light, yet blue light is used to cure light-activated composites.

CONTRAST RATIO

Once a, b, and S are obtained, the light reflectance (R) for a specimen of any thickness (X) in contact with a backing of any reflectance (R_g) can be calculated using the following formula:

$$R = [1 - R_g\ (a - b\ \mathrm{ctgh}\ bSX)]/(a + b\mathrm{ctgh}\ bSX - R_g)$$

An estimate of the opacity of a 1-mm-thick specimen can then be calculated from the contrast ratio (C) as follows:

$$C = R_O / R$$

where R_0 is the computed light reflectance of the specimen with a black backing.

Masking Ability

Dental restorations are often used to resolve esthetic problems, even when carious lesions are not present. This is the case in patients presenting staining due to intrinsic or extrinsic factors (examples of which are staining by antibiotics and smoking habits, respectively) or in restorations where an opaque reinforcing structure is required, as in the case of metallic or highly crystalline ceramic posts. The masking ability of restorative materials depends on their optical constants, as previously described, and on their thickness. In Figure 4-34 examples of materials with the same thickness but different optical properties are shown against a black and white background to demonstrate variations in the masking ability.

Thermal Properties

Temperature

The temperature of a substance can be measured with a thermometer or a thermocouple. An important application of temperature measurement in dentistry is the measurement of heat during cavity preparation or during light activation of resin composites. Examples of the effect of handpiece rotational speed and coolants on temperature in tooth structure during cavity preparation are shown in Figure 4-38.

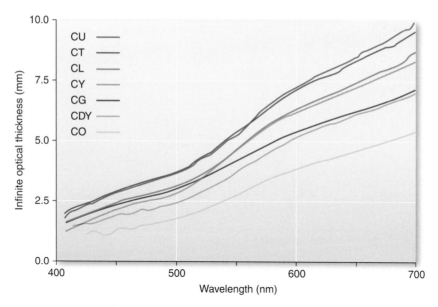

FIGURE 4.37 **Infinite optical thickness versus wavelength for shades of a composite, C.** Shades are U, universal; T, translucent; L, light; Y, yellow; G, gray; DY, dark yellow; and O, opaque. *(From Yeh CL, Miyagawa Y, Powers JM: J. Dent. Res. 61, 797, 1982.)*

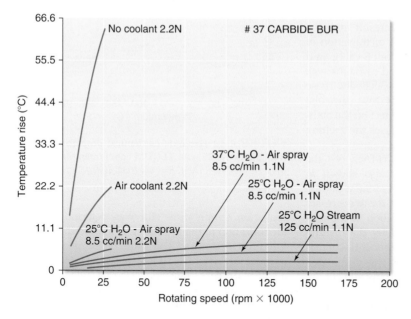

FIGURE 4.38 **Temperature rises developed by carbide burs during cutting of tooth tissue, operated at different speeds and with and without coolants.** *(Modified from Peyton FA: J. Am. Dent. Assoc. 56, 664, 1958.)*

The temperature was measured by a thermocouple inserted into a small opening that extended into the dentoenamel junction. The tooth was then cut in the direction of the thermocouple and the maximum temperature recorded.

Transition Temperatures

The arrangement of atoms and molecules in materials is influenced by the temperature; as a result, thermal techniques are important in understanding the properties of dental materials.

Differential thermal analysis (DTA) has been applied to study the components of dental waxes. The DTA curve of a mixture of paraffin and carnauba wax is shown in Figure 4-39. The thermogram was obtained when the difference in temperature between the wax and a standard was recorded under the same heating conditions in which thermocouples were used. The difference in temperature was recorded as a function of the temperature of the surroundings. A decrease in the value of ΔT indicated an endothermic process in the specimen. The endotherms

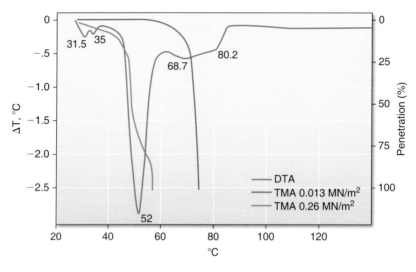

FIGURE 4.39 **Thermograms of a 75% paraffin and 25% carnauba wax mixture.**

at 31.5 and 35° C are solid-solid transitions occurring in the paraffin wax as the result of a change of crystal structure. The endotherm at 52° C represents the solid-liquid transition of paraffin wax, whereas the endotherms at 68.7 and 80.2° C result from the melting of carnauba wax. The heat of transition of the two solid-solid transitions is about 8 cal/g, and the melting transition of paraffin and carnauba wax is approximately 39 and 11 cal/g, respectively. These and other thermograms show that 25% carnauba wax added to paraffin wax has no effect on the melting point of paraffin wax but increases the melting range about 28° C.

Thermomechanical analysis (TMA) of the carnauba-paraffin wax mixture is also shown in Figure 4-39. The percent penetration of the wax mixture by a cylindrical probe is shown for two stresses of 0.013 and 0.26 MPa. The penetration of the wax at the lower stress was controlled by the melting transition of the carnauba wax component, whereas the penetration at the higher stress was dominated by the solid-solid and solid-liquid transitions of the paraffin wax components. About 44% penetration, which is related to flow, occurred before the melting point of the paraffin wax was reached.

Other properties correlate with thermograms. The coefficient of thermal expansion of paraffin wax increases from about $300 \times 10^{-6}/$ C to $1400 \times 10^{-6}/$ C just before the solid-solid transition, and the flow increases greatly in this temperature range.

Dynamic mechanical analysis (DMA) of a dimethacrylate copolymer is shown in Figure 4-40. A thin film of the copolymer was subjected to a sinusoidal tensile strain at a frequency of 11 Hz. As temperature was increased, values of modulus of elasticity (E′) and loss tangent (tan δ) were obtained. The glass

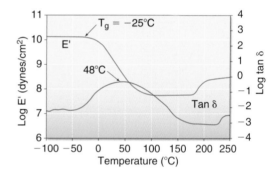

FIGURE 4.40 **Dynamic mechanical properties of a 75 wt% Bis-GMA/25 wt% TEGDM copolymer.** *(From Wilson TW, Turner DT: J. Dent. Res. 66, 1032, 1987.)*

transition temperature (T_g) was determined from identification of the beginning of a rapid decrease in E′ with temperature. The value of Tg identifies the temperature at which a glassy polymer transforms to a softer, rubbery state upon heating, which in turn relates to the increase in the number of degrees of freedom given to the molecules by the increased entropy. A lower value of T_g can result from a lower degree of conversion of double bonds, less crosslinked, more flexible networks or from saturation by water. As discussed later, the value of the coefficient of thermal expansion of a polymer changes at T_g.

Heat of Fusion

The heat of fusion, L, is the heat in calories, or joules, J, required to convert 1 g of a material from solid to liquid state at the melting temperature. The equation for the calculation of heat of fusion is $L = Q/m$, where Q is the total heat absorbed and m is the

TABLE 4.9   Heat of Fusion (L) of Some Materials

Materials	Temperature (° C)	Heat of Fusion (cal/g [J/g])
METALS		
Mercury	−39	3 [12]
Gold	1063	16 [67]
Silver	960	26 [109]
Platinum	1773	27 [113]
Copper	1083	49 [205]
Cobalt	1495	58 [242]
Chromium	1890	75 [314]
Aluminum compounds	660	94 [393]
Alcohol	−114	25 [104]
Paraffin	52	35 [146]
Beeswax	62	42 [176]
Glycerin	18	47 [196]
Ice	0	80 [334]

TABLE 4.10   Thermal Conductivity (K) of Various Materials

Material	Thermal Conductivity	
	cal/sec/cm²/ (° C/cm)	J/sec/cm² (° C/cm)
METALS		
Silver	1.006	4.21
Copper	0.918	3.84
Gold	0.710	2.97
Platinum	0.167	0.698
Dental amalgam	0.055	0.23
Mercury	0.020	0.084
NONMETALS		
Gypsum	0.0031	0.013
Zinc phosphate cement	0.0028	0.012
Resin composite	0.0026	0.011
Porcelain	0.0025	0.010
Enamel	0.0022	0.0092
Dentin	0.0015	0.0063
Zinc oxide–eugenol cement	0.0011	0.0046
Acrylic resin	0.0005	0.0021
Beeswax	0.00009	0.0004

mass of the substance melted. Therefore, in practical applications it is apparent that the larger the mass of material being melted, the more heat required to change the total mass to liquid. The heat of fusion is closely related to the melting or freezing point of the substance, because when the change in state occurs, it is always necessary to apply additional heat to the mass to cause liquefaction, and as long as the mass remains molten, the heat of fusion is retained by the liquid. When the mass is frozen, or solidified, the heat that was retained in the liquid state is liberated. The difference in energy content is necessary to maintain the kinetic molecular motion, which is characteristic of the liquid state.

The values for heat of fusion of some common substances (given in round numbers) are listed in Table 4-9. It may be seen that the values for heat of fusion of gold and the metals used for dental gold alloys (silver and copper) are below those of many other metals and compounds. This is true also for the specific heat of gold and its alloys.

Thermal Conductivity

The thermal conductivity, K, of a substance is the quantity of heat in calories, or joules, per second passing through a body 1-cm thick with a cross-section of 1 cm² when the temperature difference is 1° C. The units are cal/sec/cm²/(° C/cm). The conductivity of a material changes slightly as the surrounding temperature is altered, but generally the difference resulting from temperature changes is much less than the difference that exists between different types of materials.

Several important applications of thermal conductivity exist in dental materials. For example, a large amalgam filling or gold crown in proximity to the pulp may cause the patient considerable discomfort when hot or cold foods produce temperature changes; this effect is mitigated when adequate tooth tissue remains or cavity liners are placed between the tooth and filling for insulation. Cavity liners are relatively poor thermal conductors and insulate the pulp area.

A better understanding of the conductivities of various restorative materials is desirable to develop an appropriate degree of insulation for the pulp tissue, comparable with that in the natural tooth. The conductivity of certain dental materials is listed in Table 4-10. Nonmetallic materials have lower thermal conductivity than metals, and are therefore good insulators. Dental cements have a thermal conductivity similar to that of dentin and enamel. Note that the thermal conductivity of a liner or base is important in reducing the thermal transfer to the pulp, and that the temperature difference across an insulator depends on the extent of the heating or cooling period and the magnitude of the temperature difference.

Specific Heat

The specific heat, Cp, of a substance is the quantity of heat needed to raise the temperature of 1 g of the substance 1° C. Water is usually chosen as the standard substance and 1 g as the standard mass. The heat required to raise the temperature of 1 g of water from 15 to 16° C is 1 cal, which is used as the basis for the definition of the heat unit. Most substances are more readily heated, gram for gram, than water.

Obviously the total heat required to raise the temperature of a substance 1° C depends on the total mass and the specific heat. For example, 100 g of water requires more calories than 50 g of water to raise the temperature 1° C. Likewise, because of the difference in specific heat of water and alcohol, 100 g of water requires more heat than 100 g of alcohol to raise the temperature the same amount. In general, the specific heat of liquids is higher than those of solids. Some metals have specific heat values of less than 10% that of water.

During the melting and casting process, the specific heat of the metal or alloy is important because of the total amount of heat that must be applied to the mass to raise the temperature to the melting point. Fortunately, the specific heat of gold and the metals used in gold alloys is low, so prolonged heating is unnecessary. The specific heat of both enamel and dentin is higher than that of metals used for fillings, as shown in Table 4-11.

Thermal Diffusivity

The thermal diffusivity, Δ, is a measure of transient heat-flow and is defined as the thermal conductivity, K, divided by the product of the specific heat, Cp, times the density, ϱ:

$$\Delta = K / (Cp\, p)$$

The units of thermal diffusivity are mm^2/sec.

The thermal diffusivity describes the rate at which a body with a nonuniform temperature approaches equilibrium. For a gold crown or a dental amalgam, the low specific heat combined with the high thermal conductivity creates a thermal shock more readily than normal tooth structure does. Values of thermal diffusivity of some materials are listed in Table 4-12. These values may vary somewhat with composition of the particular restorative material.

As mentioned in the discussion of thermal conductivity, thickness of the material is important. A parameter governing lining efficiency (Z) is related

TABLE 4.11   Specific Heat (Cp) of Various Materials

Material	Specific Heat (cal/g/° C [J/g/° C])
SOLIDS	
Gold	0.031 [0.13]
Platinum	0.032 [0.13]
Silver	0.056 [0.23]
Copper	0.092 [0.38]
Enamel	0.18 [0.75]
Quartz	0.19 [0.79]
Aluminum	0.21 [0.88]
Porcelain	0.26 [1.09]
Dentin	0.28 [1.17]
Acrylic resin	0.35 [1.46]
LIQUIDS	
Water	1.000 [4.18]
Paraffin	0.69 [2.88]
Glycerin	0.58 [2.42]
Alcohol (ethyl)	0.547 [2.29]
Mercury	0.033 [0.14]

to thickness (T) and thermal diffusivity (Δ) as follows:

$$Z = T / (\Delta)^{\frac{1}{2}}$$

Coefficient of Thermal Expansion

The change in length $(l_{final} - l_{original})$ per unit length of a material for a 1° C change in temperature is called the *linear coefficient of thermal expansion*, α, and is calculated as follows:

$$(l_{final} - l_{original}) / [l_{original} \times (°C_{final} - °C_{original})] = \alpha$$

The units are represented by the notation /° C, and because the values are usually small they are expressed in exponential form such as $22 \times 10^{-6}/°C$. A less common practice is to report the change in parts per million (ppm) and the previous number would be expressed as 22 ppm.

The linear coefficients of thermal expansion for some materials important in restorative dentistry are given in Table 4-13. Although the coefficient is a material constant, it does not remain constant over wide temperature ranges. For example, the linear coefficient of thermal expansion of a dental wax may have an average value of $300 \times 10^{-6}/°C$ up to 40° C, whereas it may have an average value of $500 \times 10^{-6}/°C$ from 40 to 50° C. The coefficient of thermal

TABLE 4.12   Thermal Diffusivity (Δ) of Various Materials

Material	Thermal Diffusivity (mm^2/sec)
Pure gold (calculated)	119.0
Amalgam	9.6
Resin composite	0.675
Porcelain	0.64
Enamel	0.469
Zinc oxide–eugenol cement	0.389
Zinc phosphate cement	0.290
Dental compound	0.226
Zinc polyacrylate cement	0.223
Glass ionomer cement	0.198
Dentin	0.183
Acrylic resin	0.123

TABLE 4.13   Linear Coefficient (α) of Thermal Expansion of Various Materials

Material	Coefficient ($\times 10^{-6}$/° C)
Inlay waxes	350-450
Silicone impression material	210
Polysulfide impression material	140
Pit and fissure sealants	71-94
Acrylic resin	76.0
Mercury	60.6
Resin composites	14-50
Zinc oxide–eugenol cement	35
Amalgam	22-28
Silver	19.2
Copper	16.8
Gold	14.4
Porcelain	12.0
Tooth (crown portion)	11.4
Glass ionomer (type 2)	10.2-11.4

expansion of a polymer changes as the polymer goes from a glassy state to a softer, rubbery material. This change in the coefficient corresponds to the glass transition temperature (T_g).

Either the linear or volumetric coefficient of thermal expansion may be measured, and for most materials that function as isotropic solids, the volumetric thermal coefficient may be considered to be three times the linear thermal coefficient.

Both linear expansion and volume expansion are important in restorative materials and processes. It is obvious that with a reduction of temperature, or cooling, there is a contraction of the substance that is equal to the expansion that results from heating. Accordingly, tooth structure and restorative materials in the mouth will expand when warmed by hot foods and beverages but will contract when exposed to cold substances. Such expansions and contractions may break the marginal seal of a filling in the tooth, particularly if the difference between the coefficient of expansion of the tooth and the restorative material is large. The high coefficient of expansion of pattern waxes is an important factor in the construction of properly fitting restorations. The change in volume as a result of cooling is responsible for the shrinkage spots or surface cracks that often develop in gold alloy castings during solidification. Compensation for the contraction that occurs during the cooling of gold alloys must be made if accurate gold castings are to result. The values in Table 4-13 show that with comparable temperature changes, materials such as acrylic resin and amalgam expand more than tooth tissue, whereas ceramic expands less. The coefficient of

inlay pattern wax is exceptionally high when compared with that of other materials.

Of particular importance in casting investments is the property of thermal expansion of three crystalline polymorphic forms of silica. As a principal ingredient in dental investments that are to be heated before a metal casting is made, the amount of expansion at various temperatures is critical and important. This quality of silica compounds in relation to use in casting investments was described in 1932. Curves in Figure 4-41 illustrate the relative percentage of thermal expansion of the four forms of silica at different temperatures below about 800° C. Of the crystalline forms, cristobalite shows the greatest expansion at the lowest temperature and quartz requires a higher temperature to develop an equal amount of expansion as cristobalite. Fused silica has long been recognized as having an exceedingly low thermal expansion.

Electrical Properties

Electrical Conductivity and Resistivity

The ability of a material to conduct an electric current may be stated as either specific conductance or conductivity, or conversely, as the specific resistance or resistivity. *Resistivity* is the more common term. The resistance of a homogeneous conductor of uniform cross section at a constant temperature varies directly with the length and inversely with the cross-sectional area of the specimen, according to the equation:

$$R = \rho l / A$$

in which R is the resistance in ohms, ρ (rho) is the resistivity, l is the length, and A is the section area. The resistivity depends on the nature of the material. If a unit cube of 1-cm edge length is employed, the l and A are equal to unity, and in this case $R = \rho$. The resistivity is expressed as ohm-centimeters where R is in ohms, l is in centimeters, and A is in square centimeters.

The change in electrical resistance has been used to study the alteration in internal structure of various alloys as a result of heat treatment. An early investigation of the gold-copper alloy system by electrical conductivity methods revealed a change in internal crystal structure with an accompanying change in conductivity. The correlation of these conductivity studies with related changes in other properties established the fundamental basis of structural changes associated with heat-treatment operations on dental gold alloys.

Values for the resistivity of human tooth structure are shown in Table 4-14. Resistivity is important in the investigation of the pain perception threshold resulting from applied electrical stimuli and of displacement of fluid in teeth caused by ionic movements. The electrical resistance of normal and carious teeth has been observed to differ, with less resistance offered by the carious tissue. Sound enamel is a relatively poor conductor of electricity, whereas dentin is somewhat better (see Table 4-14).

The conductivity of materials used to replace tooth tissue is of concern in restorative dentistry. The effectiveness of insulating cement bases and other nonmetallic restorative materials is not yet established. Several studies have measured the resistivity of dental cements (see Table 4-14). The zinc oxide–eugenol cements have the highest resistivity, followed by the zinc polyacrylate and zinc phosphate cements. The glass ionomer cements are the most conductive of the cements and have values most similar to dentin.

Dielectric Constant

A material that provides electrical insulation is known as a *dielectric*. Values of the dielectric constant for human dentin and several dental cements are listed in Table 4-15. The dielectric constant of a dental cement generally decreases as the material hardens. This decrease reflects a change from a paste that is relatively ionic and polar to one that is less so. As shown by the high values of permittivity of the glass ionomer and zinc polyacrylate cements in Table 4-15, these cements have a high ionic content and are quite polar compared with zinc oxide–eugenol cements and human dentin.

The problem of electrical insulation is made more complex by the presence of galvanic currents in the mouth, resulting from cells formed from metallic restorations. Recent studies indicate that a cement base does not effectively insulate the pulp from the electric current developed in a metallic restoration in the mouth. How much insulation is essential or how to effectively restore the tooth to its original status of equilibrium is currently not known.

Electromotive Force

Working with metals and alloys for dental restorations or with instruments that are susceptible to corrosion necessitates some understanding of the relative position of the metal in the electromotive force series. The electromotive series is a listing of electrode potentials of metals according to the order of their decreasing tendency to oxidize in solution.

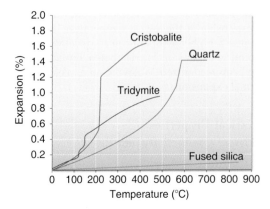

FIGURE 4.41 **Thermal expansion curves for four types of silica.** *(Modified from Volland RH, Paffenbarger GC: J. Am. Dent. Assoc. 19, 185, 1932.)*

TABLE 4.14 Values of Resistivity (r) of Human Tooth Structure and Several Dental Cements

Material	Resistivity (ohm · cm)
HUMAN ENAMEL	
Bjorn (1946)	$2.9\text{-}3.6 \times 10^6$
Mumford (1967)	$2.6\text{-}6.9 \times 10^6$
Human Dentin	
Bjorn (1946)	$0.7\text{-}6.0 \times 10^4$
Mumford (1967)	$1.1\text{-}5.2 \times 10^4$
Dental Cement	
Glass ionomer	$0.8\text{-}2.5 \times 10^4$
Zinc oxide–eugenol	$10^9\text{-}10^{10}$
Zinc polyacrylate	$0.4\text{-}4 \times 10^5$
Zinc phosphate	2×10^5

This serves as the basis of comparison of the tendency of metals to oxidize in air. Those metals with a large negative electrode potential are more resistant to tarnish than those with a high positive electrode potential. In general, the metals above copper in the series, such as aluminum, zinc, and nickel, tend to oxidize relatively easily, whereas those below copper, such as silver, platinum, and gold, resist oxidation. A list of oxidation-reduction potentials for some common corrosion reactions in water and in salt water is given in Table 4-16. The values of electrode potential and the order of the series change when measured in a saline solution rather than water. The electrode

potentials of some dental alloys measured in artificial saliva at 35° C are listed in Table 4-17.

Likewise, it is possible to determine from the electromotive force series that the reduction of the oxides of gold, platinum, and silver to pure metal can be accomplished more readily than with those metals that have a higher electromotive force value.

Galvanism

The presence of metallic restorations in the mouth may cause a phenomenon called *galvanic action*, or galvanism. This results from a difference in potential between dissimilar fillings in opposing or adjacent teeth. These fillings, in conjunction with saliva or bone fluids such as electrolytes, make up an electric cell. When two opposing fillings contact each other, the cell is short-circuited, and if the flow of current occurs through the pulp, the patient experiences pain and the more anodic restoration may corrode. A single filling plus the saliva and bone fluid may also constitute a cell of liquid junction type. As shown in Figure 4-42, ions capable of conducting electricity can easily migrate through dentin and around the margins of a restoration.

Studies have indicated that relatively large currents will flow through metallic fillings when they

TABLE 4.15 Dielectric Constant (ε_r) for Human Dentin and Several Dental Cements

Material	Dielectric Constant
Human dentin	8.6
Dental cements (set)	
Glass ionomer	2 to 7×10^5
Zinc oxide–eugenol	10
Zinc polyacrylate	4×10^3 to 2×10^5

TABLE 4.16 Oxidation-Reduction Potentials for Corrosion Reactions in Water and Salt Water

Metal	Corrosion Reaction	In Water, Electrode Potential at 25° C (Volts versus Normal Hydrogen Electrode)	In Salt Water, Electrode Potential at 25° C (Volts versus 0.1 N Calomel Scale)
Aluminum	$Al \rightarrow Al^{3+} + 3e$	+1.662*	+0.83
Zinc	$Zn \rightarrow Zn^{2+} + 2e$	+0.763	+1.10
Chromium	$Cr \rightarrow Cr^{3+} + 3e$	+0.744	+0.4 to −0.18
Iron	$Fe \rightarrow Fe^{2+} + 2e$	+0.440	+0.58
Cobalt	$Co \rightarrow Co^{2+} + 2e$	+0.277	—
Nickel	$Ni \rightarrow Ni^{2+} + 2e$	+0.250	+0.07
Tin	$Sn \rightarrow Sn^{2+} + 2e$	+0.136	+0.49
Hydrogen	$H_2 \rightarrow 2H^+ + 2e$	0.000	—
Copper	$Cu \rightarrow Cu^{2+} + 2e$	−0.337	+0.20
	$4(OH^-) \rightarrow O_2 + 2H_2O + 4e$	−0.401	—
Mercury	$2Hg \rightarrow Hg_2^{2+} + 2e$	−0.788	—
Silver	$Ag \rightarrow Ag^+ + e$	−0.799	+0.08
Palladium	$Pd \rightarrow Pd^{2+} + 2e$	−0.987	—
Platinum	$Pt \rightarrow Pt^{2+} + 2e$	−1.200	—
	$2H_2o \rightarrow O_2 + 4H^+ + 4e$	−1.229	—
Gold	$Au \rightarrow Au^{3+} + 3e$	−1.498	—

Modified from Flinn RA, Trojan PK: Engineering Materials and Their Applications, ed 4, Boston, Houghton Mifflin, 1990.
*A positive value indicates a strong tendency for the metal to go into solution. Higher positive values are more anodic, whereas higher negative values are more cathodic.

TABLE 4.17 Galvanic Series of Some Dental Alloys in Artificial Saliva at 35° C

Material	Volts[*]
Tin crown form	+0.048
Hydrogen/H	0.000
Amalgam	
Conventional spherical	−0.023
Dispersed high-copper	−0.108
Nickel-chromium alloy	−0.126 to 0.240
Cobalt-chromium alloy	−0.292
Gold alloy	
Au-Cu-Ag	−0.345
Au-Pt-Pd-Ag	−0.358 to -0.455

Modified from Arvidson K, Johansson EG: Scand. J. Dent. Res. 85, 485, 1977.
[*]High positive sign indicates a strong tendency for the metal to go into solution.

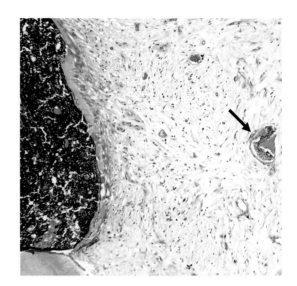

FIGURE 4.42 **Human pulp capped with calcium hydroxide cement.** Observation period: 70 days. A thin bond of hard tissue lined by cells is covering most of the exposure site (rank B). Calcified tissue in relation to displaced calcium hydroxide cement particles (*arrow*) (hematoxylin-eosin, original magnification ×100). *(From Hörsted-Bindslev P, Vilkinis V, Sidlauskas A: Oral Surg. Oral Med. Oral Pathol. Oral Radiol. Endod. 96(5), pp. 591-600, 2003.)*

are brought into contact. The current rapidly falls off if the fillings are maintained in contact, probably as a result of polarization of the cell. The magnitude of the voltage, however, is not of primary importance, because indications support the fact that the sensitivity of the patient to the current has a greater influence on whether pain is felt. Although most patients feel pain at a value between 20 and 50 μamp, some may feel pain at 10 μamp, whereas others do not experience it until 110 μamp are developed. This is a possible explanation for the fact that some patients are bothered by galvanic action and others are not, despite similar conditions in the mouth.

The galvanic currents developed from the contact of two metallic restorations depend on their composition and surface area. An alloy of stainless steel develops a higher current density than either gold or cobalt-chromium alloys when in contact with an amalgam restoration. As the size of the cathode (such as a gold alloy) increases relative to that of the anode (such as an amalgam), the current density may increase. The larger cathode, likewise, can enhance the corrosion of the smaller anode. Current densities associated with non-γ_2-containing amalgams appear to be less than those associated with the γ_2-containing amalgams.

Electrochemical Corrosion

The corrosion and electrochemical behavior of restorative materials have received new interest with the study of multiphase systems such as gold alloys and amalgam. For example, the corrosion of γ, γ_1, and γ_2 phases in amalgam has been studied by electrochemical analysis. Anodic and cathodic polarization measurements indicated no strongly passive behavior of these phases in artificial saliva. The dental amalgam specimens became pitted at the boundaries between the phases or in γ_2 phase. Other studies, however, indicate that amalgam alloys exhibit decreasing electrochemical potentials, resulting in noble values when stored in neutral solutions. The addition of copper to amalgam alloys to form copper-tin compounds during hardening has improved the resistance of amalgam to chloride and galvanic corrosion. As shown in Figure 4-43, the anodic activity of AgSn amalgam is quite different from AgSn + AgCu amalgams. The AgSn + AgCu amalgam remains passive under the testing conditions, whereas the AgSn amalgam does not.

Studies of corrosion of surgical stainless steel and stainless steel orthodontic brackets have been reported. Corrosion of these alloys and others can result in decreased mechanical properties and the formation of corrosion products, which in some instances accumulate in the human organs. As shown previously in Table 4-16, corrosion can be affected by the environment, and certain metals such as cobalt and copper corrode more rapidly in a saline solution containing serum albumin and fibrinogen proteins.

Zeta-Potential

A charged particle suspended in an electrolytic solution attracts ions of opposite charge to those at its surface. The layer formed by these ions is called

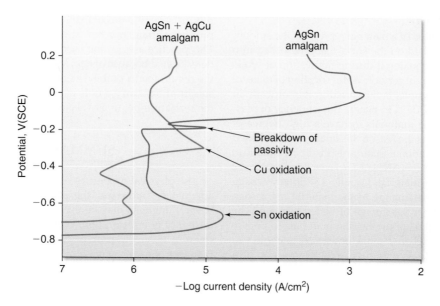

FIGURE 4.43 **Anodic polarization curves of two types of amalgam in synthetic saliva.** *(Modified from Fairhurst CW, Marek M, Butts MB, et al: J. Dent. Res. 57,725, 1978.)*

the *Stern layer.* To maintain the electrical balance of the suspending fluid, ions of opposite charge are attracted to the Stern layer. The potential at the surface of that part of the diffuse double layer of ions is called the *electrokinetic* or *zeta-potential.*

Electrophoresis may be used to increase the stability of colloids, stimulate adsorption of ions, and characterize particle surfaces. Effects of pH, surface-active agents, and enzymes on zeta-potential are important. Zeta-potential may affect the near-surface mechanical properties (such as wear) of a material. The zeta-potentials of some materials are listed in Table 4-18.

Other Properties

Certain properties often are highly important in the selection and manipulation of materials for use either in the mouth or for laboratory applications. Five such properties are tarnish and discoloration, water sorption, solubility and disintegration, setting time, and shelf life.

Tarnish and Discoloration

Discoloration of a restorative material from any cause is a very troublesome quality. The tarnish of metal restorations from oxide, sulfide, or any other materials causing a surface reaction is a critical quality of metal restorations in the mouth and of laboratory and clinical instruments. The process of steam sterilization of surgical instruments has long presented a serious problem of tarnish and corrosion. Many nonmetallic materials such as cements and

TABLE 4.18 Zeta-Potential (ζ) of Some Dental Materials

Material	Zeta-Potential (mV)
Hydroxyapatite	−9.0 to −10.9
Tooth structure*	
Calculus	−15.3
Cementum	
Exposed	−6.96
Unexposed	−9.34
Dentin	−6.23
Enamel	−9.04 to −10.3

Modified from O'Brien WJ (Ed.): 1997. Dental Materials and Their Selection, ed 2, Carol Stream, Quintessence.
Measured in Hanks' balanced salt solution at 30° C.

composite restorations have displayed a tendency to discolor in service because colored substances penetrate the materials and continue chemical reactions in the composites.

Various in vitro tests have been proposed to study tarnish, particularly that of crown and bridge and partial denture alloys. Testing generally relies on controlled exposure of the alloy to a solution rich in sulfides, chlorides, and phosphates. Most recently the discoloration of alloys exposed to such solutions has been evaluated by spectrophotometric methods to determine a color-difference parameter discussed earlier in this chapter.

Water Sorption

Water sorption of a material represents the amount of water adsorbed on the surface and absorbed into the body of the material during fabrication or while the restoration is in service. Water sorption of denture acrylic, for example, is measured gravimetrically in $\mu g/mm^3$ after 7 days in water. The tendency of plastic denture base materials to have a high degree of water sorption is the reason this quality was included in American National Standards Institute/American Dental Association (ANSI/ADA) specification No. 12 for this type of material. Usually a serious warpage and dimensional change in the material are associated with a high percentage of water sorption. The tendency of alginate impression materials to imbibe water if allowed to remain immersed and then to change dimensions requires careful disinfection procedures and pouring within the manufacturer's recommended time.

Setting Time

Setting time characteristics are associated with the reaction rates and affect the practical applications of many materials in restorative dentistry. Materials such as cements, impression materials, dental plaster, stone, and casting investments depend on a critical reaction time and hardening rate for their successful application. From the practical standpoint of manipulation and successful application, the time required for a material to set or harden from a plastic or fluid state may be its most important quality. The setting time does not indicate the completion of the reaction, which may continue for much longer times. The time varies for different materials, depending on the particular application, but duplication of results from one lot to another or from one trade brand of material to another is highly desirable. The influence of manipulative procedures on the setting time of various types of materials is important to the dentist and the assistant.

Shelf Life

Shelf life is a term applied to the general deterioration and change in quality of materials during shipment and storage. The temperature, humidity, and time of storage, as well as the bulk of material involved and the type of storage container, are significant factors that vary greatly from one material to another. A material that has exceptionally good properties when first produced may be quite impractical if it deteriorates badly after a few days or weeks. These qualities are discussed in chapters dealing with gypsum materials and impression materials. Some studies of these qualities of various materials have been made in recent years, and through accelerated aging tests, improvements in quality can sometimes be made. Radiographic film, anesthetics, and a few other products carry dates of expiration beyond which the product should not be expected to be serviceable. This practice assures the user that the material is not deteriorated because of age. Most materials that meet the requirements of the American Dental Association specifications carry a date of production as a part of the serial number or as a separate notation.

SUMMARY

The physical properties of oral restorations must adequately withstand the stresses of mastication. Several methods may be used to ensure proper performance of a restoration. With a constant force, the stress is inversely proportional to the contact area; therefore, stresses may be reduced by increasing the area over which the force is distributed. In areas of high stress, materials having high elastic moduli and strength properties should be used if possible. If a weaker material has desirable properties, such as esthetic qualities, one may minimize the stress by increasing the bulk of the material when possible or ensuring proper occlusion on the restoration.

Restorations and appliances should be designed so the resulting forces of mastication are distributed as uniformly as possible. Also, sharp line angles, nonuniform areas, and notched, scratched, or pitted surfaces should be avoided to minimize stress concentrations. For example, joints between abutments and pontics of fixed partial dentures should be properly radiused to distribute stress during function. Implant screws should not be scratched or notched when inserted.

Restorative materials are generally weaker in tension than in compression. Restorations should be designed to minimize areas of high tension. Material flaws can further contribute to areas prone to failure. Fatigue is also an important consideration. For example, repeated flexure of an improperly loaded implant-supported restoration can concentrate stresses in the abutment screw or implant body, leading to fatigue fracture.

The dentist is often concerned not so much with the fracture of an appliance as with the deflection that occurs when a force is applied. This is the case with a fixed partial denture, which may be cast as a single unit or may consist of soldered units. As discussed earlier in this chapter, the deflection of a beam, or in this case a fixed partial denture, supported on each end with a concentrated load in the center depends directly on the cube of the beam length and indirectly on the cube of the beam thickness. Doubling the length of the beam, therefore, increases the deflection by eight times. This also indicates that decreasing the thickness of the beam by one half increases the deflection by eight times. If too much bulk were required to develop the stiffness desired, changing to a material with a higher elastic modulus, or stiffness, would be beneficial. If repeated failures occur, consider increasing the occlusogingival dimension of the proximal connectors, balancing the occlusion over a larger surface area, and narrowing the occlusal table.

These isolated examples of applied knowledge of biting forces and stresses in dental structures indicate why an understanding of this subject is necessary to the practicing dentist.

In summary, three interrelated factors are important in the long-term function of dental restorative materials: (1) material choice, (2) component geometry (e.g., to minimize stress concentrations), and (3) component design (e.g., to distribute stresses as uniformly as possible). It should be noted that failures can and do occur. In such instances, a failure analysis should be performed by answering several questions: (1) Why did it fail? (2) How did it fail? (3) Did the material or design fail? and (4) How can this failure be prevented in the future? Lastly, remember that dental material behavior depends on interrelated physical, chemical, optical, mechanical, thermal, electrical, and biological properties, and improvement of one specific property often leads to a reduction in another property.

SELECTED PROBLEMS

Mechanical Properties

PROBLEM 1

With an average occlusal force of 565 N on the first or second molar, how is it possible for a patient to fracture a gold alloy fixed dental prosthesis (FDP) in service when the alloy has a tensile strength of 690 MPa?

Solution

The stress produced by the occlusal force is a function of the cross section of the FDP and the size of the contact area over which the force is applied. When the contact area from the opposing tooth is very small and located near a portion of the FDP having a small cross section, bending produces tensile stresses that can exceed the tensile strength of the gold alloy. For example, in problem 1, relating the occlusal force of 565 N to the tensile strength of 690 MPa indicates that a minimum area of 0.82 mm² is necessary in this FDP.

PROBLEM 2

Why is the yield strength of a restorative material such an important property?

Solution

The yield strength defines the stress at the point at which the material changes from elastic to plastic behavior. In the elastic range, stresses and strains return to zero after biting forces are removed, whereas in the plastic range some permanent deformation results on removal of the force. Significant permanent deformation may result in a functional failure of a restoration even though fracture does not occur.

PROBLEM 3

Why is the elongation value for a casting alloy not always an indication of the burnishability of the margins of the casting?

Solution

Although the elongation of an alloy gives an indication of its ductility, or ability to be drawn into a wire without fracturing, to burnish a margin of a casting, sufficient force must be applied to exceed the yield strength. Therefore, alloys with high yield strengths are difficult to burnish even though they have high values for elongation.

PROBLEM 4

Why does a mesio-occlusal-distal (MOD) amalgam fail in tension when compressive biting forces are applied from the opposing teeth?

Solution

The compressive load produces bending of the MOD amalgam, which results in compressive stress on the occlusal surface and tensile stresses at the base of the restoration. Amalgam is a brittle solid with much lower tensile than compressive strength, and therefore fails first at the base of the restoration, with the crack progressing to the occlusal surface of the amalgam.

PROBLEM 5

Because the modulus of nickel-chromium alloys is about twice that of gold alloys, why is it not correct to reduce the thickness by half and have the same deflection in bending?

Solution

Although the deflection in the bending equation is directly proportional to the modulus, it is inversely proportional to the cube of the thickness. Therefore, only minimal reductions in thickness are possible for the nickel-chromium alloy to maintain the same deflection.

PROBLEM 6

How is it possible to use a single elastomeric impression material and yet have the correct viscosity for use in the syringe and the tray?

Solution

Correct compounding of the polymer and filler produces a material that has the quality described as *shear thinning*. Such a material decreases in viscosity at high shear rates, such as during spatulation or syringing, and has a higher viscosity at low shear rates, as when it is placed and used as a tray material.

PROBLEM 7

After an orthodontic elastic band is extended and placed, the force applied decreases with time more than expected for the distance the tooth moves. Why?

Solution

Latex rubber bands behave elastically and viscoelastically. It is principally the viscous deformation that is not recoverable that accounts for the greater than expected decrease in force as the band shortens from the movement of the tooth. This effect is even more pronounced when plastic rather than latex bands are used.

PROBLEM 8

If dental manufacturers showed you the compliance versus time curve for their elastomeric impression material and pointed out that it had a high elastic compliance, moderate viscoelastic compliance, and a very low viscous compliance, how would you characterize the product?

Solution

The material would be highly flexible, should recover from deformation moderately rapidly, and the recovery from deformation should be nearly complete.

PROBLEM 9

Why is wear a matter of concern when selecting materials and designing restorations?

Solution

The wear of dental materials can be brought about, for example, by restorations with different hardness values put in opposing contact, a problem that is even more evident in patients with parafunctional habits. For that reason, the selection of materials to be put in highly solicited occlusal areas has to be judicious. The resistance to wear of composites in posterior restorations has improved over the past few years with the development of polymers that attain greater conversion, but mainly due to modifications in the filler systems.

SELECTED PROBLEMS

Colloidal State, Membranes, Surface Tension, Contact Angle, Adhesion, Capillary Rise

PROBLEM 1

Why is mercury difficult to handle without contamination in the operatory?

Solution

The high surface tension of mercury and high contact angles on most surfaces cause mercury to cohere and roll off most surfaces. The vapor pressure of mercury at room temperature is high enough so that its concentration in air can be toxic. The solution is to use precapsulated amalgam systems.

PROBLEM 2

Gold inlay castings made with the lost wax process were rough. What could have been the problem?

Solution

There could be several causes for the rough castings. A detergent or wetting agent may not have been used on the wax pattern prior to the investing procedure. Wax patterns are not readily wetted by the water-based gypsum investment unless a wetting agent is used; if one is not used, rough internal mold surfaces produce rough castings.

On the other hand, too much wetting agent placed on the wax will interfere with the setting of the investment and a rough surface will result. The wetting agent is painted on the wax pattern and the excess is removed by painting with a dry brush. Very little wetting agent is needed.

PROBLEM 3

The bond between a pit-and-fissure material that had just been removed from the refrigerator and etched enamel was found to be poor. Why?

Solution

The bonding of pit-and-fissure sealants to enamel depends on the capillary penetration of the sealant into the fine microscopic spaces produced by etching. The rate of capillary penetration is dependent upon the wetting and viscosity of the sealant. At lower temperatures, the viscosity of sealants is too high for rapid penetration. Therefore it is necessary to allow a refrigerated sealant to warm to room temperature before application.

PROBLEM 4

An addition silicone impression was poured in high-strength stone, but it was difficult to reproduce the fine margins of cavity preparations. What might have been the problem?

Solution

In all probability, a hydrophobic addition silicone impression material was used, and wetting of the surface by the mix of high-strength stone was troublesome. Check the manufacturer's literature, and likely there will be no indication that it is a hydrophilic type. Manufacturers will specify whether an addition silicone impression material is hydrophilic, but not whether it is hydrophobic.

PROBLEM 5

A complete-denture patient is having difficulty with retention of a maxillary denture. What factors should you check to improve the retention?

Solution

Make sure there is adequate extension at the periphery so that on movement the seal is not broken.

The fit, especially at the periphery, is important because it will control the thickness of the saliva film between the denture and the tissue and the force needed to dislodge the denture. The thinner the film of saliva, the greater the retention.

SELECTED PROBLEMS

Corrosion, Optical Properties, and Thermal Properties

PROBLEM 1

A hole was drilled in a gold crown to facilitate an endodontic procedure. Subsequently, the hole was filled with a dental amalgam. After several months the amalgam appeared discolored and corroded. What caused this problem, and how could it have been avoided?

Solution

The dental amalgam is anodic to the gold alloy. Furthermore, the surface area of the gold restoration is much larger than that of the amalgam. Both of these factors will cause the amalgam to corrode by galvanic action. The hole should be filled with gold foil to minimize corrosion.

PROBLEM 2

A ceramic veneer to be bonded on an anterior tooth matches the color of the shade guide but not the adjacent tooth. What most likely caused this problem, and how could it have been avoided?

Solution a

If different light sources are used to match metameric shades, the color could appear correct when observed under one light but not under the other. Be sure to match teeth and shade guides under appropriate lighting conditions.

Solution b

Ceramic is a translucent material, the color of which can be affected by the color of the cement retaining the restoration, particularly if the veneer lacks an opaque layer. Select a resin cement of an appropriate shade to bond the veneer.

PROBLEM 3

A glaze applied to a ceramic restoration cracks on cooling. What caused the glaze to crack, and how can this problem be avoided?

Solution

Ceramics have a low thermal diffusivity and are subject to cracking as a result of thermal shock. Be sure to cool a ceramic restoration as recommended by the manufacturer to minimize larger thermal gradients.

PROBLEM 4

A denture cleaned in hot water distorted and no longer fits the patient's mouth. Why?

Solution

If the temperature of the denture during cleaning exceeds the glass transition temperature of the resin, then distortion can occur readily. Be sure to use cool water before cleaning a denture.

Bibliography—Mechanical Properties

Forces on Dental Structures

Black GV: An investigation of the physical characters of the human teeth in relation to their diseases, and to practical dental operations, together with the physical characters of filling materials, *Dent. Cosmos* 37:469, 1895.

Burstone CJ, Baldwin JJ, Lawless DT: The application of continuous forces in orthodontics, *Angle Orthod* 31:1, 1961.

Dechow PC, Carlson DS: A method of bite force measurement in primates, *J Biomech* 16:797, 1983.

Koolstra JH, van Euden TM: Application and validation of a three-dimensional mathematical model of the human masticatory system in vivo, *J Biomech* 25:175, 1992.

Korioth TW, Versluis A: Modeling the mechanical behavior of the jaws and their related structures by finite element (FE) analysis, *Crit Rev Oral Biol Med* 8:90, 1997.

Kuhlberg AJ, Priebe D: Testing force systems and biomechanics—measured tooth movements from differential moment closing loops, *Angle Orthod* 73:270, 2003.

Magne P, Versluis A, Douglas WH: Rationalization of incisor shape: experimental-numerical analysis, *J Prosthet Dent* 81:345, 1999.

Plesh O, Bishop B, McCall WD Jr: Kinematics of jaw movements during chewing at different frequencies, *J Biomech* 26:243, 1993.

Southard TE, Southard KA, Stiles RN: Factors influencing the anterior component of occlusal force, *J Biomech* 23:1199, 1990.

Stress Analysis and Design of Dental Structures

Brunski JB: Biomechanical factors affecting the bone-dental implant interface, *Clin Mater* 10:153, 1992.

Craig RG, Farah JW: Stress analysis and design of single restorations and fixed bridges, *Oral Sci Rev* 10:45, 1977.

Farah JW, Craig RG: Distribution of stresses in porcelain-fused-to-metal and porcelain jacket crowns, *J Dent Res* 54:255, 1975.

Farah JW, Powers JM, Dennison JB, et al: Effects of cement bases on the stresses and deflections in composite restorations, *J Dent Res* 55:115, 1976.

Hart RT, Hennebel VV, Thonpreda N, et al: Modeling the biomechanics of the mandible: a three-dimensional finite element study, *J Biomech* 25:261, 1992.

Hylander WL: Mandibular function in galago crassicaudatus and macaca fascicularis: an in vivo approach to stress analysis of the mandible, *J Morph* 159:253, 1979.

Kohn DH: Overview of factors important in implant design, *J Oral Implantol* 18:204, 1992.

Ko CC, Kohn DH, Hollister SJ: Micromechanics of implant/tissue interfaces, *J Oral Implantol* 18:220, 1992.

Korioth TW, Hannam AG: Deformation of the human mandible during simulated tooth clenching, *J Dent Res* 73:56, 1994.

Meredith N: A review of nondestructive test methods and their application to measure the stability and osseointegration of bone anchored endosseous implants, *Crit Rev Biomed Eng* 26:275, 1998.

Sakaguchi RL, Borgersen SE: Nonlinear finite element contact analysis of dental implant components, *Int J Oral Maxillofac Implants* 8:655, 1993.

Sakaguchi RL, Borgersen SE: Nonlinear contact analysis of preload in dental implant screws, *Int J Oral Maxillofac Implants* 10:295, 1995.

Sakaguchi RL, Brust EW, Cross M, et al: Independent movement of cusps during occlusal loading, *Dent Mater* 7:186, 1991.

Sakaguchi RL, Cross M, Douglas WH: A simple model of crack propagation in dental restorations, *Dent Mater* 8:131, 1992.

Tantbirojn D, Versluis A, Pintado MR, et al: Tooth deformation patterns in molars after composite restoration, *Dent Mater* 20:535, 2004.

General Biomechanics

Bronzino JD, editor: *The Biomechanical Engineering Handbook*, Boca Raton, 1995, CRC Press.

Dowling NE: *Mechanical behavior of materials*, ed 2, Englewood Cliffs, NJ, 1999, Prentice-Hall.

Flinn RA, Trojan PK: *Engineering materials and their applications*, ed 4, New York, 1995, Wiley.

Fung YC: *Biomechanics, mechanical properties of living tissues*, ed 2, New York, 1993, Springer-Verlag.

Fung YC: *Biomechanics, motion, flow, stress, and growth*, New York, 1990, Springer-Verlag.

Hayashi K, Kamiya A, Ono K, editors: *Biomechanics, functional adaptation and remodeling*, Tokyo, 1996, Springer-Verlag.

Park JB, Lakes RS: *Biomaterials: an introduction*, New York, 1992, Plenum Press.

von Recum AF, editor: *Handbook of biomaterials evaluation: scientific, technical, and clinical testing of implant materials*, Philadelphia, 1999, Taylor and Francis.

Fracture Toughness

Baran GR, McCool JI, Paul D, et al: Weibull models of fracture strengths and fatigue behavior of dental resins in flexure and shear, *J Biomed Mater Res* 43:226, 1998.

de Groot R, Van Elst HC, Peters MC: Fracture mechanics parameters for failure prediction of composite resins, *J Dent Res* 67:919, 1988.

Dhuru VB, Lloyd CH: The fracture toughness of repaired composite, *J Oral Rehabil* 13:413, 1986.

El Mowafy OM, Watts DC: Fracture toughness of human dentin, *J Dent Res* 65:677, 1986.

Ferracane JL, Antonio RC, Matsumoto H: Variables affecting the fracture toughness of dental composites, *J Dent Res* 66:1140, 1987.

Fujishima A, Ferracane JL: Comparison of four modes of fracture toughness testing for dental composites, *Dent Mater* 12:38, 1996.

Hassan R, Vaidyanathan TK, Schulman A: Fracture toughness determination of dental amalgams through microindentation, *J Biomed Mater Res* 20:135, 1986.

Lloyd CH: The fracture toughness of dental composites. II. The environmental and temperature dependence of the stress intensification factor (K_{IC}), *J Oral Rehabil* 9:133, 1982.

Lloyd CH: The fracture toughness of dental composites. III. The effect of environment upon the stress intensification factor (K_{IC}) after extended storage, *J Oral Rehabil* 11:393, 1984.

Lloyd CH, Adamson M: The fracture toughness (K_{IC}) of amalgam, *J Oral Rehabil* 12:59, 1985.

Lloyd CH, Iannetta RV: The fracture toughness of dental composites. I. The development of strength and fracture toughness, *J Oral Rehabil* 9:55, 1982.

Mecholsky JJ Jr: Fracture mechanics principles, *Dent Mater* 11:111, 1995.

Mueller HJ: Fracture toughness and fractography of dental cements, lining, build-up, and filling materials, *Scanning Microsc* 4:297, 1990.

Pilliar RM, Smith DC, Maric B: Fracture toughness of dental composites determined using the short-rod fracture toughness test, *J Dent Res* 65:1308, 1986.

Roberts JC, Powers JM, Craig RG: Fracture toughness of composite and unfilled restorative resins, *J Dent Res* 56:748, 1977.

Roberts JC, Powers JM, Craig RG: Fracture toughness and critical strain energy release rate of dental amalgam, *J Mater Sci* 13:965, 1978.

Rosenstiel SF, Porter SS: Apparent fracture toughness of metal ceramic restorations with different manipulative variables, *J Prosthet Dent* 61:185, 1989.

Rosenstiel SF, Porter SS: Apparent fracture toughness of all-ceramic crown systems, *J Prosthet Dent* 62:529, 1989.

Scherrer SS, Denry IL, Wiskott HW: Comparison of three fracture toughness testing techniques using a dental glass and a dental ceramic, *Dent Mater* 14:246, 1998.

Taira M, Nomura Y, Wakasa K, et al: Studies on fracture toughness of dental ceramics, *J Oral Rehabil* 17:551, 1990.

Uctasli S, Harrington E, Wilson HJ: The fracture resistance of dental materials, *J Oral Rehabil* 22:877, 1995.

Shear Strength

Black J: "Push-out" tests, *J Biomed Mater Res* 23:1243, 1989.

Johnston WM, O'Brien WJ: The shear strength of dental porcelain, *J Dent Res* 59:1409, 1980.

Drummond JL, Sakaguchi RL, Racean DC, et al: Testing mode and surface treatment effects on dentin bonding, *J Biomed Mater Res* 32:533, 1996.

Bending and Torsion

Asgharnia MK, Brantley WA: Comparison of bending and torsion tests for orthodontic wires, *Am J Orthod* 89:228, 1986.

Brantley WA, Augat WS, Myers CL, et al: Bending deformation studies of orthodontic wires, *J Dent Res* 57:609, 1978.

Dolan DW, Craig RG: Bending and torsion of endodontic files with rhombus cross sections, *J Endod* 8:260, 1982.

Magne P: Efficient 3D finite element analysis of dental restorative procedures using micro-CT data, *Dent Mater* 23:539–548, 2007.

Viscosity

Combe EC, Moser JB: The rheological characteristics of elastomeric impression materials, *J Dent Res* 57:221, 1978.

Herfort TW, Gerberich WW, Macosko CW, et al: Viscosity of elastomeric impression materials, *J Prosthet Dent* 38:396, 1977.

Koran A, Powers JM, Craig RG: Apparent viscosity of materials used for making edentulous impressions, *J Am Dent Assoc* 95:75, 1977.

Vermilyea SG, Powers JM, Craig RG: Rotational viscometry of a zinc phosphate and a zinc polyacrylate cement, *J Dent Res* 56:762, 1977.

Vermilyea SG, Powers JM, Koran A: The rheological properties of fluid denture-base resins, *J Dent Res* 57:227, 1978.

Viscoelasticity

Cook WD: Permanent set and stress relaxation in elastomeric impression materials, *J Biomed Mater Res* 15:449, 1981.

Duran RL, Powers JM, Craig RG: Viscoelastic and dynamic properties of soft liners and tissue conditioners, *J Dent Res* 58:1801, 1979.

Ferracane JL, Moser JB, Greener EH: Rheology of composite restoratives, *J Dent Res* 60:1678, 1981.

Goldberg AJ: Viscoelastic properties of silicone, polysulfide, and polyether impression materials, *J Dent Res* 53:1033, 1974.

Lee JK, Choi JY, Lim BS, et al: Change of properties during storage of a UDMA/TEGDMA dental resin, *J Biomed Mater Res B Appl Biomater* 68:216, 2004.

Morris HF, Asgar K, Tillitson EW: Stress-relaxation testing. Part I: A new approach to the testing of removable partial denture alloys, wrought wires, and clasp behavior, *J Prosthet Dent* 46:133, 1981.

Park JB, Lakes RS: *Biomaterials: An introduction*, New York, 1992, Plenum Press.

Ruyter IE, Espevik S: Compressive creep of denture base polymers, *Acta Odont Scand* 38:169, 1980.

Tolley LG, Craig RG: Viscoelastic properties of elastomeric impression materials: polysulphide, silicone and polyether rubbers, *J Oral Rehabil* 5:121, 1978.

Wills DJ, Manderson RD: Biomechanical aspects of the support of partial dentures, *J Dent* 5:310, 1977.

Xu HH, Liao H, Eichmiller FC: Indentation creep behavior of a direct-filling silver alternative to amalgam, *J Dent Res* 77:1991, 1998.

Dynamic Properties

Impact resistance of plastics and electrical insulating material, D 256–92. In *ASTM Standards 1993*, vol 8.01, Philadelphia, 1993, American Society for Testing and Materials.

Koran A, Craig RG: Dynamic mechanical properties of maxillofacial materials, *J Dent Res* 54:1216, 1975.

Sakaguchi RL, Shah NC, Lim BS, et al: Dynamic mechanical analysis of storage modulus development in light-activated polymer matrix composites, *Dent Mater* 18:197, 2002.

Rubinstein M, Colby RH: Networks and gelation. In *Polymer Physics*, New York, 2008, Oxford University Press.

Graessley WW: Linear Viscoelasticity. In *Polymeric Liquids and Networks: Dynamics and Rheology*, New York, 2008, Taylor and Francis group.

Macosko CW: Linear Viscoelasticity. In *Rheology: Principles, Measurements and Applications*, New York, 1994, Wiley-VCH.

Properties of Composite Materials

Bayne SC, Thompson JY, Swift EJ Jr, et al: A characterization of first-generation flowable composites, *J Am Dent Assoc* 129:567, 1998.

Braem MJ, Davidson CL, Lambrechts P, et al: In vitro flexural fatigue limits of dental composites, *J Biomed Mater Res* 28:1397, 1994.

Braem M, Van Doren VE, Lambrechts P, et al: Determination of Young's modulus of dental composites: a phenomenological model, *J Mater Sci* 22:2037, 1987.

Choi KK, Condon JR, Ferracane JL: The effects of adhesive thickness on polymerization contraction stress of composite, *J Dent Res* 79:812, 2000.

Condon JR, Ferracane JL: Reduction of composite contraction stress through non-bonded microfiller particles, *Dent Mater* 14:256, 1998.

Ferracane JL: Current trends in dental composites, *Crit Rev Oral Biol Med* 6:302, 1995.

Ferracane JL, Berge HX, Condon JR: In vitro aging of dental composites in water—effect of degree of conversion, filler volume, and filler/matrix coupling, *J Biomed Mater Res* 42:465, 1998.

Ferracane JL, Condon JR: In vitro evaluation of the marginal degradation of dental composites under simulated occlusal loading, *Dent Mater* 15:262, 1999.

Goldberg AJ, Burstone CJ, Hadjinikolaou I, et al: Screening of matrices and fibers for reinforced thermoplastics intended for dental applications, *J Biomed Mater Res* 28:167, 1994.

McCabe JF, Wang Y, Braem M: Surface contact fatigue and flexural fatigue of dental restorative materials, *J Biomed Mater Res* 50:375, 2000.

Peutzfeldt A: Resin composites in dentistry: the monomer systems, *Eur J Oral Sci* 105:97, 1997.

Sakaguchi RL, Ferracane JL: Stress transfer from polymerization shrinkage of a chemical-cured composite bonded to a pre-cast composite substrate, *Dent Mater* 14:106, 1998.

Sakaguchi RL, Wiltbank BD, Murchison CF: Contraction force rate of polymer composites is linearly correlated with irradiance, *Dent Mater* 20:402, 2004.

Sakaguchi RL, Wiltbank BD, Murchison CF: Prediction of composite elastic modulus and polymerization shrinkage by computational micromechanics, *Dent Mater* 20:397, 2004.

Sakaguchi RL, Wiltbank BD, Shah NC: Critical configuration analysis of four methods for measuring polymerization shrinkage strain of composites, *Dent Mater* 20:388, 2004.

Urabe I, Nakajima M, Sano H, et al: Physical properties of the dentin-enamel junction region, *Am J Dent* 13:129, 2000.

Van der Varst PG, Brekelmans WA, De Vree JH, et al: Mechanical performance of a dental composite: probabilistic failure prediction, *J Dent Res* 72:1249, 1993.

Tear Strength and Tear Energy

Herfort TW, Gerberich WW, Macosko CW, et al: Tear strength of elastomeric impression materials, *J Prosthet Dent* 39:59, 1978.

MacPherson GW, Craig RG, Peyton FA: Mechanical properties of hydrocolloid and rubber impression materials, *J Dent Res* 46:714, 1967.

Strength of conventional vulcanized rubber and thermoplastic elastomers, D 624–91. In *ASTM Standards 1994*, vol 9.01, Philadelphia, 1994, American Society for Testing and Materials.

Webber RL, Ryge G: The determination of tear energy of extensible materials of dental interest, *J Biomed Mater Res* 2:231, 1968.

Hardness, Friction, and Wear

Abe Y, Sato Y, Akagawa Y, Ohkawa S: An in vitro study of high-strength resin posterior denture tooth wear, *Int J Prosthodont* 10:28, 1997.

Barbakow F, Lutz F, Imfeld T: A review of methods to determine the relative abrasion of dentifrices and prophylaxis pastes, *Quint Int* 18:23, 1987.

Condon JR, Ferracane JL: Factors effecting dental composite wear in vitro, *J Biomed Mater Res* 38:303, 1997.

Condon JR, Ferracane JL: In vitro wear of composite with varied cure, filler level, and filler treatment, *J Dent Res* 76:1405, 1997.

DeBellis A: Fundamentals of Rockwell hardness testing. In *Hardness Testing Reprints, WD-673*, Bridgeport, Conn, 1967, Wilson Instrument Division.

DeLong R, Douglas WH, Sakaguchi RL, et al: The wear of dental porcelain in an artificial mouth, *Dent Mater* 2:214, 1986.

DeLong R, Sakaguchi RL, Douglas WH, et al: The wear of dental amalgam in an artificial mouth: a clinical correlation, *Dent Mater* 1:238, 1985.

Doerner MF, Nix WD: A method for interpreting the data from depth-sensing indentation measurements, *J Mater Res* 1:601, 1986.

Douglas WH, Sakaguchi RL, DeLong R: Frictional effects between natural teeth in an artificial mouth, *Dent Mater* 1:115, 1985.

Draughn RA, Harrison A: Relationship between abrasive wear and microstructure of composite resins, *J Prosthet Dent* 40:220, 1978.

Ferracane JL, Mitchem JC, Condon JR, Todd R: Wear and marginal breakdown of composites with various degrees of cure, *J Dent Res* 76:1508, 1997.

Hu X, Harrington E, Marquis PM, et al: The influence of cyclic loading on the wear of a dental composite, *Biomaterials* 20:907, 1999.

Hu X, Marquis PM, Shortall AC: Two-body in vitro wear study of some current dental composites and amalgams, *J Prosthet Dent* 82:214, 1999.

Knibbs PJ: Methods of clinical evaluation of dental restorative materials, *J Oral Rehabil* 24:109, 1997.

Koczorowski R, Wloch S: Evaluation of wear of selected prosthetic materials in contact with enamel and dentin, *J Prosthet Dent* 81:453, 1999.

Lysaght VE: How to make and interpret hardness tests on plastics. In *Hardness Testing Reprints, WD-673*, Bridgeport, Conn, 1967, Wilson Instrument Division.

Lysaght VE: *Indentation hardness testing*, New York, 1949, Reinhold.

Lysaght VE, DeBellis A: Microhardness testing. In *Hardness Testing Reprints, WD-673*, Bridgeport, Conn, 1967, Wilson Instrument Division.

Powers JM, Craig RG: Wear of dental tissues and restorative materials. June 4–6, 1979, *Proceedings of National Symposium on Wear and Corrosion*, Washington, DC, 1979, American Chemical Society.

Powers JM, Fan PL, Craig RG: *Wear of dental restorative resins*. In Gebelein CG, Koblitz FF, editors: *Biomedical and dental applications of polymers: Polymer science and technology*, vol 14, New York, 1981, Plenum Press.

Roberts JC, Powers JM, Craig RG: Wear of dental amalgam, *J Biomed Mater Res* 11:513, 1977.

Teoh SH, Ong LF, Yap AU, et al: Bruxing-type dental wear simulator for ranking of dental restorative materials, *J Biomed Mater Res* 43:175, 1998.

Tirtha R, Fan PL, Dennison JB, et al: in vitro depth of cure of photo-activated composites, *J Dent Res* 61:1184, 1982.

Turssi C, Purquerio B, Serra M: Wear of dental resin composites: insights into underlying processes and assessment methods. A review, *J Biomed Mater Res B Appl Biomater* 65B:280, 2003.

Wu W, McKinney JE: Influence of chemicals on wear of dental composites, *J Dent Res* 61:1180, 1982.

Yap AU, Ong LF, Teoh SH, et al: Comparative wear ranking of dental restoratives with the BIOMAT wear simulator, *J Oral Rehabil* 26:228, 1999.

Van Meerbeek B, Willems G, Celis JP, et al: Assessment by nano-indentation of the hardness and elasticity of resin-dentin bonding area, *J Dent Res* 72:1434, 1993.

Willems G, Celis JP, Lambrechts P, et al: Hardness and young's modulus determined by nanoindentation technique of filler particles of dental restorative materials compared with human enamel, *J Biomed Mater Res* 27:747, 1993.

Xu HH, Smith DT, Jahanmir S, et al: Indentation damage and mechanical properties of human enamel and dentin, *J Dent Res* 77:472, 1998.

Specifications

Council on Scientific Affairs: *Clinical products in dentistry; a desktop reference*, Chicago, 1996, American Dental Association.

United States General Services Administration: *Index of Federal Specifications and Standards*, Washington, DC, 1994, Superintendent of Documents, U.S. Government Printing Office.

Colloidal State, Surface Properties, Adhesion

Baier RE, Meyer AE: Surface analysis. In von Recum AF, editor: *Handbook of biomaterials evaluation*, New York, 1986, Macmillan.

Baran G, O'Brien WJ: Wetting of amalgam alloys by mercury, *J Am Dent Assoc* 94:897, 1977.

Craig RG, Berry GC, Peyton FA: Wetting of poly(methyl methacrylate) and polystyrene by water and saliva, *J Phys Chem* 64:541, 1960.

Dental composites and adhesives in the 21st century: The Gunnar Ryge Memorial Symposium, *Quint Int* 24(9):605, 1993.

Iler RK: *The chemistry of silica-solubility, polymerization, colloid and surface properties, and biochemistry*, New York, 1979, John Wiley & Sons.

Myers CL, Ryge G, Heyde JB, et al: In vivo test of bond strength, *J Dent Res* 42:907, 1963.

Norman AL: Frictional resistance and dental prosthetics, *J Prosthet Dent* 14:45, 1964.

O'Brien WJ: Surface energy of liquids isolated in narrow capillaries, *J Surface Sci* 19:387, 1970.

O'Brien WJ: Capillary action around dental structures, *J Dent Res* 52:544, 1973.

O'Brien WJ: *Capillary effects in adhesion, Proceedings of Conference on Dental Adhesive Materials*, New York, 1973, New York University Press.

O'Brien WJ, Craig RG, Peyton FA: Capillary penetration around a hydrophobic filling material, *J Prosthet Dent* 19:400, 1968.

O'Brien WJ, Craig RG, Peyton FA: Capillary penetration between dissimilar materials, *J Colloid Interface Sci* 26:500, 1968.

O'Brien WJ, Fan PL, Apostolidis A: Penetrativity of sealants and glazes, *Oper Dent* 3:51, 1978.

Rosales JI, Marshall GW, Marshall SJ, et al: Acid-etching and hydration influence on dentin roughness and wettability, *J Dent Res* 78:1554, 1999.

Shaw DJ: *Electrophoresis*, New York, 1969, Academic Press.

Somorjai GA: *Introduction to surface chemistry and catalysis*, New York, 1994, John Wiley & Sons.

van Meerbeek B, Williams G, Celis JP, et al: Assessment by mono-indentation of the hardness and elasticity of the resin-dentin bonding area, *J Dent Res* 72:1434, 1993.

van Pelt AWJ: *Adhesion of oral streptococci to solids*, Groningen, The Netherlands, 1985, Drukkerij Van Denderen B.V.

Willems G, Celis JP, Lambrechts P, et al: Hardness and Young's modulus determined by nanoindentation technique of filler particles of dental restorative materials compared with human enamel, *J Biomed Mater Res* 27:747, 1993.

Williams BF, von Fraunhofer JA, Winter GB: Tensile bond strength between fissure sealants and enamel, *J Dent Res* 53:23, 1974.

Yoshida Y, van Meerbeek B, Nakayama Y, et al: Evidence of chemical bonding at biomaterial-hard tissue interfaces, *J Dent Res* 79:709, 2000.

Yoshida Y, van Meerbeek B, Snowwaert J, et al: A novel approach to AFM characterization of adhesive tooth-biomaterials interfaces, *J Biomed Mater Res* 47:85, 1999.

Color and Optical Properties

Asmussen E: Opacity of glass-ionomer cements, *Acta Odontol Scand* 41:155, 1983.

Baran GR, O'Brien WJ, Tien T-Y: Colored emission of rare earth ions in a potassium feldspar glass, *J Dent Res* 56:1323, 1977.

Cho MS, Yu B, Lee YK: Opalescence of all-ceramic core and veneer materials, *Dent Mater* 25:695, 2009.

Colorimetry, official recommendations of the International Commission on Illumination (CIE), Publication CIE No 15 (E-1.3.1), 1971.

Corciolani G, Vichi A, Louca C, Ferrari M: Influence of layering thickness on the color parameters of a ceramic system, *Dent Mater* 26:737, 2010.

Hall JB, Hefferren JJ, Olsen NH: Study of fluorescent characteristics of extracted human teeth by use of a clinical fluorometer, *J Dent Res* 49:1431, 1970.

Heffernan MJ, Aquilino SA, Diaz-Arnold AM, Haselton DR, Stansford CM, Vargas MA: Relative translucency of six all ceramics. Part I: core materials, *J Prosthet Dent* 88:4, 2000.

Heffernan MJ, Aquilino SA, Diaz-Arnold AM, Haselton DR, Stansford CM, Vargas MA: Relative translucency of six all ceramics. Part II: core and veneer materials, *J Prosthet Dent* 88:10, 2000.

Johnston WM, Ma T, Kienle BH: Translucency parameter of colorants for maxillofacial prostheses, *Int J Prosthodont* 8:79, 1995.

Johnston WM, O'Brien WJ, Tien T-Y: The determination of optical absorption and scattering in translucent porcelain, *Color Res Appl* 11:125, 1986.

Johnston WM, O'Brien WJ, Tien T-Y: Concentration additivity of Kubelka-Munk optical coefficients of porcelain mixtures, *Color Res Appl* 11:131, 1986.

Jorgenson MW, Goodkind RJ: Spectrophotometric study of five porcelain shades relative to the dimensions of color, porcelain thickness, and repeated firings, *J Prosthet Dent* 42:96, 1979.

Judd DB: Optical specification of light-scattering materials, *J Res Nat Bur Standards* 19:287, 1937.

Judd DB, Wyszecki G: *Color in business, science, and industry*, ed 3, New York, 1975, John Wiley & Sons.

Kiat-amnuay S, Lemon JC, Powers JM: Effects of opacifiers on color stability of pigmented maxillofacial silicone A-2186 subjected to artificial aging, *J Prosthodont* 11:109, 2002.

Koran A, Powers JM, Raptis CN, Yu R: Reflection spectrophotometry of facial skin, *J Dent Res* 60:979, 1981.

Kubelka P: New contributions to the optics of intensely light-scattering materials, Part I, *Opt Soc Am J* 38:448, 1948.

Kubelka P, Munk F: Ein Beitrag zur Optik der Farbanstriche, *Z Tech Phys* 12:593, 1931.

Lee Y-K, Lim B-S, Powers JM: Color changes of dental resin composites by a salivary enzyme, *J Biomed Mater Res* 70B:66, 2004.

Miyagawa Y, Powers JM: Prediction of color of an esthetic restorative material, *J Dent Res* 62:581, 1983.

Miyagawa Y, Powers JM, O'Brien WJ: Optical properties of direct restorative materials, *J Dent Res* 60:890, 1981.

Nickerson D: The specification of color tolerances, *Textile Res* 6:509, 1936.

Noie F, O'Keefe KL, Powers JM: Color stability of resin cements after accelerated aging, *Int J Prosthodont* 8:51, 1995.

O'Brien WJ, Johnston WM, Fanian F: Double-layer color effects in porcelain systems, *J Dent Res* 64:940, 1985.

O'Brien WJ, Johnston WM, Fanian F, et al: The surface roughness and gloss of composites, *J Dent Res* 63:685, 1984.

O'Keefe KL, Powers JM, Noie F: Effect of dissolution on color of extrinsic porcelain colorants, *Int J Prosthodont* 6:558, 1993.

Panzeri H, Fernandes LT, Minelli CJ: Spectral fluorescence of direct anterior restorative materials, *Aust Dent J* 22:458, 1977.

Paravina RD, Ontiveros JC, Powers JM: Curing-dependent changes in color and translucency parameter of composite bleach shades, *J Esthet Restor Dent* 14:158, 2002.

Paravina RD, Ontiveros JC, Powers JM: Accelerated aging effects on color and translucency of bleaching-shade composites, *J Esthet Restor Dent* 16:117, 2004.

Paravina RD, Powers JM, editors: *Esthetic color training in dentistry*, St. Louis, 2004, Mosby.

Powers JM, Capp JA, Koran A: Color of gingival tissues of blacks and whites, *J Dent Res* 56:112, 1977.

Powers JM, Koran A: Color of denture resins, *J Dent Res* 56:754, 1977.

Powers JM, Yeh CL, Miyagawa Y: Optical properties of composite of selected shades in white light, *J Oral Rehabil* 10:319, 1983.

Ragain JC, Johnston WM: Accuracy of Kubelka-Munk reflectance theory applied to human dentin and enamel, *J Dent Res* 80:449, 2001.

Ruyter IE, Nilner K, Moller B: Color stability of dental composite resin material for crown and bridge veneers, *Dent Mater* 3:246, 1987.

Seghi RR, Johnston WM, O'Brien WJ: Spectrophotometric analysis of color differences between porcelain systems, *J Prosthet Dent* 56:35, 1986.

Specifying color by the Munsell system, D1535–68 (1974). In ASTM Standards, 1975, Part 20, Philadelphia, 1975, American Society for Testing and Materials.

Sproull RC: Color matching in dentistry. Part III. Color control, *J Prosthet Dent* 31:146, 1974.

Van Oort RP: *Skin color and facial prosthetic—a colorimetric study*, doctoral dissertation, The Netherlands, 1982, Groningen State University.

Wyszecki G, Stiles WS: *Color science*, New York, 1967, John Wiley & Sons.

Yeh CL, Miyagawa Y, Powers JM: Optical properties of composites of selected shades, *J Dent Res* 61:797, 1982.

Vichi A, Ferrari M, Davidson CL: Influence og ceramic and cement thickness on the masking of various types of opaque posts, *J Prosthet Dent* 83:412, 2000.

Thermal Properties

Antonucci JM, Toth EE: Extent of polymerization of dental resins by differential scanning calorimetry, *J Dent Res* 62:121, 1983.

Brady AP, Lee H, Orlowski JA: Thermal conductivity studies of composite dental restorative materials, *J Biomed Mater Res* 8:471, 1974.

Brauer GM, Termini DJ, Burns CL: Characterization of components of dental materials and components of tooth structure by differential thermal analysis, *J Dent Res* 49:100, 1970.

Brown WS, Christiansen DO, Lloyd BA: Numerical and experimental evaluation of energy inputs, temperature gradients, and thermal stress during restorative procedures, *J Am Dent Assoc* 96:451, 1978.

Brown WS, Dewey WA, Jacobs HR: Thermal properties of teeth, *J Dent Res* 49:752, 1970.

Civjan S, Barone JJ, Reinke PE, et al: Thermal properties of nonmetallic restorative materials, *J Dent Res* 51:1030, 1972.

Craig RG, Eick JD, Peyton FA: Properties of natural waxes used in dentistry, *J Dent Res* 44:1308, 1965.

Craig RG, Peyton FA: Thermal conductivity of tooth structure, dental cements, and amalgam, *J Dent Res* 40:411, 1961.

Craig RG, Powers JM, Peyton FA: Differential thermal analysis of commercial and dental waxes, *J Dent Res* 46:1090, 1967.

Craig RG, Powers JM, Peyton FA: Thermogravimetric analysis of waxes, *J Dent Res* 50:450, 1971.

Dansgaard W, Jarby S: Measurement of nonstationary temperature in small bodies, *Odont Tskr* 66:474, 1958.

de Vree JH, Spierings TA, Plasschaert AJ: A simulation model for transient thermal analysis of restored teeth, *J Dent Res* 62:756, 1983.

Fairhurst CW, Anusavice KJ, Hashinger DT, et al: Thermal expansion of dental alloys and porcelains, *J Biomed Mater Res* 14:435, 1980.

Henschel CJ: Pain control through heat control, *Dent Dig* 47:294, 444, 1941.

Lisanti VF, Zander HA: Thermal conductivity of dentin, *J Dent Res* 29:493, 1950.

Lloyd CH: The determination of the specific heats of dental materials by differential thermal analysis, *Biomaterials* 2:179, 1981.

Lloyd CH: A differential thermal analysis (DTA) for the heats of reaction and temperature rises produced during the setting of tooth coloured restorative materials, *J Oral Rehabil* 11:111, 1984.

McCabe JF, Wilson HJ: The use of differential scanning calorimetry for the evaluation of dental materials. I. Cements, cavity lining materials and anterior restorative materials, *J Oral Rehabil* 7:103, 1980.

McCabe JF, Wilson HJ: The use of differential scanning calorimetry for the evaluation of dental materials. II. Denture base materials, *J Oral Rehabil* 7:235, 1980.

McLean JW: Physical properties influencing the accuracy of silicone and thiokol impression materials, *Br Dent J* 110:85, 1961.

Murayama T: *Dynamic mechanical analysis of polymeric materials*, New York, 1978, Elsevier Science.

Pearson GJ, Wills DJ, Braden M, et al: The relationship between the thermal properties of composite filling materials, *J Dent* 8:178, 1980.

Peyton FA: Temperature rise and cutting efficiency of rotating instruments, *NY J Dent* 18:439, 1952.

Peyton FA: Effectiveness of water coolants with rotary cutting instruments, *J Am Dent Assoc* 56:664, 1958.

Peyton FA, Morrant GA: High speed and other instruments for cavity preparation, *Int Dent J* 9:309, 1959.

Peyton FA, Simeral WG: The specific heat of tooth structure, *Alum Bull U Mich School Dent* 56:33, 1954.

Powers JM, Craig RG: Penetration of commercial and dental waxes, *J Dent Res* 53:402, 1974.

Powers JM, Hostetler RW, Dennison JB: Thermal expansion of composite resins and sealants, *J Dent Res* 58:584, 1979.

Rootare HM, Powers JM: Determination of phase transitions in gutta-percha by differential thermal analysis, *J Dent Res* 56:1453, 1977.

Soderholm KJ: Influence of silane treatment and filler fraction on thermal expansion of composite resins, *J Dent Res* 63:1321, 1984.

Souder WH, Paffenbarger GC: *Physical properties of dental materials*, National Bureau of Standards Circular No C433, Washington, DC, 1942, U.S. Government Printing Office.

Soyenkoff BC, Okun JH: Thermal conductivity measurements of dental tissues with the aid of thermistors, *J Am Dent Assoc* 57:23, 1958.

Tay WM, Braden M: Thermal diffusivity of glass-ionomer cements, *J Dent Res* 66:1040, 1987.

Walsh JP, Symmons HF: A comparison of the heat conduction and mechanical efficiency of diamond instruments, stones, and burs at 3,000 and 60,000 rpm, *NZ Dent J* 45:28, 1949.

Watts DC, Smith R: Thermal diffusivity in finite cylindrical specimens of dental cements, *J Dent Res* 60:1972, 1981.

Watts DC, Smith R: Thermal diffusion in some polyelectrolyte dental cements: the effect of powder/liquid ratio, *J Oral Rehabil* 11:285, 1984.

Wilson TW, Turner DT: Characterization of polydimethacrylates and their composites by dynamic mechanical analysis, *J Dent Res* 66:1032, 1987.

Electrical and Electrochemical Properties

Arvidson K, Johansson EG: Galvanic series of some dental alloys, *Scand J Dent Res* 85:485, 1977.

Bergman M, Ginstrup O, Nilner K: Potential and polarization measurements in vivo of oral galvanism, *Scand J Dent Res* 86:135, 1978.

Bjorn H: Electrical excitation of teeth, *Svensk Tandlak T* 39(Suppl), 1946.

Braden M, Clarke RL: Dielectric properties of zinc oxide-eugenol type cements, *J Dent Res* 53:1263, 1974.

Braden M, Clarke RL: Dielectric properties of polycarboxylate cements, *J Dent Res* 54:7, 1975.

Cahoon JR, Holte RN: Corrosion fatigue of surgical stainless steel in synthetic physiological solution, *J Biomed Mater Res* 15:137, 1981.

Clark GC, Williams DF: The effects of proteins on metallic corrosion, *J Biomed Mater Res* 16:125, 1982.

Fairhurst CW, Marek M, Butts MB, et al: New information on high copper amalgam corrosion, *J Dent Res* 57:725, 1978.

Gjerdet NR, Brune D: Measurements of currents between dissimilar alloys in the oral cavity, *Scand J Dent Res* 85:500, 1977.

Holland RI: Galvanic currents between gold and amalgam, *Scand J Dent Res* 88:269, 1980.

Maijer R, Smith DC: Corrosion of orthodontic bracket bases, *Am J Orthod* 81:43, 1982.

Marek M, Hochman R: *The corrosion behavior of dental amalgam phases as a function of tin content*, Washington, DC, April 12–15, 1973, microfilmed paper no. 192, delivered at the Annual Meeting of the International Association for Dental Research, Dental Materials Group.

Mohsen NM, Craig RG, Filisko FE: The effects of different additives on the dielectric relaxation and the dynamic mechanical properties of urethane dimethacrylate, *J Oral Rehabil* 27:250, 2000.

Mumford JM: Direct-current electrodes for pulp testing, *Dent Pract* 6:236, 1956.

Mumford JM: *Direct-current paths through human teeth*, master's thesis Ann Arbor, Mich, 1957, University of Michigan School of Dentistry.

Mumford JM: Electrolytic action in the mouth and its relationship to pain, *J Dent Res* 36:632, 1957.

Mumford JM: Resistivity of human enamel and dentin, *Arch Oral Biol* 12:925, 1957.

Mumford JM: Path of direct current in electric pulp-testing, *Br Dent J* 106:23, 1959.

O'Brien WJ: Electrochemical corrosion of dental gold castings, *Dent Abstracts* 7:46, 1962.

Phillips LJ, Schnell RJ, Phillips RW: Measurement of the electric conductivity of dental cement. III. Effect of increased contact area and thickness: values for resin, calcium hydroxide, zinc oxide–eugenol, *J Dent Res* 34: 597, 1955.

Phillips LJ, Schnell RJ, Phillips RW: Measurement of the electric conductivity of dental cement. IV. Extracted human teeth; in vivo tests; summary, *J Dent Res* 34:839, 1955.

Rootare HM, Powers JM: Comparison of zeta-potential of synthetic fluorapatite obtained by stepwise and continuous methods of streaming, *J Electrochem Soc* 126:1979, 1905.

Schreiver W, Diamond LE: Electromotive forces and electric currents caused by metallic dental fillings, *J Dent Res* 31:205, 1952.

Shaw DJ: *Electrophoresis*, New York, 1969, Academic Press.

Tay WM, Braden M: Dielectric properties of glass ionomer cements, *J Dent Res* 60:1311, 1981.

Wilson AD, Kent BE: Dental silicate cements. V. Electrical conductivity, *J Dent Res* 47:463, 1968.

Zitter H, Plenk H Jr: The electrochemical behavior of metallic implant materials as an indicator of their biocompatibility, *J Biomed Mater Res* 21:881, 1987.

Other Properties

German RM, Wright DC, Gallant RF: In vitro tarnish measurements on fixed prosthodontic alloys, *J Prosthet Dent* 47:399, 1982.

Koran A, Powers JM, Lepeak PJ, et al: Stain resistance of maxillofacial materials, *J Dent Res* 58:1455, 1979.

Mesu FP: Degradation of luting cements measured in vitro, *J Dent Res* 61:655, 1982.

Raptis CM, Powers JM, Fan PL, et al: Staining of composite resins by cigarette smoke, *J Oral Rehabil* 9:367, 1982.

Solovan DF, Powers JM: Effect of denture cleansers on partial denture alloys and resilient liners, *J Mich Dent Assoc* 60:135, 1978.

Walls AW, McCabe JF, Murray JJ: An erosion test for dental cements, *J Dent Res* 64:1100, 1985.

Wilson AD, Merson SA, Prosser HJ: A sensitive conductimetric method for measuring the material initially water-leached from dental cements. I. Zinc polycarboxylate cements, *J Dent* 8:263, 1980.

Websites

Academy of Dental Materials:
www.academydentalmaterials.org

American Dental Association: specifications and technical reports: http://www.ada.org/830.aspx

Biomaterials Database (University of Michigan): http://www.lib.umich.edu/node/21861

Efunda, Engineering Fundamentals: efunda.com

Houston Biomaterials Research Center: www.db.uth.tmc.edu/biomaterials

International/American Association for Dental Research: www.iadr.org

National ESCA and Surface Analysis Center for Biomedical Problems: http://www.nb.uw.edu/

Society for Biomaterials: www.biomaterials.org

Surfaces in Biomaterials Foundation: www.surfaces.org

The Dental Advisor: www.dentaladvisor.com

Testing of Dental Materials and Biomechanics

In Chapter 4, we introduced fundamental concepts in biomechanics and physical properties of dental materials. The data presented were collected with a variety of test instruments. In this chapter we describe the individual tests in more detail.

COMPRESSIVE STRENGTH

When an object is tested in compression, failure might occur as a result of complex stresses in the object. The forces of compression applied to each end of the specimen are resolved into forces of shear along a cone-shaped area at each end and, as a result of the action of the two cones on the cylinder, into tensile forces in the central portion of the mass. Because of this resolution of forces in the body, it has become necessary to adopt standard sizes and dimensions to obtain reproducible test results. Figure 5-1 shows that if a test specimen is too short, the force distributions become more complicated as a result of the cone formations overlapping in the ends of the cylinder. If the specimen is too long, buckling may occur. Therefore, the cylinder should have a length twice that of the diameter for the most satisfactory results.

Compressive strength is most useful for comparing materials that are brittle and generally weak in tension. Compressive strength is therefore a useful property for the comparison of dental amalgam, resin composites, and cements and for determining the qualities of other materials such as plaster and investments. Typical values of compressive strength of some restorative dental materials are given in Table 5-1.

FLEXURE

The bending, or flexural, properties of many materials are often more important than their tensile or compressive properties. The flexural properties of stainless steel wires, endodontic files and reamers, and hypodermic needles are especially important. For example, American National Standards Institute/American Dental Association (ANSI/ADA) specification No. 28 for endodontic files and reamers requires flexure tests.

Flexural properties are measured by bending a beam-shaped specimen. In a single cantilever beam configuration, the beam is fixed at one end and a force is applied at a prescribed distance from the fixed end. In a dual cantilever beam configuration, both ends of the beam are fixed and a load is placed on the center of the beam. In a three-point or four-point flexural configuration, the beam is supported on two rollers and a load is applied to the top of the beam. Specimens are subjected to conditions that resemble pure bending, and beam theory is used to analyze the data. As the force is increased and the specimen is bent, corresponding values for the angle of bending and the bending moment (force × distance) are recorded. Graphic plots of the bending moment versus the angle of bending are similar in appearance to stress-strain curves. As an example, a series of plots for various sizes of endodontic reamers is shown in

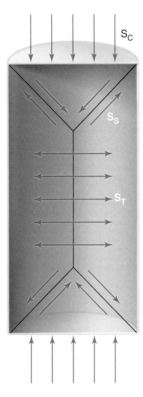

FIGURE 5.1 **Complex stress pattern developed in cylinder subjected to compressive stress. Compressive stress (S_C), Shear stress (S_S), Tensile stress (S_T).**

TABLE 5.1   Compressive Strength of Selected Dental Materials

Material	Compressive Strength (MPa)
Enamel	384
Dentin	297
Amalgam	189
Calcium hydroxide liner	8
Feldspathic porcelain	149
High-strength stone	81
Resin composite	225
Zinc phosphate cement	110

Figure 5-2. An instrument will be permanently bent if the bending angle exceeds the value at the end of the linear portion of the curve. The larger instruments are stiffer, as shown by the initial steeper slope. The initial linear portion of the curve is shorter for the larger instruments and thus the deviation from linearity occurred at lower angular bends.

FLEXURAL STRENGTH

The flexural strength of a material is obtained when one loads a simple single beam, simply supported (not fixed) at each end, with a load applied in the middle (Figures 5-3 and 5-4). Such a test is called a *three-point bending (3PB)* or *flexure test* and the maximum stress measured in the test is called *flexural strength*. The flexural strengths for several dental materials are shown in Table 5-2. This test determines not only the strength of the material indicated but also the amount of distortion expected. The flexural strength test is a part of ANSI/ADA specification No. 12 (ISO 1567) for denture base resins. The flexural strength and accompanying deformation are important also in long fixed partial denture spans in which the occlusal stress may be severe.

The equation for the maximum stress developed in a rectangular beam loaded in the center of the span is as follows:

$$\text{Stress} = 3 \times \text{Load} \times \text{Length} / (2 \times \text{Width} \times \text{Thickness}^2)$$

or

$$\sigma = 3Pl / 2bd^2$$

The resulting deformation or displacement in such a beam or bridge can be calculated from the following equation:

$$\text{Deformation} = \text{Load} \times \text{Length}^3 / 4 \times \text{Elastic modulus} \times \text{Width} \times \text{Thickness}^3$$

or

$$\delta = Pl / 4Ebd^3$$

Four-point bending is often preferred to three-point bending when measuring flexural modulus

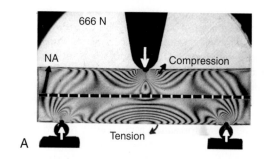

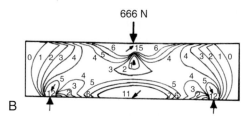

FIGURE 5.4 **Photo-elastic analysis of flexural strength test. A,** Photo-elastic model with isochromatic fringes. **B,** Drawing to illustrate isochromatic fringe order. Neutral axis (NA).

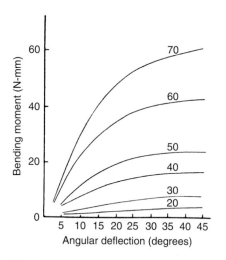

FIGURE 5.2 **Bending moment–angular deflection curves for endodontic reamers sizes 20 through 70.**

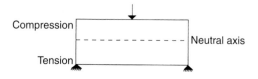

FIGURE 5.3 **Schematic of a three-point bending test.** The three points are the two supports at the bottom and the central loading point on the top.

TABLE 5.2 Flexural Strength of Selected Dental Materials

Material	Flexural Strength (MPa)
Resin composite	139
Lathe-cut amalgam	124
Feldspathic porcelain	65
High-strength stone	17
Resin-modified glass ionomer	42-68
Resin cement	66-121

and flexural strength. If an easily deformed material is tested with inadequately rounded loading and support elements, the elements can cause localized deformation. This is undesirable because the beam theory used to calculate deflection assumes uniform beam deformation without localized stresses and constraints. A four-point bend fixture uses two loading elements instead of the one used in a three-point bend fixture. The two loading elements apply a more uniform load to the beam that prevents V-shaped buckling of the beam, and stress concentrations in the midline when a single loading element is used. In this configuration, a larger, more representative area of the specimen is tested.

PERMANENT BENDING

During fabrication, many dental restorations are subjected to permanent bending. The adjustment of removable partial denture clasps and the shaping of orthodontic wires are two examples of such bending operations. Comparisons of wires and needles of different compositions and diameters subjected to repeated 90-degree bends are often made. The number of bends a specimen will withstand is influenced by its composition and dimensions, as well as its treatment in fabrication. Such tests are important because this information is not readily related to standard mechanical test data such as tensile properties or hardness. Severe tensile and compressive stresses can be introduced into a material subjected to permanent bending. It is partly for this reason that tensile and compressive test data for a material are so important.

DIAMETRAL TENSILE STRENGTH

An alternative method of testing brittle materials, in which the ultimate tensile strength of a brittle material is determined through compressive testing, is popular because of its relative simplicity and reproducibility. The method is described in the literature as the *diametral compression test for tension* or *the Brazilian method*. In this test, a disk of the brittle material is compressed diametrically in a testing machine until fracture occurs, as shown in Figure 5-5. The compressive stress applied to the specimen introduces a tensile stress in the material in the plane of the force application of the test machine because of the Poisson effect. The tensile stress (σ_x) is directly proportional to the load (P) applied in compression through the following formula:

$$\sigma_x = 2P / \pi DT$$

Note that this test is designed for brittle materials. If the specimen deforms significantly before failure

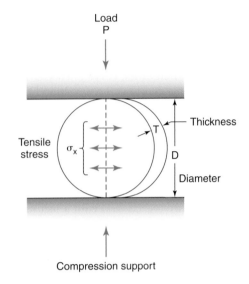

FIGURE 5.5 How a compressive force develops tensile stress in brittle materials.

TABLE 5.3   Tensile Strength of Selected Dental Materials

Material	Diametral Tensile Strength (MPa)	Ultimate Tensile Strength (MPa)
Enamel	—	10
Dentin	—	106
Amalgam	54	32
Calcium hydroxide liner	1	2.3
Feldspathic porcelain	—	25
High-strength stone	8	6
Zinc phosphate cement	8	10

or fractures into more than two equal pieces, the data may not be valid. Some materials exhibit different diametral tensile strengths when tested at different rates of loading and are described as being strain-rate sensitive. The diametral tensile test is not valid for these materials. Values of diametral and ultimate tensile strengths for some dental materials are listed in Table 5-3.

SHEAR STRENGTH

The shear strength is the maximum stress that a material can withstand before failure in a shear mode of loading. It is particularly important in the study of interfaces between two materials, such as ceramic-metal or an implant-bone interface. One method of testing the shear strength of dental materials is the

TABLE 5.4   Values of Shear Strength Tested by the
Punch Method for Some Restorative Dental Materials

Material	Shear Strength (MPa)
Enamel	90
Dentin	138
Acrylic denture resin	122
Amalgam	188
Porcelain	111
Zinc phosphate cement	13

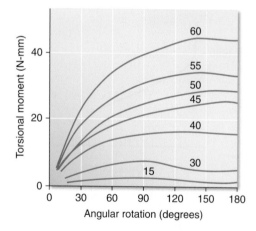

FIGURE 5.6 **Torsional moment–angular rotation curves for endodontic files sizes 15 through 60.**

punch or push-out method, in which an axial load is applied to push one material through another. The shear strength (τ) is calculated by the following formula:

$$\text{Shear strength } (\tau) = F/\pi dh$$

where F is the compressive force applied to the specimen, d is the diameter of the punch, and h is the thickness of the specimen. Note that the stress distribution caused by this method is not pure shear and that results often differ because of differences in specimen dimensions, surface geometry, composition and preparation, and mechanical testing procedure. However, it is a simple test to perform and has been used extensively. Alternatively, shear properties may be determined by subjecting a specimen to torsional loading. Shear strengths of some dental materials are listed in Table 5-4. The specifics of shear testing for adhesive interfaces is discussed in detail in the bond strength methods section of this chapter.

TORSION

Another mode of loading important to dentistry is torsion or twisting. For example, when an endodontic file is clamped at the tip and the handle is rotated, the instrument is subjected to torsion. Because most endodontic files and reamers are rotated in the root canal during endodontic treatment, their properties in torsion are of particular interest. ANSI/ADA specification No. 28 for endodontic files and reamers describes a test to measure resistance to fracture by twisting with a torque meter. Torsion results in a shear stress and a rotation of the specimen. In these types of applications, we are interested in the relation between torsional moment (M_t = shear force × distance) and angular rotation π. A series of graphs in which the torsional moment was measured as a function of angular rotation are shown in Figure 5-6. In this example, the instruments were twisted clockwise, which results in an untwisting of the instrument. As was the case with bending, the curves

appear similar to stress-strain curves, with an initial linear portion followed by a nonlinear portion. The instruments should be used clinically so that they are not subjected to permanent angular rotation; thus the degrees of rotation should be limited to values within the linear portion of the torsional moment–angular rotation curves. The larger instruments are stiffer in torsion than the smaller ones, but their linear portion is less. The irregular shape of the curves at high angular rotation results from the untwisting of the instruments. Torsion is also an important consideration for threaded fasteners such as those used in implant restorations. Use of a torque gage is recommended for tightening abutment screws to prevent overloading the screw and possible torsional failure in the shank of the screw.

FATIGUE STRENGTH

Based on the previous discussions, an object that is subjected to a stress below the yield stress and subsequently relieved of this stress should return to its original form without any change in its internal structure or properties. A few cycles of loading and unloading do not appreciably affect a material. However, when this stress is repeated many times, the strength of the material may be drastically reduced and ultimately cause failure. *Fatigue* is defined as a progressive fracture under repeated loading. Fatigue tests are performed by subjecting a specimen to alternating stress applications below the yield strength until fracture occurs. Tensile, compressive, shear, bending, and torsional fatigue tests can all be performed.

The *fatigue strength* is the stress level at which a material fails under repeated loading. Failure under repeated or cyclic loading is therefore dependent on

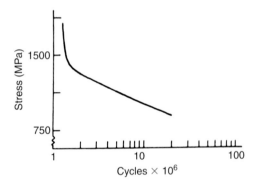

FIGURE 5.7 **Flexural fatigue curve for a cobalt-chromium-nickel alloy used for partial dentures.**

the magnitude of the load and the number of loading repetitions. Fatigue data are often represented by an S-N curve, a curve depicting the stress (or strain) (S) at which a material will fail as a function of the number of loading cycles (N). An example of an S-N curve is shown in Figure 5-7. When the stress is sufficiently high, the specimen will fracture at a relatively low number of cycles. As the stress is reduced, the number of cycles required to cause failure increases. Therefore, when specifying fatigue strength, the number of cycles must also be specified. For some materials, a stress at which the specimen can be loaded an infinite number of times without failing is eventually approached. This stress is called the *endurance limit*.

The determination of fatigue properties is of considerable importance for dental restorations subjected to cyclic forces during mastication. Stress applications during mastication may approach 300,000 flexures per year. Because dental materials can be subjected to moderate stresses repeated a large number of times, it is important in the design of a restoration to know what stress it can withstand for a predetermined number of cycles. Restorations should be designed with a safety margin so the clinical cyclic stresses are below the fatigue limit.

Fatigue fractures develop from small cracks that coalesce and ultimately lead to a macroscopic crack and catastrophic failure. Areas of stress concentration, such as surface defects and notches, are particularly dangerous and can lead to catastrophic failure. Fatigue properties are mostly dependent on the microstructure of the material, and the history of fabrication and treatment; therefore, they do not always directly correlate to other mechanical properties. Also, the environment plays a role, because the medium in which the material is submersed when in use may also cause degradation. Elevated temperatures, humidity, aqueous media, biological substances, and pH deviations away from neutral can all reduce fatigue properties. As a result, fatigue data, which are typically presented based on

tests in laboratory air at room temperature, are not always relevant to the service conditions in the oral cavity. The higher temperature, humidity, saline environment with proteins, and fluctuating pH all tend to reduce fatigue strength from its level in the laboratory.

FRACTURE TOUGHNESS

A fracture toughness test is usually performed using flexure bars with a notch, at the tip of which a crack with a nanometer-sized tip is introduced. In this configuration, materials can be characterized by the energy release rate, G, and the stress intensity factor, K. The energy release rate is a function of the energy involved in crack propagation, whereas the stress intensity factor describes the stresses at the tip of a crack. The stress intensity factor changes with crack length and stress according to the following formula:

$$K = Y\sigma a^{\frac{1}{2}}$$

where Y is a function that is dependent on crack size and geometry. A material fractures when the stress intensity reaches a critical value, K_c. This value of the stress intensity at fracture is called the *fracture toughness*. Fracture toughness gives a relative value of a material's ability to resist crack propagation. The units of K_c are units of stress (force/length^2) × units of length$^{\frac{1}{2}}$, or force × length$^{-\frac{3}{2}}$, and are typically reported as MN m$^{-\frac{3}{2}}$ or MPa m$^{\frac{1}{2}}$.

FRACTOGRAPHIC ANALYSIS

Fractographic analysis has been used in engineering for many years to help define the cause of failures and aid in structural design, as well as to improve existing materials. Its use in dentistry is relatively recent, but advances in the field have helped identify the role of residual stresses, temperature, and preexisting flaws on the longevity of dental restorations.

Brittle materials are easier to analyze with fractography because they typically fail catastrophically. The typical features of crack propagation (Figure 5-8) are readily identified and the origin of the fracture can be determined. The origin of fracture is the point at which the worst combination of flaw severity (determined by flaw size and shape) and stress demands are present. Differences in processing of ceramics, for example, may lead to significantly different structures, as shown in Figure 5-9, with a homogenous structure produced by effective processing. Flaw growth is observed from cumulative mistakes during processing. Flaws larger than the ones observed in Figure 5-9, *B*, are considered critical. In Figure 5-9, *D*, the problem is maximized by the presence of a very sharp flaw that concentrates stresses.

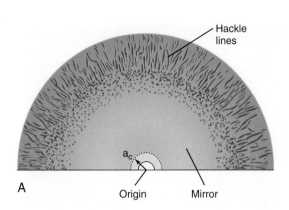 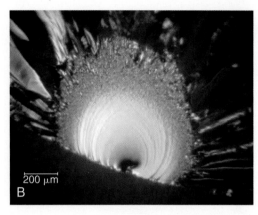

FIGURE 5.8 **Typical features of a brittle fracture surface. A,** Drawing of a fracture surface. **B,** The photograph shows a fracture surface in a quartz rod that failed catastrophically. It is possible to identify a mirror-like region, with hackle lines pointing to the origin of fracture. *(Part B From Quinn GD: Fractography of Ceramics and Glasses, NIST, U.S. Department of Commerce, Special publication 960-16, 2007).*

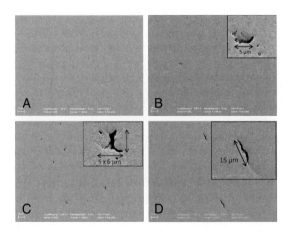

FIGURE 5.9 **Scanning electron micrographs of ceramic materials. A,** Shows a well processed material, with little to no flaws present. The sequence from **B** through **D** shows materials with increasingly bigger/sharper flaws, resulting from poor processing. *(Courtesy of Scherrer SS, University of Geneva)*

In the clinical situation, poor prosthesis design may also lead to failure, even if a preexisting flaw is not present. Fractographic analysis allows the origin to be identified, but in these cases, the fracture patterns are much more complex. In Figure 5-10 chipping caused a catastrophic failure at a margin where the porcelain structure was excessively thin.

TEAR STRENGTH AND TEAR ENERGY

Tear strength is a measure of the resistance of a material to tearing forces. Tear strength is an important property of dental polymers used in thin

sections, such as flexible impression materials in interproximal areas, maxillofacial materials, and soft liners for dentures. Specimens for tear strength testing are usually crescent-shaped and notched. The tear strength of the notched specimen is calculated by dividing the maximum load by the thickness of the specimen. The unit of tear strength is N/m.

Because of the viscoelastic nature of the materials tested, tear strength depends on the rate of loading. Rapid loading rates result in higher values of tear strength. Clinically, the rapid (or snap) removal of an alginate impression is recommended to maximize the tear strength and also to minimize permanent deformation. Typical values of tear strength are listed in Table 5-5 for some dental materials.

The *tear energy* (T) is a measure of the energy per unit area of newly torn surface and is determined from the load *(F)* required to propagate a tear in a trouser-shaped specimen as follows:

$$T = (F / t)(\lambda + 1)$$

where t is the specimen thickness and λ is an extension ratio. Typical values of tear energy determined for some dental impression materials and maxillofacial materials are listed in Table 5-6.

HARDNESS

Hardness testing is done by applying a standardized force or weight to an indenter. This produces a symmetrically shaped indentation that can be measured under a microscope for depth, area, or width of the indentation produced. The indentation dimensions are then related to tabulated hardness values. With a fixed load applied to a standardized indenter, the dimensions of the indentation vary inversely with

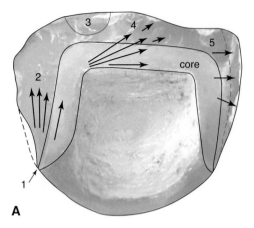
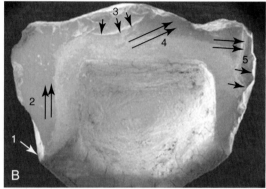

FIGURE 5.10 **Determination of origin of fracture in a ceramic restoration.** Sketched illustration of the stereo findings (A) as well as a summary image of SEM mapping the general direction of crack propagation of the recovered broken Procera AllCeram crown part (B). *(From Scherrer SS, et al: Dent. Mater. 24, 1107-1113, 2008.)*

TABLE 5.5   Tear Strength of Selected Dental Materials

Material	Tear Strength (KN/m)
Denture liners	2.6-45
Agar duplicating materials	0.22
Impression materials	
Agar	1.0
Alginate	0.47
Polysulfide	3.6
Polyvinylacetate-polyethylene mouth protectors	114

TABLE 5.6   Tear Energy* (*T*) of Some Dental Materials

Material	Tear Energy (J/m² [Mergs/cm²])
IMPRESSION MATERIALS	
Addition silicone	390-1150 [0.39-1.15]
Alginate	66 [0.066]
Polyether	640 [0.64]
Polysulfide	1100-3000 [1.1-3.0]
MAXILLOFACIAL MATERIALS	
Polyurethane	1800 [1.8]
Polyvinylchloride	11,000 [11]
Silicone	660 [0.66]

*Crosshead speed, 2 cm/min.

the resistance to penetration of the material tested. Thus lighter loads are used for softer materials.

Brinell Hardness Test

The Brinell hardness test is one of the oldest methods used to test metals and alloys used in dentistry. The method depends on the resistance to the penetration of a small steel or tungsten carbide ball, typically 1.6 mm in diameter, when subjected to a load of 123 N. In testing the Brinell hardness of a material, the penetrator remains in contact with the specimen tested for a fixed time of 30 seconds, after which it is removed and the indentation diameter is carefully measured. A diagram showing the principle of Brinell hardness testing, together with a microscopic view of the indentations into a gold alloy, is shown in Figure 5-11. Because the Brinell hardness test yields a relatively large indentation area, this test is good for determining average

hardness values and poor for determining very localized values.

Knoop Hardness Test

The Knoop hardness test was developed to fulfill the needs of a micro-indentation test method. This test method is suitable for thin plastic or metal sheets or brittle materials where the applied load does not exceed 3.6 kgf (kilogram-force; 35 N). The Knoop method is designed so that varying loads may be applied to the indenting instrument. The resulting indentation area, therefore, varies according to the load applied and the nature of the material tested. The advantage of this method is that materials with a great range of hardness can be tested simply by varying the test load. Because very light load applications produce extremely delicate micro-indentations, this

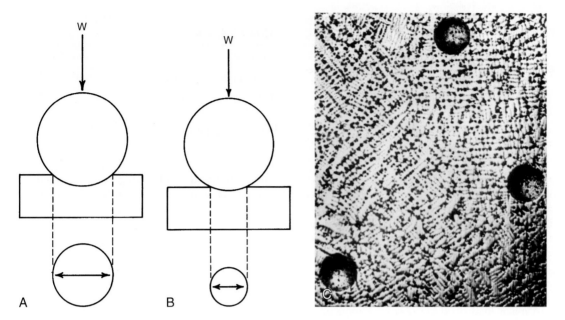

FIGURE 5.11 **Brinell hardness test. A,** Indentation in soft material. **B,** Indentation in harder material. **C,** Microscopic view of indentations.

TABLE 5.7   Knoop Hardness Number (KHN) of Selected Dental Materials

Material	KHN (kg/mm^2)
Enamel	343
Dentin	68
Cementum	40
Cobalt-chromium partial denture alloy	391
Denture acrylic	21
Feldspathic porcelain	460
Silicon carbide abrasive	2480
Zinc phosphate cement	38

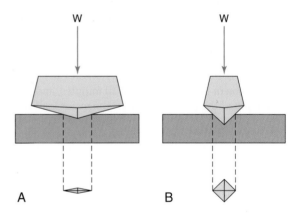

FIGURE 5.12 **A,** Principle of the Knoop hardness measurement. **B,** The diamond pyramid (Vickers) indentation test.

method of testing can be used to examine materials that vary in hardness over an area of interest. The main disadvantages of the method are the need for a highly polished and flat test specimen and the time required to complete the test operation, which is considerably greater than that required for some other less precisely controlled methods. The KHN (Knoop hardness number) values of some dental materials are listed in Table 5-7.

Vickers Hardness Test

The Vickers hardness test uses a square-based diamond indenter. The method is similar in principle to the Knoop and Brinell tests, except that a 136-degree diamond pyramid-shaped indenter is forced into the material with a definite load application. The indenter produces a square indentation, the diagonals of which are measured as shown in Figure 5-12.

Rockwell Hardness Test

The Rockwell hardness test was developed as a rapid method for hardness determinations. A ball or metal cone indenter is normally used, and the depth of the indentation is measured with a sensitive dial micrometer. The indenter balls or cones are of several different diameters, as well as different load

TABLE 5.8   Indentation Depth and Percent Recovery of Some Dental Polymers

Material	Indentation Depth (μm)	% Recovery
Acrylic denture teeth	93	88
Pit and fissure sealants	85-158	74-86
Resin composite	56-72	70-83

TABLE 5.9   Values of Shore A Hardness for Selected Dental Polymers

Material	Shore A Hardness
Resilient denture liners	48-85
Polyvinylacetate-polyethylene mouth protector	67
Silicone maxillofacial elastomer	25

applications (60 to 150 kgf [588 to 1470 N]), with each combination described as a special Rockwell scale, Rockwell A to G, denoted R_A, R_B, and so on.

The superficial Rockwell method has been used to test plastics used in dentistry. This method uses a relatively light (30 kgf [294 N]) load and a large-diameter (12.7 mm) ball in comparison with the standard Rockwell methods. The test is made by first applying a preload (minor load) of 3 kgf (29.4 N). A major load of 30 kgf (294 N) then is applied to the specimen for 10 minutes before a reading is taken. Because dental plastics are viscoelastic, recovery of the indentation occurs once the major load has been removed. The percent recovery can be determined on the same specimen by the following equation:

$$\text{Percent recovery} = [\,(A - B)\,/\,A\,] \times 100\%$$

where A is the depth of the indentation caused by application of the major load for 10 minutes, and B is the depth of the indentation after the major load has been removed for 10 minutes. Values of indentation depth and percent recovery for some dental plastics are listed in Table 5-8. The advantages of the Rockwell hardness test are that hardness is read directly and it is good for testing viscoelastic materials. The disadvantages are that a preload is needed, greater time is required, and the indentation may disappear immediately on removal of the load.

Barcol Hardness Test

The Barcol hardness test is one method used to study the depth of cure of resin composites. The Barcol indenter is a spring-loaded needle with a diameter of 1 mm that is pressed against the surface to be tested. The reading on the scale decreases as the indenter penetrates the surface. Depth of cure of a resin composite is tested by preparing specimens varying in thickness from 0.5 to 6.0 mm or more in increments of 0.5 mm. Then the top surface of a specimen is activated by a light-curing unit. The Barcol hardness of the top surface is compared with that of the bottom surface. The depth of cure is defined as the maximum thickness at which the Barcol reading of the bottom surface does not change by more than

10% of the reading of the top surface. Research has shown that a 10% decrease in Barcol hardness of a resin composite results in a 20% decrease in the flexural strength.

Shore A Hardness Test

The hardness measurements described previously cannot be used to determine the hardness of elastomers, because the indentation disappears after the removal of the load. An instrument called a *Shore A durometer* is used in the rubber industry to determine the relative hardness of elastomers, where hardness is measured in terms of material elasticity. The instrument consists of a blunt-pointed indenter 0.8 mm in diameter that tapers to a cylinder of 1.6 mm. The indenter is attached by a lever to a scale that is graduated from 0 to 100 units. If the indenter completely penetrates the specimen, a reading of 0 is obtained, and if no penetration occurs, a reading of 100 units results. Because elastomers are viscoelastic, an accurate reading is difficult to obtain because the indenter continues to penetrate the elastomer as a function of time. The usual method is to press down firmly and quickly on the indenter and record the maximum reading as the Shore A hardness. The test has been used to evaluate soft denture liners, mouth protectors, and maxillofacial elastomers, values of which are listed in Table 5-9.

NANO-INDENTATION

Traditional indentation tests use loads as high as several kilograms and result in indentations as large as 100 μm. Although valuable for screening materials and determining relative values among different materials, these tests are subject to limitations. Many materials have microstructural constituents or, in the case of microfilled composites, filler phases substantially smaller than the dimensions of the indenter. To accurately measure the properties of these microphases, it is necessary to be able to create indentations of a smaller size scale and to spatially control the location of the indentations. These techniques,

TABLE 5.10 Properties of Tooth Tissues from Nano-indentation Tests

Tissue	Nano-hardness		Dynamic Hardness		Elastic Modulus
	GPa	kg/mm²	GPa	kg/mm²	GPa
Enamel	4.48 (0.44)*	457 (45)	2.90 (0.23)	295 (23)	87.7 (5.9)
DEJ	2.37	242			53.2
Dentin	0.70 (0.12)	71 (12)	0.55 (0.09)	56 (9)	24.0 (3.9)

Modified from Urabe I, Nakajima M, Sano H, et al: Am. J. Dent. 13,129, 2000.
*Numbers in parentheses represent standard deviations.
DEJ, Dentin-enamel junction.

commonly referred to as *nano-indentation*, are able to apply loads in the range of 0.1 to 5000 mg-f (miligram-force), resulting in indentations approximately 1 μm in size. In addition, indentation depth is continuously monitored, eliminating the need to image the indentation to compute mechanical properties. Although most commonly used to measure hardness of micron-sized phases, the technique is also useful for measuring elastic modulus. For brittle materials, yield strength and fracture toughness may be determined.

The nano-hardness, dynamic hardness, and elastic moduli values of human enamel and dentin are listed in Table 5-10, along with the nano-hardness and elastic modulus for the region of the dentin-enamel junction. The nano-hardness of dentin of 71 kg/mm² (696 MPa) agrees well with the Knoop value of 68 kg/mm² (666 MPa) reported in Table 5-7; however, the nano-hardness of 457 kg/mm² (4.48 GPa) for enamel is considerably higher than the Knoop value of 343 kg/mm² (3.36 GPa). This difference may result from the much smaller indentation used in the nano-indentation test in relation to the size of the enamel rods. The dynamic hardness values are lower than those for the corresponding nano-hardness because they are calculated from the maximum displacement, whereas the nano-hardness values are calculated from the permanent deformation. The elastic moduli of 87.7 and 24.0 GPa for enamel and dentin by nano-indentation are in reasonable agreement with the values from compressive test specimens of 84.1 and 18.3 GPa, respectively. Of special interest is the elastic modulus of 53.2 GPa for the region of the dentin-enamel junction, which is intermediate to the values for enamel and dentin. The nano-indentation test is especially useful in studying this small region, which was not possible with compressive or tensile tests.

Nano-DMA (dynamic mechanical analysis) is possible with some nano-indenters by measuring the resistance to the indentation force during force removal. This method enables the measurement of storage and loss modulus in viscoelastic materials. DMA is described more fully later in this chapter.

TABLE 5.11 Two-Body Abrasion of Restorative Dental Materials

Material	Two-body abrasion (10⁻⁴ mm³/mm of travel)
AMALGAM	
Spherical	7.0
AgSn / AgCu	5.6
COMPOSITE RESIN	
Glass filled	7.7
Glass filled – no silane	13.8
Quartz filled	3.8
Quartz filled – no silane	5.6
Microfilled	12.0
Diacrylate resin	17.0
Pit and fissure sealant	21.5
Unfilled acrylic resin	13.3

WEAR

Wear has been studied by (1) service or clinical testing, (2) simulated service measurements, (3) model systems using various wear machines, (4) measurements of related mechanical properties such as hardness, and (5) examination of the amount and type of surface failure from a single or low number of sliding strokes.

Two-body abrasion tests have been used to rank the wear resistance of restorative materials. As shown in Table 5-11, the resistance of composite resins to abrasion depends on the nature of the filler particles (glass or quartz) and on silanation of the filler. Three-body abrasion tests are often used to compare the abrasion resistance of tooth structure with that of dentifrices and prophylaxis materials. Enamel is about 5 to 20 times more resistant to abrasion than dentin. Cementum is the least resistant to abrasion. Measurements of enamel loss during a 30-second prophylaxis have shown that fluoride is removed from the enamel surface and have allowed estimation of the removal of enamel to be 0.6 to 4 μm, depending on the abrasive.

Unfortunately, a 1:1 ratio between wear observed clinically and that measured in the laboratory seldom exists. Thus most tests strive to rank materials in an order that is seen clinically. Traditional wear tests measure the volume of material lost but do not reveal mechanisms of wear, whereas a single-pass sliding technique may characterize modes of surface failure. In general, wear data do not correlate well with other mechanical property data, making it more difficult to infer wear properties from other simpler laboratory tests.

SETTING TIME

Definition and Importance

The time required for the reaction to be completed is called the *final setting time*. If the rate of the reaction is too fast or the material has a short setting time, the mixed mass may harden before the operator can manipulate it properly. On the other hand, if the rate of reaction is too slow, an excessively long time is required to complete the operation. Therefore, a proper setting time is one of the most important characteristics of materials such as gypsum.

Working time refers to the time after which the material cannot be manipulated without creating distortion in the final product. An example from gypsum is the elapsed time at which the semifluid mass can no longer flow easily into the fine details of an impression. An example from impression materials is the elapsed time at which the paste becomes too rigid to record the details of the hard and soft tissues.

The *final setting time* is defined as the time at which a material such as alginate can be withdrawn without distortion or tearing. For gypsum, it is the time when it can be separated from the impression without fracture. The *initial setting time* is the time at which a certain arbitrary stage of firmness is reached in the setting process.

Measurement

The initial setting time is usually measured arbitrarily by some form of penetration test, although occasionally other types of test methods have been designed. For example, the loss of gloss from the surface of the mixed mass of model plaster or dental stone is an indication of this stage in the chemical reaction and is sometimes used to indicate the initial set of the mass. Similarly, the setting time may be measured by the temperature rise of the mass, because the chemical reaction is exothermic.

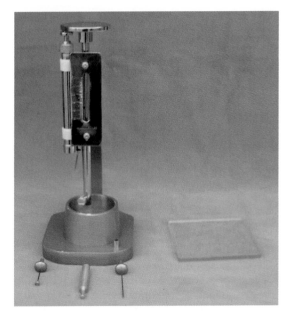

FIGURE 5.13 **Vicat penetrometer used to determine initial setting time of gypsum products.**

The Vicat apparatus shown in Figure 5-13 is commonly used to measure the initial setting time of gypsum products. It consists of a rod weighing 300 g with a needle of 1-mm diameter. A ring container is filled with the mix, the setting time of which is to be measured. The rod is lowered until it contacts the surface of the material, then the needle is released and allowed to penetrate the mix. When the needle fails to penetrate to the bottom of the container, the material has reached the Vicat or the initial setting time. Other types of instruments, such as Gillmore needles, can be used to obtain the initial and final setting times of gypsum materials.

DYNAMIC MECHANICAL ANALYSIS

Through dynamic mechanical analysis (DMA), some very useful properties of materials can be measured, such as the *dynamic elastic modulus (E')* and the *glass transition temperature* (T_g) in polymers. The calculation of these values is described in testing standard ASTM D 4092 (ASTM International). The test can be carried out in several conformations: tensile, flexure in single or dual cantilever, three-point bending, compression or shear and is suitable for liquids or solids (in the form of bars or powder), increasing the scope of application to many different materials. A sinusoidal strain is applied to the material at a given frequency, while the temperature is ramped up or down over time through a range, typically between −50 and 220° C for most polymers, between 25 and 600° C for most glasses and ceramics, and between 50 and 600° C for metals. As the test progresses, the resulting force is registered by a transducer and a stress-strain plot is generated. The complex modulus (E*) is calculated from the slope of this curve and from E*, storage (E′) and loss (E″) moduli are obtained, as previously explained in Chapter 4.

The ratio between E′ and E″ provides the loss factor, tan δ. In an increasing temperature ramp, the typical evolution of properties is as follows: as molecular motion is favored by the increase in temperature, loss or viscous modulus increases and storage or elastic modulus decreases. The temperature at which the maximum in the tan delta peak is observed is the T_g and defines the point at which the material transitions from an elastic to a rubbery state. Through analysis of the breadth of the tan delta peak, it is also possible to gain insight into the degree of homogeneity of the material's structure. Broader tan delta peaks indicate more heterogeneous materials, and the presence of two tan delta peaks in the same run is strong evidence for the presence of two phases within the structure. Even though virtually all materials used in dentistry have T_gs well above room or body temperatures, a good correlation between other mechanical properties and T_g makes it a useful predictor of the strength and structure of materials.

RHEOLOGY

Rheology is the study of deformation and flow of materials. Similar to DMA, this test involves the application of an oscillatory shear deformation (strain) to the material, placed between circular plates (parallel or in a cone-plate configuration), at a determined frequency, usually under isothermal conditions. In this case, the complex shear modulus (G*) is calculated and resolved into storage (G′) and loss (G″) shear moduli. As previously discussed in Chapter 4, the relationship between shear modulus and shear rate (or frequency) provides the viscosity. Viscometers are a very simple version of a rheometer. Working and setting times in cements and direct filling composites have been transitionally determined through rheology, with the increase in viscosity monitored during setting.

More recently, the determination of gel point in polymers has been accomplished with this technique. The *gel point* defines the point in conversion at which the material transitions from a viscous liquid into a viscoelastic solid and can be correlated to the crossover between G′ and G″ development curves during polymerization. At the crossover, elastic properties start to predominate over the viscous

response, and that is a reflection of polymeric network development. This is especially important during the polymerization of dental composites, occurring under confinement by the adhesion to the cavity walls. For the conventional dimethacrylates found in most commercial formulations, vitrification follows shortly after gelation as represented by the reaction kinetics plot. At this point, stresses at the bonded interface become more significant, and therefore, materials with delayed gelation are desirable. This technique is then very practical for the design of new materials.

DIFFERENTIAL SCANNING CALORIMETRY

Differential scanning calorimetry (DSC) is another tool to determine a series of temperature transitions in materials, such as the T_g and melting temperature (T_m). The calorimeter measures the difference in heat flow between the sample and a blank reference, either during a temperature sweep or through the course of nonisothermal phenomena, such as polymerization and the melting of metals, respectively. During a temperature sweep experiment, endotherm peaks are observed as the material goes through its glass transition and melting. The endotherm is brought about by the sudden increase in the number of molecular degrees of freedom at those transitions, which require energy gain from the environment. For dynamic exothermic reactions, as is the case for active polymerizations, the heat released by the material during isothermal experiments can be correlated to the amount of reacted vinyl double bonds and the degree of conversion in real time. This method measures an indirect manifestation of the reaction (enthalpy) and is therefore not accurate in evaluating chemical structure.

SPECTROMETRIC TECHNIQUES

Fourier-transformed infrared (FTIR) spectroscopy is a very useful tool for molecular characterization and for following chemical reactions. Each chemical bond between the atoms of a material has one specific vibrational characteristic, which produces interference in electromagnetic waves, at highly specific wavelengths. As light is transmitted through the sample, chemical bonds can be identified with the use of an infrared (IR) bench detector. The Fourier transform algorithm produces a spectrum with characteristic bands over a wavelength range, providing a very accurate picture of molecular structure. Using this method, newly synthesized materials can be characterized and reactions can be followed through the appearance or disappearance of determined bands. This is of particular interest for polymerization reactions, for example, of vinyl monomers, in which the C-H stretch vibration of the carbon double bond can be followed. The mid and near-IR spectra of Bis-GMA, a very commonly used monomer in dental restorative materials, are shown in Figure 5-14, *A* and *B*. This bond has peaks both in the mid-IR (400-4000 cm^{-1}) and in the near-IR regions (4000-7000 cm^{-1}). Other peaks of interest include the C-H stretch vibration of aromatic rings. Sampling in the mid-IR region is somewhat complicated because typically absorptions are very high, requiring the use of thin samples. The other concern is that water and carbon dioxide both have very strong absorptions in this region, and therefore, the system needs to be purged with an inert gas to allow accurate measurements. For dental composites, another drawback is a very broad band from glass particles that shadows many bands of interest in mid-IR. This requires the use of salt plates as substrates. In the near-IR region, absorptions are relatively weaker, so relatively thick samples can be used. In addition, glass or carbon dioxide show no absorption in this region, eliminating the need for purging and allowing the use of samples sandwiched between glass slides for more convenient specimen preparation. That also allows the use of fiber optics for remote monitoring of double-bond conversion.

Spectroscopic techniques can be combined with other test instruments to monitor conversion or molecular characterization simultaneously with the development of other properties. For example, near-IR spectroscopy can be combined with rheometry to determine the exact polymer conversion at the onset of gelation. The same is true for volumetric shrinkage and shrinkage stress measurements, described in the section, METHODS FOR MEASURING SHRINKAGE AND STRESS DURING CURE OF RESIN COMPOSITES, below.

PYCNOMETRY

Pycnometry is a technique used to determine material densities. Water pycnometry is based on the Archimedes principle and relies on the buoyancy of a material in water. That is considered to be a crude measurement because small pores entrapped in the material are not occupied by the water molecules and dissolved oxygen is not purged from the sample, so values tend to be underestimated. Gas pycnometry, on the other hand, uses the difference in volume occupied by the material and helium gas molecules in a chamber of known volume. If the material's mass is known, the density is then calculated through the simple relation d = m/V (*d* = density; *m* = mass; *V* = volume). Because helium molecules are much smaller than water, they can occupy voids in the material and also displace some of the dissolved oxygen and moisture, providing a true, accurate measurement of density. It is also possible to calculate volumetric shrinkage in polymerizations, by equating the densities of the material in the monomeric and polymeric states.

BOND STRENGTH TEST METHODS

Bond strength tests are abundant in the dental literature in part because they are relatively easy to perform and are not equipment intensive. They, however, present several limitations that reduce their usefulness as a selection criterion in clinical practice. These drawbacks are briefly explained below.

Stresses at the interface are not uniformly distributed— Bond strength is reported as the nominal stress value (in MPa), that is, the failure load (in Newtons) divided by the entire bonded area (in mm^2). This is often not accurate because the stress distribution at the interface is very heterogeneous. Debonding occurs due to stress concentration around a critical

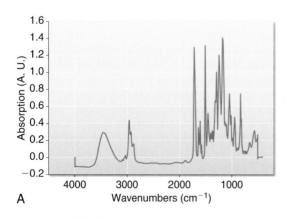

A

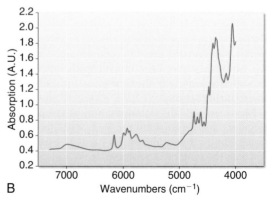

B

FIGURE 5.14 **Infrared spectra of Bis-GMA in the, A, mid-IR and in the, B, near-IR regions.**

size flaw, or void, at the interface that causes a crack to propagate. The actual stress level that initiates crack propagation can be several times higher than the nominal (or average) value. Therefore, nominal bond strength does not represent the failure stress (Figure 5-15).

High incidence of mixed and cohesive failures—Tensile stress concentration in the tooth substrate during load application may cause the crack to propagate into dentin or enamel, preventing the assessment of the interfacial strength.

Results of different studies are not comparable—Bond strength values for a specific material can vary a lot among studies due to differences in the bonding substrate, specimen preparation, storage conditions, and loading method. Unfortunately, there is very little standardization among research laboratories. Comparisons among different studies must be done very carefully.

Bond strength tests lack clinical significance—Based on what was described above, a threshold bond strength value that can be associated with a good clinical performance cannot be determined. Nevertheless, similar trends can be found in the literature for some adhesive systems. Systems that show poor performance *in vitro* generally have poor clinical performance.

Interfacial bond strength can be tested by a variety of methods. Using the dimensions of the bonded area, bond strength methods can be categorized as *macro* (4-28 mm²) or *micro* (approximately 1 mm²). The interface can be loaded either in tension or shear.

Macroshear Bond Strength Tests

In a macroshear bond strength test, a composite cylinder is built on the bonding substrate. After a predetermined storage time, the specimen is positioned in a universal testing machine where a single-edged

chisel, a flat-end rod, or a wire loop is attached to the actuator used to dislodge the composite cylinder from the substrate.

It is important to note that in shear tests, it is a tensile stress that actually causes debonding. In other words, the term *shear test* refers to the loading mode, and not to the stress causing interfacial failure. When the loading distance from the interface increases, tensile stress also increases due to creation of a bending moment in the composite cylinder.

The location and configuration of the loading device influences the stress distribution at the bonded interface and therefore affects the bond strength. Computer simulation using finite element analysis shows that, for a nominal stress of 15 MPa, the maximum tensile stress at the interface is 178 MPa when a chisel is used for loading. With the wire loop, the maximum tensile stress is 69 MPa. The higher the stress concentration at the load application area, the lower the bond strength. Therefore, the use of a knife-edge chisel results in lower bond strength values than the wire loop, where the load is distributed over a larger area. Typical dentin bond strength values with macroshear tests are 10 to 50 MPa. Cohesive and mixed failures are very frequent, and may affect up to 55% of the specimens.

Another aspect of interest is the elastic modulus of the composite used for the specimen cylinder. The larger the mismatch between the elastic modulus of the composite and the elastic modulus of the substrate, the higher the stress concentration at the interface. This lowers the measured bond strength.

Macrotensile Bond Strength Tests

Stress distribution in tensile tests is much more uniform than in shear tests. This provides a more faithful estimate of the stress level that initiated

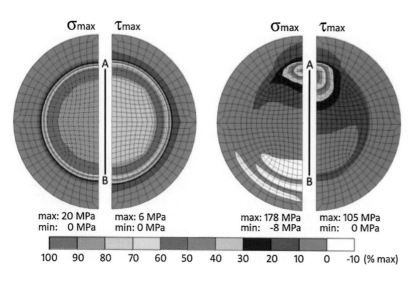

FIGURE 5.15 **Stress distributions (maximum principal stress, σmax, and maximum shear stress, τmax) at the dentin side of dentin/composite interfaces loaded in tension (*left*) or shear, using a 0.2-mm chisel applied at 0.2 mm from the interface (*right*). Line A–B indicates the diameter of the bonding area.** *(From Braga RR, Meira JB, Boaro LC, et al: Dent. Mater. 26(2), e38, 2010.)*

debonding. In macrotensile bond strength tests, a perpendicular alignment of the bonded interface to the loading axis is very important. Otherwise, bending stresses will develop. Specimen preparation is thus more difficult for tensile bond strength tests than shear bond tests.

As for the shear test, a mismatch between the elastic modulii of the composite and the substrate also influences bond strength. Typical dentin bond strengths are about 10 MPa. Cohesive and mixed failures may occur in 35% of the specimens.

Microtensile Bond Strength Tests

Microtensile tests use beam-shaped or hourglass-shaped specimens with a cross-sectional area of approximately 1 mm². This method provides a much lower incidence of mixed and cohesive failures compared to other methods (less than 20%). Specimen preparation is more labor intensive than with *macro* tests, because it involves sectioning of a large bonded interface into thin slices with diamond disks. The slices are trimmed to obtain hourglass specimens or further sectioned to obtain beams. Depending on the test conditions or materials, a significant number of pretest failures may occur. There is no consensus among researchers on the statistical management of these pretest failures.

Several testing fixtures are available for microtensile testing. The specimen can be glued using cyanoacrylate adhesive or actively or passively attached to the testing fixture with grips. The grip method interferes with the stress distribution in the specimen. Dentin bond strength values vary between 30 to 50 MPa. Values from this method are much higher than those found with macrotensile tests because the critical size for flaws is smaller in a microinterface. Fracture mechanics theory shows the size of the critical flaw is inversely related to the intensity of the stress necessary to initiate crack propagation.

One aspect concerning the preparation of enamel/composite specimens is the inclusion of defects at the periphery of the bonded interface during sectioning with diamond disks. These defects concentrate stress and initiate debonding at relatively low loads and contribute to a "false" low strength.

Microshear Bond Strength Tests

Composite cylinders are built on the substrate using silicone tubes 0.5 mm in height and 0.7 mm in diameter. Typically, up to six tube segments are bonded to a surface and filled with composite. The test procedure is similar to that for macroshear tests. Similarly, all the problems related to stress distribution also apply.

Bond strength values are about 20 MPa and the incidence of mixed and cohesive failures is 50%.

Push-out Tests

Another option for testing bond strength is the push-out test. When used to test bond strength of adhesives to dentin, a 1 to 2-mm thick dentin slice is bored to create a tapered cylindrical hole. The internal surface of the hole is treated with an adhesive and the hole is filled with composite. After storage, the composite cylinder is pushed though the dentin from the smaller diameter side, and bond strength is calculated by dividing the extrusion force by the lateral area of the tapered cylinder. This method simulates the clinical condition more closely than in shear/tensile tests because it includes constraint of the curing composite and the associated polymerization stress. Some authors refer to this method as a *micro* push-out test when it involves disks of radicular dentin and the root canal is filled with the tested material.

METHODS FOR MEASURING SHRINKAGE AND STRESS DURING CURE OF RESIN COMPOSITES

There are several methods described in the literature for measuring the contraction that accompanies the setting of resin composite restorative materials. Some of them record the total change in volume during cure, whereas others measure specific phases of cure. In resin composites, the shrinkage that occurs after development of a measurable stiffness of the paste is referred to as *post-gel shrinkage*. Some methods are also affected by the constraint imposed on the specimen, which defines the shrinkage force vectors. Finally, some methods record the linear shrinkage, whereas others record volumetric shrinkage. Linear shrinkage values can be converted to volumetric shrinkage by simply multiplying the linear value by three, if the material is isotropic. Data from different methods cannot be directly compared because of these issues, although dimensional change during cure is a basic material property. Some of the most frequently used methods are described below.

Mercury Dilatometer

The mercury dilatometer method uses the variation in height of a mercury column caused by composite shrinkage to calculate total volumetric shrinkage. The composite specimen is placed on a glass slide and immersed in mercury filling a glass capillary tube. A linear variable differential transformer (LVDT) probe floats on the surface, at the top of the mercury column. After probe stabilization, the composite is light cured from below, through the glass slide, and the change in height of the column is monitored in real time. One disadvantage of this method is the temperature sensitivity of the mercury in the column. To correct for this, a thermocouple monitors the temperature variation of the mercury caused by the heat liberated by the curing lamp and the corresponding variation in column height is adjusted at the end of the test run. Shrinkage values are calculated using the initial mass of the specimen and the composite's specific gravity.

Bonded Disk

For the bonded disk method, a disk of resin composite, 8 × 1.5 mm, is placed into a brass ring of approximately 16 mm in diameter and 1.5 mm in height that is bonded to a glass slide. The composite, which does not touch the brass ring, is covered with a microscope cover slip (approximately 0.1 mm thick). An LVDT probe is placed in contact with the center of the cover slip (Figure 5-16). The composite specimen is light activated from below the specimen, through the glass slide. As the composite cures and shrinks, it pulls the cover slip down and its deflection in monitored by the LVDT probe. Displacement

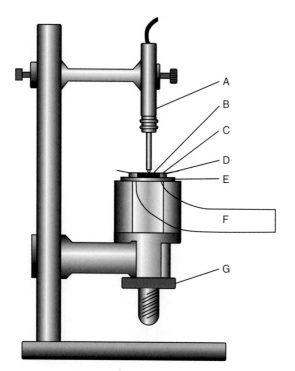

FIGURE 5.16 **Schematic cross section of the shrinkage test assembly.** *A*, Transducer; *B*, test specimen; *C*, cover slip; *D*, brass support ring; *E*, rigid glass plate; *F*, light optic; and *G*, height adjustment screw. *(From Watts DC, Cash AJ: Dent. Mater. 7,281, 1991.)*

data (in μm) is obtained from the signal output of the transducer (in mV) and applying it to a calibration curve. Shrinkage is calculated by dividing the measured deflection of the cover slip by the initial height of the composite. Because the composite specimen must exhibit some stiffness to deflect the cover slip, this method likely measures post-gel shrinkage. However, the values recorded are usually higher than those obtained by other post-gel methods.

AcuVol

AcuVol is a video-imaging device developed for measuring composite shrinkage that uses a CCD (charge-coupled device) camera to capture and analyze profiles of the specimen. A 12 μL composite specimen is shaped into a hemisphere and positioned on a Teflon pedestal. The tip of the curing light source is placed 1 mm above the specimen. Shrinkage-time curves are obtained from a single view or with the specimen rotating on the pedestal (multiview mode). Multiview mode allows for correction of asymmetries on the specimen surface. The measured values express the total volumetric shrinkage of the composite and are quite similar to those obtained with a mercury dilatometer.

Managing Accurate Resin Curing (MARC) Test

The managing accurate resin curing (MARC) test measures composite shrinkage in a constrained configuration (Figure 5-17). The internal walls of a glass ring, 5 mm in diameter and 2 mm in height, are etched with hydrofluoric acid. The volume and density of the ring is measured, and it is then coated with ceramic primer and a layer of unfilled resin. The ring is filled with composite and, after curing, the specimen is again measured for volume and density. The volume of the cured composite is calculated by the difference between the volumes of the glass ring filled with composite and the empty ring. Polymerization shrinkage is calculated as the percent variation between the internal volume of the glass ring and the volume of the cured composite.

Cavity Configuration Factor (C-Factor)

When a resin composite or glass ionomer cement cures while bonded to the walls of a cavity preparation and its setting reaction is accompanied by volumetric shrinkage and elastic modulus development, stresses arise in the material, at the tooth/restoration interface and in the tooth structure. Stresses are induced into the tooth from resistance to material shrinkage. These stresses are of clinical relevance because it may create interfacial gaps or, if the bond

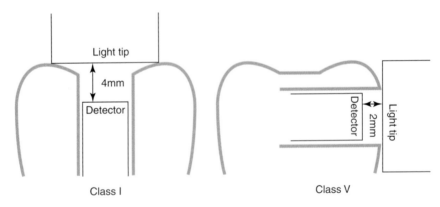

FIGURE 5.17 MARC (Managing Accurate Resin Curing). Schematics of the location of the light detectors placed in simulated Class I and Class V preparation sites. The teeth were placed inside a mannequin simulation head. *(From Price RBT, Felix CM, Whalen JM: J. Can. Dent. Assoc. 76:a94, 2010.)*

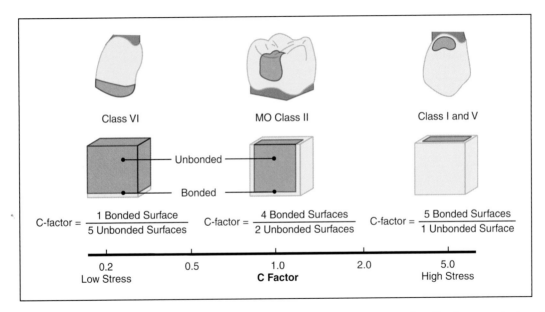

FIGURE 5.18 C-factor. Relation between model rectangular preparations, corresponding C-values, standard cavity preparations, and cylindrical test specimens. *(Modified from Feilzer AJ, De Gee AJ, Davidson CL: J. Dent. Res. 66(11), 1636-1639, 1987.)*

is sufficiently strong, cause tooth deformation or cuspal deflection. Unfortunately, polymerization stress cannot be directly measured on restored teeth. Only the effects of contraction stresses can be evaluated, for example, by *in vitro* microleakage, and bond strength and cuspal deflection tests.

Composite polymerization stress is defined by a combination of properties of the tooth and the restorative materials involved: the geometry (or anatomy) of the tooth and the restoration, the quality of the bonded interface and the restorative technique used (bulk or incremental filling and curing protocol). Among the factors related to the geometry of the restoration, the *cavity configuration factor (C-factor)*,

defined as the ratio of bonded-to-unbonded areas of the restoration, is an index used to express the level of constraint imposed on the shrinking restorative material (Figure 5-18). This index was developed based on laboratory experiments in which the shrinkage force generated by cylindrical specimens of composite was determined for different aspect ratios (i.e., height to diameter). For a given material and laboratory configuration, the higher the specimen's C-factor, the higher the calculated nominal stress.

Based on those findings, a class I restoration represents a less favorable situation than a class II configuration because of its larger C-factor. A class I cavity has a greater bonded-to-unbounded surface area than a typical class II cavity. Similarly, box-shaped class V restorations should generate higher stresses than saucer-shaped cavities. Such assumptions seem valid in broad terms. However, the applicability of the C-factor to clinical situations, though widespread, must be considered carefully because the complexity of the clinical situation does not allow for the prediction of stress levels based solely on the C-factor.

Another important aspect related to the stress distribution in a restored tooth is the amount of remaining tooth structure. In a large class II restoration, the reduced stiffness of the cavity walls increases stress concentration in the tooth. A small class II with similar bonded-to-unbonded area, on the other hand, shows higher stresses at the bonded interface and in the composite. Therefore, two restorations with the same C-factor may present very dissimilar stress distributions and, possibly, different clinical outcomes. Although some *in vitro* studies were able to verify a significant effect of C-factor on interfacial bond strength and microleakage, others were not. Even within the same study, the influence of C-factor on interfacial integrity may vary depending on the adhesive system tested. A long-term clinical study also failed to verify a significant effect of the C-factor on the longevity of class I composite restorations.

STRESS ANALYSIS AND DESIGN OF DENTAL STRUCTURES

The mechanical properties of dental restoration materials must be able to withstand the stresses and strains caused by the repetitive forces of mastication. The design of dental restorations is particularly important to leverage the best properties of a restorative material. Appropriate designs do not result in stresses or strains that exceed the strength properties of a material under clinical conditions.

Stresses in dental structures have been studied by such techniques as brittle coatings analysis, strain gauges, holography, two- and three-dimensional photoelasticity, finite element analysis, and other numerical methods. Stress analysis studies of inlays, crowns, bases supporting restorations, fixed bridges, complete dentures, partial dentures, endodontic posts, and implants have been reported, as well as studies of teeth, bone, and oral soft tissues. The stress analysis literature is too extensive and beyond the scope of this text to review. Only a brief summary of finite element analysis is provided here.

Finite Element Analysis

The finite element method or analysis (FEM or FEA) is a numerical method and offers considerable advantages over physical modeling methods

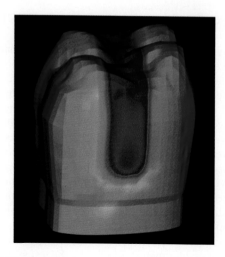

FIGURE 5.19 **Finite element analysis of stresses resulting from polymerization shrinkage of a class II composite restoration.** *(Courtesy of Dr. Svenn Borgersen, Eagan, MN.)*

(Figure 5-19). The method is useful for analyzing complex geometries, and it can determine stresses and strains throughout a three-dimensional object. In this method, a finite number of discrete structural elements are interconnected at a finite number of points or nodes. These finite elements are formed when the original structure is divided into a number of appropriately shaped sections, where each element is assigned the mechanical properties of the material to be simulated. The information needed to calculate the stresses and displacements in a finite element model is (1) the node and element description, (2) the elastic moduli and Poisson's ratio for the materials associated with each element, (3) the type of boundary constraints, (4) the description of the forces applied to the external nodes, and (5) a description of the mechanical behavior of the material, such as linearly elastic, nonlinearly elastic, viscoelastic, isotropic, anisotropic, and orthotropic.

Note that finite element methods are purely numerical and are based on many limiting assumptions. Finite element analysis is used in the design of physical experiments, including specimen size and fixture design. It is also useful for interrogating results from physical experiments. FEA simulations can reduce the number of physical experiments and optimize design by predicting results and performance. When doing a finite element analysis, it is important to understand the materials being evaluated and how to assess the simulation data. It is a powerful tool, but one that can be easily abused if the concepts are not fully understood and if the numerical model is not validated through physical experiments or other methods.

POLYMERIZATION STRESS TEST

The polymerization *in vitro* stress test was designed to evaluate the stresses developed at the bonded interface due to resin composite polymerization while bonded to cavity walls. The basic principle is common to all tests: the composite or resin is bonded to two surfaces, under variable degrees of constraint, and allowed to cure. As polymerization takes place, the inherent shrinkage that follows pulls the two bonded surfaces together, much like what would happen in a cavity preparation. Load and/or displacement is exerted on the bonding substrate, and the stress is calculated using the initial cross sectional area of the specimen. One important consideration in these methods is the system compliance, which defines the amount of deformation allowed by the test system as stresses are developed. This depends on the elastic modulus of the bonding substrate, as well as the stiffness of the test instrument. The cavity configuration factor can also be relatively easily accommodated in all systems, though with limitations, by adjusting the rod diameter and the height of the specimen. Even though all tests are useful for ranking materials in terms of the stress developed, they do not simulate the clinical condition, and direct correlations with *in vivo* observations should be made carefully.

Tensilometer

With the tensilometer test apparatus, the material is bonded between two rods, with steel, glass, and polymethyl methacrylate (in decreasing order of elastic modulus) being the most common materials (Figure 5-20). The rods are connected to a universal testing machine or system (UTS) with closed loop

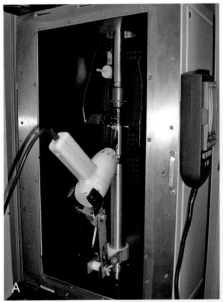
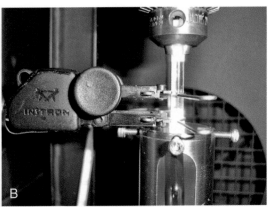
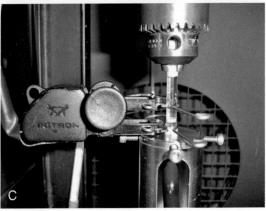

FIGURE 5.20 Tensilometer for measuring polymerization stress during cure of composites, showing the light source, test specimen, and extensometer for measuring displacement.

feedback control, where one rod is connected to the crosshead and the other rod is fixed. This is the only system in which an extensometer is attached to the specimen to maintain a constant distance between the two bonded interfaces during the test. The compliance of the system is very low and this can be further controlled by adjusting the elastic modulus of the rods. The load cell in the universal testing machine then records the load exerted by the material during polymerization under these confined conditions, and stress is calculated by dividing that load by the initial cross-sectional area of the specimen.

Tensometer

Similar to procedures using the tensilometer, with the tensometer the test material is bonded between two glass rods. One rod is fixed to the base of the instrument, and the second rod is attached to a cantilever beam (Figure 5-21). As the material polymerizes, it causes a deflection in the beam, registered by

a linear variable differential transformer. A load cell is not present in this system. A calibration curve of pressure x displacement is created prior to testing. Then, by applying the calibration curve and deflecting beam theory, stress is calculated and corrected for by the cross-sectional area of the specimen. An extensometer is not used in this case, and the system compliance is controlled by the elastic modulus of the cantilever beam and/or by the location of the glass rod in relation to the fulcrum of the beam. Fiber-optic cables provide a remote degree of conversion monitoring through the near-IR spectrometric techniques, described earlier in this chapter, for measuring the extent of polymerization and stress development in real time.

Crack Analysis

Localized contraction stresses can be calculated by analyzing the propagation of initial indentations made in a brittle material. Using an indenter, initial

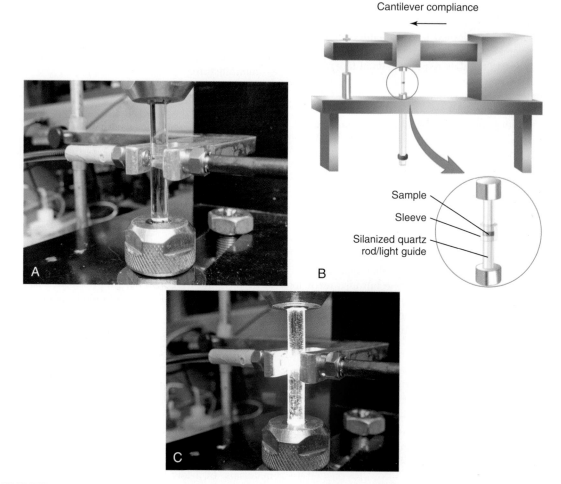

FIGURE 5.21 **ADAF Tensometer for measuring polymerization stress during cure of composites.** Test configuration before light exposure (A); during light exposure (C); illustration of test device (B) and enlargement of region shown in parts A and C.

cracks are made adjacent to a hole in a brittle material that simulates dental enamel, such as a glass or ceramic. As the bonded composite in the hole is polymerized, tensile stresses develop and the crack lengthens. The lengths of the cracks are measured before and after polymerization, and the resulting stress is calculated from the changes in crack length and the known fracture toughness of the brittle substrate.

SPECIFICATIONS FOR RESTORATIVE MATERIALS

The properties described in this and other chapters serve as the basis for a series of specifications that have been developed for restorative materials, instruments, and equipment. One group is the American National Standards Institute (ANSI)/American Dental Association Standards Committee on Dental Products. Standards developed and approved by this committee are reviewed by the Council on Scientific Affairs of the ADA, which has responsibility for adopting specifications. Presently, 68 specifications have been adopted (see Appendix Table 1). A larger group called *Federal Specifications and Standards* is designed to regulate requirements of federal government service agencies for the purchase and use of materials. Specifications of this type have been available for the past half century, and additional specifications continue to be added in each group. A series of similar specifications is available for products in Australia, Japan, and several other countries. In 1963, a program for international specifications was established that combined the efforts of the FDI World Dental Federation and the International Organization for Standardization (ISO). The practice of using physical test controls through methods of applied specifications is well established and will likely continue. Both the dental student and the practitioner must not only recognize that specifications for certain materials are available but also learn to some extent the qualities that are controlled by each specification. Through the specifications the quality of each product is maintained and improved.

AMERICAN DENTAL ASSOCIATION SPECIFICATIONS

The first of the American Dental Association Specifications was for amalgam alloy, formulated and reported in 1930. Since that time other specifications have been or are being formulated, as indicated in Appendix Table 1.

Copies of the specifications and worksheets to assist in the recording of the required data are available from the Council on Scientific Affairs of the American Dental Association in Chicago. The website of the Council lists the trade names and manufacturers of accepted dental products. This publication can also be obtained from the American Dental Association.

An examination of each specification reveals a general pattern of standardization common to each material.

1. These features include an item on the scope and classification of the material, which defines the application and general nature of each material.
2. Each specification includes information on other applicable specifications.
3. The requirements of each material consider such factors as uniformity, color, or general working characteristics of the material, as well as the general limitations of test values.
4. The methods of sampling, inspection, and testing procedures include details of specimen preparation and physical tests to be performed.
5. Each specification includes information on preparation for delivery, with instructions concerning packaging, instructions for use, and marking with lot numbers and the date of manufacture.
6. Each specification includes notes that provide additional information on intended uses, and references to the literature or other special items.

The important features of each of these specifications are described appropriately in later chapters.

AMERICAN DENTAL ASSOCIATION ACCEPTANCE PROGRAM

The American Dental Association, through the Council on Scientific Affairs, maintains an acceptance program for consumer products, such as denture adherents, dental floss, and toothbrushes.

INDEX OF FEDERAL SPECIFICATIONS AND STANDARDS

The Index of Federal Specifications and Standards includes specifications for a number of restorative dental materials not described elsewhere. These specifications are used primarily by the federal services to maintain some quality control of dental products and are valuable for suppliers of these materials. In a few instances, reference is made to specific federal specifications and standards in later chapters.

SELECTED PROBLEMS

PROBLEM 1

How does the snap removal of an alginate impression maximize its tear strength?

Solution

As with other impression materials, the viscoelastic nature of the material makes the rate of deformation a very important factor in determining its final strength. With the rapid removal of the impression, not enough time is allowed at the deformed state, and that increases not only the tear strength but also maximizes dimensional stability.

PROBLEM 2

Why is it important to know materials properties under different kinds of loading (tension, compression, shear)?

Solution

Because in the oral cavity materials are going to be subjected to complex forms of loading and both the choice of material and design of the restoration should balance the type of mechanical solicitation with the material that is expected to behave the best under that situation.

PROBLEM 3

In resin composites, why is the degree of polymer conversion a useful property? How does it correlate with other properties of the material?

Solution

The degree of conversion, assessed either directly through spectrometric techniques or indirectly through dynamic scanning calorimetry, relates with the strength and shrinkage of the material. In general terms, the higher the conversion, the greater the resistance to wear, general mechanical properties and volumetric shrinkage. That also increases the stress at the bonded interface in a restoration, which could increase the incidence of gaps and recurrent caries. A lot of research has been done to try and minimize such stresses while maintaining high conversion to keep mechanical properties acceptable during use.

Bibliography

Dynamic Mechanical Analysis and Rheology

Rubinstein M, Colby RH: Networks and gelation. In Polymer Physics, New York, 2008, Oxford University Press.

Graessley WW: Linear viscoelasticity. In *Polymeric Liquids and Networks: Dynamics and Rheology*, New York, 2008, Taylor and Francis Group.

Macosko CW: Linear viscoelasticity. In *Rheology: Principles, Measurements and Applications*, New York, 1994, Wiley-VCH.

Menard KP: *Dynamic Mechanical Analysis: a Practical Introduction*, Boca Raton, 2008, Taylor & Francis.

Chiou BS, English RJ, Khan SA: UV cross-linking of thiolene polymers: A rheological study, *Photopolymerization* 673:150–166, 1997.

Chiou BS, Khan SA: Real-time FTIR and in situ rheological studies on the UV curing kinetics of thiol-ene polymers, *Macromolecules* 30(23):7322–7328, 1997.

Cook WD, Brockhurst P: The Oscillating Rheometer — What Does It Measure, *J Dent Res* 59(5):795–799, 1980.

Winter HH: Can the gel point of crosslinking polymers be detected by the G′-G″ crossover? *Pol Eng Scie* 27:1698, 1987.

Botella A, Dupuy J, Roche AA, et al: Photo-rheometry/NIR spectrometry: An in situ technique for monitoring conversion and viscoelastic properties during photopolymerization, *Macr Rapid Comm* 25:1155, 2004.

Odian G: *Principles of polymerization*. New York, 2004, Wiley-Interscience, p 11–114.

Ferracane JL, Moser JB, Greener EH: Rheology of composite restoratives, *Journal of Dental Research* 60(9):1678–1685, 1981.

Urabe I, Nakajima S, Sano H, Tagami J: Physical properties of the dentin-enamel junction region, *Am J Dent* 13(3):129–135, 2000.

Spectrometric Techniques

Silverstein R, Webster F, Kiemle D: *Spectrometric identification of organic compounds*, Hoboken, NJ, 2005, John Wiley & sons, p 72–79.

Ferracane JL, Greener EH: Fourier transform infrared analysis of degree of polymerization in unfilled resins– methods comparison, *J Dent Res* 63(8):1093–1095, 1984.

Stansbury JW, Dickens SH: Determination of double bond conversion in dental resins by near infrared spectroscopy, *Dent Mater* 17(1):71–79, 2001.

Wells-Gray EM, Kirkpatrick SJ, Sakaguchi RL: A dynamic light scattering approach for monitoring dental composite curing kinetics, *Dent Mater* 26(7):634–642, 2010 Jul:Epub 2010 Apr 7.

Pycnometry

Viana M, Jouannin P, Pontier C, Chulia D: About pycnometric density measurements, *Talanta* 57:583, 2002.

Polymerization Stress Tests

Condon JR, Ferracane JL: Assessing the effect of composite formulation on polymerization stress, *J Am Dent Assoc* 131(4):497–503, 2000.

Condon JR, Ferracane JL: Reduced polymerization stress through non-bonded nanofiller particles, *Biomaterials* 23(18):3807–3815, 2002.

Feilzer AJ, De Gee AJ, Davidson CL: Setting stress in composite resin in relation to configuration of the restoration, *J Dent Res* 66(11):1636–1639, 1987.

Ferracane JL, Mitchem JC: Relationship between composite contraction stress and leakage in Class V cavities, *Am J Dentistry* 16(4):239–243, 2003.

Lu H, Stansbury JW, Bowman CN: Towards the elucidation of shrinkage stress development and relaxation in dental composites, *Dent Mater* 20(10):979–986, 2004.

Lu H, Stansbury JW, Dickens SH, et al: Probing the origins and control of shrinkage stress in dental resin composites. II. Novel method of simultaneous measurement of polymerization shrinkage stress and conversion, *J Biomed Mater Res B Appl Biomater* 71(1):206–213, 2004.

Lu H, Stansbury JW, Dickens SH, et al: Probing the origins and control of shrinkage stress in dental resin-composites: I. Shrinkage stress characterization technique, *J Mater Sci Mater Med* 15(10):1097–1103, 2004.

Pfeifer CS, Ferracane JL, Sakaguchi RL, Braga RR: Factors affecting photopolymerization stress in dental composites, *J Dent Res* 87(11):1043–1047, 2008 Nov.

Pfeifer CS, Ferracane JL, Sakaguchi RL, Braga RR: Photoinitiator content in restorative composites: influence on degree of conversion, reaction kinetics, volumetric shrinkage and polymerization stress, *Am J Dent* 22(4):206–210, 2009 Aug.

Sakaguchi RL, Wiltbank BD, Murchison CF: Contraction force rate of polymer composites is linearly correlated with irradiance, *Dent Mater* 20(4):402–407, 2004.

Sakaguchi RL, Wiltbank BD, Murchison CF: Prediction of composite elastic modulus and polymerization shrinkage by computational micromechanics, *Dent Mater* 20(4):397–401, 2004 May.

Sakaguchi RL, Wiltbank BD, Murchison CF: Cure induced stresses and damage in particulate reinforced polymer matrix composites: a review of the scientific literature, *Dent Mater* 21(1):43–46, 2005 Jan.

Stansbury JW, Trujillo-Lemon M, Lu H, et al: Conversion-dependent shrinkage stress and strain in dental resins and composites, *Dent Mater* 21(1):56–67, 2005.

Yamamoto T, Ferracane JL, Sakaguchi RL, Swain MV: Calculation of contraction stresses in dental composites by analysis of crack propagation in the matrix surrounding a cavity, *Dent Mater* 25(4):543–550, 2009 Apr:Epub 2008 Dec 18.

Yamamoto T, Nishide A, Swain MV, et al: Contraction stresses in dental composites adjacent to and at the bonded interface as measured by crack analysis, *Acta Biomater* 7(1):417–423, 2011 Jan:Epub 2010 Aug 4.

Fracture Toughness and Fractographic Analysis

Quinn GD: Fractographic analysis of Ceramics and glasses: NIST Practice Guide. Materials Science and Engineering Laboratory, National Institute of Standards and Technology, *Special Publications* 2007. Available for download at http://www.nist.gov/manuscript-publication-search.cfm?pub_id=850928.

Lohbauer U, Amberger G, Quinn GD, Scherrer SS: Fractographic analysis of a dental zirconia framework: a case study on design issues, *J Mech Behav Biomed Mater* 3(8): 623–629, 2010.

Quinn JB, Quinn GD, Kelly JR, Scherrer SS: Fractographic analyses of three ceramic whole crown restoration failures, *Dent Mater* 21(10):920–929, 2005.

Scherrer SS, Kelly JR, Quinn GD, Xu K: Fracture toughness (KIc) of a dental porcelain determined by fractographic analysis, *Dent Mater* 15(5):342–348, 1999.

Scherrer SS, Quinn GD, Quinn JB: Fractographic failure analysis of a Procera AllCeram crown using stereo and scanning electron microscopy, *Dent Mater* 24(8):1107–1113, 2008.

Scherrer SS, Quinn JB, Quinn GD, Wiskott HW: Fractographic ceramic failure analysis using the replica technique, *Dent Mater* 23(11):1397–1404, 2007.

Rodrigues SA Jr, Scherrer SS, Ferracane JL, Della Bona A: Microstructural characterization and fracture behavior of a microhybrid and a nanofill composite, *Dent Mater* 24(9):1281–1288, 2008.

Bond Strength Methods, Volumetric Shrinkage Methods, C-factor

Armstrong A, Geraldeli S, Maia R, et al: Adhesion to tooth structure: A critical review of "micro" bond strength test methods, *Dent Mater* 26:e50–e62, 2010.

Braga RR, Boaro LC, Kuroe T, et al: Influence of cavity dimensions and their derivatives (volume and 'C' factor) on shrinkage stress development and microleakage of composite restorations, *Dent Mater* 22:818–823, 2006.

Braga RR, Meira JB, Boaro LC, Xavier TA: Adhesion to tooth structure: A critical review of "macro" test methods, *Dent Mater* 26:e38–e49, 2010.

Choi KK, Ryu GJ, Choi SM, Lee MJ, et al: Effects of cavity configuration on composite restoration, *Oper Dent* 29:462–469, 2004.

Feilzer AJ, De Gee AJ, Davidson CL: Setting stress in composite resin in relation to configuration of the restoration, *J Dent Res* 66:1636–1639, 1987.

Pfeifer CSC, Braga RR, Cardoso PEC: Influence of cavity dimensions, insertion technique and adhesive system on microleakage of Class V restorations, *JADA* 137:197–202, 2006.

Price RB, Felix CM, Whalen JM: Factors Affecting the Energy Delivered to Simulated Class I and Class V Preparations, *J Can Dent Assoc* 76:a94, 2010.

Price RB, Riskalla AS, Hall GC: Effect of stepped light exposure on the volumetric polymerization shrinkage and bulk modulus of dental composites and an unfilled resin, *Amer J Dent* 13:176–180, 2000.

Sakaguchi RL, Wiltbank BD, Shah NC: Critical configuration analysis of four methods for measuring polymerization shrinkage strain of composites, *Dent Mater* 20:388–396, 2004.

Sharp LJ, Choi IB, Lee TE, et al: Volumetric shrinkage of composites using video-imaging, *J Dent* 31:97–103, 2003.

Shiraia K, De Munck J, Yoshida Y, et al: Effect of cavity configuration and aging on the bonding effectiveness of six adhesives to dentin, *Dent Mater* 21:110–124, 2005.

van Dijken JW: Durability of resin composite restorations in high C-factor cavities: A 12-year follow-up, *J Dent* 38:469–474, 2010.

Van Meerbeek B, Peumans M, Poitevin A, et al: Relationship between bond-strength tests and clinical outcomes, *Dent Mater* 26:e100–e121, 2010.

Versluis A, Tantbirojn D, Pintado MR, et al: Residual shrinkage stress distributions in molars after composite restoration, *Dent Mater* 20:554–564, 2004.

Watts DC, Cash AJ: Determination of polymerization shrinkage kinetics in visible-light-cured materials: methods development, *Dent Mater* 7:281–287, 1991.

Witzel MF, Ballester RY, Meira JB, et al: Composite shrinkage stress as a function of specimen dimensions and compliance of the testing system, *Dent Mater* 23:204–210, 2007.

6

Biocompatibility and Tissue Reaction to Biomaterials

Biocompatibility is formally defined as the ability of a material to elicit an appropriate biological response in a given application in the body. Inherent in this definition is the idea that a single material may not be biologically acceptable in all applications. For example, a material that is acceptable as a full cast crown may not be acceptable as a dental implant. Also implicit in this definition is an expectation for the biological performance of the material. In a bone implant, the expectation is that the material will allow the bone to integrate with the implant. Thus an appropriate biological response for the implant is osseointegration. In a full cast crown, the expectation is that the material will not cause inflammation of pulpal or periodontal tissues, but osseointegration is not an expectation. Whether or not a material is biocompatible therefore depends on the physical function for which the material will be used and the biological response that will be required from it. Using this definition, it makes little sense to say that any given material is or is not biocompatible—how the material will be used must be defined before that can be assessed.

In that regard, biocompatibility is much like color. Color is a property of a material interacting with its environment (light), and the color of a material depends on the light source and the observer of the light. Similarly, biocompatibility is a property of a material interacting with its environment. The biological response will change if changes occur in the host, the application of the material, or the material itself (Figure 6-1).

Dentistry shares concerns about biocompatibility with other fields of medicine, such as orthopedics, cardiology, and vascular biology, among others. In the development of any biomaterial, one must consider the strength, esthetics, and functional aspects of the material, as well as its biocompatibility. Furthermore, demands for appropriate biological responses are increasing as materials are expected to perform more sophisticated functions in the body for longer time periods. Thus considerations of biocompatibility are important to manufacturers, practitioners, scientists, and patients. The field of biocompatibility is interdisciplinary and draws on knowledge from materials science, bioengineering, biochemistry, molecular biology, tissue engineering and other fields.

This chapter briefly surveys the tests used for evaluating biocompatibility of dental materials and how well they correlate with one another, overviews the specifications that govern such testing, and describes the strengths and weaknesses of the testing methods. The majority of the chapter is devoted to a discussion of the biocompatibility of the various materials used in dentistry within the framework of these principles.

MEASURING BIOCOMPATIBILITY

Measuring the biocompatibility of a material is not simple, and the methods of measurement are evolving rapidly as more is known about the interactions between dental materials and oral tissues and as technologies for testing improve. Historically, new materials were simply tested in humans to assess their biocompatibility. However, this practice has not been acceptable for many years, and current materials must be extensively screened for biocompatibility before they are used in humans. Several varieties of tests are currently used to ensure that new materials are biologically acceptable. These tests are classified as in vitro, animal, and usage tests. These three testing types include clinical trials, which is really a special case of a usage test in humans. This section discusses examples of each type of test, their advantages and disadvantages, how the tests are used together, and standards that rely on these tests to regulate the use of materials in dentistry.

In Vitro Tests

In vitro tests for biocompatibility, done outside a living organism, require placement of a material or a component of a material in contact with a cell, enzyme, or some other isolated biological system. The contact can be either direct, when the material contacts the cell system without barriers, or indirect, when there is a barrier of some sort between the material and the cell system. Direct tests can be further subdivided into those in which the material is physically present with the cells and those in which some extract from the material contacts the cell system.

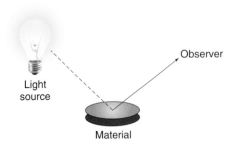

FIGURE 6.1 **Biocompatibility.** Like color, biocompatibility is not a property of just a material, but rather a property of how a material interacts with its environment. A material's color depends on the character of the light source, how the light interacts with the material, and how the observer interprets the reflected light. In this sense, the material's color depends on its environment. The biocompatibility of a material is similar in the sense that it depends on its environment as well as the nature of the material.

In vitro tests can be roughly subdivided into those that measure cytotoxicity or cell growth, those that measure some metabolic or other cell function, and those that measure the effect on the genetic material in a cell (mutagenesis assays). Often there is overlap in what a test measures. In vitro tests have a number of significant advantages over other types of biocompatibility tests (Table 6-1). They are relatively quick, generally cost less than animal or usage tests, can be standardized, are well suited to large-scale screening, and can be tightly controlled to address specific scientific questions. The overriding disadvantage of in vitro tests is their questionable relevance to the final in vivo use of the material (see later section on correlation between tests on page 114). Another significant disadvantage includes the lack of inflammatory and other tissue-protective mechanisms in the in vitro environment. It should be emphasized that in vitro tests alone cannot entirely predict the overall biocompatibility of a material.

Standardization of in vitro tests is a primary concern. Two types of cells can be used for in vitro assays. *Primary cells* are those cells taken directly from an animal and cultured. These cells will grow for only a limited time in culture but usually retain many of the characteristics of cells in vivo. *Continuously grown cells* or *cell lines* are cells that have been transformed previously to allow them to grow more or less indefinitely in culture. Because of this transformation, these cells do not retain all in vivo characteristics, but they do consistently exhibit those features that they do retain. Primary cell cultures seem to be more relevant than continuous cell lines for measuring cytotoxicity of materials. However, primary cells, being from a single individual, have limited genetic variability, may harbor viral or bacterial agents that alter their behavior, and often rapidly lose their in vivo functionality once placed in culture. Furthermore, the genetic and metabolic stability of continuous cell lines contributes significantly toward standardizing assay methods. In the end, both primary and continuous cells both play important roles in in vitro testing; and both should be used to assess materials.

Cytotoxicity Tests

Cytotoxicity tests assess cell death caused by a material by measuring cell number or growth before and after exposure to that material. Control materials should be well defined and commercially available to facilitate comparisons among other testing laboratories. *Membrane permeability* tests are used to measure cytotoxicity by the ease with which a dye can pass through a cell membrane, because membrane permeability is equivalent to or very nearly equivalent to cell death (Figures 6-2 and 6-3).

TABLE 6.1   Advantages and Disadvantages of Biocompatibility Tests

Test	Advantages	Disadvantages
In vitro tests	Quick to perform	Relevance to in vivo is questionable
	Least expensive	
	Can be standardized	
	Large-scale screening	
	Good experimental control	
	Excellence for mechanisms of interactions	
In vivo tests	Allows complex systemic interactions	Relevance to use of material is questionable
	Response more comprehensive than in vitro tests	Expensive
	More relevant than in vitro tests	Time consuming
		Legal/ethical concerns
		Difficult to control
		Difficult to interpret and quantify
Usage tests	Relevance to use of material is assured	Very expensive
		Very time consuming
		Major legal/ethical issues
		Can be difficult to control
		Difficult to interpret and quantify

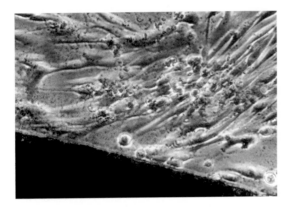

FIGURE 6.2 **Noncytotoxic interaction.** Light microscopic view of a noncytotoxic interaction between a material (*dark image at bottom of the picture*) and periodontal ligament fibroblasts in a cell culture (in vitro) test. The morphology of the fibroblasts indicates that they are alive and are not suffering from a toxic response (see Figure 6-3 for contrast). The material in this case was a calcium hydroxide pulp-capping agent.

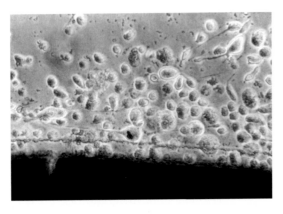

FIGURE 6.3 **Cytotoxic interaction.** Light microscopic view of a cytotoxic interaction between a material (*dark image at the bottom of the picture*) and periodontal ligament fibroblasts in a cell culture test. The fibroblasts are rounded and detached (see Figure 6-2 for contrast), indicating that they are either dead or dying. The material is a type of calcium hydroxide pulp-capping agent, different from the one shown in Figure 6-2.

Tests for Cell Metabolism or Cell Function

Some in vitro tests for biocompatibility use the biosynthetic or enzymatic activity of cells to assess cytotoxic response. Tests that measure deoxyribonucleic acid (DNA) synthesis or protein synthesis are common examples of this type of test. A commonly used enzymatic test for cytotoxicity is the MTT (MTT [3-(4,5-dimethylthiazol-2-yl)-2,5-diphenyl tetrazolium bromide] test, as well as the NBT (nitroblue tetrazolium), XTT [2,3-Bis-(2-methoxy-4-nitro-5-sulfophenyl)-2H-tetrazolium-5-carboxanilide salt], and WST (a water-soluble tetrazolium), all being colorimetric assays based on different tetrazolium salts. Alamar Blue tests quantitatively measure cell

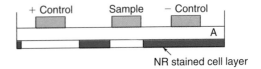

FIGURE 6.4 **Agar overlay method.** The agar overlay method has been used to evaluate the cytotoxicity of dental materials. The cell layer, which has been previously stained with neutral red (*NR*), is covered with a thin layer of agar (*A*). Samples are placed on top of the agar for a time. If the material is cytotoxic, it will injure the cells and the neutral red will be released, leaving a zone of inhibition.

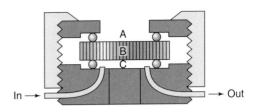

FIGURE 6.5 **Dentin disk barrier test method.** A dentin disk is used as a barrier in cytotoxicity tests that attempt to predict the toxicity of materials placed on dentin in vivo. The material is placed on one side (*A*) of the dentin disk (*B*) in the device used to hold the dentin disk. Collection fluid (cell culture medium or saline) is on the other side of the disk (*C*). Cells can also be grown on the collection side. Components of the material may diffuse through the dentin and the effect of the medium on cell metabolism can then be measured. To assess the rate of diffusion, the collection fluid can be circulated into and out of the collection chamber (*C*).

proliferation using a fluorescent indicator that allows continuous monitoring of cells over time.

Tests That Use Barriers (Indirect Tests)

Because direct contact often does not exist between cells and materials during in vivo use, several in vitro barrier tests have been developed to mimic in vivo conditions. These tests include an agar overlay method, which uses agar to form a barrier between the cells and the material, and the Millipore filter assay, in which a monolayer of cells is grown on a filter that is turned over so that test materials are placed on the filter and leachable diffusion products are allowed to interact with the cells. The agar diffusion and Millipore filter tests can provide, at best, a qualitative cytotoxic ranking among materials (Figure 6-4).

A number of studies have shown that dentin forms a barrier through which toxic materials must diffuse to reach pulp tissue, with the thickness of the dentin directly correlating with the protection offered to the pulp. These assays, which incorporate dentin disks between the test sample and the cell assay system, have the added advantage of directional diffusion between the restorative material and the culture medium (Figure 6-5).

Other Assays for Cell Function

In vitro assays to measure immune function or other tissue reactions have also been used. These assays measure cytokine production by lymphocytes and macrophages, lymphocyte proliferation, chemotaxis, or T-cell rosetting to sheep red blood cells. Other tests measure the ability of a material to alter the cell cycle or activate complement. The in vivo significance of these assays is yet to be ascertained, but many show promise for being able to reduce the number of animal tests required to assess the biocompatibility of a material.

Mutagenesis Assays

Mutagenesis assays assess the effect of a biomaterial on a cell's genetic material. There are a wide range of mechanisms by which a material can affect a cell's genes. Genotoxic mutagens directly alter cell DNA through various types of mutations. Each chemical may be associated with a specific type of DNA mutation. Genotoxic chemicals may be mutagens in their native states, or may require activation or biotransformation to be mutagens, in which case they are called *promutagens*. Epigenetic mutagens do not alter the DNA themselves, but support tumor growth by altering the cell's biochemistry, altering the immune system, acting as hormones, or by other mechanisms. *Carcinogenesis* is the ability to cause cancer in vivo. Mutagens may or may not be carcinogens, and carcinogens may or may not be mutagens. Thus quantitation and relevance of tests that measure mutagenesis and carcinogenesis are extremely complex. A number of government-sponsored programs evaluate the ability of in vitro mutagenesis assays to predict carcinogenicity.

The Ames test is the most widely used short-term mutagenesis test and the only short-term one that is considered thoroughly validated. It looks at the conversion of a mutant stock of *Salmonella typhimurium* back to a native strain, because chemicals that increase the frequency of reversion back to the native state have a high probability of being carcinogenic in mammals. A second test for mutagenesis is the Styles' cell transformation test. This test on mammalian cells offers an alternative to bacterial tests (Ames test), which may not be relevant to mammalian systems. However, because the Ames test is widely used, extensively described in the literature, and technically easier to conduct in a testing laboratory than the other test, it is most often conducted in a screening program.

Animal Tests

Animal tests for biocompatibility, usually involving mammals such as mice, rats, hamsters, or guinea pigs, are distinct from usage tests (which are also often done in animals) in that the material is not placed in the animal with regard to its final use. The use of an animal allows for the complex interactions between the material and a functioning, complete biological system to occur. This is extremely difficult to mimic in a cell-culture system. Thus the biological responses in animal tests are more comprehensive and may be more relevant than in vitro tests, and these features are the major advantages of these tests (see Table 6-1). The main disadvantages of animal tests are that they can be difficult to interpret and control, are expensive, time consuming, and often involve significant ethical concerns and oversight. Furthermore, the relevance of the test to the in vivo use of a material is often unclear, especially in estimating the appropriateness of an animal species to represent a human. A variety of animal tests have been used to assess biocompatibility.

The *mucous membrane irritation test* determines whether a material causes inflammation to mucous membranes or abraded skin. In a *skin sensitization test*, materials are injected intradermally to test for development of skin hypersensitivity reactions, followed by secondary treatment with adhesive patches containing the test substance. *Implantation tests* are used to evaluate materials that will contact subcutaneous tissue or bone. The location of the implantation site is determined by the use of the material and may include connective tissue, bone, or muscle. Although amalgam and alloys are tested because the margins of the restorative materials contact the gingiva, most subcutaneous tests are used for materials that will directly contact soft tissue during implantation, as well as endodontic and periodontal treatment materials.

Usage Tests

Usage tests may be done in animals or in human study participants. They are distinct from other animal tests because they require that the material be placed in a situation identical to its intended clinical use. The usefulness for predicting biocompatibility is directly proportional to the fidelity with which the test mimics the clinical use of the material in every regard, including time, location, environment, and placement technique. For this reason, usage tests in animals usually employ larger animals that have similar oral environments to humans, such as dogs, mini-swine or monkeys. When humans are used, the usage test is termed a *clinical trial*. The overwhelming advantage for usage tests is their relevance (see Table 6-1). These tests are the gold standard, in that they give the ultimate answer to whether or not a material will be biocompatible and clinically useful. One might ask, then, why bother with in vitro or animal tests at all. The answer is in the significant disadvantages of the usage test. These tests are extremely expensive, last for long periods, involve many ethical and often legal concerns, are exceptionally difficult to control and interpret accurately, and may harm the test participants. Additionally, statistical analysis of these tests is often a daunting process. In dentistry, dental pulp, periodontium, and gingival or mucosal tissues are the main targets of usage tests.

Dental Pulp Irritation Tests

Generally, materials to be tested on the dental pulp are placed in class 5 cavity preparations in intact, noncarious teeth. At the conclusion of the study, the teeth are removed and sectioned for microscopic examination, with tissue necrotic and inflammatory reactions classified according to the intensity of the response. Although most dental-pulp irritation tests have involved intact, noncarious teeth, without inflamed pulps, there has been increased concern that inflamed dental pulp tissue may respond differently than normal pulps to liners, cements, and restorative agents. So, usage tests on teeth with induced pulpitis, which allow evaluation of the type and amount of reparative dentin formed, will likely continue to be developed and refined.

Dental Implants in Bone

At present, the best predictors for success of implants are careful patient selection and ideal clinical conditions. The following terms are used to define various degrees of success: *early implant success* for implants surviving 1 to 3 years, *intermediate implant success* for implants surviving 3 to 7 years, and *long-term success* for implants surviving more than 7 years. As such, there are three commonly used tests to predict implant success: (1) penetration of a periodontal probe along the side of the implant, (2) mobility of the implant, and (3) radiographs indicating either osseous integration or radiolucency around the implant. A bone implant is considered successful if it exhibits no mobility, no radiographic evidence of peri-implant radiolucency, has minimal vertical bone loss and is completely encased in bone, and has an absence of persistent peri-implant soft-tissue complications. Any fibrous capsule formation is a sign of irritation and chronic inflammation, which is likely to lead to micromotion of the implant and ultimately to loosening and failure.

Mucosa and Gingival Usage Tests

Tissue response to materials with direct contact of gingival and mucosal tissues is assessed by placement in cavity preparations with subgingival extensions. The material's effect on gingival tissues are observed and responses are categorized as slight, moderate, or severe, depending on the number of mononuclear inflammatory cells (mainly lymphocytes and neutrophils) in the epithelium and adjacent connective tissues. A difficulty with this type of study is the frequent presence of some degree of preexisting inflammation in gingival tissue due to the presence of bacterial plaque, surface roughness of the restorative material, open or overhanging margins, and over- or under-contouring of the restoration.

Correlation Among In Vitro, Animal, and Usage Tests

In the field of biocompatibility, some scientists question the usefulness of in vitro and animal tests in light of the apparent lack of correlation with usage tests and the clinical history of materials. However, lack of correlation is not surprising in light of differences among these tests. in vitro and animal tests often measure aspects of biological response that are more subtle or less prominent than those observed during a material's clinical use. Furthermore, barriers between the material and tissues may exist in usage tests or clinical use, but may not exist in the in vitro or animal tests. Thus it is important to remember that each type of test has been designed to measure different aspects of biological response to a material, and correlation is not always to be expected.

The best example of a barrier that occurs in use but not during in vitro testing is the dentin barrier. When restorative materials are placed in teeth, dentin will generally be interposed between the material and the pulp. The dentin barrier, although possibly only a fraction of a millimeter thick, is effective in modulating the toxic effect of a dental material. This dentin barrier effect is illustrated by the following classic study (Table 6-2). Three methods were used to evaluate the following materials: ZOE (zinc oxide eugenol) cement; resin composite; and silicate cement. The evaluation methods included (1) four different cell culture tests, (2) an implantation test, and (3) a usage test in class 5 cavity preparations in monkey teeth. The results of the four cell culture tests were relatively consistent, with silicate having only a

TABLE 6.2   Comparison of Reactions of Three Materials by Screening and Usage Tests

Material	Cell Culture	Implantation in Connective Tissue	Pulp Response
Silicate	+	+	+ +
Resin composite	+ +	+ +	+
ZOE	+ + +	+	0

From Mjör IA, Hensten-Pettersen A, Skogedal O: Int. Dent. J. 27,127, 1977.
+ + +, Severe; + +, moderate; +, slight; 0, no reaction.
ZOE, Zinc oxide–eugenol.

slight effect on cultured cells, composite a moderate effect, and ZOE a severe effect. These three materials were also embedded subcutaneously in connective tissue in polyethylene tubes (secondary test), and observations were made at 7, 30, and 90 days. Reactions at 7 days could not be determined because of inflammation caused by the operative procedure. At 30 days, ZOE caused a more severe reaction than silicate cement. The inflammatory reactions at 90 days caused by ZOE and silicate were slight, whereas the reaction to resin composites was moderate. When the three materials were evaluated in class 5 cavity preparations under prescribed conditions of cavity size and depth (usage test), the results were quite different from those obtained by the other methods. The silicate was found to have the most severe inflammatory reaction, the composite had a moderate to slight reaction, and the ZOE had little or no effect.

Apparent contradictions in this study are explained by considering the components that were released from the materials and the environments into which they were released. The silicate cement released hydrogen ions that were probably buffered in the cell culture and implantation tests but were not adequately buffered by the dentin in the usage tests. Microleakage of bacteria or bacterial products may have added to the inflammatory reaction in those usage tests. Thus this material appeared to be the most toxic in the usage test. The composites released low-molecular-weight resins, and the ZOE released eugenol and zinc ions. In the cell culture tests, these compounds had direct access to cells and probably caused the moderate to severe cytotoxicity. In the implantation tests, the released components may have caused some cytotoxicity, but the severity may have been reduced because of the capacity of the surrounding tissue to disperse the toxins. In usage tests, these materials probably were less toxic because the diffusion gradient of the dentin barrier reduced concentrations of the released molecules to low levels. The slight reaction observed with the composites may also have been caused in part by microleakage around these restorations. The ZOE did not show this reaction, however, because the eugenol and zinc probably killed bacteria in the cavity, and the ZOE may have reduced microleakage.

Another example of the lack of correlation of usage tests with implantation tests is the inflammatory response of the gingiva at the gingival and interproximal margins of restorations that accumulate bacterial plaque and calculus. Plaque and calculus cannot accumulate on implanted materials and therefore the implantation test cannot hope to duplicate the usage test. However, connective tissue implantation tests are of great value in demonstrating the cytotoxic effects of materials and evaluating materials that will be used in contact with alveolar bone and apical periodontal connective tissues. In these cases, the implant site and the usage sites are sufficiently similar to compare the test results of the two sites.

Using In Vitro, Animal, and Usage Tests Together

For about 25 years, scientists, industry, and the government have recognized that the most accurate and cost-effective means to assess biocompatibility of a new material is a combination of in vitro, animal, and usage tests. Implicit in this philosophy is the concept that no single test will be adequate to completely characterize biocompatibility of a material. The ways in which these tests are used together, however, are controversial and have evolved over many years as knowledge has increased and new technologies were developed. This evolution can be expected to continue as materials are asked to perform more sophisticated functions for longer periods.

Early combination schemes proposed a pyramid testing protocol, in which all materials were tested at the bottom of the pyramid and materials were "weeded out" as the testing continued toward the top of the pyramid (Figure 6-6). Tests at the bottom of the pyramid were "unspecific toxicity" tests of any type (in vitro or animal) with conditions that did not necessarily reflect those of the material's use. The next tier shows specific toxicity tests that presumably dealt with conditions more relevant to the use of the material. The final tier was a clinical trial of the material. Later, another pyramid scheme was proposed that divided tests into initial, secondary, and usage tests. The philosophy was similar to the first scheme, except that the types of tests were broadened to encompass biological reactions other than toxicity, such as immunogenicity and mutagenicity. The concept of a usage test in an animal was also added (versus a clinical trial in a human). There are several important features of these early schemes. First, only materials that "passed" the first tier of tests were graduated to the second tier, and only those that passed the second tier were graduated to the clinical trials.

Presumably, then, this scheme funneled safer materials into the clinical trials area and eliminated unsafe materials. This strategy was welcomed because clinical trials are the most expensive and time-consuming aspect of biocompatibility testing. Second, any material that survived all three tiers of tests was deemed acceptable for clinical use. Third, each tier of the system put a great deal of weight on the tests used to accurately screen in or out a material. Although still used in principle today, the inability of in vitro and animal tests to unequivocally

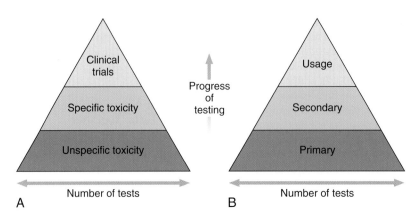

FIGURE 6.6 **Early and contemporary strategies for the use of biocompatibility tests to assess the safety of materials.** Testing begins at the bottom of the pyramid and works up. The number of tests needed decreases with the progress of testing because unacceptable materials are theoretically eliminated in the early testing stages. **A,** The earliest strategy, in which the testing strategy is focused on toxicity only. *Unspecific toxicity* refers to tests not necessarily related to the use of the material, whereas tests under *specific toxicity* are more relevant. Clinical trials are equivalent to usage tests in this scheme. **B,** The contemporary strategy used in most standards documents.

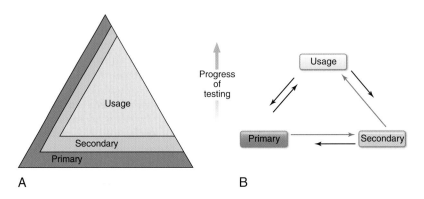

FIGURE 6.7 **Two suggested future strategies for biocompatibility testing of materials. A,** The pyramid scheme of Figure 6-6 is retained, but it is acknowledged that primary and secondary tests will play a continuing (but decreased) role as the progress of the testing continues. **B,** The usage test has the most stature and the most common progression of tests is from primary to secondary to usage, but the need to go through several iterations between testing types is acknowledged. Furthermore, the ongoing nature of biocompatibility is recognized by the need to use primary and secondary tests after clinical evaluation of a material. In this scheme the order of testing is ultimately determined as the testing and clinical use of the material continues to provide new data.

screen materials in or out has led to development of newer schemes in biocompatibility testing.

Two newer testing schemes have evolved in the past 5 years with regard to using combinations of biocompatibility tests to evaluate materials (Figure 6-7). Both of these newer schemes accommodate several important ideas. First, all tests (in vitro, animal, and usage) continue to be of value in assessing biocompatibility of a material during its development and even in its clinical service. For example, tests of inflammatory response in animals may be useful not only during the development of a material, but also if a problem is noted with the material after it has been on the market for a time. Second, these new schemes recognize the inability of current testing methods to accurately and absolutely screen in or out a material. Finally, they incorporate the philosophy that assessing the biocompatibility of a material is an ongoing process. Undoubtedly, we will see still newer strategies in the use of combinations of biocompatibility tests as the roles of materials change and the technologies for testing improve.

Standards That Regulate the Measurement of Biocompatibility

The first efforts of the American Dental Association (ADA) to establish guidelines for dental materials came in 1926 when scientists at the National Bureau of Standards (NBS), now the National Institute of

Science and Technology (NIST), developed specifications for dental amalgam. Unfortunately, recommendations on materials and conditions for biological compatibility have not kept pace with the technological development of dental materials. Reasons for this are (1) the fast advance of cellular and molecular biology, (2) the variety of tests available for assessing biocompatibility of materials, and (3) the lack of standardization of these tests.

Standardization is a difficult and lengthy process, made more difficult by disagreement on the appropriateness and significance of particular tests. One of the early attempts to develop a uniform test for all materials was the study by Dixon and Rickert in 1933, in which the toxicity of most dental materials in use at that time was investigated by implanting the materials into pockets in subdermal tissue. Small, standard-sized pieces of gold, amalgam, gutta-percha, silicates, and copper amalgam were sterilized and placed in uniformly sized pockets within skeletal muscle tissue. Biopsy specimens were evaluated microscopically after 6 months. Other early attempts to standardize techniques were carried out by Mitchell (1959) on connective tissue and by Massler (1958) on tooth pulp. Not until the passage of the Medical Device Bill by Congress in 1976 was biological testing for all medical devices (including dental materials) given a high priority. In 1972 the ADA Council on Dental Materials, Instruments, and Equipment (now the Council on Scientific Affairs) approved specification No. 41 for Recommended Standard Practices for Biological Evaluation of Dental Materials. The committee that developed this document recognized the need for standardized methods of testing and for sequential testing of materials to reduce the number of compounds that would need to be tested clinically. In 1982, an addendum was made to this document, and it was further updated to its present form in 2005.

ANSI/ADA Specification 41

Three categories of tests are described in the 2005 ANSI/ADA (American National Standards Institute/American Dental Association) specification: initial, secondary, and usage tests. This document uses the testing scheme shown in Figure 6-6, *B*. The initial tests include in vitro assays for cytotoxicity, red blood cell membrane lysis (hemolysis), mutagenesis and carcinogenesis at the cellular level, and in vivo acute physiological distress and death at the level of the organism. Based on the results of these initial tests, promising materials are tested by one or more secondary tests in small animals (in vivo) for inflammatory or immunogenic potential (e.g., dermal irritation, subcutaneous and bony implantation, and hypersensitivity tests). Finally, materials that pass secondary tests and still hold potential are subjected

to one or more in vivo usage tests, first in larger animals, often primates, and finally, with Food and Drug Administration approval, in humans. The ANSI/ADA specification No. 41, 1982 addendum, added two assays for mutagenesis—the Ames test and the Styles' cell transformation test. The standard was most recently revised to conform to the ISO (International Organization for Standardization) standard below, and was released as ANSI/ADA specification No. 41, Recommended Standard Practices for Biological Evaluation of Dental Materials (2005).

ISO 10993

In the 1980s, international efforts were initiated by several organizations to develop international standards for biomedical materials and devices. Several multinational working groups, including scientists from ANSI and the ISO, were formed to develop standard ISO 10993, published in 1992. Revision of the dental components of this document resulted in ISO 7405:2008 "Preclinical evaluation of biocompatibility of medical devices used in dentistry—Test methods for dental materials." This is the most recent ISO standard available for biocompatibility testing of dental materials.

The standard divides tests into *initial* and *supplementary* tests to assess the biological reaction to materials. Initial tests are tests for cytotoxicity, sensitization, and systemic toxicity. Some of these tests are done in vitro, others in animals in nonusage situations. Most of the supplementary tests, to assess things such as chronic toxicity, carcinogenicity, and biodegradation, are done in animal systems, many in usage situations. Significantly, although guidelines for the selection of tests are given in part 1 of the standard and are based on how long the material will be present; whether it will contact body surface only, blood, or bone; and whether the device communicates externally from the body, the ultimate selection of tests for a specific material is left up to the manufacturer, who must present and defend the testing results.

BIOCOMPATIBILITY OF DENTAL MATERIALS

Reactions of Pulp

Microleakage

There is evidence that restorative materials may not bond to enamel or dentin with sufficient strength to resist the forces of contraction during polymerization, wear, or thermal cycling. If a bond does not form, or debonding occurs, bacteria, food debris, or saliva may be drawn into the gap between the restoration and the tooth by capillary action.

This effect has been termed *microleakage*. The importance of microleakage in pulpal irritation has been extensively studied. Several early studies reported that various dental restorative materials irritated pulp tissue in animal tests. However, several other studies hypothesized that the products of microleakage, not the restorative materials, caused the irritation. Subsequently, numerous studies showed that bacteria present under restorations and in dentinal tubules might be responsible for pulpal irritation. Other studies showed that bacteria or bacterial products such as lipopolysaccharides could cause pulp irritation within hours of being applied to dentin.

Finally, a classic animal study shed light on the roles of restorative materials and microleakage on pulpal irritation. Amalgam, composite, zinc phosphate cement, and silicate cement were used as restorative materials in class 5 cavity preparations in monkey teeth. The materials were placed directly on pulp tissues. Half of the restorations were surface-sealed with ZOE cement. Although some irritation was evident in all restorations at 7 days, after 21 days, the sealed restorations showed less pulpal irritation than those not sealed, presumably because microleakage had been eliminated. Only zinc phosphate cement elicited a long-term inflammatory response. Furthermore, the sealed teeth exhibited a much higher rate of dentin bridging under the material. Only amalgam seemed to prevent bridging. This study suggests that microleakage plays a significant role in pulpal irritation, but that the materials can also alter normal pulpal and dentinal repair.

Recently, the concept of *nanoleakage* has been put forward. Like microleakage, nanoleakage refers to the leakage of saliva, bacteria, or material components through the interface between a material and tooth structure. However, nanoleakage refers specifically to dentin bonding, and may occur between mineralized dentin and a bonded material in the very small spaces of demineralized collagen matrix into which the bonded material did not penetrate. Thus nanoleakage can occur even when the bond between the material and dentin is intact. It is not known how significant a role nanoleakage plays in the biological response to materials, but it is thought to play at least some role and it is suspected of contributing to the hydrolytic degradation of the dentin-material bond, leading ultimately to much more serious microleakage.

The full biological effects of restorative materials on the pulp are still not clear. Restorative materials may directly affect pulpal tissues, or may play an auxiliary role by causing sublethal changes in pulpal cells that make them more susceptible to bacteria or neutrophils. It is clear, however, that the design of tests measuring pulpal irritation to *materials* must include provisions for eliminating bacteria, bacterial products, and other microleakage. Furthermore, the role of dentin in mitigating the effects of microleakage remains to be fully understood. Recent research has focused on the effects that resin components have on the ability of odontoblasts to form secondary dentin. Other research has established the rates at which these components traverse the dentin (see the next section on dentin bonding).

Although it is true that the majority of studies in this arena have in the past focused on the damaging effects of materials on the cells of the pulp and dentin, more recent evidence suggests that there are potentially beneficial effects that may derive from these interactions. Subtoxic exposure to certain dental materials, such as acid etchants, bonding resins, liners and bases, cements, and restorative materials, may solubilize molecules sequestered within the dentin during tooth development. These molecules include growth factors and other proteins and enzymes capable of stimulating existing odontoblasts or signaling undifferentiated cells to migrate to the site and begin the process of dentinal regeneration. These events may occur whether or not the material produces a sealed margin with the tooth, and is likely moderated by the health of the tooth in terms of the level of inflammation and the presence of bacterial infection. The exciting aspect of acquiring this new knowledge is the potential to design dental materials capable of initiating the tooth repair process in a systematic rather than random way. This is discussed at greater length in Chapter 16, Tissue Engineering.

Dentin Bonding

Traditionally, the strength of bonds to enamel have been higher than those to dentin. Bonding to dentin has proved more difficult because of its composition (being both organic and inorganic), wetness, and lower mineral content. The wettability of demineralized dentin collagen matrix has also been problematic. Because the dentinal tubules and their resident odontoblasts are extensions of the pulp, bonding to dentin also involves biocompatibility issues.

After being cut, such as in a cavity preparation, the dentin surface that remains is covered by a 1- to 2-μm layer of organic and inorganic debris. This layer has been named the *smear layer* (Figure 6-8). In addition to covering the surface of the dentin, the smear layer debris is also deposited into the tubules to form dentinal plugs. The smear layer and dentinal plugs, which appear impermeable when viewed by electron microscopy, reduce the flow of fluid (convective transport) significantly. However, research has shown that diffusion of molecules as large as albumin (66 kDa) will occur through the smear layer. The presence of this smear layer is important to the strength of bonds to restorative materials and to the biocompatibility of those bonded materials.

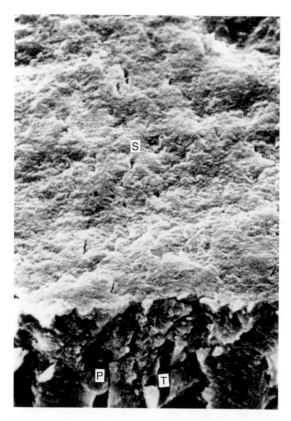

FIGURE 6.8 **Scanning electron micrograph of cut dentin.** When a dentin surface is cut with a bur, a layer of debris, called the *smear layer (S)*, remains on the surface. The smear layer consists of organic and inorganic debris that covers the dentinal surface and the tubules *(T)*. Often, the debris fills the distal part of the tubules in a smear plug *(P)*. *(From Brännström M: Dentin and Pulp in Restorative Dentistry. Dental Therapeutics AB, Stockholm, 1981.)*

Numerous studies have shown that removing the smear layer improves the strength of the bond between dentin and restorative materials with contemporary dentin bonding agents, although earlier research with older bonding agents showed the opposite effect. A variety of agents have been used to remove the smear layer, including acids, chelating agents such as ethylenediamine tetraacetic acid (EDTA), sodium hypochlorite, and proteolytic enzymes. Removing the smear layer increases the wetness of the dentin and requires that the bonding agent be able to wet dentin and displace dentinal fluid. The precise mechanism by which bonding occurs remains unclear. However, it appears that the most successful bonding agents are able to penetrate into the layer of collagen that remains after acid etching. There, they create a *hybrid layer* of resin and collagen in intimate contact with dentin and dentinal tubules. The strength of the collagen itself has also been shown to be important to bond strengths.

From the standpoint of biocompatibility, the removal of the smear layer may pose a threat to the pulp for three reasons. First, its removal juxtaposes resin materials and dentin without a barrier, and therefore increases the risk that these materials can diffuse and cause pulpal irritation. Second, the removal of the smear layer makes any microleakage more significant because a significant barrier to the diffusion of bacteria or bacterial products toward the pulp is removed. Third, the acids used to remove the smear layer are a potential source of irritation themselves. Nevertheless, removal of the smear layer is now a routine procedure because superior bond strengths are achieved. Some recent techniques that etch and "bond" direct pulp exposures make biocompatibility of the bonding agents even more critical, because the dentinal barrier between the materials and the pulp is totally absent.

Biocompatibility of acids used to remove the smear layer has been extensively studied. Numerous acids, including phosphoric, hydrochloric, citric, and lactic acids, have been used to remove the smear layer. The effect of these acids on pulp tissues depends on a number of factors, including thickness of dentin between the restoration and the pulp, strength of the acid, and degree of etching. Most studies have shown that dentin is a very efficient buffer of protons, and that most of the acid never reaches the pulp if sufficient dentin remains. A dentin thickness of 0.5 mm has proved adequate in this regard. Citric or lactic acids are not as well buffered, probably because these weak acids do not dissociate as efficiently. Usage tests that have studied the effects of acids have shown that phosphoric, pyruvic, and citric acids produce moderate pulpal inflammatory responses, but this resolves after 8 weeks. Recent research has shown that in most cases the penetration depth of acid into the dentin is less than 100 μm. However, the possibility of adverse effects of these acids cannot be ruled out, because odontoblastic processes in the tubules may be affected even though the acids do not reach the pulp itself.

The more positive aspect of this dissolution of the dentin by acids used in dentin bonding agents may be the release of potentially bioactive molecules entrapped during development. Significant research has shown that extracted dentin matrix proteins, which contain a large variety of phosphorylated and nonphosphorylated proteins, proteoglycans, metalloproteinases, and a variety of growth factors, may be released from intact dentin by basic and acidic chemicals, including acid etchants used in dental adhesives. Studies have shown that many of these molecules may serve as cell signaling agents to recruit undifferentiated cells or as direct stimulants to up-regulate the production of extracellular matrix as a step in the process of dentin remineralization.

The specific role for each of the molecules in this process is not currently known, nor is it known what the desirable concentration of a specific protein or combination of molecules is to produce optimal results. However, the fact that these naturally present molecules may be released by routine dental restorative procedures and serve as participants in the repair process provides an opportunity for the development and design of future materials.

Bonding Agents

Numerous bonding agents have been developed and are applied to cut dentin during restoration of the tooth. There have been a number of studies of biocompatibility of these bonding systems. Many of these reagents are cytotoxic to cells in vitro if tested alone. However, when placed on dentin and rinsed with water between applications of subsequent reagents as prescribed by the manufacturer, cytotoxicity is reduced. Longer-term in vitro studies suggest, however, that components of the bonding agents may penetrate up to 0.5 mm of dentin and cause significant suppression of cellular metabolism for up to 4 weeks after application. This suggests that residual unbound constituents may cause adverse reactions.

Hydroxyethyl methacrylate (HEMA), a hydrophilic resin contained in several bonding systems, is at least 100 times less cytotoxic in tissue culture than Bis-GMA. Studies using long-term in vitro systems have shown, however, that adverse effects of resins occur at much lower concentrations (by a factor of 100 or more) when exposure times are increased to 4 to 6 weeks. Many cytotoxic effects of resin components are reduced significantly by the presence of a dentin barrier. However, if the dentin in the floor of the cavity preparation is thin (<0.1 mm), there is some evidence that HEMA is cytotoxic in vivo. Further, studies have shown that HEMA is capable of diffusing through dentin, presumably via the dentinal tubules, even in opposition to an outward flow of fluid driven by normal pulpal pressure. What effect HEMA may then have on the pulp cells in situ is not known, but HEMA has been shown to stimulate the expression of growth factors in mouse odontoblast-like cells.

Other studies have established the in vitro cytotoxicity of most of the common resins in bonding agents, such as Bis-GMA, triethylene glycol dimethacrylate, urethane dimethacrylate (UDMA), and others. Combinations of HEMA and other resins found in dentin bonding agents may act synergistically to cause cytotoxic effects in vitro. There have been very few clinical studies of diffusion of hydrophilic and hydrophobic resin components through dentin. These studies indicated that some diffusion of these components occurs in vivo as well. Interestingly, there has been one report that some resin components

enhance the growth of oral bacteria. If substantiated, this would cause concern about the ability of resin-based materials to increase plaque formation.

Finally, studies have also shown the release of matrix metalloproteinases (MMPs) from dentin by virtue of its interaction with the acid components in dentin adhesives may cause degradation of the adhesive bond by enzymatic action on the exposed collagen within the hybrid layer. The application of an MMP inhibitor, such as chlorhexidine, has been shown to minimize this effect, and has been recommended for maintaining the durability of the dentin bond. However, the overall effect of chlorhexadine on pulp cells has yet to be determined.

Resin-Based Materials

For tooth restorations, resin-based materials have been used as cements and restorative materials. Because they are a combination of organic and inorganic phases, these materials are called *resin composites.* in vitro, freshly set chemically cured and light-cured resins often cause moderate cytotoxic reactions in cultured cells over 24 to 72 hours of exposure, although several newer systems seem to have minimal toxicity. The cytotoxicity is significantly reduced 24 to 48 hours after setting and by the presence of a dentin barrier. Several studies have shown that some materials are persistently cytotoxic in vitro even up to 4 weeks, whereas others gradually improve, and a few newer systems show little toxicity even initially. In all cases, cytotoxicity is thought to be mediated by resin components released from the materials. Evidence indicates that the light-cured resins are less cytotoxic than chemically cured systems, but this effect is highly dependent on the curing efficiency of the light and the type of resin system. in vivo, usage tests have been used to assess the biological response to resin composites. The pulpal inflammatory response to chemically and light-activated resin composites was low to moderate after 3 days when they were placed in cavities with approximately 0.5 mm of remaining dentin. Any reaction diminished as the postoperative periods increased to 5 to 8 weeks and was accompanied by an increase in reparative dentin (Figure 6-9). With a protective liner or a bonding agent, the reaction of the pulp to resin composite materials is minimal. The longer-term effects of resins placed directly on pulpal tissue are not known, but are suspected to be less favorable.

Amalgam and Casting Alloys

Dental amalgam has been used extensively for dental restorations. Biocompatibility of amalgam is thought to be determined largely by the corrosion products released while in service. Corrosion, in turn, depends on the type of amalgam, whether it contains the γ_2 phase, and its composition. In cell

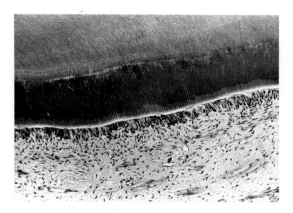

FIGURE 6.9 **Light micrograph of the dentinal and pulpal response to unlined composite at 5 to 8 weeks in a monkey.** The primary dentin is the lighter layer seen at the top. The tubules are evident. Secondary dentin is occurring (*the dark, wide middle layer*), and it is closely approximated by intact odontoblasts in the pulp. Few inflammatory cells are present. The response seen in this micrograph is indicative of a favorable response to the material. *(Courtesy of A.K. Avery, Ann Arbor, Michigan.)*

culture screening tests, free or nonreacted mercury from amalgam is toxic. With the addition of copper, amalgams become toxic to cells in culture, but low-copper amalgam that has set for 24 hours does not inhibit cell growth.

Implantation tests show that low-copper amalgams are well tolerated, but high-copper amalgams cause severe reactions when in direct contact with tissue. Unreacted mercury or copper leaching out from these high-copper alloys has usually been the constituent leading to adverse response. An in vitro study of the effects of particulate amalgams and their individual phases on macrophages showed that all particles except the γ_2 are effectively phagocytized by macrophages. Cell damage was seen in treated cultures exposed to particulate γ_1. In usage tests, the response of the pulp to amalgam in shallow cavities or in deeper but lined cavities is minimal, and amalgam rarely causes irreversible damage to the pulp. However, pain results from using amalgams in deep, unlined cavity preparations (0.5 mm or less remaining dentin), with an inflammatory response occurring after 3 days.

This pain may be related to the high thermal and electrical conductivity of the material, which is significantly mitigated by the presence of a barrier of remaining dentin or an insulating lining material. Thus, in cavities with less than 0.5 to 1.0 mm of dentin remaining in the floor, the cavity preparation should be lined for two reasons. First, the transfer of hot and cold stimuli, primarily from food and drink, through the amalgam may be substantial. Second, margins of newly placed amalgam restorations show significant microleakage. Marginal leakage of salivary and microbial products is probably enhanced by the natural daily thermal cycle in the oral cavity, which may expand and contract the marginal gap leading to a percolation of fluids. Although long-term sealing of the margins occurs through the buildup of corrosion products, the timeframe over which this occurs is somewhat a function of the composition of the amalgam, being longer for the high-copper amalgams in use today.

Usage tests reported that after 3 days, the pulpal response to high-copper amalgams appears similar to that elicited by low-copper amalgams in deep, unlined cavities. At 5 weeks they provoke only slight pulpal response. At 8 weeks the inflammatory response was reduced. Bacterial tests on the high-copper amalgam pellets have revealed little inhibitory effect on serotypes of *Streptococcus mutans*, thus suggesting that metallic elements were not released in amounts necessary to kill these microorganisms. Although the high-copper amalgams seem biologically acceptable in usage tests, liners are suggested for all deep cavities. Again, this may be related more to a need for thermal and electrical insulation than a concern over toxicity. Further, the diffusion of released metallic elements into the tooth structure produces discoloration, and may be minimized by the presence of an intervening liner. There are also reports of inflammatory reactions of the dentin and pulp, similar to the reactions to many other restorative materials. Mercury has been found in the lysosomes of macrophages and fibroblasts in some patients with lesions.

Although not a commonly used material, amalgams based on gallium rather than mercury have been developed to provide direct restorative materials that are mercury-free. In cell culture, these alloys appear to be no more cytotoxic than traditional high-copper amalgams. These restorations release significant amounts of gallium in vitro, but the biological significance of this release is not known. In implantation tests, gallium alloys caused significant foreign body reaction. Clinically, these materials show much higher corrosion rates than standard amalgams. This leads to surface roughness and discoloration. There are few reports of pulpal responses to these materials.

Cast alloys have been used for single restorations, fixed partial dentures, ceramic-metal crowns, and removable partial dentures. The gold content in these alloys ranges from 0 wt% to 85 wt%. These alloys contain several other noble and non-noble metals that may have an adverse effect on cells if they are released from the alloys. However, metal ions released from these materials are most likely to contact gingival and mucosal tissues, whereas the pulp is more likely to be affected by the cement retaining the restoration.

Glass Ionomers

Glass ionomer has been used as a cement (luting agent), liner, base, and restorative material. Light-cured ionomer systems have been introduced; these systems use HEMA or other monomers or oligomers as additives or as pendant chains on the polyacrylic acid main chain. In screening tests, freshly prepared ionomer is mildly cytotoxic, but this effect is reduced over time. The fluoride release from these materials, which is probably of some therapeutic value, has been implicated in this cytotoxicity in vitro. Some researchers have reported that certain systems are more cytotoxic than others, and though the reasons for this are not clear, presumably it is related to the composition of the glasses used in the material, which may contain aluminum, calcium, manganese, zinc, strontium, and other metallic elements.

The overall pulpal biocompatibility of glass ionomer materials has been attributed to the weak nature of the polyacrylic acid, as well as to its high molecular weight. Thus polyacrylic acid is unable to diffuse through dentin due to its large size. In usage tests the pulp reaction to these cements is mild, and histological studies show that any inflammatory infiltrate from ionomer is minimal or absent after 1 month. There have been several reports of pulpal hyperalgesia for short periods (days) after placing glass ionomers in cervical cavities. This effect is probably the result of increased dentin permeability after acid etching. In any case, glass ionomer has not been shown to be well tolerated when placed directly upon living pulp tissue as a direct pulp capping agent.

As previously discussed with dentin bonding agents, acid dental materials have the capacity for demineralizing dentin and therefore releasing bioactive molecules present within this tissue. Although this effect has not been shown specifically for glass ionomers to date, it seems reasonable to assume that it does occur clinically. In a recent study in nonhuman primates, dentin matrix proteins were shown to enhance the formation of reactionary dentin over exposed pulps, compared with calcium hydroxide or resin-modified glass ionomer. Although the response to resin-modified glass ionomer was less consistent than calcium hydroxide, in many cases it did result in new dentin formation, even when directly exposed to the pulp. It is important to note that the natural tooth repair process producing reactionary dentin does occur, following an initial inflammatory reaction, under glass ionomer when the material is placed over an existing dentin surface. Thus it is possible that the repair process is again aided by the presence of the bioactive molecules released from the dentin by the mild demineralization produced by the material under these conditions.

Liners, Varnishes, and Nonresin Cements

Calcium hydroxide cavity liners come in many forms, ranging from saline suspensions with a very alkaline pH (above 12) to modified forms containing zinc oxide, titanium dioxide, and resins. Resin-containing preparations can be polymerized chemically, but light-activated systems are also available. The high pH of calcium hydroxide in suspension leads to extreme cytotoxicity in screening tests. Calcium hydroxide cements containing resins cause mild-to-moderate cytotoxic effects in tissue culture in both the freshly set and long-term set conditions. Inhibition of cell metabolism is reversible in tissue culture by high levels of serum proteins, suggesting that protein binding or buffering in inflamed pulp tissue may play an important role in detoxifying these materials in vivo. The initial response after exposing pulp tissue to these highly alkaline aqueous pulp-capping agents is necrosis to a depth of 1 mm or more. The alkaline pH also helps to coagulate any hemorrhagic exudate of the superficial pulp.

Shortly after necrosis occurs, neutrophils infiltrate into the subnecrotic zone. After 5 to 8 weeks, only a slight inflammatory response remains. Within weeks to months, however, the necrotic zone undergoes dystrophic calcification, which appears to be a stimulus for dentin bridge formation.

When resins are incorporated into the compound, these calcium hydroxide compounds become less irritating and are able to stimulate reparative dentin bridge formation more quickly than the $Ca(OH)_2$ suspension alone. Significantly, this occurs with no zone of necrosis, and reparative dentin is laid down adjacent to the liner (Figure 6-10). This indicates that replacement odontoblasts form the dentin bridge in contact with the liner. However, some of these materials evidently break down with time and create a gap between the restoration and the cavity wall. Resin-containing calcium hydroxide pulp capping agents are the most effective liners now available for treating pulp exposures, and after treatment, the uninfected pulp undergoes a relatively uncomplicated wound-healing process.

Recent evidence suggests that calcium hydroxide placed on residual dentin in a tooth preparation may also have a stimulating effect on dentin remineralization through the solubilization of noncollagenous proteins, including growth factors such as transforming growth factor-beta-1 (TGF-β1), and glycosaminoglycans from the dentin. Mineral trioxide aggregate (MTA) has the same effect, and possibly to an even greater degree. This is perhaps not surprising because the main soluble component from MTA has been shown to be calcium hydroxide. Thus when placed in contact with dentin, these materials may cause the release of these bioactive molecules, which then serve as signaling agents to recruit undifferentiated cells to the wound site.

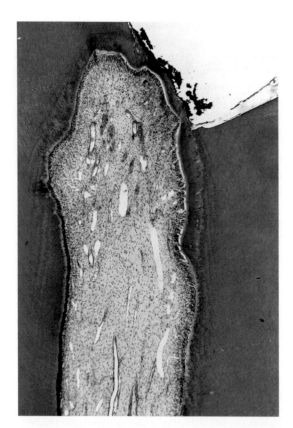

FIGURE 6.10 **Light micrograph of a dentin bridge that has formed between a material and the pulp in a monkey.** Initially, the pulp of the tooth was purposely exposed *(top right)* with a bur. The exposure was covered with a calcium hydroxide pulp-capping agent for 5 weeks before histological evaluation. A layer of secondary dentin has formed at the site of the pulp exposure, forming a dentin bridge. Some inflammatory cells are evident under the bridge, but the pulpal response is generally favorable. *(Courtesy of D.R. Heys, Ann Arbor, Michigan.)*

These cells may then differentiate to odontoblast-like cells that begin the process of dentin bridge formation described above. Evidence exists both in cell culture and in situ that pulp cells exposed to MTA undergo proliferation and migration, followed by differentiation to odontoblast-like cells. Further, studies have shown that MTA-derived products can stimulate osteoblast-like cells and fibroblasts to express proteins, such as osteonectin, osteocalcin, and osteopontin, which are involved with extracellular matrix formation and mineralization. Thus, the mode of dentin bridge formation under materials such as calcium hydroxide and MTA may be more complex than simply a reaction to an elevated pH stimulus.

Numerous investigators have analyzed the effects of applying thin liners such as resin-based copal *varnishes* and polystyrenes under restorations.

These materials are not generally used under resin-based materials, because resin components dissolve the thin film of varnish. Because liners are used in such thin layers, they do not provide thermal insulation, but initially isolate the dentinal tubule contents from the cavity preparation. They may also reduce penetration of bacteria or chemical substances for a time. However, because of the thinness of the film and formation of pinpoint holes, the integrity of these materials is not as reliable as that of other cavity liners applied in a greater thickness.

Zinc phosphate has been widely used as a cement for seating castings and fixing orthodontic bands, and as a thermal insulating base under metallic dental restorations, because the thermal conductivity of this cement is approximately equal to that of enamel and is considerably less than that of metals. In vitro screening tests indicate that zinc phosphate cement elicits strong-to-moderate cytotoxic reactions that decrease with time. Leaching of zinc ions and a low pH may explain these effects. The dilution of leached cement products by dentin filtration has been shown to protect the pulp from most of these cytotoxic effects. Focal necrosis, observed in implantation tests with zinc phosphate cements injected into rat pulp, confirm the cytotoxic effects of this cement when it contacts pulp tissue. In usage tests in deep cavity preparations, moderate-to-severe localized pulpal damage is produced within 3 days, probably because of the initial low pH (4.2 at 3 minutes). However, the pH of the set cement approaches neutrality after 48 hours. By 5 to 8 weeks, only mild chronic inflammation is present, and reparative dentin has usually formed. Because of the initially painful and damaging effects on the pulp by this cement when placed in deep cavity preparations, the placement of a protective layer of a dentin bonding agent, ZOE, varnish, or calcium hydroxide, is recommended in preparations with minimal remaining dentin covering the pulp.

Zinc polyacrylate cements (polycarboxylate cements) were developed to combine the strength of zinc phosphate cements with the adhesiveness and biocompatibility of ZOE cements. In short-term tissue culture tests, cytotoxicity of freshly set and completely set cements has correlated with both the release of zinc and fluoride ions into the culture medium and with a reduced pH. Some researchers suggest that this cytotoxicity is an artifact of tissue culture because the phosphate buffers in the culture medium facilitate zinc ion leaching from the cement. Supporting this theory, cell growth inhibition can be reversed if EDTA, which chelates zinc, is added to the culture medium. Furthermore, inhibition of cells decreases as the cement sets. The polymer component of the cement may also be of concern, because concentrations of polyacrylic acid above 1% appear to be cytotoxic in tissue culture tests. On the other hand, subcutaneous and bone implant tests over a 1-year period have not indicated long-term cytotoxicity of these cements. Thus other mechanisms such as buffering and protein-binding of these materials may neutralize these effects in vivo over time. Polyacrylate cements evoke a pulpal response similar to that caused by ZOE, with a slight-to-moderate response after 3 days and only mild, chronic inflammation after 5 weeks. Reparative dentin formation is minimal with these cements, and thus they are recommended only in cavities with intact dentin in the floors of the cavity preparations.

ZOE cements have been used in dentistry for many years. in vitro, eugenol from ZOE fixes cells, depresses cell respiration, and reduces nerve transmission with direct contact. Surprisingly, it is relatively innocuous in usage tests with class 5 cavity preparations. This is not contradictory for a number of reasons. The effects of eugenol are dose dependent and diffusion through dentin dilutes eugenol by several orders of magnitude. Thus, although the concentration of eugenol in the cavity preparations just below the ZOE has been reported to be 10^{-2} M (bactericidal), the concentration on the pulpal side of the dentin may be 10^{-4} M or less. This lower concentration reportedly suppresses nerve transmission and inhibits synthesis of prostaglandins and leukotrienes (antiinflammatory). In addition and as described before, ZOE may form a temporary seal against bacterial invasion. In cavity preparations in primate teeth (usage tests), ZOE caused only a slight-to-moderate inflammatory reaction within the first week. This was reduced to a mild, chronic inflammatory reaction, with some reparative dentin formation (within 5 to 8 weeks), when cavities were deep. For this reason, it has been used as a negative control substance for comparison with restorative procedures in usage tests.

Bleaching Agents

Bleaching agents have been used on nonvital and vital teeth for many years, but their use on vital teeth has increased astronomically in recent years. These agents usually contain some form of peroxide (generally carbamide or hydrogen peroxide) in a gel that can be applied to the teeth either by a dentist or at home by a patient. The agents may be in contact with teeth for several minutes to several hours depending on the formulation of the material. Home bleaching agents may be applied for weeks to even months in some cases. in vitro studies have shown that peroxides can rapidly (within minutes) traverse the dentin in sufficient concentrations to be cytotoxic. The cytotoxicity depends to a large extent on the concentration of the peroxide in the bleaching agent. Other studies have even shown that peroxides can rapidly penetrate intact enamel and reach the pulp in a few

minutes. In vivo studies have demonstrated adverse pulpal effects from bleaching, and most reports agree that a legitimate concern exists about the long-term use of these products on vital teeth. In clinical studies, the occurrence of tooth sensitivity is very common with the use of these agents, although the cause of these reactions is not known. Bleaching agents will also chemically burn the gingiva if the agent is not sequestered adequately in the bleaching tray. This is not a problem with a properly constructed tray, and long-term, low-dose effects of peroxides on the gingival and periodontal tissues are not known.

Reaction of Other Oral Soft Tissues to Restorative Materials

Restorative materials may cause reactions in the oral soft tissues such as the gingiva. It is not clear how much of the in vivo cytotoxicity observed is caused by the restorative materials and how much is caused by products of bacterial plaque that accumulate on teeth and restorations. In general, conditions that promote retention of plaque, such as rough surfaces or open margins, increase inflammatory reactions around these materials. However, released products from restorative materials also contribute either directly or indirectly to this inflammation. This is particularly true in areas where the washing effects of saliva are minimal, such as in interproximal areas, in deep gingival pockets, or under removable appliances. Several studies have documented increased inflammation or recession of gingiva adjacent to restorations where plaque indexes are low. In these studies, released products from materials could cause inflammation in the absence of plaque or could inhibit formation of plaque and cause inflammation in gingiva. in vitro research has shown that components from dental materials and plaque may synergize to enhance inflammatory reactions.

Cements exhibit some soft-tissue cytotoxicity in the freshly set state, but this decreases substantially over time. The buffering and protein-binding effects of saliva appear to mitigate these cytotoxic effects.

Resin composites in direct contact with fibroblasts are initially very cytotoxic in vitro. This cytotoxicity most likely results from unpolymerized components in the air-inhibited layer that leach out from the materials. Other in vitro studies, which have aged the composites in artificial saliva for up to 6 weeks, have shown that toxicity diminishes with some materials but remains high for others. Some of the newer composites with non-Bis-GMA and non-UDMA matrices have significantly lower cytotoxicity in vitro, presumably because of lower amounts of leached components. Polished composites show markedly less cytotoxicity in vitro, although some materials are persistently toxic even in the polished state.

Recently, there has been significant controversy about the ability of bisphenol A and bisphenol A dimethacrylate to cause estrogen-like responses in vitro. These compounds are basic components of many commercial composites. However, there is no evidence that xenoestrogenic effects are a concern in vivo from any commercial resin. Relatively little is known about other in vivo effects of released components of composites on soft tissues, although the concerns are similar to those regarding denture base resin and soft liners (see later discussion in this section on page 127). There is some evidence that methacrylate-based composite components may cause significant rates of hypersensitivity, although few clinical trials exist.

Amalgams have been used for 150 years; about 200 million amalgams are inserted each year in the United States and Europe. In spite of its substantial history, however, periodically concern arises about the biocompatibility of amalgam. Allergic reactions to amalgam restorations are rare, although there are case reports of allergic contact dermatitis, gingivitis, stomatitis, and remote cutaneous reactions. This is not surprising, because there is no material that 100% of the population is immune to 100% of the time. Such responses usually disappear in a few days or, if not, on removal of the amalgam or with use of a cavity liner. Other local or systemic effects from mercury contained in dental amalgam have not been demonstrated. No well-conducted scientific study has conclusively shown that dental amalgam, placed and used correctly, produces any ill effects.

In patients with oral lesions near *amalgam* sites, positive patch tests have been reported. However, the appropriate patch test has still not been determined. Amalgam restorations carried into the gingival crevice may cause inflammation of the gingiva because of products of corrosion or bacterial plaque. Seven days after placing an amalgam, a few inflammatory cells appear in the gingival connective tissue, and hydropic degeneration of some epithelial cells may be seen. Some proliferation of epithelial cells into the connective tissue may also occur by 30 days, and chronic mononuclear cell infiltration of connective tissue is evident. Increased vascularity persists, with more epithelial cells invaginating into the connective tissue. Some of these changes may be a chronic response of the gingiva to plaque on the margins of the amalgam. Nevertheless, corrosion products from amalgam cannot be ruled out at this time because implanted amalgams produce similar responses in connective tissues in animals. In addition, although copper enhances the physical properties of amalgam and is bactericidal, it is also toxic to host cells and causes severe tissue reactions in implantation tests. With the increased use of more corrosion-resistant amalgams, the volume of corrosion products and subsequent reactions are reduced. Animal implantation studies have shown severe reactions to gallium-based alloys that have been used as amalgam replacements.

There is a report in the literature in which amalgam and resin composite restorations were placed in cavity preparations in monkey central incisors that had been extracted for less than 1 hour. The cavities, with depths of about 2 mm, were placed halfway between the cementoenamel junction and the root tip. The teeth were immediately replanted after restoration, and the animals were sacrificed at intervals up to 6 months. Repair of the periodontal ligament (PDL) took place in a normal fashion except for the presence of an intense inflammatory infiltrate in the PDL adjacent to the amalgams through 2 weeks. A similar effect was observed through 3 to 6 months with the resin composites. This result suggests that resin composites and amalgam release cytotoxic materials that cause tissue responses, at least at sites of implantation. For materials that are placed where they are rinsed in saliva, these cytotoxic agents are probably washed away before they harm the gingiva.

However, rough surfaces on these types of restorations have been associated with increased inflammation in vivo. Usage tests in which restorations were extended into the gingival crevice have shown that finished materials gave a much milder inflammatory response than unfinished materials. The detrimental effect of surface roughness has been attributed to the increased plaque retention on these surfaces. However, rough surfaces on alloy restorations also caused increased cytotoxic effects in vitro, where plaque was absent. This and other in vitro studies again would suggest that the cytotoxic response to alloys may be associated with release of elements from the alloys, and that the increased surface area of a rough surface may enhance release of these elements.

Implantation studies have shown that amalgam is reasonably well tolerated by soft and hard tissue. In a rabbit muscle implantation model, biological reactions to amalgams were found to depend on the time of implantation. All amalgams were strongly toxic 1 hour after setting. After 7 days, only high-copper amalgam showed any reaction.

In another series of studies, low- and high-copper amalgam powders and various phases of amalgam were implanted subcutaneously in guinea pigs. After 1.5 to 3 months, fine secondary particles containing silver and tin were distributed throughout the lesions. These gave rise to macroscopic tattooing of the skin. Secondary material and small, degrading, primary particles from both types of amalgam were detected in the submandibular lymph nodes. Elevated mercury levels were detected in the blood, bile, kidneys, liver, spleen, and lungs, with the highest concentrations found in the renal cortex.

In another study, primates received occlusal amalgam fillings or maxillary bone implants of amalgam for 1 year. Amalgam fillings caused deposition of mercury in the spinal ganglia, anterior pituitary, adrenal, medulla, liver, kidneys, lungs, and intestinal lymph glands. Maxillary amalgam implants released mercury into the same organs, except for the liver, lungs, and intestinal lymph glands. Organs from control animals were devoid of precipitate. However, neither of these studies, nor any other, has demonstrated any changes in biochemical function of any of the laden organs.

Note that studies using powdered amalgam likely overestimate the amount of breakdown products, and therefore biological response, because the surface area of powders can be 5 to 10 times the surface area of a solid component. It must also be emphasized that any reaction to amalgam, whether in cell culture, local tissue response, or systemic response, does not necessarily imply a reaction to mercury. Such reactions could be in response to some other constituent of the amalgam or corrosion product. For example, in vitro cell culture testing that measured fibroblasts affected by various elements and phases of amalgams has shown that pure copper and zinc show greater cytotoxicity than pure silver and mercury. Pure tin has not been shown to be cytotoxic (Figure 6-11). The γ_1 phase is moderately cytotoxic. Cytotoxicity is decreased by the addition of 1.5% and 5% tin (Figure 6-12). However, the addition of 1.5% zinc to γ_1 containing 1.5% tin increases cytotoxicity to the same level as that of pure zinc. Whenever zinc is present, higher cytotoxicity is revealed. High-copper amalgams show the same cytotoxicity as a zinc-free, low-copper amalgam. The addition of selenium does not reduce amalgam cytotoxicity, and excessive additions of selenium increase cytotoxicity. The cytotoxicity of amalgams decreases after 24 hours, possibly from the combined effects of surface oxidation and further amalgamation. The results of this study suggest that the major contributor to the cytotoxicity of amalgam alloy powders is probably copper, whereas that for amalgam is zinc.

Casting alloys have a long history of in vivo use with a generally good record of biocompatibility. Some questions about the biological liability of elemental release from many of the formulations developed in the past 10 years have arisen, but there is no clinical evidence that elemental release is a problem, aside from hypersensitivity. Nickel allergy is a relatively common problem, occurring in 10% to 20% of females. It is a significant risk from nickel-based alloys, because release of nickel ions from these alloys is generally higher than for high-noble or noble alloys. Stainless steels, commonly used in preformed pediatric crowns, also contain a significant concentration of Ni in their composition. Palladium sensitivity has also been a concern in some countries,

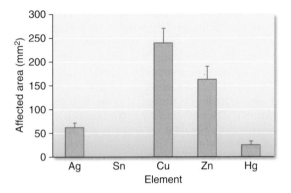

FIGURE 6.11 **Quantitative representation of the affected areas of fibroblasts reveals the magnitude of cytotoxicity of amalgam elements.** Standard deviations are represented by vertical bars. *Ag,* Silver; *Sn,* tin; *Cu,* copper; *Zn,* zinc; *Hg,* mercury. *(From Kaga M, Seale NS, Hanawa T, et. al: Dent. Mater. 7, 68, 1991.)*

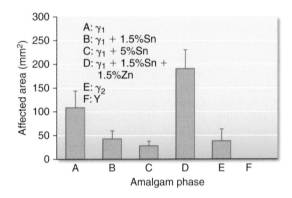

FIGURE 6.12 **Quantitative representation of the affected areas of fibroblasts reveals the magnitude of cytotoxicity of amalgam phases.** Standard deviations are represented by vertical bars. *(From Kaga M, Seale NS, Hanawa T, et. al: Dent. Mater. 7, 68, 1991.)*

although the incidence of true palladium allergy is one third that of nickel allergy. However, it has been clinically documented that patients with palladium allergy are virtually always allergic to nickel. The converse is not true, however.

In vitro, there have been numerous articles published on the effects of metal ions on cells in the gingival tissues, such as epithelial cells, fibroblasts, and macrophages. For the most part, the concentrations of metal ions required to cause problems with these cells in vitro are greater than those released from most casting alloys. However, some recent research has shown that extended exposures to low doses of metal ions may also have biological liabilities. These new data are noteworthy because the low-dose concentrations approach those known to be released from some alloys. Clinical significance of this research, however, is not known.

Denture base materials, especially methacrylates, have been associated with immune hypersensitivity reactions of gingiva and mucosa more than any other dental material. The greatest potential for hypersensitization is for dental and laboratory personnel who are exposed repeatedly to a variety of unreacted components. Hypersensitivity has been documented to the acrylic and diacrylic monomers, certain curing agents, antioxidants, amines, and formaldehyde. For patients, however, most of these materials have undergone the polymerization reaction, and the incidence of hypersensitization is quite low. Screening tests for sensitization potential include testing the unreacted ingredients, the polymeric substance after reaction, and oil, saline, or aqueous extracts of the polymer using the in vitro tests previously described. In addition to hypersensitivity, visible light-cured denture base resins and denture base resin sealants have been shown to be cytotoxic to epithelial cells in culture.

Soft-tissue responses to *soft denture liners* and *denture adhesives* are of concern because these materials are used in intimate contact with the gingiva. Plasticizers, incorporated into some materials to make them soft and flexible, are released in vivo and in vitro. Cell culture tests have shown that some of these materials are extremely cytotoxic and affect a number of cellular metabolic reactions. In animal tests, several of these materials have caused significant epithelial changes, presumably from the released plasticizers. In usage, the effects of the released plasticizers are probably often masked by the inflammation already present in the tissues onto which these materials are placed. Denture adhesives have been evaluated in vitro and show severe cytotoxic reactions. Several had substantial formaldehyde content. The adhesives also allowed significant microbial growth. Newer formulations that add antifungal or antibacterial agents have not yet been shown to be clinically effective.

Reaction of Bone and Soft Tissues to Implant Materials

Interest in the biocompatibility of implant materials has grown because the use of implants in clinical practice has increased dramatically in the past 10 years. Successful dental implant materials either promote osseointegration or biointegration (see Dental and Orofacial Implants, Chapter 15).

Reactions to Ceramic Implant Materials

Ceramic materials may be conveniently divided into two groups: bioactive materials and nonbioactive ceramics. Most ceramic implant materials have very low toxic effects on tissues, because they are in an oxidized state and are corrosion resistant.

As a group, not only are they minimally toxic but they also are nonimmunogenic and noncarcinogenic. However, mechanically, they are brittle and lack impact and shear strength. Additionally, nonbioactive ceramic materials generally invoke fibrous encapsulation as mentioned above.

Reactions to Implant Metals and Alloys

Pure metals and alloys are the oldest type of oral implant materials. All metal implants share the quality of strength. Initially, metallic implant materials were selected on the basis of ease of fabrication. Over time, however, biocompatibility with bone and soft tissue and the longevity of the implant have become more important. Although a variety of implant materials have previously been used (including stainless steel and chromium-cobalt-molybdenum), the only metallic dental implant materials in common use today are titanium-based alloys.

Titanium is a pure metal when initially cast. However, in less than a second the surface forms a thin conformal layer of various titanium oxides. This oxide layer is corrosion resistant and allows bone to osseointegrate. A major disadvantage of this metal is that it is difficult to cast. It has been wrought into various forms, but this process introduces metallic impurities into the surface that may adversely affect bone cell response unless extreme care is taken during manufacturing. Titanium implants have been used with success as root forms to support a prosthesis. With frequent recall and good oral hygiene, implants have been maintained in healthy tissue for longer than three decades. Titanium-aluminum-vanadium alloys (Ti-6Al-4V) have been used successfully in this regard as well. This alloy is significantly stronger than commercially pure titanium, has better fatigue resistance, but has the same desirable stiffness and thermal properties as the commercially pure CP metal. Although titanium and titanium alloy implants have corrosion rates that are markedly less than other metallic implants, they do release titanium into the body. Currently there is no evidence that released titanium ions are a problem locally or systemically. However, questions remain about the liability of released aluminum and vanadium from alloys.

In soft tissue, the bonds epithelium form to titanium is morphologically similar to that formed with the tooth, but this interface has not been fully characterized. Connective tissue apparently does not bond to the titanium, but does form a tight seal that seems to limit ingress of bacteria and bacterial products. Techniques are being developed to limit downgrowth of the epithelium and loss of bone height around the implant, because this will ultimately cause implant failure. Peri-implantitis is now a documented disease around implants and involves many of the same bacteria as periodontitis. The role of the implant material or its released components in the progression of peri-implantitis is not known.

Reactions to Resorbable Materials

Initially, the choice of materials for use as implants in the oral cavity depended on the commercial availability of the material, with most materials aiming to minimize the immune response to the implanted material. With the survival of implanted materials for decades or more, the predominant thought began to shift in emphasis from achieving exclusively such benign (or tolerated) tissue response to instead producing bioactive materials that could elicit a controlled action and reaction in the physiological environment. Continuing in this vein, were the development of resorbable biomaterials that exhibit clinically appropriate, controlled chemical breakdown and resorption. In these materials, the problem of a tissue-material interface is resolved, because the materials provoke a physiologic response to replace the material with regenerated tissues. One of the earliest examples of these materials was the development of resorbable sutures. These materials were composed of a co-polymer of polylactic acid (PLA) and polyglycolic acid (PGA). When implanted in the body, they undergo a hydrolytic decomposition into CO_2 and H_2O. By the mid-1980s, clinical use of resorbable polymeric sutures was commonplace. Resorbable fracture fixation plates and screws, guided tissue membranes, and controlled drug-release systems have rapidly followed. Although generally well-tolerated by tissues in vivo, the resorbability of these materials depends on the volume of material implanted and because these materials degrade into acidic byproducts, the subsequent drop in pH in the surrounding tissues may invoke an inflammatory response. Other polymeric materials such as polycaprolactone, and hyaluronan derivatives, as well as natural polymers such as cross-linked collagen, starch, and cellulose are currently being investigated for their ability to resorb in vivo after serving their function as an implant.

SUMMARY

Biocompatibility of a dental material depends on its composition, location, and interactions with the oral cavity. Metal, ceramic, and polymer materials elicit different biological responses because of differences in composition. Furthermore, diverse biological responses to these materials depend on whether they release their components and whether those components are toxic, immunogenic, or mutagenic at the released concentrations. The location of a material in the oral cavity partially determines its biocompatibility. Materials that are biocompatible in contact with the oral mucosal surface may cause adverse reactions if they are implanted beneath it. Materials that are toxic in direct contact with the pulp may be essentially innocuous if placed on dentin or enamel. Finally, interactions between the material and the body influence the biocompatibility of the material. A material's response to changes in pH, application of force, or the effect of biological fluids can alter its biocompatibility. Surface features of a material may promote or discourage attachment of bacteria, host cells, or biological molecules. These effects also determine whether the material will promote plaque retention, integrate with bone, or adhere to dentin.

SELECTED PROBLEMS

PROBLEM 1

You have a group of six materials, all of which can be classified as posterior composites, but each of which has a slightly different formula. How would you determine which of these freshly set materials is the least toxic using the least expensive, least time-consuming tests?

Solution

You could choose a direct in-vitro cell culture test to evaluate the materials. With that test, the materials are formed into disks of equal dimensions. The disks should be stabilized on the bottoms of cell culture wells. Cells are then placed into the wells with the materials and are incubated in an appropriate incubation medium and environment for 24 hours or more. Then the disks and wells are observed and photographed under phase-contrast microscopy, taking special note of cytopathic effects around each disk to determine semiquantitative results.

PROBLEM 2

If you have the same situation presented in Problem 1, but you want to quantify your results, what are your options?

Solution

You could choose the same test model as that used in the solution for Problem 1, but you would measure the cellular response quantitatively rather than by visual observation. There are two primary options: (1) measure the membrane permeability of the cells that remain around the disks using neutral red or ^{51}Cr or (2) measure some aspect of cellular biosynthesis or metabolism (MTT test, DNA synthesis, protein synthesis, total protein). You could also choose another test model such as that in which samples are extracted for 1 to 3 days in given volumes of solvent and then the cells are treated with serial dilutions of the elutants.

PROBLEM 3

If you are presented with the same situation described in Problem 1, but want to know the effect of the setting reaction or time on the toxicity of the material, how would you proceed?

Solution

You could form the material into disks and allow it to set for varying periods (from 1 to several days). Then the set disk for each period would be placed into a tissue culture well or extracted with a solvent that is placed into the tissue culture well. Thereafter your options would be the same as those presented in the solutions for Problems 1 or 2.

PROBLEM 4

You read a research paper on the in vitro cytotoxicity of composites that shows that some composites are initially very cytotoxic but improve with time of elution into artificial saliva, whereas others continue to be toxic. How can you interpret these results in terms of clinical use of the composites?

Solution

Extrapolation of in vitro tests to clinical situations is always difficult, but one interpretation could be that the composites that improve with time in vitro pose lower long-term risks clinically than those that continue to be cytotoxic. This line of reasoning may be dangerous, however, if the material is designed to release a substance that is cytotoxic in vitro but therapeutic in vivo. Such is the case for fluoride release from some composites and glass ionomer cements.

PROBLEM 5

If you have a series of composites and you want to rank them according to the toxicity they may have specifically for pulpal tissues, what would you do?

Solution

You should choose a test model in which dentin is interspaced between material and cell test system. The dentin barrier may alter the effects of released components from the material and change the response of pulpal cells. Without such a barrier, the composites may appear more cytotoxic in vitro than they would be clinically.

PROBLEM 6

One of your six composite materials is associated fairly consistently with pulpitis when used by you and your fellow clinicians. The cytotoxicity test that you chose indicates that this material is not much more toxic than the other materials. What additional testing could help you better understand what is causing the pulpitis?

Solution

The pulpitis may be caused by microleakage of bacteria or by the material's ability to cause a chronic inflammatory (versus toxicity) response. If the facilities are available, you may do in vitro chemotaxis tests, using human peripheral leukocytes with the test sample to determine which materials might be responsible for the inflammation. Tests on monocytes could also be done, using materials or material components at nontoxic concentrations. If the material does not show an inflammatory response in these tests, then usage tests in animals could be used to verify the pulpitis in vivo in a more controlled environment. Then, if usage tests in animals substantiate the pulpitis, you should be highly suspicious of microleakage of environmental materials or bacteria products. To confirm this suspicion, additional usage tests could be performed in which the margins of the restoration are surface-sealed to prevent microleakage.

PROBLEM 7

You have a new polymeric substance that you believe might function well as a root cylinder implant. What kinds of tests should you conduct to answer questions of safety according to the Food and Drug Administration (FDA) standards, and how long would this take?

Solution

Initial tests should include cytotoxicity tests, a hemolysis test, a test for mutagenesis or gene toxicity, and probably an oral LD_{50} test. (All tests except mutagenesis can be performed and analyzed in about 2 to 3 weeks if run concurrently. The mutagenesis tests may require between 1 and 3 months for performance analysis.) Secondary tests might include implantation into bone and soft tissue of small animals, tests for mucous membrane irritation, and hypersensitivity tests. If done concurrently, about 1 month would elapse before histological preparation of tissue would begin. Time required for histology and reading of slides may vary, depending on the size of the project. Usage tests (percutaneous implants) in jaws of larger animals may require that the implants remain in place for 1 to 2 years, followed by histological processing and evaluation.

PROBLEM 8

You are a dentist who has been practicing for 20 years, and you like to do a lot of your own laboratory work. You have noticed that when you handle methacrylate denture base and monomer, a rash develops on your hands. What is the problem, and what can you do about it?

Solution

You are probably hypersensitive to the monomer and should wear rubber gloves when around monomer and freshly polymerized methacrylate. Try to avoid any contact because monomer can penetrate latex rubber.

PROBLEM 9

A dental patient comes to you with concerns about the estrogenicity of dental composites you have placed. What would you tell her?

Solution

First, it is true that some starting components (bisphenol A and its dimethacrylate) show estrogenic types of reactions in in vitro tests. However, the concentrations of these compounds in today's commercially available resins are *very* low. Second, there is no verifiable clinical evidence that these compounds or others are released in sufficient concentrations to cause estrogenic reactions. For example, the concentration of bisphenol A required to cause an estrogenic response is 1000 times greater than that of the naturally occurring hormone estradiol. Finally, there are no documented cases of these materials having any estrogenic type of reactions in dental patients, despite the placement of millions of these restorations.

Bibliography

Abdul Razak AA: Mercury toxicity and its implications—a review of the literature, *Dent J Malays* 10:5, 1988.

AAMI Standards and Recommended Practices: Biological Evaluation of Medical Devices, *Association for the Advancement of Medical Instrumentation*, vol 4, 1994, Arlington, VA.

Addy M, Martin MV: Systemic antimicrobials in the treatment of chronic periodontal diseases: a dilemma, *Oral Dis* 9:38, 2003.

al-Dawood A, Wennberg A: Biocompatibility of dentin bonding agents, *Endod Dent Traumatol* 9:1, 1993.

American Dental Association (ADA) Council on Scientific Affairs: Dental amalgam: update on safety concerns, *J Am Dent Assoc* 129:494, 1998.

Aoba T, Fejerskov O: Dental fluorosis: chemistry and biology, *Crit Rev Oral Biol Med* 13:155, 2002.

Autian J, Dillingham E: Toxicogenic potentials of biomaterials and methods for evaluating toxicity, *Med Instrum* 7:125, 1973.

Banerjee R, Nageswari K, Puniyani RR: Hematological aspects of biocompatibility—review article, *J Biomater Appl* 12:57, 1997.

Barile FA: *In vitro cytotoxicity: mechanisms and methods*, Boca Raton, 1994, CRC Press.

Bauer JG, First HA: The toxicity of mercury in dental amalgam, *J Calif Dent Assoc* 10:47, 1982.

Beltran-Aguilar ED, Goldstein JW, Lockwood SA: Fluoride varnishes. A review of their clinical use, cariostatic mechanism, efficacy and safety, *J Am Dent Assoc* 31:589, 2000.

Bergenholtz G: In vivo pulp response to bonding of dental restorations, *Trans Acad Dent Mater* 123, 1998.

Berkenstock OL: Issues concerning possible cobalt-chromium carcinogenicity: a literature review and discussion, *Contemp Orthop* 24:265, 1992.

Bouillaguet S, Wataha JC: Future directions in bonding resins to the dentine-pulp complex, *J Oral Rehabil* 31:385, 2004.

Bouillaguet S, Ciucchi B, Holz J: Potential risks for pulpal irritation with contemporary adhesive restorations: an overview, *Acta Med Dent Helv* 1:235, 1996.

Brackett WW, Tay FR, Brackett MG, et al: The effect of chlorhexidine on dentin hybrid layers in vivo. *Oper Dent* 32:107–111, 2007.

Brannstrom M: *Dentin and pulp in restorative dentistry*, London, 1982, Wolfe Medical.

Brodin P: Neurotoxic and analgesic effects of root canal cements and pulp-protecting dental materials, *Endod Dent Traumatol* 4:1, 1988.

Browne RM: Animal tests for biocompatibility of dental materials—relevance, advantages and limitations, *J Dent* 22:S21, 1994.

Browne RM: The in vitro assessment of the cytotoxicity of dental materials—does it have a role? *Int Endod J* 21:50, 1988.

Brune D: Metal release from dental biomaterials, *Biomaterials* 7:163, 1986.

Carrilho MR, Geraldeli S, Tay F, et al: In vivo preservation of the hybrid layer by chlorhexidine, *J Dent Res* 86:529–533, 2007.

Chai J: Some myths and legends about dental implants, *Ann Acad Med Singapore* 24:43, 1995.

Clarkson TW: The toxicology of mercury, *Crit Rev Clin Lab Sci* 34:369, 1997.

Cook SD, Dalton JE: Biocompatibility and biofunctionality of implanted materials, *Alpha Omegan* 85:41, 1992.

Counter SA, Buchanan LH: Mercury exposure in children: a review, *Toxicol Appl Pharmacol* 15:209, 2004.

Cox CF, Hafez AA: Biocomposition and reaction of pulp tissues to restorative treatments, *Dent Clin North Am* 45:31, 2001.

Cox CF, Keall CL, Keall HJ, Ostro EO: Biocompatibility of surface-sealed dental materials against exposed pulps, *J Prosthet Dent* 57:1, 1987.

Cox CF, Suzuki S, Suzuki SH: Biocompatibility of dental adhesives, *J Calif Dent Assoc* 23:35, 1995.

Cox CF: Evaluation and treatment of bacterial microleakage, *Am J Dent* 7:293, 1994.

Dadoun MP, Bartlett DW: Safety issues when using carbamide peroxide to bleach vital teeth—a review of the literature, *Eur J Prosthodont Restor Dent* 11:9, 2003.

Dahl JE, Pallesen U: Tooth bleaching—a critical review of the biological aspects, *Crit Rev Oral Biol Med* 14:292, 2003.

Davies JE: In vitro assessment of bone biocompatibility, *Int Endod J* 21:178, 1988.

Dodes JE: Amalgam toxicity: a review of the literature, *Oper Dent* 13:32, 1988.

Dunne SM, Gainsford ID, Wilson NH: Current materials and techniques for direct restorations in posterior teeth. Part 1: Silver amalgam, *Int Dent J* 47:123, 1997.

Duque C, Hebling J, Smith AJ, et al: Reactionary dentinogenesis after applying restorative materials and bioactive dentin matrix molecules as liners in deep cavities prepared in nonhuman primate teeth, *J Oral Rehabil* 33:452–461, 2006.

Ecobichon DJ: *The basis of toxicity testing*, Boca Raton, 1992, CRC Press.

Edgerton M, Levine MJ: Biocompatibility: its future in prosthodontic research, *J Prosthet Dent* 69:406, 1993.

Eggleston DW: Dental amalgam: a review of the literature, *Compendium* 10:500, 1989.

Eley BM, Cox SW: "Mercury poisoning" from dental amalgam—an evaluation of the evidence, *J Dent* 16:90, 1988.

Eliades T, Athanasiou AE: In vivo aging of orthodontic alloys: implications for corrosion potential, nickel release, and biocompatibility, *Angle Orthod* 72:222, 2002.

Enwonwu CO: Potential health hazard of use of mercury in dentistry:critical review of the literature, *Environ Res* 42:257, 1987.

Ferracane JL: Elution of leachable components from composites, *J Oral Rehabil* 21:441, 1994.

Ferracane JL, Cooper PR, Smith AJ: Can interaction of materials with the dentin-pulp complex contribute to dentin regeneration? *Odontology* 98:2–14, 2010.

Fry BW: Toxicology of fluorides, *Symp Pharmacol Ther Toxicol Group* 21:26, 1974.

Fung YK, Molvar MP: Toxicity of mercury from dental environment and from amalgam restorations, *J Toxicol Clin Toxicol* 30:49, 1992.

Gerzina TM, Hume WR: Diffusion of monomers from bonding resin-resin composite combinations through dentine in vitro, *J Dent* 24:125–128, 1996.

Geurtsen W, Leyhausen G: Biological aspects of root canal filling materials—histocompatibility, cytotoxicity, and mutagenicity, *Clin Oral Investig* 1:5, 1997.

Geurtsen W, Leyhausen G: Chemical-biological interactions of the resin monomer triethyleneglycol-dimethacrylate (TEGDMA), *J Dent Res* 80:2046, 2001.

Geurtsen W: Biocompatibility of resin-modified filling materials, *Crit Rev Oral Biol Med* 11:333, 2000.

Geurtsen W: Biocompatibility of root canal filling materials, *Aust Endod J* 27:12, 2001.

Geurtsen W: Substances released from dental resin composites and glass ionomer cements, *Eur J Oral Sci* 106:687, 1998.

Glantz PO, Mjor IA: On amalgam toxicity, *Int J Technol Assess Health Care* 6:363, 1990.

Glantz PO: Intraoral behaviour and biocompatibility of gold versus non precious alloys, *J Biol Buccale* 12:3, 1984.

Gochfeld M: Cases of mercury exposure, bioavailability, and absorption, *Ecotoxicol Environ Saf* 56:174, 2003.

Goldberg M, Smith AJ: Cells and extracellular matrices of dentin and pulp: a biological basis for repair and tissue engineering, *Crit Rev Oral Biol Med* 15:13–27, 2004.

Goldstein GR, Kiremidjian-Schumacher L: Bleaching: is it safe and effective, *J Prosthet Dent* 69:325, 1993.

Graham L, Cooper PR, Cassidy N, et al: The effect of calcium hydroxide on solubilisation of bi-active dentin matrix components, *Biomater* 27:2865–2873, 2006.

Grimaudo NJ: Biocompatibility of nickel and cobalt dental alloys, *Gen Dent* 49:498, 2001.

Gross UM: Biocompatibility—the interaction of biomaterials and host response, *J Dent Educ* 52:798, 1988.

Haeffner-Cavaillon N, Kazatchkine MD: Methods for assessing monocytic cytokine production as an index of biocompatibility, *Nephrol Dial Transplant* 9:112, 1994.

Hammesfahr PD: Biocompatible resins in dentistry, *J Biomater Appl* 1:373, 1987.

Hanks CT, Wataha JC, Sun Z: In vitro models of biocompatibility: a review, *Dent Mater* 12:186, 1996.

Hanson M, Pleva J: The dental amalgam issue. A review, *Experientia* 15:9, 1991.

Hauman CH, Love RM: Biocompatibility of dental materials used in contemporary endodontic therapy: a review. Part 1. Intracanal drugs and substances, *Int Endod J* 36:75, 2003.

Hauman CH, Love RM: Biocompatibility of dental materials used in contemporary endodontic therapy: a review. Part 2. Root-canal-filling materials, *Int Endod J* 36:147, 2003.

Hayden J Jr: Considerations in applying to man the results of drug effects observed in laboratory animals, *J Am Dent Assoc* 95:777, 1977.

Haywood VB, Heymann HO: Nightguard vital bleaching: how safe is it? *Quint Int* 22:515, 1991.

Hensten-Pettersen A: Comparison of the methods available for assessing cytotoxicity, *Int Endod J* 21:89, 1988.

Hensten-Pettersen A: Skin and mucosal reactions associated with dental materials, *Eur J Oral Sci* 106:707, 1998.

Hodgson E, Levi PE, editors: *A textbook of modern toxicology*, New York, 1987, Elsevier Science.

Horsted-Bindslev P: Amalgam toxicity—environmental and occupational hazards, *J Dent* 32:359, 2004.

Hubbard MJ: Calcium transport across the dental enamel epithelium, *Crit Rev Oral Biol Med* 11:437, 2000.

Hume WR, Gerzia TM: Bioavailability of components of resin-based materials which are applied to teeth, *Crit Rev Oral Biol Med* 7:172, 1996.

Hume WR, Massey WL: Keeping the pulp alive: the pharmacology and toxicology of agents applied to dentine, *Aust Dent J* 35:32, 1990.

Hume WR: A new technique for screening chemical toxicity to the pulp from dental restorative materials and procedures, *J Dent Res* 64:1322, 1985.

International Standards Organization: *Biological evaluation of medical devices*, ISO 10993, ed 1, Geneva, 1992, Switzerland, ISO.

International Standards Organization: Preclinical evaluation of biocompatibility of medical devices used in dentistry—Test methods for dental materials, ISO 7405:1997, Geneva, Switzerland, 1997, ISO.

Jansen JA, Caulier H, Van't Hof MA, Naert I: Evaluation of Ca-P coatings in animal experiments: importance of study design, *J Invest Surg* 9:463, 1996.

Jarup L: Hazards of heavy metal contamination, *Br Med Bull* 68:167, 2003.

Jones PA, Taintor JF, Adams AB: Comparative dental material cytotoxicity measured by depression of rat incisor pulp respiration, *J Endod* 5:48, 1979.

Jontell M, Okiji T, Dahlgren U, et al: Immune defense mechanisms of the dental pulp, *Crit Rev Oral Biol Med* 9:179, 1998.

Jorge JH, Giampaolo ET, Machado AL, et al: Cytotoxicity of denture base acrylic resins: a literature review, *J Prosthet Dent* 90:190, 2003.

Kanca J III: Pulpal studies: biocompatibility or effectiveness of marginal seal, *Quint Int* 21:775, 1990.

Kawahara H, Yamagami A, Nakamura M: Biological testing of dental materials by means of tissue culture, *Int Dent J* 18:443, 1968.

Kirkpatrick CJ, Bittinger F, Wagner M, et al: Current trends in biocompatibility testing, *Proc Inst Mech Eng [H]* 212:75, 1998.

Kuratate M, Yoshiba K, Shigetani Y, et al: Immunohistochemical analysis of nestin, osteopontin, and proliferating cells in the reparative process of exposed dental pulp capped with mineral trioxide aggregate, *J Endod* 34:970–974, 2008.

Laurencin CT, Pierre-Jacques HM, Langer R: Toxicology and biocompatibility considerations in the evaluation of polymeric materials for biomedical applications, *Clin Lab Med* 10:549, 1990.

Leggat PA, Kedjarune U, Smith DR: Toxicity of cyanoacrylate adhesives and their occupational impacts for dental staff, *Ind Health* 42:207, 2004.

Leggat PA, Kedjarune U: Toxicity of methyl methacrylate in dentistry, *Int Dent J* 53:126, 2003.

Lemons J, Natiella J: Biomaterials, biocompatibility, and peri-implant considerations, *Dent Clin North Am* 30:3, 1986.

Levy M: Dental amalgam: toxicological evaluation and health risk assessment, *J Can Dent Assoc* 61:667, 1995.

Lewis B: Formaldehyde in dentistry: a review for the millennium, *J Clin Pediatr Dent* 22:167, 1998.

Li Y: Tooth bleaching using peroxide-containing agents: current status of safety issues, *Compend Contin Educ Dent* 19:783, 1998.

Li Y: Peroxide-containing tooth whiteners: an update on safety, *Compend Contin Educ Dent Suppl* 28:S4, 2000.

Lutz J, Kettemann M, Racz I, Noth U: Several methods utilized for the assessment of biocompatibility of perfluorochemicals, *Artif Cells Blood Substit Immobil Biotechnol* 23:407, 1995.

Mackenzie R, Holmes CJ, Jones S, et al: Clinical indices of in vivo biocompatibility: the role of ex vivo cell function studies and effluent markers in peritoneal dialysis patients, *Kidney Int Suppl* 88:S84, 2003.

Mackert JR, Bergland A: Mercury exposure from dental amalgam filling: absorbed dose and the potential for adverse health effects, *Crit Rev Oral Biol Med* 8:410, 1997.

Mackert JR Jr, Wahl MJ: Are there acceptable alternatives to amalgam, *J Calif Dent Assoc* 32:601, 2004.

Mackert JR Jr: Dental amalgam and mercury, *J Am Dent Assoc* 122:54, 1991.

Mackert JR Jr: Side-effects of dental ceramics, *Adv Dent Res* 6:90, 1992.

Mantellini MG, Botero T, Yaman P, et al: Adhesive resin and the hydrophilic monomer HEMA induce VEGF expression on dental pulp cells and macrophages, *Dent Mater* 22:434–440, 2006.

Masuda-Murakami Y, Kobayashi M, Wang X, et al: Effects of mineral trioxide aggregate on the differentiation of rat dental pulp cells, *Acta Histochem* 112(5):452–458, 2010.

Marigo L, Vittorini Orgeas G, Piselli D, et al: Pulpo-dentin protection: the biocompatibility of materials most commonly used in restorative work. A literature review, *Minerva Stomatol* 48:373, 1999.

Marshall MV, Cancro LP, Fischman SL: Hydrogen peroxide: a review of its use in dentistry, *J Periodontol* 66:786, 1995.

Meryon SD: The influence of dentine on the in vitro cytotoxicity testing of dental restorative materials, *J Biomed Mater Res* 18:771, 1984.

Messer RL, Bishop S, Lucas LC: Effects of metallic ion toxicity on human gingival fibroblasts morphology, *Biomaterials* 20:1647, 1999.

Mjör IA, Hensten-Pettersen A, Skogedal O: Biologic evaluation of filling materials: a comparison of results using cell culture techniques, implantation tests and pulp studies, *Int Dent J* 27:124, 1977.

Mjor IA: Current views on biological testing of restorative materials, *J Oral Rehabil* 17:503, 1990.

Moienafshari R, Bar-Oz B, Koren G: Occupational exposure to mercury. What is a safe level, *Can Fam Physician* 45:43, 1999.

Mongkolnam P: The adverse effects of dental restorative materials—a review, *Aust Dent J* 37:360, 1992.

Mutter J, Naumann J, Sadaghiani C, et al: Amalgam studies: disregarding basic principles of mercury toxicity, *Int J Hyg Environ Health* 207:391, 2004.

Natiella JR: The use of animal models in research on dental implants, *J Dent Educ* 52:792, 1988.

National Institutes of Health: Consensus development statement on dental implants, *J Dent Educ* 52:824, 1988:June 13–15, 1988.

Nicholson JW, Braybrook JH, Wasson EA: The biocompatibility of glass-poly(alkenoate) (glass-ionomer) cements: a review, *J Biomater Sci Polym Ed* 2:277, 1991.

Nicholson JW: Glass-ionomers in medicine and dentistry, *Proc Inst Mech Eng [H]* 212:121, 1998.

Northup SJ: Strategies for biological testing of biomaterials, *J Biomater Appl* 2:132, 1987.

Osborne JW, Albino JE: Psychological and medical effects of mercury intake from dental amalgam. A status report for the American Journal of Dentistry, *Am J Dent* 12:151, 1999.

Pariente JL, Bordenave L, Bareille R, et al: Cultured differentiated human urothelial cells in the biomaterials field, *Biomaterials* 21:835, 2000.

Peterson DE: Oral toxicity of chemotherapeutic agents, *Semin Oncol* 19:478, 1992.

Pierce LH, Goodkind RJ: A status report of possible risks of base metal alloys and their components, *J Prosthet Dent* 62:234, 1989.

Pillai KS, Stanley VA: Implications of fluoride—an endless uncertainty, *J Environ Biol* 23:81, 2002.

Pizzoferrato A, Ciapetti G, Stea S, et al: Cell culture methods for testing biocompatibility, *Clin Mater* 15:173, 1994.

Polyzois GL: In vitro evaluation of dental materials, *Clin Mater* 16:21, 1994.

Pretorius E, Naude H: Dental amalgam and mercury toxicity: should dentists be concerned, *SADJ* 58:366, 2003.

Ratcliffe HE, Swanson GM, Fischer LJ: Human exposure to mercury: a critical assessment of the evidence of adverse health effects, *J Toxicol Environ Health* 25:221, 1996.

Ratner BD: Replacing and renewing: synthetic materials, biomimetics, and tissue engineering in implant dentistry, *J Dent Educ* 65:1340, 2001.

Reinhardt JW: Risk assessment of mercury exposure from dental amalgams, *J Public Health Dent* 48:172, 1988.

Rogers KD: Status of scrap (recyclable) dental amalgams as environmental health hazards or toxic substances, *J Am Dent Assoc* 119:159, 1989.

Rubel DM, Watchorn RB: Allergic contact dermatitis in dentistry, *Australas J Dermatol* 41:63, 2000.

Santerre JP, Shajii L, Leung BW: Relation of dental composite formulations to their degradation and the release of hydrolyzed polymeric-resin-derived products, *Crit Rev Oral Biol Med* 12:136, 2001.

Santini A: Biocompatibility of dentine-bonding agents. 1. Factors associated with function, *Prim Dent Care* 5:15, 1998.

Santini A: Biocompatibility of dentine-bonding agents. 2. Pulpal considerations, *Prim Dent Care* 5:69, 1998.

Schmalz G: Concepts in biocompatibility testing of dental restorative materials, *Clin Oral Investig* 1:154, 1997.

Schmalz G: The biocompatibility of non-amalgam dental filling materials, *Eur J Oral Sci* 106:696, 1998.

Schmalz G: Use of cell cultures for toxicity testing of dental materials—advantages and limitations, *J Dent* 22:S6, 1994.

Schuster GS, Lefebvre CA, Wataha JC, et al: Biocompatibility of posterior restorative materials, *J Calif Dent Assoc* 24:17, 1996.

Schuurs AH: Reproductive toxicity of occupational mercury. A review of the literature, *J Dent* 27:249, 1999.

Shabalovskaya SA: On the nature of the biocompatibility and on medical applications of NiTi shape memory and superelastic alloys, *Biomed Mater Eng* 6:267, 1996.

Sidhu SK, Schmalz G: The biocompatibility of glass-ionomer cement materials. A status report for the American Journal of Dentistry, *Am J Dent* 14:387, 2001.

Smith AJ: Vitality of the dentin-pulp complex in health and disease: growth factors as key mediators, *J Dent Educ* 67:678–689, 2003.

Smith GE: Is fluoride a mutagen, *Sci Total Environ* 68:79, 1988.

Smith GE: Toxicity of fluoride-containing dental preparations: a review, *Sci Total Environ* 43:41, 1985.

Soderholm KJ, Mariotti A: Bis-GMA–based resins in dentistry: are they safe? *J Am Dent Assoc* 130:201, 1999.

Stadtler P: Dental amalgam. III: Toxicity, *Int J Clin Pharmacol Ther Toxicol* 29:168, 1991.

Stanley HR: Biological evaluation of dental materials, *Int Dent J* 42:37, 1992.

Stanley HR: Effects of dental restorative materials: local and systemic responses reviewed, *J Am Dent Assoc* 124:76, 1993.

Stanley HR: Local and systemic responses to dental composites and glass ionomers, *Adv Dent Res* 6:55, 1992.

Stanley HR: Pulpal responses to ionomer cements—biological characteristics, *J Am Dent Assoc* 120:25, 1990.

Tomson PL, Grover LM, Lumley PJ, et al: Dissolution of bio-active dentine matrix components by mineral trioxide aggregate, *J Dent* 35:636–642, 2007.

van der Bijl P, Dreyer WP, van Wyk CW: Mercury in dentistry: a review, *J Dent Assoc S Afr* 42:537, 1987.

van Zyl I: Mercury amalgam safety: a review, *J Mich Dent Assoc* 81:40, 1999.

Veron MH, Couble ML: The biological effects of fluoride on tooth development: possible use of cell culture systems, *Int Dent J* 42:108, 1992.

Wahl MJ: Amalgam—resurrection and redemption. Part 2: The medical mythology of anti-amalgam, *Quint Int* 32:696, 2001.

Ward RA: Phagocytic cell function as an index of biocompatibility, *Nephrol Dial Transplant* 9:46, 1994.

Wataha JC, Hanks CT, Craig RG: Precision of and new methods for testing in vitro alloy cytotoxicity, *Dent Mater* 8:65–71, 1992.

Wataha JC, Hanks CT, Strawn SE, et al: Cytotoxicity of components of resins and other dental restorative materials, *J Oral Rehabil* 21:453, 1994.

Wataha JC, Hanks CT: Biological effects of palladium and risk of using palladium in dental casting alloys, *J Oral Rehabil* 23:309, 1996.

Wataha JC: Biocompatibility of dental casting alloys: a review, *J Prosthet Dent* 83:223, 2000.

Wataha JC: Principles of biocompatibility for dental practitioners, *J Prosthet Dent* 86:203, 2001.

Watts A, Paterson RC: Initial biological testing of root canal sealing materials—a critical review, *J Dent* 20:259, 1992.

Whitford GM: Fluoride in dental products: safety considerations, *J Dent Res* 66:1056, 1987.

Whitford GM: The physiological and toxicological characteristics of fluoride, *J Dent Res* 69:539, 1990.

Williams DF: In Williams DF, editor: *Fundamental aspects of biocompatibility, Toxicology of ceramics,* vol 2, Boca Raton, 1981, CRC Press.

Ziff MF: Documented clinical side-effects to dental amalgam, *Adv Dent Res* 6:131, 1992.

General Classes of Biomaterials

Dental biomaterials are generally categorized into four classes: metals, polymers, ceramics and composites. The four classes are distinctly different from each other in terms of density, stiffness, translucency, processing method, application, and cost. One class, composites, is a combination of two or more classes that produces materials that can be engineered for specific applications. For some applications, such as intracoronal restorations, several classes offer suitable materials. For other applications, such as endosseus implants, only one class is appropriate. Requirements such as esthetics, stiffness, and osseointegration dictate the choice of material class. Restoration design and material class are always coordinated to achieve the best patient outcome.

This chapter is organized into four sections by the class of material. Fundamental concepts of each class are presented here. Additional detail is provided in other chapters when specific applications are discussed.

METALS AND ALLOYS

Metals and alloys are used in almost all aspects of dental practice, including the dental laboratory, direct and indirect dental restorations, implants, and instruments used to prepare teeth. Metals and alloys have optical, physical, chemical, thermal, and electrical properties that are unique among the basic types of materials and suitable for many dental applications. Although tooth-colored materials are often desired for restorations, metals provide strength, stiffness, and longevity for long-term dental applications that are often not achievable with other classes of materials. Evidence in the scientific literature of clinical performance is the most extensive for this material class.

As a class, metals are ductile and malleable and therefore exhibit elastic and plastic behavior; they are good electrical and thermal conductors, higher in density than other classes, exhibit good toughness, are opaque, and can be polished to a luster. Metals may be cast, drawn, or machined to create dental restorations and instruments.

CHEMICAL AND ATOMIC STRUCTURE OF METALS

A metal is any element that ionizes positively in solution. As a group, metals constitute nearly two thirds of the periodic table (Figure 7-1). During ionization, metals release electrons. This ability to exist as free, positively charged, stable ions is a key factor in the behavior of metals and is responsible for many metallic properties that are important in dentistry. Another important group of elements shown in Figure 7-1 are the metalloids, including carbon, silicon, and boron. Although metalloids do not always form free positive ions, their conductive and

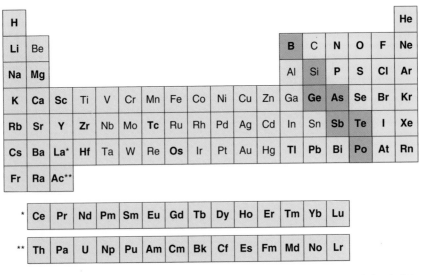

FIGURE 7.1 **Periodic table of elements.** The periodic table of the elements can be subdivided into metals *(blue backgrounds)*, metalloids *(purple backgrounds)*, and nonmetals *(yellow backgrounds)*. Elements in non-bolded type are used in dental alloys or as pure metals. The metals are elements that ionize positively in solution and comprise the majority of elements in the periodic table. Note that not all elements are shown. Hydrogen is often included in Group IA (left column) because it forms compounds with oxidation numbers of both +1 and −1. Also, under very high pressures, hydrogen exhibits the properties of a metal. The single asterisk indicates the insertion point in the table for the lanthanide series of elements, whereas the double asterisk indicates the insertion point for the actinide series of elements. Reference: The American Chemical Society.

electronic properties make them important components of many dental alloys.

Atomic Structure

At the atomic level, pure metals exist as crystalline arrays (Figure 7-2) that are continuous in three dimensions. In these arrays, the nuclei and core electrons occupy the atomic center with the ionizable electrons floating freely among the atomic positions. The mobility of the valence electrons is responsible for many properties of metals, such as electrical conductivity. It is important to note that the positively charged atomic centers are held together by the electrons and their positive charge is simultaneously neutralized by the negative electrons. Thus pure metals have no net charge.

The relationships between the atomic centers in a metallic crystalline array are not always uniform in all directions. The distances in the x, y (horizontal), and z (vertical) axes may be the same or different, and the angles between these axes may or may not be 90 degrees. In all, six crystal systems occur (Figure 7-3), and they can be further divided into 14 crystalline arrays. Metallic nuclei may occur at the center of faces or vertices of the crystal. Within each array, the smallest repeating unit that captures all the relationships among atomic centers is called a *unit cell* (see Figure 7-2). The unit cells for the most common arrays in dental metals are shown in

Figure 7-4. In the body-centered cubic (BCC) array, all angles are 90 degrees and all atoms are equidistant from one another in the horizontal and vertical directions. Metallic atoms are located at the corners of the unit cell, and one atom is at the center of the unit cell (hence the name *body-centered cubic*). This is the crystal structure of iron and is common for many iron alloys. The face-centered cubic (FCC) array has 90-degree angles and atomic centers that are equidistant horizontally and vertically (as does the BCC), but atoms are located in the centers of the faces with no atom in the center of the unit cell (hence the name *face-centered cubic*). Most pure metals and alloys of gold, palladium, cobalt, and nickel exhibit the FCC array. Titanium exhibits the more complex hexagonal close-pack array. In this array, the atoms are equidistant from each other in the horizontal plane, but not in the vertical direction.

In a metallic crystal, the atomic centers are positively charged because the free valence electrons float in the crystal. Although we might expect the atomic centers to repel each other, the freely floating electrons bind the centers together and create a strong force between the atomic centers. This is known as the *metallic bond* and is a fundamentally important type of primary bond. The metallic bond is fundamentally different from other primary bonds, such as covalent bonds that occur in organic compounds, and ionic bonds that occur in ceramics.

Physical Properties of Metals

All properties of metals result from the metallic crystal structure and metallic bonds. In general, metals have high densities that result from the efficient packing of atomic centers in the crystal lattice. Metals

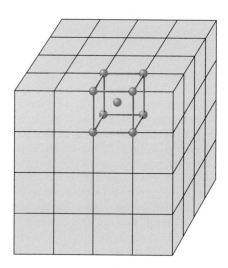

FIGURE 7.2 **A typical metallic crystal lattice, in this case a body-centered cubic lattice.** Every lattice has a unit cell *(shown in bold)* that extends (repeats) in three dimensions for large distances. Electrons are only relatively loosely bound to atomic nuclei and core electrons. The nuclei occupy specific sites *(shown as dots in the unit cell)* in the lattice, whereas the electrons are relatively free to move about the lattice. In reality, the metal atoms are large enough to touch each other.

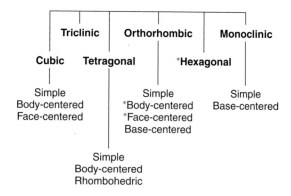

Triclinic	Orthorhombic	Monoclinic
Cubic Tetragonal	*Hexagonal	
Simple Body-centered Face-centered	Simple *Body-centered *Face-centered Base-centered	Simple Base-centered
	Simple Body-centered Rhombohedric	

FIGURE 7.3 **Lattice structures.** All metals occur in one of the lattice structures shown. There are six families of lattices, four of which can be subdivided. Each family is defined by the distances between vertices and the angles at the vertices. The body-centered cubic, face-centered cubic, and hexagonal lattices *(asterisks)* are the most common in dental alloys and pure metals.

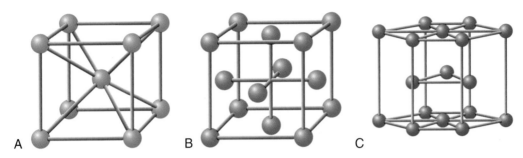

FIGURE 7.4 **The three most common crystal lattice unit cells in dental metals and alloys. A,** Body-centered cubic cell; **B,** face-centered cubic cell; and **C,** hexagonal close-packed cell. The atoms *(circles)* in all three cases would be larger and touching each other. They were drawn smaller to make the structures easier to visualize.

are electrically and thermally conductive because of the mobility of the valence electrons in the crystal lattice. The opacity and reflective nature of metals result from the ability of the valence electrons to absorb and emit light. Melting occurs as the metallic bond energy is overcome by the applied heat. Interestingly, the number of valence electrons per atomic center influences the melting point somewhat. As the number of valence electrons increases, the metallic bond develops some covalent character that contributes to higher melting points. This phenomenon occurs for iron (Fe^{3+}) and nickel (Ni^{2+}).

The corrosion properties of metals depend on the ability of atomic centers and electrons to be released in exchange for energy. The amount of energy required depends on the strength of the metallic force, which is related to the freedom of the valence electron, and the energy that the released ion can gain by solvating in solution. For metals such as sodium and potassium, the metallic bond is weaker because the valence electrons are loosely held, and the energy of solvation is high. Thus these metals corrode into water with explosive energy release. For metals such as gold and platinum, the metallic bond is stronger; valence electrons are more tightly held, and solvation energies are relatively low. Thus gold and platinum are far less likely to corrode. The corrosion of metals always involves oxidation and reduction. The released ion is oxidized because the electrons are given up, and the electrons (that cannot exist alone) are gained by some molecules in the solution (that are therefore reduced).

Because the distances between metal atoms in a crystal lattice may be different in the horizontal and vertical directions (see Figure 7-4), properties such as conductivity of electricity and heat, magnetism, and strength may also vary by direction if a single crystal is observed. These directional properties of metals and metalloids have been exploited in the semiconductor industry to fabricate microchips for computers. However, in dentistry, a single crystal

is rarely observed. Rather, a collection of randomly oriented crystals, each called a *grain,* generally make up a dental alloy. In this case, the directional properties are averaged across the material. In general, a fine-grained structure is desirable to encourage alloys with uniform properties in any direction. Nonuniformity of directional properties is termed *anisotropy.*

Like the physical properties, the mechanical properties of metals are also a result of the metallic crystal structure and metallic bonds. Metals generally have good ductility (ability to be drawn into a wire) and malleability (ability to be hammered into a thin sheet) relative to polymers and ceramics. To a large extent, these properties result from the ability of the atomic centers to slide against each other into new positions within the same crystal lattice. Because the metallic bonds are essentially nondirectional, such sliding is possible.

If the metallic crystals were perfect, calculations have shown that the force required to slide the atoms in the lattice would be hundreds of times greater than experiments indicate. Less force is necessary because the crystals are not perfect; they have flaws called *dislocations.* Dislocations allow the atomic centers to slide past each other one plane at a time (Figure 7-5). Because movement can occur one plane at a time, the force required is much less than if the forces of all the planes have to be overcome simultaneously. An analogy is moving a large heavy rug by forming a small fold or kink in the rug and pushing the fold from one end of the rug to the other. Dislocations are of several types, but all serve to allow the relatively easy deformation of metals. All methods for increasing the strength of metals act by impeding the movement of dislocations.

Metals fracture when the atomic centers cannot slide past one another freely. For example, this failure can happen when impurities block the flow of dislocations (Figure 7-6). The inability of the dislocation to be moved through the solid results in the lattice rupturing locally. Once this small crack is started, it

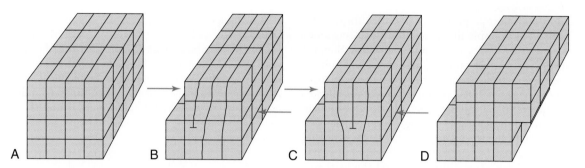

FIGURE 7.5 **Sketches representing a crystal and slip mechanisms resulting from movement of a dislocation.** By the dislocation moving through the metal one plane at a time (**A** to **B** to **C** to **D**), far less energy is necessary to deform the metal. Furthermore, the movement occurs without fracture or failure of the crystal lattice.

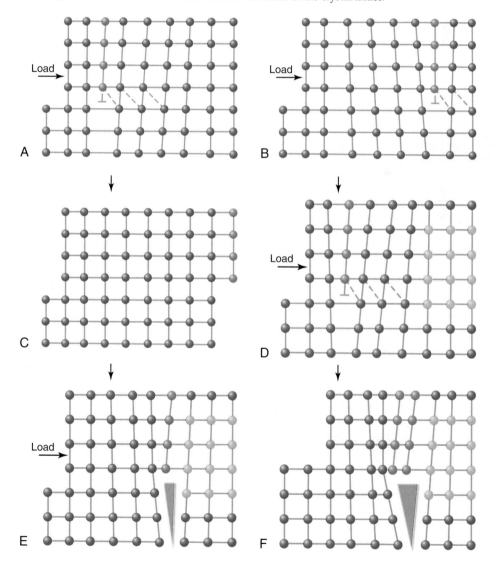

FIGURE 7.6 **Sketches showing plastic shearing with crack formation at the site of an impurity** *(orange circles)*. Without the impurity (**A, B, C**), the load forces the dislocations completely through the lattice without fracture (note the progression of red circles from left to right). However, when the impurity is present (**D, E, F**), it stops the progress of the dislocation. As other dislocations build up, the lattice below them cannot accommodate and a crack forms in the lattice (**E**). In **E**, note the broken bonds between atoms. Once formed, a crack can grow rapidly and relatively easily and lead to catastrophic failure.

takes little force to propagate the crack through the lattice. An example illustrates this idea. Consider a plate of steel 15 cm wide and 6 mm thick. Suppose it has a 5-cm crack running into one side. The force required to make the crack run the remaining 10 cm would be about 1800 Newtons (N). Without the aid of the crack, 2.2 million Newtons (MN) would be required if the steel were the best commercial grade available. If the steel were a single, flawless crystal, 44 MN would be necessary! The fracture of metals depends heavily on dislocations and the local rupture of the crystal lattice.

POLYMERS

Polymers are commonly used for applications such as tooth restoratives, sealants, cements, orthodontic space maintainers and elastics, obturators for cleft palates, impressions, provisional restorations, root canal filling materials, denture bases, and athletic mouth protectors. In addition, polymers are typically one of the components of the fourth class of material, composites, which are discussed later in this chapter. As a class, polymers are formable, can be made translucent or opaque, low in density, low in hardness, and are poor conductors of temperature and electricity. Of the four classes of materials presented, polymers have the lowest stiffness, lowest functional stability, and the lowest melting or glass transition point.

Basic Nature of Polymers

Chemical Composition

The term *polymer* denotes a molecule that is made up of many (poly) parts (mers). The *mer* ending represents the simplest repeating chemical structural unit from which the polymer is composed. Thus poly(methyl methacrylate) is a polymer having chemical structural units derived from methyl methacrylate, as indicated by the simplified reaction and structural formula I.

The molecules from which the polymer is constructed are called *monomers* (one part). Polymer molecules may be prepared from a mixture of different types of monomers. They are called *copolymers* if they contain two or more different chemical units and *terpolymers* if they contain three different units, as indicated by the structural formulas, II and III.

II

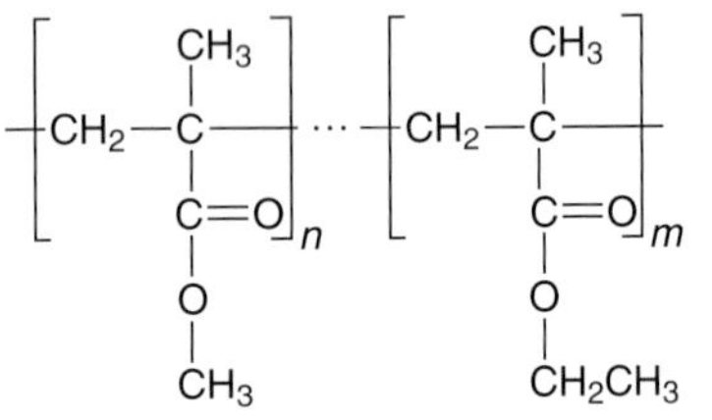

Methyl methacrylate–ethyl methacrylate copolymer

III

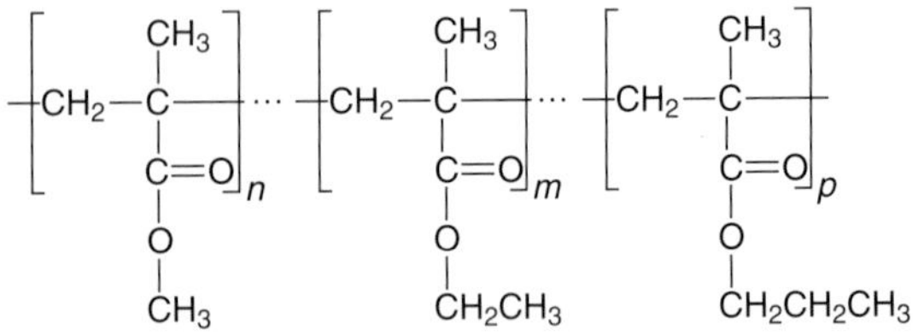

Methyl-, ethyl-, propyl methacrylate copolymer or terpolymer

As a convenience in expressing the structural formulas of polymers, the *mer* units are enclosed in brackets, and subscripts such as n, m, and p represent the average number of the various mer units that make up the polymer molecules. Notice that in normal polymers the mer units are spaced in a random orientation along the polymer chain. It is possible, however, to produce copolymers with mer units arranged so that a large number of one mer type are connected to a large number of another mer type. This special type of polymer is called a *block polymer*. It also is possible to produce polymers having mer units with a special spatial arrangement with respect

I

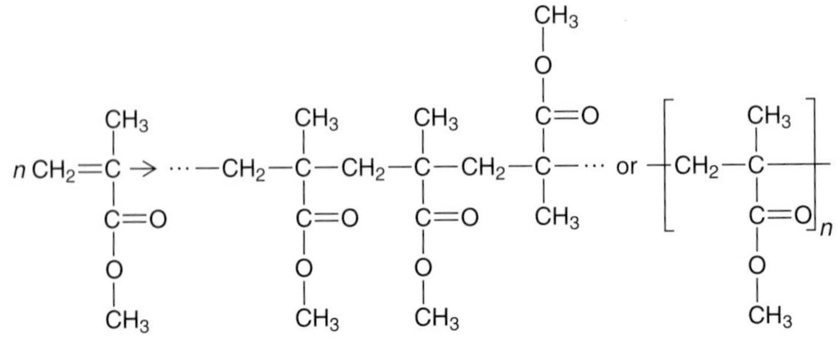

Methyl methacrylate   **Poly (methyl methacrylate)**

to the adjacent units; these are called *stereospecific* polymers.

The mers of the polymers are joined through covalent, C–C, bonds. Typically, during the polymerization process, C=C double bonds are converted to C–C single bonds and a mer is attached to one of the carbon atoms that was part of the C=C double bond. The next section describes various network configurations for mers, including cross-linking, in which chains are linked in a nonlinear configuration.

Molecular Weight

The molecular weight of the polymer molecule, which equals the molecular weight of the various mers multiplied by the number of the mers, may range from thousands to millions of molecular weight units, depending on the preparation conditions. The higher the molecular weight of the polymer made from a single monomer, the higher the degree of polymerization. The term *polymerization* is often used in a qualitative sense, but the *degree of polymerization* is defined as the total number of mers in a polymer molecule. In general, the molecular weight of a polymer is reported as the average molecular weight because the number of repeating units may vary greatly from one molecule to another. As would be expected, the fraction of low-, medium-, and high-molecular-weight molecules in a material, or in other words, the molecular weight distribution, has as pronounced an effect on the physical properties as does the average molecular weight. Therefore, two poly(methyl methacrylate) specimens can have the same chemical composition but greatly different physical properties because one of the specimens has a high percentage of low-molecular-weight molecules, whereas the other has a high percentage of high-molecular-weight molecules. Variation in the molecular weight distribution may be obtained by altering the polymerization procedure. These materials therefore do not possess any precise physical constants, such as melting point, as do ordinary small molecules. For example, the higher the molecular weight, the higher the softening and melting points and the stiffer the polymer.

Spatial Structure

In addition to chemical composition and molecular weight, the physical or spatial structure of the polymer molecules is also important in determining the properties of the polymer. There are three basic types of structures: linear, branched, and cross-linked. They are illustrated in Figure 7-7 as segments of linear, branched, and cross-linked polymers. The linear homopolymer has mer units of the same type, and the random copolymer of the linear type has the two mer units randomly distributed along the chain. The linear block copolymer has segments, or blocks,

along the chain whereas the mer units are the same. The branched homopolymer again consists of the same mer units, whereas the graft-branched copolymer consists of one type of mer unit on the main chain and another mer for the branches. The cross-linked polymer shown is made up of a homopolymer cross-linked with a single cross-linking agent.

The linear and branched molecules are separate and discrete, whereas the cross-linked molecules are a network structure that may result in the creation of one giant polymeric molecule. The spatial structure of polymers affects their flow properties, but generalizations are difficult to make because either the interaction between linear polymer molecules or the length of the branches on the branched molecules may be more important in a particular example. In general, however, the cross-linked polymers flow at higher temperatures than linear or branched polymers. Another distinguishing feature of some cross-linked polymers is that they do not absorb liquids as readily as either the linear or branched materials.

Thermoplastics and Thermosets

An additional method of classifying polymers other than by their spatial structure is according to whether they are thermoplastic or thermosetting. The term *thermoplastic* refers to polymers that may be softened by heating and solidify on cooling, the process being repeatable. Typical examples of polymers of this type are poly(methyl methacrylate), polyethylene-polyvinylacetate, and polystyrene. The term *thermosetting or thermoset* refers to polymers that solidify during fabrication but cannot be softened by reheating. These polymers generally become nonfusible because of a cross-linking reaction and the formation of a spatial structure. Typical dental examples are cross-linked poly(methyl methacrylate), silicones, *cis*-polyisoprene, and dimethacrylates.

Polymers as a class have unique properties, and by varying the chemical composition, molecular weight, molecular-weight distribution, or spatial arrangement of the mer units, the physical and mechanical properties of polymers may be altered. Additional discussion of polymers in included in Chapter 9.

CERAMICS

The term *ceramic* refers to any product made essentially from a nonmetallic inorganic material usually processed by firing at a high temperature to achieve desirable properties. They are oxides of metals. As a class, ceramics are hard, low in toughness compared to metals, stiff, poor thermal and electrical conductors, and can be cast or machined to fabricate dental restorations. The translucency and opacity of

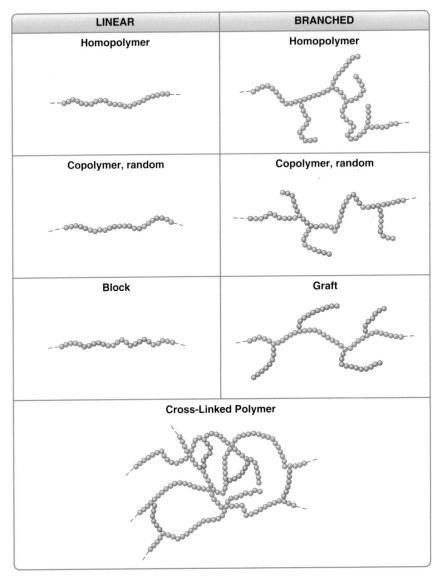

FIGURE 7.7 **Linear, branched, and cross-linked homopolymers and copolymers.** *Red circles*, one type of mer unit; *blue circles*, another type of mer unit; *dashed lines*, continuation of the polymer segment.

a dental ceramic can be modified for applications where color and translucency are critical. Ceramics demonstrate little plastic behavior and are thus considered brittle. Their stress-strain curves are generally linear with no plastic strain. Ceramics are used in restorative dentistry as full- and partial-coverage crowns, denture teeth, and as particulate fillers for resin matrix composite filling materials.

The more restrictive term *porcelain* refers to a specific compositional range of ceramic materials made by mixing kaolin, quartz, and feldspar, and firing at high temperature. Dental ceramics for *ceramic-metal* restorations belong to this compositional range and are commonly referred to as *dental porcelains.* Dental porcelain is used as veneers on metal frameworks (metal ceramic restoration) and on minimally prepared anterior teeth, and for denture teeth.

The laboratory portion of a ceramic restoration is usually made in a commercial dental laboratory by a skilled technician working with specialized equipment to the shape and shade specifications provided by the dentist. Skilled technicians and artisans are also employed by the manufacturers of artificial denture teeth to produce the many forms, types, and shades necessary in this application of porcelain. Computer-aided design and manufacturing or milling (CAD-CAM) is the basis for the acquisition of digital images of tooth preparations and computer-aided design of restorations. Portable milling machines under digital control mill machineable ceramic blanks to create final restorations. Additional discussion of digital impressioning can be found in Chapter 14.

The properties of dental ceramics depend on their composition, microstructure, and flaw population. The nature and amount of reinforcing crystalline phase present dictate the material's strength and resistance to crack propagation as well as its optical properties.

Ceramics are brittle and contain at least two populations of flaws: fabrication defects and surface cracks. The fracture mechanisms involve crack propagation from these flaws. Fabrication defects are created during processing and consist of inclusions at the condensation stage or voids generated during sintering. Inclusions are often linked to improper cleaning of the metal framework or use of unclean instruments. Porosity on the internal side of clinically failed glass-ceramic restorations has been identified as the fracture initiation site. Microcracks also develop upon cooling in feldspathic porcelains and can be due to thermal contraction mismatch between the leucite crystals and the glassy matrix or to thermal shock if the porcelain is cooled too rapidly.

Surface cracks are induced by machining or grinding. The average natural flaw size varies from 20 to 50 μm. Usually, failure of the ceramic originates from the most severe flaw.

Dental ceramics are subjected to repeated (cyclic) loading in a humid environment (chewing), conditions that are ideal for the extension of the preexisting defects or cracks. This phenomenon, called *slow crack growth,* can contribute to a severe reduction of the survival probability of ceramic restorations.

COMPOSITES

Composites are a combination of two or more classes of materials. In dentistry, the most common composite is a combination of a polymer and ceramic, where the polymer is used to bind ceramic particles. The polymer functions as the matrix in dental composites and the particles are reinforcing materials. Polymer matrix composites, also known as *resin composites*, are used as sealants, intracoronal and extracoronal restorations, provisional restorations, veneers, denture teeth, cements, and core buildups. As a class, dental composites are formable, can be made to be machineable, opaque or translucent, moderate in stiffness and hardness, thermal and electrical insulators, and sparingly soluble. Many advances have been made recently in particle technology (see Chapter 9).

In a composite the properties are intermediate between the two compositional materials. A benefit of combining two material classes is the ability to fabricate a new material that has desirable handling properties that are not achievable with one material alone. For example, individual ceramic particles are not condensable or packable, but the addition of a polymer to bind them enables the composite to be used as a paste. Use of a polymer alone will not achieve sufficient stiffness and stability, which are properties contributed by the ceramic particles. Resin composites continue to increase in popularity as concern rises over the health and environmental effects of mercury in amalgam. The polymer used in many dental composites, bisphenol A glycidyl methacrylate (Bis-GMA), has come under close scrutiny because of a perceived connection with bisphenol A, which has been shown to have some health risks. To date, no significant health risks have been associated with Bis-GMA used in dental resin composites.

In industries and professions other than dentistry, other classes are combined to form composites, such as metal-ceramic composites used in aerospace. A commonly used material in the construction industry, concrete, is a composite of sand, gravel, and Portland cement. As with dental resin composites, the cement in concrete is the binder for the sand and gravel particles. Composites differ from alloys in that, at the microscopic level, the individual components of the composite are visible.

In the case of concrete, a limiting factor is the adhesion between the Portland cement and sand-gravel particles. At the surface, the cement washes away with use, leaving the particles incompletely surrounded by cement. These particles are then easily dislodged, leaving a void in the surface of the concrete. In dental resin composites, coupling agents are used to enhance the adhesion between the ceramic particles and polymer matrix, thereby increasing its wear resistance and long-term surface integrity.

Considerable attention has been devoted to polymerization shrinkage of restorative composites. During polymerization, a volumetric contraction of the polymer matrix occurs that results in strain within the matrix. This contraction strain is coupled with the increase in elastic modulus as the composite cures. The combination of contraction strain and development of elastic modulus produces stress within the composite because the periphery of the restoration is constrained by adhesion to the enamel and dentin cavity walls. Methods to reduce residual stress include the use of polymers with reduced shrinkage during cure, incremental placement of the material in the tooth preparation, modulated intensities of curing light sources, and placement of liners along cavity walls. More detail on the measurement of polymerization shrinkage can be found in Chapter 5 and the mechanism for polymerization can be found in Chapter 9.

SELECTED PROBLEMS

PROBLEM 1

In the metallic crystal lattice, the valence electrons are relatively unbound to their atomic centers. What properties of metals result from this configuration?

Solution

The loose valence electrons are mobile and allow metals to readily conduct heat and electricity. The electrons can also accommodate shifts of the nuclear centers that often make the metals malleable and ductile. The high reflectivity (mirror-like surface) of a polished metallic surface occurs because the valence electrons reflect light that hits the surface.

PROBLEM 2

A person hands you two samples of the same metal. In the first sample *(A)*, she tells you that there are absolutely no flaws in the crystal structure of the metal. In the second sample *(B)*, there are numerous crystal flaws. How do the strengths of *A* and *B* compare, and why?

Solution·

A will be stronger by at least one order of magnitude. Without flaws, no dislocation-mediated sliding can take place and the total of the metallic bonds must be overcome at once. With flaws present, the metal can deform one row of atoms at a time, and thus the deformation occurs at a lower stress (see Figure 7-5).

PROBLEM 3

If you are given a single crystal of a pure metal with a hexagonal close-packed lattice in the shape of a cube 3 mm on a side, and you test the compressive strength in the horizontal and vertical directions, will the strengths be the same? If you take a sample, the same size, that is made of a collection of microscopic crystals, what will be the result of measured strengths?

Solution

For the single crystal, the strengths will not be the same vertically and horizontally because the distribution of the atoms in a crystal lattice is not isotropic (independent of direction). Because the metal sample is a pure single crystal, the strength in the horizontal and vertical directions will depend on the conformation of atoms in those directions. Because the conformation of atoms in the hexagonal close-packed lattice is different in the horizontal and vertical directions, the horizontal and vertical strengths will vary. For the sample with many smaller crystals,

the strength will be the same (at least theoretically) in either direction because the different crystals are oriented randomly with respect to one another, and any directional difference in properties is averaged out over the sample.

PROBLEM 4

You are given two wires of the same diameter and length. One is wrought and the other is cast. Which will have the greatest percentage of elongation?

Solution

Chances are that the cast wire will have the greatest elongation. By mechanically working a wire to its wrought form, the dislocations that allow elongation are "used up" and therefore further stress will result in fracture, not elongation. On the other hand, the tensile strength of the wrought wire is probably greater because it resists the deformation leading to fracture.

PROBLEM 5

A patient showed considerable wear of enamel on the teeth in occlusion with porcelain crowns. Explain.

Solution

Dental porcelain is harder than tooth enamel and can wear it away. Ceramic-metal restorations with metal lingual surfaces on anterior crowns result in less wear. However, because the porcelain crowns are already cemented, the use of an occlusal splint in the case of bruxism may be indicated.

PROBLEM 6

Two specimens of poly(methyl methacrylate) were listed by the manufacturer to be 100% pure, which was true, yet one had a significantly lower softening temperature than the other. Why?

Solution

The two specimens could have had different average molecular weights, different molecular-weight distributions, or different spatial structures (linear, branched, or cross-linked).

PROBLEM 7

Two denture-base poly(methyl methacrylate) products were heated. It was found that one specimen softened and flowed, whereas the second decomposed rather than melted. What is the most likely reason for this observation?

Solution

The first poly(methyl methacrylate) sample was most likely a linear polymer and thus thermoplastic, whereas the second was a cross-linked poly(methyl methacrylate) that was not thermoplastic.

PROBLEM 8

An experimenter determined the degree of polymerization of a poly(methyl methacrylate) material and used this information to calculate the degree of conversion. Would this procedure give a correct result?

Solution

No. The degree of polymerization measures the number of mer units in the polymer molecule, whereas the degree of conversion measures the number of unreacted carbon double bonds.

PROBLEM 9

Because composites are blends of one or more classes of materials, the resulting product exhibits properties that are a weighted average of the two or more components. Is this an accurate statement?

Solution

The properties are not a simple weighted average of the proportions of the two or more components. A volume fraction approach to calculating properties will achieve reasonable results, but interactions between components will not be accounted for.

PROBLEM 10

Metal alloys are blends of two or more elements, so they should be considered as composites. Is this a true statement?

Solution

No. At the microscopic level, the individual elements are not distinguishable, so a metal alloy is not a composite.

PROBLEM 11

Composites are plagued with loss of the reinforcing particulate filler when the surface is worn or when the material absorbs water. Is this a true statement?

Solution

No. A silane coupling agent enhances the bond between the polymer matrix and the reinforcing filler to prevent the loss of filler particles.

Bibliography

Anusavice KJ: Phillips' Science of Dental Materials, ed 11, St. Louis, 2003, Saunders.

Asmussen E: NMR—analysis of monomers in restorative resins, Acta Odontol Scand 33:129, 1975.

Brauer GM, Antonucci JM: Dental applications. In Encyclopedia of polymer science and engineering, vol 4, ed 2 New York, 1986, Wiley.

Brodbelt RHW, O'Brien WJ, Fan PL: Translucency of dental porcelain, J Dent Res 59:70, 1980.

Craig RG: Chemistry, composition, and properties of composite resins, Dent Clin North Am 25:219, 1981.

Craig RG: Photopolymerization of dental composite systems. In Leinfelder KF, Taylor DF, editors: Posterior composites, Chapel Hill, NC, 1984, Proceedings of the International Symposium on Posterior Composite Resins.

Denry IL: Recent advances in ceramics for dentistry, Crit Rev Oral Bio Med 7(2):134, 1996.

Dieter G: Mechanical metallurgy, ed 3, New York, 1986, McGraw-Hill.

Flinn RA, Trojan PK: Engineering materials and their applications, ed 4, New York, 1990, John Wiley & Sons.

Fontana MG: Corrosion engineering, ed 3, New York, 1986, McGraw-Hill.

Garvie RC, Hannink RH, Pascoe RT: Ceramic steel? Nature 258:703, 1975.

Gettleman L: Noble alloys in dentistry, Current Opinion Dent 2:218, 1991.

Hodson JT: Some physical properties of three dental porcelains, J Prosthet Dent 9:235, 1959.

Höland W, Beall G: Glass-ceramic technology, Westerville, OH, 2002, The American Ceramic Society.

Kelly JR, Nishimura I, Campbell SD: Ceramics in dentistry: historical roots and current perspectives, J Prosthet Dent 75:18, 1996.

Kelly JR, Tesk JA, Sorensen JA: Failure of all-ceramic fixed partial dentures in vitro and in vivo: analysis and modeling, J Dent Res 74:1253, 1995.

Kingery WD, Bowen HK, Uhlmann DR: Introduction to ceramics, ed 2, New York, 1976, John Wiley & Sons.

Lawn BR, Pajares A, Zhang Y, et al: Materials design in the performance of all-ceramic crowns, Biomaterials 25(14): 2885, 2004.

Malhotra ML: Dental gold casting alloys: a review, Trends Tech Contemp Dent Lab 8:73, 1991.

May K, Russell M, Razzoog M, Lang B: Precision of fit: the Procera AllCeram crown, J Prosth Dent 80:394, 1998.

O'Brien WJ: Recent developments in materials and processes for ceramic crowns, J Am Dent Assoc 110:547, 1985.

O'Brien WJ: Dental materials and their selection, ed 2, Carol Stream, IL, 1997, Quintessence.

Paravina RD, Powers JM, editors: *Esthetic color training in dentistry*, St. Louis, 2004, Mosby.

Powers JM, Wataha JC: *Dental materials: properties and manipulation*, ed 9, St. Louis, Mosby.

Rekow ED: A review of the developments in dental CAD/CAM systems, *Curr Opin Dent* 2:25, 1992.

Ruyter IE: Monomer systems and polymerization. In Vanherle G, Smith DC, editors: *International Symposium on Posterior Composite Resin Dental Restorative Materials*, Netherlands, *Peter Szulc Publ* 6:109, 1985.

Seghi R, Sorensen J: Relative flexural strength of six new ceramic materials, *Int J Prosthodont* 8(3):239, 1995.

Zhang Y, Lawn BR: Long-term strength of ceramics for biomedical applications, *J Biomed Mater Res* 69B(2):166, 2004.

Preventive and Intermediary Materials

Prevention is a foundation of dentistry. Low-level fluorides in water supplies have provided tremendous benefit in reducing the incidence of dental caries in children. Fluorides can be introduced into community water supplies to ensure systemic ingestion during early life, when the teeth are forming. Fluoride can also be provided as a dietary supplement to inhibit caries where drinking water is not fluoridated. Patients who are at high risk for developing caries in spite of receiving systemic fluoride can be given various topical applications such as toothpastes, mouth rinses, gels, and varnishes. A combination of systemic and topical fluoride applications has contributed to a dramatic reduction in the prevalence of smooth surface caries over the past 50 years. Pits and fissures on the occlusal surfaces of posterior teeth, however, are more resistant to fluoride uptake because of the irregular morphology of the occlusal surface. This, combined with the retention of food and the difficulty of proper brushing in the posterior segment, can lead to the start of a carious lesion. A preventive therapy consisting of a sealant to fill in the irregularities can reduce the risk of caries by creating a smoother surface that is easier to clean and less likely to retain food and harbor bacteria.

PIT AND FISSURE SEALANTS

The most common sealants are based on Bis-GMA resin and are light cured, although some self-cured products are still available. The expanded name for Bis-GMA is 2,2-bis[4(2-hydroxy-3-methacryloyloxypropyloxy)-phenyl] propane. The chemistry of Bis-GMA sealants is the same as that described for resin composites in Chapter 9. The principal difference is that sealants are much more fluid to enable them to penetrate the pits, fissures, and etched areas on the enamel, which promote retention of the sealant. The viscous Bis-GMA resin is mixed with a diluent, such as triethylene glycol dimethacrylate, to produce a reasonably low viscosity, flowable resin. An alternative but similar oligomer base is urethane dimethacrylate; some materials are formulated from a combination of the two base resins. To provide stiffness to the material and improve wear resistance, filler particles of fumed silica or silanated inorganic glasses can be added to form low-viscosity composites.

Light-Cured Sealants

Today, most sealants are light cured, activated by a diketone and an aliphatic amine. The complete reactions for resin composites are given in Chapter 9. Light-cured sealants are supplied in light-tight containers and should have a shelf-life of more than 12 months. The sealant is applied to the pit and fissure with an appropriate applicator and is cured by exposing it to light for 20 seconds, with the end of the light source positioned about 1 to 2 mm from the surface. Sealants are applied in thin sections so depth of cure should be adequate with 20-second exposure times, even for opaque materials. The advantage in using a light-cured sealant is that the working time can be completely controlled by the operator.

Air Inhibition of Polymerization

During polymerization there is a surface layer of air inhibition that varies in depth with different commercial products. Sufficient material must be applied to completely coat all pits and fissures with a layer thick enough to ensure complete polymerization after removal of the tacky surface layer. The uncured, air inhibited, layer can be easily removed after curing using an abrasive slurry of pumice, applied on a cotton pellet or with a prophylaxis cup in a rotary handpiece. This is more effective than wiping or rinsing.

Properties of Sealants

Reports of the physical properties of sealants are scarce because specimen preparation with such low-viscosity materials is difficult. Because sealants are completed circumscribed by enamel and are not subjected to occlusal stresses, the mechanical properties of sealants are less important than those for resin composite restoratives. By adding ceramic or glass filler particles up to 40% by weight, as in the restorative composites, all properties except tensile strength show improvement. The modulus of elasticity shows the most dramatic improvement, and the increased rigidity makes the filled material less subject to deflection under occlusal stress. Filler is also added with the hope of improving wear resistance and making the material more visible on clinical inspection (Figure 8-1).

Optimal adhesion of the sealant to enamel occurs when the sealant has a high surface tension, good wetting, and a low viscosity. These properties permit the sealant to flow easily along the enamel surface. The surface wettability is demonstrated by the contact angle of a drop of liquid on the enamel surface. A drop that spreads readily produces a low contact angle. This highly wetted surface is conducive to a strong adhesive bond. Polymer tags form when the resin flows into the surface irregularities created by acid etching and are responsible for the mechanical bond that retains the sealant to enamel. Functional durability of the sealant bond is related to stresses induced by shrinkage of the resin during curing, thermal cycling, deflection from occlusal forces, water sorption, and abrasion, with total failure manifested by the clinical loss of material.

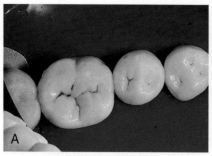
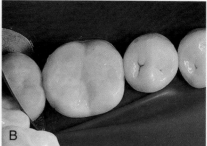

FIGURE 8.1 **Typical molar with stained fissures and no diagnosable caries. A,** Before sealing, and **B,** after sealing with a natural-colored sealant material. *(From Hatrick CD, Eakle WS, Bird WF: Dental materials: clinical applications for dental assistants and dental hygienists, ed 2, Saunders, St. Louis, 2011.)*

Sealant materials have a variety of features that must be selected carefully by the healthcare provider. Most current materials are light-cured rather than self-cured because of the ease and controlled rate of cure. Tooth-colored or clear resins are available that are very natural looking on the tooth surface, but they are also available in opaque or tinted materials to make the recall examination process easier (Figure 8-2). A new class of color-reversible, photosensitive sealants has recently been developed. They are very similar to the light-cured sealants in resin composition and filler loading. In addition, photosensitive pigments are added that are normally colorless but change to green or pink when exposed to the dental curing light. The color change lasts for about 5 to 10 minutes after exposure, to help determine whether the sealant adequately covers the pit and fissures. The color change can be repeated at recall visits with another exposure to a dental curing light.

An increasing number of sealants are marketed with the claim that they release fluoride. The release is highest in the first 24 hours after placement and then tapers to a low maintenance level, which may or may not be sufficient to provide extended clinical protection against caries.

Clinical Studies

Many clinical studies using Bis-GMA resins have been documented. In earlier studies on effectiveness of treatment with sealant in newly erupting teeth, a light-cured sealant demonstrated a retention rate of 42% and an effectiveness of 35% in caries reduction after 5 years. In a similar study, a filled resin sealant showed a retention rate of 53% and a clinical effectiveness of 54% after 4 years. Results involving a quicker-setting unfilled resin sealant with very good penetration showed a retention rate of 80% and an effectiveness of 69% after 3 years. The longest published study on sealant effectiveness is a 15-year evaluation of a self-cured unfilled material, which

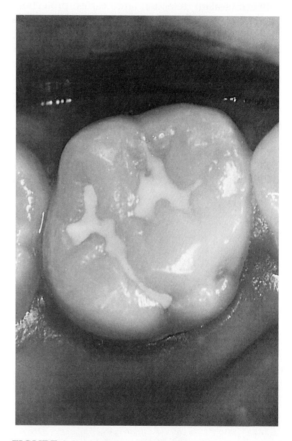

FIGURE 8.2 **Maxillary molar tooth with opaque sealant that has been in place for 5 years.**

showed 27.6% complete retention and 35.4% partial retention.

In pair-wise comparisons, the treated first molars had 31.3 decayed and filled primary tooth surfaces (dfs) and the untreated controls had 82.8 dfs. In a more current 4-year study comparing a fluoride-releasing sealant with one that did not have fluoride, retention rates were 91% for the fluoride material (77% complete and 14% partial) and 95% for the nonfluoride sealant (89% complete and 6% partial).

Although the retention was somewhat lower in the fluoride-containing sealant, the caries incidence for both groups was identical (10%). In a study conducted in private practice, the 2-year retention rates for two newer fluoride-containing resins were greater than 90%, and no caries was detected on the test teeth. In a continuing study with retreatment of all defective sealant surfaces at 6-month recalls, the teeth were maintained caries-free for a 5-year period. The retreatment rate was highest (18%) at 6 months, and then diminished as time progressed, but at each recall period at least two teeth (about 4%) required reapplication.

Almost all studies show a direct correlation between sealant retention and caries protection. Therefore, it is important to use materials that are retentive to enamel, resistant against occlusal wear, and easily applied with minimal opportunities for surface contamination. Current evidence indicates that sealants are most effective on occlusal surfaces where pits and fissures are well defined and retentive to food and in patients with elevated risk for pit and fissure caries.

Application of Sealants

The handling characteristics of a sealant depend on the composition of the material and the surface to which it is applied. Optimal preparation of both aspects will lead to close adaptation of the sealant to the tooth enamel, a strong seal against the ingress of oral fluids and debris, and long-term material retention.

Enamel Surface Preparation

The penetration of any of the sealants to the bottom of the pit is important. The wettability of the enamel by the sealant is improved by etching, and some advocate pretreatment with silanes in solution. Filling the pit or fissure without voids is critical. Air or debris can be trapped in the bottom of the fissure that prevents it from being completely filled, as shown in Figure 8-3. Control of the viscosity of the sealant is important to obtain optimum results. The viscosity determines the penetration of resin into the etched areas of enamel to provide adequate retention of the sealant. Penetration of sealant, forming tags, to a depth of 25 to 50 μm is shown in Figure 8-4.

Etching the pit and fissure surface for a specified time (15 to 30 seconds is adequate for enamel with a normal mineral and fluoride content) with a solution or a gel of 35% to 40% phosphoric acid is recommended. The acid etchant should be flushed thoroughly with water, and the area dried with warm air. Inadequate rinsing permits phosphate salts to remain on the surface as a contaminant, interfering with bond formation. The enamel surface should not be rubbed during etching and drying because the roughness developed can easily be destroyed. Isolation of the site is imperative throughout the procedure to achieve optimum tag formation and clinical success. If salivary

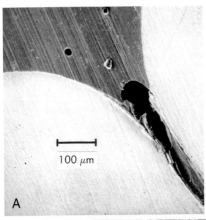

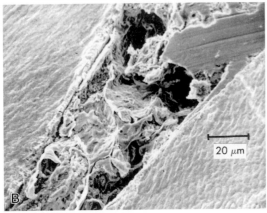

FIGURE 8.3 Section showing a fissure incompletely filled with sealant as a result of air **(A)** and debris **(B).** *(From Gwinnett AJ: J. Am. Soc. Prevent. Dent. 3,21, 1973.)*

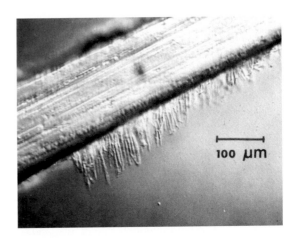

FIGURE 8.4 **Penetration of sealant into etched enamel.** These tags are responsible for the bonding to enamel. *(From Gwinnett AJ: J. Am. Soc. Prevent. Dent. 3,21, 1973.)*

contamination occurs during the treatment, the surface should be rinsed and the etch reapplied. On clinical inspection, acid-etched enamel should appear white and dull with an obviously rough texture. If the appearance is not uniform, an additional 30 seconds of etching should be done. The etched area should extend beyond the anticipated area for sealant application to secure optimum bonding along the margin and reduce the potential for early leakage, but without extensive overcoverage. A light-cured bonding agent (see Chapter 13) placed on the freshly etched enamel before placing the sealant will improve retention.

Single step etching and priming systems appear to provide a weaker bond to uncut enamel than to cut enamel walls and bevels.

SEALANT APPLICATION

Depending on its viscosity and setting time, the sealant may best be applied with a thin brush, a ball applicator, or a syringe. A buildup of excess material should be avoided because it could interfere with the occlusion. A sufficient amount of material should be placed to completely cover all exposed pits and provide a smooth transition along the inclines of the enamel cusps. Overworking of even the light-cured sealants on the tooth surface during application can introduce air voids that appear later as surface defects.

The air-inhibited surface layer should be wiped away immediately after curing and the coating inspected carefully for voids or areas of incomplete coverage. Defects can be covered at this time by repeating the entire reapplication procedure, including the acid etch, and applying fresh sealant only to those areas with insufficient coverage. After the sealant is applied and fully cured, the occlusion should be checked and adjusted if necessary, to eliminate premature contacts.

Glass Ionomers as Sealants

Because of their demonstrated ability to release fluoride and provide some caries protection on tooth surfaces at risk, glass ionomers have been suggested and tested for their ability to function as a fissure sealant. Glass ionomers are generally viscous, and it is difficult to gain penetration to the depth of a fissure. Their lack of penetration also makes it difficult to obtain mechanical retention to the enamel surface to the same degree as with Bis-GMA resins. They are also more brittle and less resistant to occlusal wear. Clinical studies using various formulations of glass ionomers have shown significantly lower retention rates than resin sealants but greater fluoride deposition in the enamel surfaces. Thus there is a greater potential for latent caries protection after sealant loss.

In areas where high-risk children do not have access to definitive treatment, a conservative caries management technique can seal remaining caries in a fluoride-rich environment and establish some degree of remineralization. Atraumatic restorative treatments (ARTs) involve opening a lesion, removing soft surface decay, and filling or sealing the surface with highly filled glass ionomer with a fast setting time. Future studies in this area may produce a new generation of sealant materials noted for their fluoride deposition rather than their mechanical obturation.

Flowable Composites as Sealants

Low-viscosity composites referred to as *flowable composites* are marketed for a wide variety of applications, such as preventive resin restorations, cavity liners, restoration repairs, and cervical restorations. The properties of flowable composites are described in Chapter 9.

Flowable composites are usually packaged in syringes or in compules (Figure 8-5) for direct application to the pit or fissure. As with lower viscosity resin sealants, trapping of air in the sealant must be avoided. Because they have higher filler content than most resin sealants, flowable composites should have

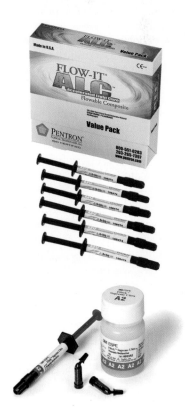

FIGURE 8.5 **Selection of flowable composite resins in syringe and compule delivery systems.** *(Courtesy of Pentron Clinical, Orange, CA)*

better wear resistance. Flowable composites appear to provide good retention and caries resistance after 24 months.

When flowable composites are used as preventive restorations, their low viscosity is a benefit in extending the restoration into adjacent fissures as a sealant. Long-term clinical efficacy of flowable composites as preventive resin restorations is yet to be established.

GLASS IONOMERS TO PREVENT THE PROGRESSION OF CARIES

The final materials that need to be considered for caries control and prevention are glass ionomers and hybrid ionomers (resin-modified glass ionomers). Because of their documented slow release of fluoride, glass ionomers are used in cervical restorations when esthetics is not critical. They are specifically recommended for patients with high caries risk (Table 8-1). A detailed description of glass ionomer chemistry can be found in Chapter 9.

Composition and Reaction

Glass ionomers are supplied as powders of various shades and a liquid. The powder is an ion-leachable aluminosilicate glass, and the liquid is a water solution of polymers and copolymers of acrylic acid. The material sets as a result of the metallic salt bridges between the Al^{++} and Ca^{++} ions leached from the glass and the acid groups on the polymers. The reaction progresses slowly, with the formation of a cross-linked gel matrix in the initial set and an aluminum ion exchange strengthening the cross-linking

in the final set. A chelation effect takes place with the calcium on the exposed tooth surface, creating an adhesive bond. The surfaces of new restorations should be protected from saliva during the initial set with a protective coating.

Properties

The properties of glass ionomers are compared qualitatively with other restorative materials in Table 8-2. Significant properties are (1) elastic modulus that is similar to dentin, (2) bond strength to dentin of 2 to 3 MPa, (3) expansion coefficient comparable to tooth structure, (4) low solubility, and (5) fairly high opacity. Fluoride in the glass releases slowly to provide an anticariogenic effect on adjacent dental plaque and tooth structure.

Although the bond strength of glass ionomers to dentin is lower than that of resin composites, clinical studies have shown that the retention of glass ionomers in areas of cervical erosion are considerably better than for composites. When the dentin is conditioned (etched) using a dilute solution (15% to 25%) of polyacrylic acid, the glass ionomer may be applied without a cavity preparation. Four-year clinical data showed a retention rate for glass ionomer cervical restorations of 75%. The surfaces of the restorations seen in the studies were noticeably rough, and some shade mismatches were present. Pulp reaction to glass ionomers is mild; if the thickness of dentin is less than 1 mm, a calcium hydroxide liner is recommended. Although the surface remains slightly rough, cervical restorations did not contribute to inflammation of gingival tissues. Fewer *Streptococcus mutans* organisms exist in plaque adjacent to glass ionomer restorations than in controls without glass ionomers.

Glass ionomers are packaged in bottles and in vacuum capsules for mechanical mixing in a mechanical mixer. In bulk dispensing, the powder and liquid are dispensed in proper amounts on the paper pad, and half the powder is incorporated to produce a

TABLE 8-1   Uses of Composites, Compomers, Hybrid Ionomers, and Glass Ionomers

Type	Uses
Hybrid/microfilled/ multipurpose composite	Classes 1, 2, 3, 4, 5, low caries–risk patient
	Classes 1, 3, 4, medium caries–risk patients
Compomer	Primary teeth, classes 1, 2 restorations in children
	Cervical lesions, classes 3, 5, medium caries–risk patients
Hybrid ionomer	Cervical lesions, classes 3, 5, primary teeth, sandwich technique, class 5, high caries–risk patients, root caries
Glass ionomer	Cervical lesions, class 5 restorations in adults where esthetics are less important, root caries

TABLE 8-2   Ranking of Selected Properties of Hybrid Ionomers and Glass Ionomers

Property	Hybrid Ionomer	Glass Ionomer
Compressive strength	Med	Low-Med
Flexural strength	Med	Low-Med
Flexural modulus	Med	Med-High
Wear resistance	Med	Low
Fluoride release	Med-High	High
Fluoride rechargability	Med-High	High
Esthetics	Good	Acceptable

homogeneous milky consistency. The remainder of the powder is added, and a total mixing time of 30 to 40 seconds is used with a typical initial setting time of 4 minutes. After placing the restorative and developing the correct contour, the surface should be protected from contamination by applying a protective barrier. Trimming and finishing should be done after 24 hours.

The liquid in the unit-dose capsule is forced into the powder by a press and is mixed by a mechanical mixer. The mixture is injected directly into the cavity preparation with a special syringe. Working time is short and critical, so it is imperative to place the material with a minimum of manipulation. If the gel stage of the reaction is disrupted during the early phase of the reaction, the physical properties will be very low and adhesion can be lost.

Optimum results are achieved if the manufacturer's instructions are followed carefully—maintaining isolation, using adequate etching procedures, protecting the restoration from saliva after placement, and delaying final finishing for a day or longer if possible.

RESIN-MODIFIED GLASS IONOMERS

Resin-modified glass ionomers, also known as *hybrid ionomers*, are used for restorations in low stress-bearing areas and are recommended for patients with high caries risk (see Table 8-2). These restorations are more esthetic than glass ionomers because of their resin content. Examples of cervical erosions, abfractions, and hybrid ionomer restorations are shown in Figure 8-6.

Composition and Reaction

The powder of resin-modified glass ionomers is similar to that of glass ionomers. The liquid contains monomers, polyacids, and water. Resin-modified glass ionomers set by a combined acid-base ionomer reaction and light-cured resin polymerization of 2-hydroxyethyl methacrylate. Placing a bonding agent before inserting a resin-modified glass ionomer is contraindicated, because it decreases fluoride uptake by the dentin and enamel.

Properties

Resin-modified ionomers bond to tooth structure without the use of a bonding agent. Typically, the tooth is conditioned (etched) with polyacrylic acid or a primer before placing the hybrid ionomer. The flexural strength of a hybrid ionomer is almost double that of a standard glass ionomer. Hybrid ionomers release more fluoride than compomers and composites but almost the same as glass ionomers. Figure 8-7 illustrates the release of fluoride ions from a standard glass ionomer and resin-modified glass ionomer over a 30-day period. There is an early period of high release, which tapers after about 10 days to 1 ppm. Glass ionomers and hybrid ionomers recharge when exposed to fluoride treatments or fluoride dentifrices. Figure 8-8 illustrates this recharge capability with a similar time-dependent release curve. In evaluating the effectiveness of this release, fluoride has been measured in plaque samples immediately adjacent to glass ionomer-based restorations (Figure 8-9). For these two materials from the same manufacturer, plaque adjacent to the resin-modified glass ionomer had significantly higher fluoride content than plaque adjacent to compomer restorations at 2 days and 21 days after insertion of the restorations.

Manipulation

An example of a hybrid ionomer packaged in capsules is shown in Figure 8-10. For hybrid ionomers packaged in bulk as powder-liquids, manipulation is like that of standard glass ionomers. Mechanical

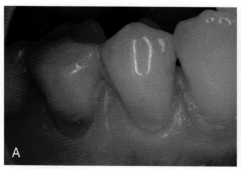
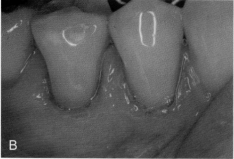

FIGURE 8.6 **Restoration of root surface lesions. A,** Abrasion/erosion lesions on the facial surface of mandibular premolars. **B,** Restorations with resin-modified glass ionomer cement and composite. *(Courtesy of Dr. Thomas J. Hilton, Portland, OR)*

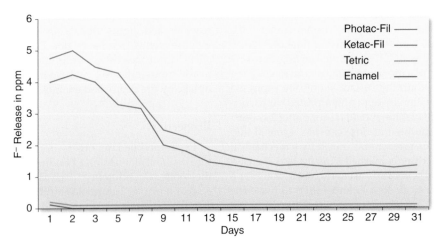

FIGURE 8.7 Fluoride release from glass ionomer cements and composite resin in distilled water over 30 days. *(Modified from Strothers, J.M., Kohn, D.H., Dennison, J.B., et. al., 1998. Dent. Mater. 14, 129.)*

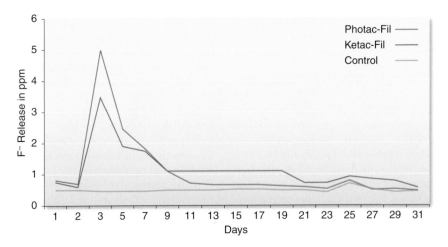

FIGURE 8.8 Fluoride re-uptake and re-release from glass ionomer cements after recharging the material with 1.1% neutral sodium fluoride gel. *(Modified from Strothers JM, Kohn DH, Dennison JB, et. al: Dent. Mater. 14, 129, 1998.)*

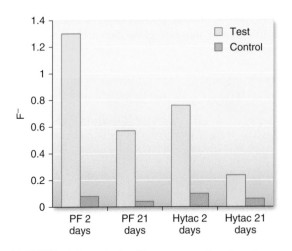

FIGURE 8.9 Total fluoride concentration in plaque (microgram fluoride per mg plaque) adjacent to resin-modified glass ionomer and compomer restorations over 21 days; restored test teeth versus nonrestored control teeth.

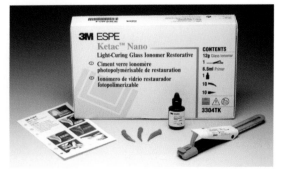

FIGURE 8.10 Resin-modified glass ionomer materials available for hand mixing or encapsulated for mechanical mixing. *(Courtesy of 3M ESPE Dental Products, St. Paul, MN)*

mixing of the unit-dose capsules provides a uniform mix that has much fewer of the larger air voids than can be introduced during hand spatulation. Optimum powder/liquid ratio is critical to the long-term maintenance of physical properties and the clinical success of restorations. Unlike glass ionomer restorations, hybrid ionomers set immediately when light-cured and can be finished 5 to 10 minutes after initial set. Color can be maintained and surface texture improved by finishing the hybrid ionomer restorations in a wet environment (water spray or water-soluble lubricant) and then recoating with a protective varnish or bonding agent. Glass ionomers are an increasingly important part of operative dentistry for both an aging population with high incidence of root caries, patients with xerostomia and reduced salivary flow, and children who have high caries risk factors.

RESIN-MODIFIED GLASS IONOMERS AS CAVITY LINERS

Resin-modified glass ionomers can also be used to line the dentin walls of a deep cavity. When used as a cavity liner, these materials provide thermal insulation. A *sandwich technique* uses a resin-modified glass ionomer to seal the dentin and provide the benefit of fluoride release over which a layer of resin composite is used to fill the remainder of the cavity. Some advocate the use of the glass ionomer as a liner to relieve stresses that result from shrinkage of the composite during cure. Glass ionomer lining cements bond to dentin with bond strengths measured in tension that vary from 2.0 to 4.9 MPa. These cements also adhere to composite restorative materials. Glass ionomer lining cements release fluoride ions and are radiopaque. More discussion of glass ionomers as cements can be found in Chapter 13.

CALCIUM HYDROXIDE CAVITY LINERS

Calcium hydroxide cements are used for lining specific areas of deep cavities or for direct pulp capping. The antibacterial action of calcium hydroxide makes these cements useful in indirect pulp-capping procedures involving carious dentin.

Calcium hydroxide cavity liners are provided as pastes that set to a hard mass when mixed. The base paste of a typical product contains calcium tungstate, tribasic calcium phosphate, and zinc oxide in glycol salicylate. The catalyst paste contains calcium hydroxide, zinc oxide, and zinc stearate in ethylene toluene sulfonamide. The ingredients responsible for setting are calcium hydroxide and a salicylate, which react to form an amorphous calcium disalicylate.

Fillers such as calcium tungstate or barium sulfate provide radiopacity.

A light-cured calcium hydroxide liner consists of calcium hydroxide and barium sulfate dispersed in a urethane dimethacrylate resin. The important properties of calcium hydroxide cements are mechanical and thermal properties, solubility, and pH. Research has also shown that these cements can create secondary dentin bridges when applied to direct pulp exposures. Calcium hydroxide (self-cured) liners have low values of tensile strength and compressive strength, or elastic modulus, compared with high-strength bases. Although setting times vary between 2.5 and 5.5 minutes, compressive strengths of these cements continue to increase over a 24-hour period. For a group of five commercial products, compressive strengths ranged from 6.5 to 14.3 MPa at 10 minutes to from 9.8 to 26.8 MPa at 24 hours. The low elastic modulus of calcium hydroxide cavity liners restricts their usage to specific areas not critical to the support of restorations.

The solubility of calcium hydroxide bases has been measured in several solvents for various periods of immersion and has been found to be significant. Some solubility of the calcium hydroxide is necessary to achieve its therapeutic properties, although an optimum value is not known. Clearly the use of acid-etching procedures and varnish in the presence of calcium hydroxide liners must be done with care. The pH of commercial products has been measured at between 9.2 and 11.7. Free calcium hydroxide in excess of that necessary to form the calcium disalicylate stimulates secondary dentin in proximity to the pulp and shows antibacterial activity. Calcium hydroxide liners are mostly used in direct pulp capping and in specific, deep spots of a cavity preparation. Light-cured resin-modified glass ionomer liners are a better choice for general lining of cavities because of their fluoride release, decreased solubility, and superior mechanical properties.

FLUORIDE VARNISHES

Fluoride-containing varnishes deliver fluoride topically to the surfaces of teeth in patients at risk for caries. The varnishes are used routinely for topical application, usually after a prophylaxis. Products contain either 5% sodium fluoride (2.26% F$^-$ or 22,600 ppm) or 1% difluorsilane (0.1% F$^-$ or 1000 ppm). The fluoride is dissolved in an organic solvent that evaporates when applied or sets when exposed to moisture, leaving a thin film of material covering all exposed tooth surfaces. The mechanism of action for a fluoride varnish is similar to that of a fluoride mouthwash. Calcium fluoride is deposited on the tooth surface and later converted through a remineralization reaction to fluorapatite.

One advantage of fluoride varnish is the extended time of exposure for the active fluoride ingredient against the tooth surface. Instead of seconds, as with a mouthwash, it may be hours before a varnish wears off. One resin-modified glass ionomer–based varnish has been reported to release fluoride for up to 6 months. Clinical trials have documented the efficacy of varnish in treating young children at risk for caries, with reductions reported as high as 70%. Another potential use for this type of material is in the prevention of root caries in an older population, which has exposed root surfaces with increasing risk as aging occurs. Semiannual application of fluoride varnishes seems to provide optimum efficacy. More research is necessary to fully document the value of using these materials in patients with moderate to high caries risk.

REMINERALIZATION

Remineralization is a natural repair process for carious lesions. Elevated levels of fluoride in toothpaste has been shown to be effective in rehardening root caries lesions that are cavitated. A 5000-ppm-F toothpaste rehardened 76% of lesions compared with 35% in a 1100-ppm-F group. The concept of the caries balance proposed by Featherstone describes three pathological factors and three protective factors for dental caries. The pathological factors are (1) acid-producing bacteria, (2) frequent consumption of fermentable carbohydrates, and (3) below normal salivary flow and function. The three protective factors are (1) a normal salivary flow and components, (2) fluoride, and (3) antibacterials. Two salivary components required for remineralization are calcium and phosphate. Fluoride enhances remineralization.

Calcium phosphate formulations have been developed for addition to toothpaste, varnishes, and gum (Figure 8-11). A calcium phosphate remineralization technology based on casein

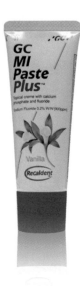

FIGURE 8.11 **Paste for remineralizing enamel.** *(Courtesy of GC America, Alsip, IL)*

phosphopeptide–amorphous calcium phosphate (CPP-ACP) was effective in remineralizing enamel subsurface lesions by stabilizing high levels of calcium and phosphate ions. When added to sugar-free gum in a randomized controlled clinical trial, an 18% reduction in caries progression after 24 months was demonstrated. In paste form, the CPP-ACP complexes have been shown to be effective in reversing early caries lesions and stabilizing the progression of caries.

A bioactive glass (calcium sodium phosphosilicate) originally developed as a bone-regenerative material, has been shown to deposit onto dentin surfaces and mechanically occlude dentinal tubules when delivered in a dentifrice. When combined with therapeutic levels of fluoride, this material increases the remineralization of caries lesions in situ.

SELECTED PROBLEMS

PROBLEM 1

What is the advantage of a fluoride varnish versus other means of applying fluoride to teeth?

Solution

Two advantages are the higher fluoride concentration used and the extended time of exposure of the teeth to the active fluoride ingredient compared with other forms of topical application.

PROBLEM 2

Why are pit and fissure sealants needed to control caries on occlusal surfaces of permanent teeth?

Solution

Pits and fissures in the occlusal surfaces of permanent teeth are susceptible to caries because their physical size and morphology provide shelter for organisms and obstruct oral hygiene procedures. As a result, fluoride treatments have not been effective in reducing caries in occlusal pits and fissures.

PROBLEM 3

When selecting a material as a pit and fissure sealant, what characteristics of a filled resin sealant are relevant?

Solution

The relevant characteristics are better physical properties and improved abrasion resistance (but with occlusal prematurities that should be adjusted after insertion); a slightly higher viscosity than an unfilled sealant but a much lower viscosity than a composite; and better control in application procedures.

PROBLEM 4

When selecting a sealant material, what characteristics of an unfilled resin sealant are relevant?

Solution

The relevant characteristics are lower viscosity; less wear resistance, but with occlusal prematurities that will wear down readily; and less control in application procedures.

PROBLEM 5

Postoperative evaluation of a freshly placed sealant revealed subsurface air voids, some communicating with the external surface. What manipulative variables can be controlled to minimize this problem?

Solution

The problem can be minimized by controlling the following variables: (1) avoid mixing or stirring the sealant if at all possible after it is dispensed for application, or use a photo-initiated resin; (2) avoid using a brush for application, which tends to carry excess material and incorporate air; (3) use a ball-tipped applicator, which permits the application of smaller increments of material to specific sites on the tooth surface with only minimal manipulation of the setting sealant; (4) avoid moisture contamination during application because it can produce subsurface voids after equilibrium is reached through water sorption; (5) avoid the use of a material beyond its shelf life or one that has been stored in a warm environment because the increase in viscosity results in air entrapment during application; and (6) avoid application of the sealant to a nonwettable or inadequately etched enamel surface.

PROBLEM 6

Six months after sealant application, a first molar was clinically evaluated at recall and found to have no sealant present. What are the possible causes for this early failure?

Solution a

One cause might be inadequately prepared enamel surface, possibly the result of (1) failure to remove pellicle and debris from the surface by omitting preoperative prophylaxis cleaning; (2) inadequate acid etching by using concentrated or diluted etchant, exposure to etchant for insufficient time, or the presence of acid-resistant enamel with a high fluoride composition; (3) insufficient rinsing of the acid etchant solution or gel, leaving contaminating salts present to reduce surface energy; (4) moisture or salivary contamination during sealant application; or (5) contamination of the etched enamel site by oil or by water in the compressed air used for drying.

Solution b

A second causative factor might be inadequately cured photo-initiated sealant, possibly the result of (1) the light wand being held too high above the tooth surface; (2) failure to make multiple light applications to completely expose the entire surface; (3) inadequate exposure time to the light source; (4) use of a sealant that has previously been exposed to light or has been used beyond its shelf life; or (5) use of an opaque or deeply colored sealant without increasing the exposure time.

PROBLEM 7

At recall evaluations, sealants may have an orange-brown stain along specific marginal areas, which is indicative of bond failure and marginal leakage. What are the causative factors for this failure?

Solution

The causative factors are inadequate enamel preparation at the failure site or contamination of the etched enamel; overextension of sealant beyond the periphery of adequately etched enamel; and functional occlusal forces, placed directly over thin extensions of sealant, producing stresses that exceed the bond strength of sealant to enamel.

PROBLEM 8

Although the bond strength of glass ionomers to dentin is lower than that of composites, clinical experience has shown that the retention of glass ionomers to areas of cervical erosion are better. Why?

Solution

Although the bond strength of glass ionomers to dentin is only 2 to 3 MPa in the setting reaction, chelation occurs with the calcium on the tooth surface, producing an adhesive bond, whereas the bond of composites to tooth structure is essentially micromechanical.

PROBLEM 9

Compared with glass ionomers and composites, what are the advantages of hybrid ionomers for low stress–bearing restorations?

Solution

The flexural strength of hybrid ionomers is about twice that of glass ionomers. They release more fluoride than composites and are more esthetic than glass ionomers.

Bibliography

Fluoride Varnishes

Banting DW, Papas A, Clark DC, et. al: The effectiveness of 10% chlorhexidine varnish treatment on dental caries incidence in adults with dry mouth, *Gerodontology* 17:67, 2000.

Beltran-Aguilar ED, Goldstein JW: Fluoride varnishes: a review of their clinical use, cariostatic mechanism, efficacy and safety, *J Am Dent Assoc* 131:589, 2000.

Petersson LG, Twetman S, Pakhomov GN: The efficiency of semiannual silane fluoride varnish applications: a two-year clinical study in preschool children, *J Public Health Dent* 58:57, 1998.

Skold L, Sundquist B, Eriksson B, et al: Four-year study of caries inhibition of intensive Duraphat application in 11-15-year-old children, *Community Dent Oral Epidemiol* 22:8, 1994.

Pit and Fissure Sealants

Arenholt-Bindslev D, Breinholt V, Preiss A, et al: Time-related bisphenol-A content and estrogenic activity in saliva samples collected in relation to placement of fissure sealants, *Clinical Oral Invest* 3:120, 1999.

Boksman L, Carson B: Two-year retention and caries rates of UltraSeal XT and FluoroShield light-cured pit and fissure sealants, *General Dent* 46:184, 1998.

Buonocore MG: Adhesive sealing of pits and fissures for caries prevention, with use of ultraviolet light, *J Am Dent Assoc* 80:324, 1970.

Charbeneau GT, Dennison JB: Clinical success and potential failure after single application of a pit and fissure sealant: a four-year report, *J Am Dent Assoc* 98:559, 1979.

Dennison JB, Powers JM: Physical properties of pit and fissure sealants (annot), *J Dent Res* 58:1430, 1979.

Dennison JB, Straffon LH: Clinical evaluation comparing sealant and amalgam after 7 years: final report, *J Am Dent Assoc* 117:751, 1988.

Feigal RJ, Hitt J, Splieth C: Retaining sealant on salivary contaminated enamel, *J Am Dent Assoc* 124:88, 1993.

Fiegal RJ, Quelhas I: Clinical trial of a self-etching adhesive for sealant application: success at 24 months with Prompt-L-Pop, *Am J Dent* 16:249, 2003.

Folke BD, Walton JL, Feigal RJ: Occlusal sealant success over ten years in a private practice: Comparing longevity of sealants placed by dentists, hygienists and assistants, *Pediatr Dent* 26:426, 2004.

Frencken JE, Makoni F, Sithole WD: Atraumatic restorative treatment and glass-ionomer sealants in a school oral health programme in Zimbabwe, *Caries Res* 30:429, 1996.

Garcia-Gordoy F, Abarzua I, De Goes MF, et al: Fluoride release from fissure sealants, *J Clin Pediatr Dent* 22:45, 1997.

Gungor HC, Altay N, Alpar R: Clinical evaluation of a poly-acid-modified resin composite-based fissure sealant: two year results, *Oper Dent* 29:254, 2004.

Handleman SL, Buonocore MG, Heseck DJ: A preliminary report on the effect of fissure sealant on bacteria in dental caries, *J Prosthet Dent* 27:390, 1972.

Hannig M, Grafe A, Atalay S, et al: Microleakage and SEM evaluation of fissure sealants placed by use of self-etching priming agents, *J Dent* 32:75, 2004.

Hori M, Yoshida E, Hashimoto M, et al: in vitro testing of all-in-one adhesives as sealants, *Am J Dent* 17:177, 2004.

Horowitz HS, Heifetz SB, Poulsen S: Retention and effectiveness of a single application of an adhesive sealant in preventing occlusal caries: final report after five years of a study in Kalispell, Montana, *J Am Dent Assoc* 95:1133, 1977.

Lygidakis NA, Oulis KI: A comparison of Fluroshield with Delton fissure sealant: four year results, *Pediatr Dent* 21:429, 1999.

Manabe A, Kaneko S, Numazawa S, et al: Detection of Bisphenol-A in dental materials by gas chromatography-mass spectrometry, *Dent Mater* 19:75, 2000.

Myers CL, Rossi F, Cartz F: Adhesive taglike extensions into acid-etched tooth enamel, *J Dent Res* 53:435, 1974.

O'Brien WJ, Fan PL, Apostolidis A: Penetrativity of sealants and glazes, *Oper Dent* 3:51, 1978.

Pahlavan A, Dennison JB, Charbeneau GT: Penetration of restorative resins into acid-etched human enamel, *J Am Dent Assoc* 93:1170, 1976.

Pardi V, Pereira AC, Mialhe FL, et al: Six-year clinical evaluation of polyacid-modified composite resin used as fissure sealant, *J Clin Pediatr Dent* 28:257, 2004.

Pereira AC, Pardi V, Mialhe FL, et al: A 3-year clinical evaluation of glass ionomer cements used as fissure sealants, *Am J Dent* 16:23, 2003.

Rueggeberg FA, Dlugokinski M, Ergle JW: Minimizing patient's exposure to uncured components in a dental sealant, *J Am Dent Assoc* 130:1751, 1999.

Simonsen RJ: Retention and effectiveness of dental sealant after 15 years, *J Am Dent Assoc* 122:34, 1991.

Steinmetz MJ, Pruhs RJ, Brooks JC, et al: Rechargeability of fluoride releasing pit and fissure sealants and restorative resin composites, *Am J Dent* 10:36, 1997.

Straffon LH, Dennison JB, More FG: Three-year evaluation of sealant: effect of isolation on efficacy, *J Am Dent Assoc* 110:714, 1985.

Symons AL, Chu CY, Meyers IA: The effect of fissure morphology and pretreatment of the enamel surface on penetration and adhesion of fissure sealants, *J Oral Rehabil* 23:791, 1996.

Tarumi H, Imazato S, Narimatsu M, et al: Estrogenicity of fissure sealants and adhesive resins determined by reporter gene assay, *J Dent Res* 79:1838, 2000.

Taylor CL, Gwinnett AJ: A study of the penetration of sealants into pits and fissures, *J Am Dent Assoc* 87:1181, 1973.

Williams B, Laxton L, Holt RD, et al: Tissue sealants: a 4-year clinical trial comparing an experimental glass polyalkenoate cement with a bis glycidyl methacrylate resin used as fissure sealants, *Br Dent J* 180:104, 1996.

Flowable Composites

Behle C: Flowable composites: properties and applications, *Pract Periodont Aesthet Dent* 10:347, 1998.

Fortin D, Vargas MA: The spectrum of composites: new techniques and materials, *J Am Dent Assoc* 131:26S, 2000.

Houpt M, Fuks A, Eidelman E: The preventive resin (composite resin/sealant) restoration: nine-year results, *Quint Int* 25:155, 1994.

Unterbrink GL, Liebenberg WH: Flowable resin composites as "filled adhesives": literature review and clinical recommendations, *Quint Int* 30:249, 1999.

Glass Ionomers and Hybrid Ionomers

Bapna MS, Mueller HJ: Leaching from glass ionomer cements, *J Oral Rehabil* 21:577, 1994.

Berry EA III, Powers JM: Bond strength of glass ionomers to coronal and radicular dentin, *Oper Dent* 19:122, 1994.

Braundau HE, Ziemiecki TZ, Charbeneau GT: Restoration of cervical contours on nonprepared teeth using glass ionomer cement: a $4\frac{1}{2}$ year report, *J Am Dent Assoc* 104:782, 1984.

Cattani-Lorente MA, Dupuis V, Moya F, et al: Comparative study of the physical properties of a polyacid-modified composite resin and a resin-modified glass ionomer, *Dent Mater* 15:21, 1999.

Council on Dental Materials: Instruments, and Equipment: Using glass ionomers, *J Am Dent Assoc* 121:181, 1990.

Croll TP: Glass ionomers in esthetic dentistry, *J Am Dent Assoc* 123:51, 1992.

Farah JW, Powers JM, editors: *Fluoride-releasing restorative materials*, *Dent Advis* 15, 1998, p 2.

Fleming GJ, Faroog AA, Barralet JE: Influence of powder/liquid mixing ratio on the performance of a restorative glass-ionomer dental cement, *Biomaterials* 24:4173, 2003.

Forss H: Release of fluoride and other elements from light-cured glass ionomer in neutral and acidic conditions, *J Dent Res* 72:1257, 1993.

Garcia R, Caffesse RG, Charbeneau GT: Gingival tissue response to restoration of deficient cervical contours using a glass-ionomer material, a 12-month report, *J Prosthet Dent* 46:393, 1981.

Heys RJ, Fitzgerald M, Heys DR, et al: An evaluation of a glass ionomer luting agent: pulpal histological response, *J Am Dent Assoc* 114:607, 1987.

Hotta M, Hirukawa H, Aono M: The effect of glaze on restorative glass-ionomer cements: evaluation of environmental durability in lactic acid solution, *J Oral Rehabil* 22:685, 1995.

Kent BE, Lewis BG, Wilson AD: The properties of a glass ionomer cement, *Br Dent J* 135:322, 1973.

Maldonado A, Swartz ML, Phillips RW: An in vitro study of certain properties of a glass ionomer cement, *J Am Dent Assoc* 96:785, 1978.

McLean JW, Wilson AD: The clinical development of the glass-ionomer cements, *Aust Dent J* 22:31, 1977.

Mitchell CA, Douglas WH: Comparison of the porosity of hand-mixed and capsulated glass-ionomer luting cements, *Biomaterials* 18:1127, 1997.

Mount GJ: The role of glass ionomer cements in esthetic dentistry: a review, *Esthet Dent Update* 4:7, 1993.

Müller J, Brucker G, Kraft E, et al: Reaction of cultured pulp cells to eight different cements based on glass ionomers, *Dent Mater* 6:172, 1990.

Quackenbush BM, Donly KJ, Croll TP: Solubility of a resin-modified glass ionomer cement, *J Dent Child* 65:310, 1998.

Strother JM, Kohn DH, Dennison JB, et al: Fluoride release and re-uptake in direct tooth colored restorative materials, *Dent Mater* 14:129, 1998.

Ribeiro AP, Serra MC, Paulillo LA, et al: Effectiveness of surface protection for resin-modified glass-ionomer materials, *Quint Int* 30:427, 1999.

Sidhu S, Watson TF: Resin-modified glass ionomer materials: a status report for the American Journal of Dentistry, *Am J Dent* 8:59, 1995.

Weidlich P, Miranda LA, Maltz M, et al: Fluoride release and uptake from glass ionomer cements and composite resins, *Braz Dent J* 11:89, 2000.

Wellbury RR, Shaw AJ, Murray JJ, et al: Clinical evaluation of paired compomer and glass ionomer restorations in primary teeth, *Br Dent J* 189:93, 2000.

Wilder AD, Boghosian AA, Bayne SC, et al: Effect of powder/liquid ratio on the clinical and laboratory performance of resin-modified glass ionomers, *J Dent* 26:369, 1998.

Ylp HK, Smales RJ: Fluoride release and uptake by aged resin-modified glass ionomers and a polyacid-modified resin composite, *Int Dent J* 49:217, 1999.

Remineralization

Baysan A, Lynch E, Ellwood R, et al: Reversal of primary root caries using dentifrices containing 5,000 and 1,100 ppm fluoride, *Caries Res* 35:41–46, 2001.

Burwell AK, Litkowski LJ, Greenspan DC: Calcium sodium phosphosilicate (NovaMin): remineralization potential, *Adv Dent Res* 21(1):35, 2009.

Featherstone JD: Prevention and reversal of dental caries: role of low level fluoride, *Community Dent Oral Epidemiol* 27:31–40, 1999.

Featherstone JDB: Remineralization, the natural caries repair process: the need for new approaches, *Adv Dent Res* 21(1):4, 2009.

Featherstone JD: The caries balance: the basis for caries management by risk assessment, *Oral Health Prev Dent* 2(Suppl 1):259–264, 2004.

Reynolds EC: Casein phosphopeptide-amorphous calcium phosphate: the scientific evidence, *Adv Dent Res* 21(1):25, 2009.

ten Cate JM: The need for antibacterial approaches to improve caries control, *Adv Dent Res* 21:8–12, 2009.

Weintraub JA, Ramos-Gomez FR, Shain SG, et al: Fluoride varnish efficacy in preventing early childhood caries, *J Dent Res* 85:172–176, 2006.

Restorative Materials—Composites and Polymers

The concept of a composite biomaterial, introduced in Chapter 4, can be described as a solid that contains two or more distinct constituent materials or phases when considered at greater than an atomic scale. In these materials, mechanical properties such as elastic modulus are significantly altered in comparison with a homogenous material consisting of either of the phases alone. Enamel, dentin, bone, and reinforced polymers are considered composites, but alloys such as brass are not. The ability to change properties of the macroscale object based on control of the individual constituents is a significant advantage in the use of composite materials.

In dentistry, the term *resin composite* generally refers to a reinforced polymer system used for restoring hard tissues, for example, enamel and dentin. The proper materials science term is *polymer matrix composite* or for those composites with filler particles often used as direct-placed restorative composites, *particulate-reinforced polymer matrix composite*. In this chapter, the term *resin composite* refers to the reinforced polymer matrix materials used as restorative materials. The class of materials called *conventional glass ionomers (GIs)* and *resin-modified glass ionomers (RMGIs)* also are included in the scientific class of composite materials, but because these are water-based materials and have a distinct acid-base setting reaction, they have been traditionally categorized as a class of their own. It is important to remember, however, that most biological materials, including enamel, dentin, bone, connective tissue, muscle, and even cells, are classified as composites within the broad range of biological engineering materials.

Resin composites are used to replace missing tooth structure and modify tooth color and contour, thus enhancing esthetics. A number of commercial resin composites are available for various applications. Traditionally some have been optimized for esthetics and others were designed for higher stress bearing areas. More recently nanocomposites have become available, which are optimized for both excellent esthetics and high mechanical properties for stress bearing areas. Glass ionomers and resin-modified glass ionomers are used selectively as filling materials, usually for small lesions, especially where one or more margins are in dentin and in areas of caries activity.

Resin-based composites were first developed in the early 1960s and provided materials with higher mechanical properties than acrylics and silicates, lower thermal coefficient of expansion, lower dimensional change on setting, and higher resistance to wear, thereby improving clinical performance. Early composites were chemically activated; the next generation were photo-activated composites initiated with ultraviolet (UV) wavelengths. These were

TABLE 9.1　Types of Restorations and Recommended Resin Composites

Type of Restoration	Recommended Resin Composite
Class 1	Multipurpose, nanocomposite, packable microfilled (posterior),* compomer (posterior)*
Class 2	Multipurpose, nanocomposite, packable, laboratory, microfilled (posterior),* compomer (posterior)*
Class 3	Multipurpose, nanocomposite, microfilled, compomer
Class 4	Multipurpose, nanocomposite
Class 5	Multipurpose, nanocomposite, microfilled, compomer
Class 6 (MOD)	Packable, nanocomposite
Cervical lesions	Flowable, compomer
Pediatric restorations	Flowable, compomer
3-unit bridge or crown	Laboratory (with fiber reinforcement)
Alloy substructure	Laboratory (bonded)
Core build-up	Core
Temporary restoration	Provisional
High caries-risk patients	Glass ionomers, hybrid ionomers (see Chapter 8)

Special microfilled composites and compomers are available for posterior use.
MOD, *Mesial-occlusal-distal.*

later replaced by composites activated in the visible wavelengths. Continued improvements in composite technology have resulted in the modern materials with excellent durability, wear-resistance, and esthetics that mimic the natural teeth. In particular, the incorporation of nanotechnology in controlling the filler architecture has made dramatic improvements in these materials. Moreover, the development of bonding agents for bonding composites to tooth structure (see Chapter 13) has also improved the longevity and performance of composite restorations. A classification of preparation type and recommended composite category is listed in Table 9-1. Characteristics of these composite categories are summarized in Table 9-2.

Glass ionomers (GIs) were also developed in the 1960s and are based on an acid-base cement-forming reaction between fluoroaluminosilicate (FAS) glass powder, similar to those used in silicate cements, and aqueous solution of polycarboxylic acids. These were less prone to dissolution than silicates, but the early materials suffered from difficulty of manipulation,

TABLE 9.2   Characteristics of Various Types of Resin Composites

Type of Composite	Size of Filler Particles (μm)	Volume of Inorganic Filler (1%)	Handling Characteristics and Properties	
			Advantages	Disadvantages
Multipurpose	0.04, 0.2-3.0	60-70	High strength, high modulus	
Nanocomposite	0.002-0.075	78.5	High polish, high strength, high modulus	
Microfilled	0.04	32-50	Best polish, best esthetics	Higher shrinkage
Packable	0.04, 0.2-20	59-80	Packable, less shrinkage, lower wear	
Flowable	0.04, 0.2-3.0	42-62	Syringeable, lower modulus	Higher wear
Laboratory	0.04, 0.2-3.0	60-70	Best anatomy and contacts, lower wear	Lab cost, special equipment, requires resin cement

technique sensitivity, and poor esthetics. Advances in these materials have continued and the modern materials have improved properties. Resin-modified glass ionomers (RMGIs) were invented in the late 1980s to preserve the advantages of fluoride release and clinical adhesion of the conventional GIs yet provide the ease of light-curing and good esthetics of resin-based materials. The use of nanotechnology in resin-modified glass ionomer has resulted in enhanced esthetics of these materials.

MULTIPURPOSE COMPOSITES

Composition

Overview and Classification

A resin composite is composed of four major components: organic polymer matrix, inorganic filler particles, coupling agent, and the initiator-accelerator system. The organic polymer matrix in most commercial composites today is a cross-linked matrix of dimethacrylate monomers. The most common monomers are aromatic dimethacrylates. The double bonds at each end of these molecules undergo addition polymerization by free-radical initiation. Although these monomers can provide an optimum of optical, mechanical, and clinical properties, they are rather viscous and have to be blended with low-molecular-weight diluents monomers so that a clinically workable consistency may be obtained upon incorporation of the fillers. More recently low-shrink composites have been introduced that contain, for example, monomers with epoxy (also known as *oxirane*) functional groups at the ends. The polymerization of these monomers is initiated by cations. Other commercial resin composites utilize various

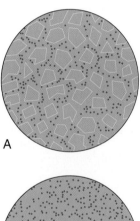

A

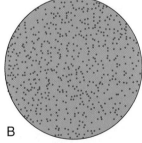

B

FIGURE 9.1 Two-dimensional diagrams of composites with, **A,** fine and, **B,** microfine particles. *(From Craig RG, Powers JM, Wataha JC: Dental Materials: Properties and Manipulation, ed 8. Mosby: St. Louis, 2004.)*

monomers and filler technology to reduce polymerization shrinkage or stress.

The dispersed inorganic filler particles may consist of one or more inorganic materials such as finely ground quartz or glass, sol-gel derived ceramics, microfine silica, or more recently nanoparticles. Two-dimensional diagrams of fine and microfine particles surrounded by polymer matrix are shown in Figure 9-1.

The coupling agent, an organosilane (often referred to as *silane*), is applied to the inorganic particles by the manufacturer to surface-treat the fillers before being mixed with the unreacted monomer mixture. Silanes are called *coupling agents,* because they form a bond between the inorganic and organic phases of the composite. One end of the molecule contains functional groups (such as methoxy), which hydrolyze and react with the inorganic filler and the other end has a methacrylate double bond that copolymerizes with the monomers.

The role of the initiator-accelerator system is to polymerize and cross-link the system into a hardened mass. The polymerization reaction can be triggered by light-activation, self-curing (chemical activation), and dual curing (chemical and light-curing).

Resin Matrix
METHACRYLATE MONOMERS

The vast majority of monomers used for the resin matrix are dimethacrylate compounds. Two monomers that have been commonly used are 2,2-*bis*[4(2-hydroxy-3-methacryloxy-propyloxy)- phenyl] propane (Bis-GMA) and urethane dimethacrylate (UDMA). Both contain reactive carbon double bonds at each end that can undergo addition polymerization initiated by free-radical initiators. The use of aromatic groups affords a good match of refractive index with the radiopaque glasses and thus provides better overall optical properties of the composites. A few products use both Bis-GMA and UDMA monomers.

The viscosity of the monomers, especially Bis-GMA, is rather high and diluents must be added, so a clinical consistency can be reached when the resin mixture is compounded with the filler. Low-molecular-weight compounds with difunctional carbon double bonds, for example, triethylene glycol dimethacrylate (TEGDMA), or Bis-EMA6 shown below, are added by the manufacturer to reduce and control the viscosity of the compounded composite.

LOW-SHRINK METHACRYLATE MONOMERS

A variety of other methacrylate monomers have been used in the newer commercial products introduced since 2008 for controlling the volumetric

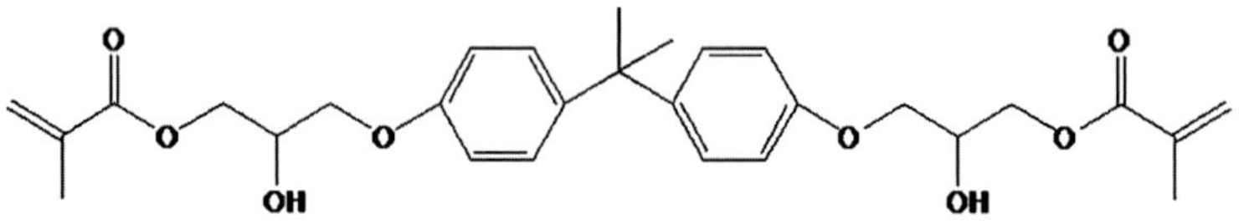

Structure of Bis-GMA.

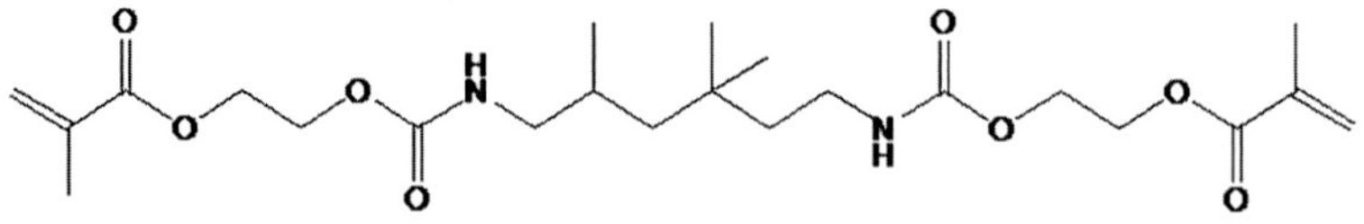

Structure of UDMA.

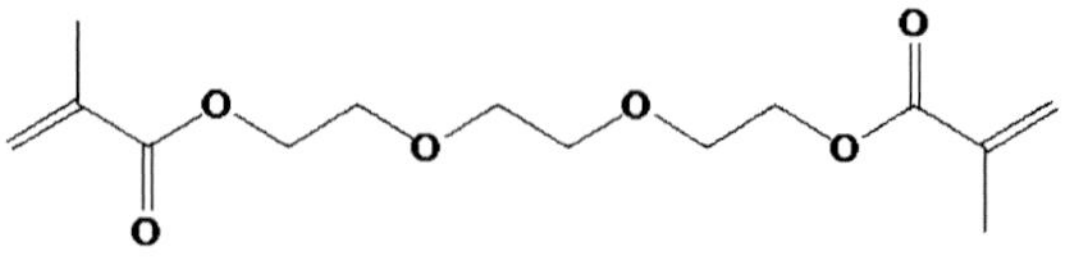

Structure of TEGDMA.

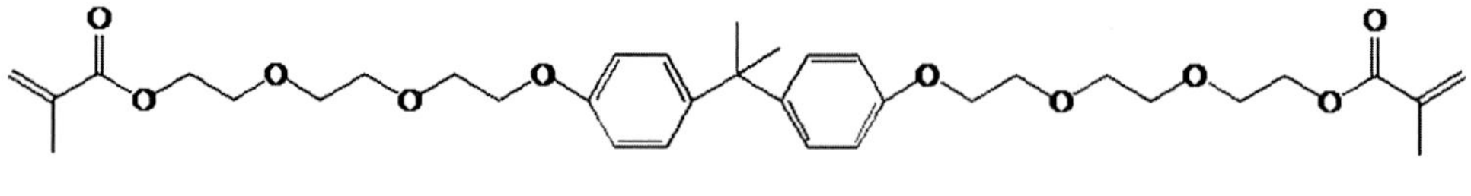

Structure of Bis-EMA6.

shrinkage and polymerization stress of composites. The general approach relies on increasing the distance between the methacrylate groups resulting in lower cross-link density or increasing the stiffness of the monomers. Some examples include the use of dimer acids, incorporation of cycloaliphatic units, and photocleavable units to relieve stress after polymerization.

The bonding agents widely used with these composites are also prepared from similar organic monomers so that they are compatible with the composites.

LOW-SHRINK SILORANE MONOMER

A new monomer system called *silorane* has been developed to reduce shrinkage and internal stress build-up resulting from polymerization. The name *silorane* was coined from its chemical building blocks *silox*ane and oxi*rane* (also known as *epoxy*). The siloxane functionality provides hydrophobicity to the composite. The oxirane functionalities undergo ring-opening cross-linking via cationic polymerization. Special initiator systems are required for the polymerization of the siloranes (described in the intiator section). Care has to be taken in choosing the filler system. If the filler surface has any residual basicity (as with some glasses and sol-gel derived systems), the composite may become unstable. Furthermore, a specific adhesive system has to be used for bonding these materials during clinical placement.

Fillers and Classification of Composites

Fillers make up a major portion by volume or weight of the composite. The function of the filler is to reinforce the resin matrix, provide the appropriate degree of translucency, and control the volume shrinkage of the composite during polymerization. Fillers have been traditionally obtained by grinding minerals such as quartz, glasses, or sol-gel derived ceramics. Most glasses contain heavy-metal oxides such as barium or zinc so that they provide radiopacity for visualization when exposed to x-rays. It is advantageous to have a distribution of filler diameters so that smaller particles fit into the spaces between larger particles and provide more efficient packing. Recently, nanofillers have been introduced into composites.

Structure of a monomer with cycloaliphatic units.

Structure of a monomer with photocleavable units.

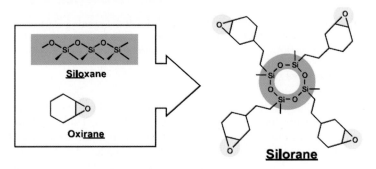

Structure of silorane.

These are described in the section on Nanofillers and Nanocomposites.

A helpful method of classifying dental composites is by the particle size, shape, and the particle-size distribution of the filler. This classification is presented below.

MACROFILLS

The early composites were macrofills. These composites contained large spherical or irregular shaped particles of average filler diameter of 20 to 30 μm. The resultant composites were rather opaque and had low resistance to wear.

HYBRID AND MICROHYBRID COMPOSITES

The hybrid composites are two types of fillers that are blended together: (1) fine particles of average particle size 2 to 4 μm and (2) 5% to 15% of microfine particles, usually silica, of particle size 0.04 to 0.2 μm. In microhybrid composites, the fine particles of a lower average particle size (0.04 to 1 μm) are blended with microfine silica. The fine particles may be obtained by grinding glass (e.g., borosilicate glass, lithium or barium aluminum silicate glass, strontium or zinc glass), quartz, or ceramic materials and have irregular shapes. The distribution of filler particles provides efficient packing so that high filler loading is possible while maintaining good handling of the composite for clinical placement. Microhybrid composites may contain 60% to 70% filler by volume, which, depending on the density of the filler, translates into 77% to 84% by weight in the composite. Most manufacturers report filler concentration in weight percent (wt%). A micrograph of a typical, fine glass filler is shown in Figure 9-2, *A*. Hybrids and microhybrids have good clinical wear resistance and mechanical properties and are suitable for stress-bearing applications. However, they lose their surface polish with time and become rough and dull.

NANOCOMPOSITES

Recently the incorporation of nanotechnology into designing and manufacturing of composites has greatly improved their properties. Nanocomposites describe this class of composites. The nanofiller technology is described in the next section.

Nanofillers and Nanocomposites

The latest advancement in composite technology has been the use of nanotechnology in development of fillers. Nanotechnology is the production of functional materials and structures in the range of 1 to 100 nanometers (nm)—the nanoscale—by various physical and chemical methods. Nanotechnology requires devices and systems to create structures

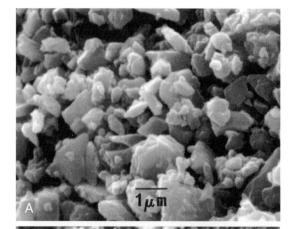
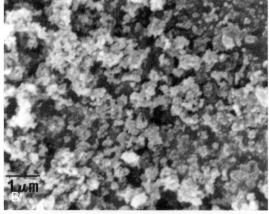
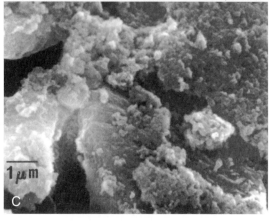

FIGURE 9.2 **Scanning electron micrographs of types of filler. A,** Fine inorganic filler; **B,** microfine silica filler; **C,** microfine silica in organic polymer filler.

that have novel properties and functions because of their small sizes. Thus it implies the ability to control and manipulate structures at the atomic and/or molecular scale. Although true nanocomposites should have all filler particles in the nanometer size, the term *nanotechnology* has some hype associated with it, and it is sometimes misused in describing a material. To date oxide nanoparticles have been the most prevalent types of nanomaterials used in dental composites. At present there are two distinct types of dental composites available that contain nanoparticles:

a. **Nanofills**—these contain nanometer sized particles (1-100 nm) throughout the resin matrix. Larger primary particles are not present.

b. **Nanohybrids**—these consist of large particles (0.4 to 5 microns) with added nanometer sized particles. Thus they are hybrid materials, not true nanofilled composites.

NANOFILL COMPOSITES

All filler particles of true nanofilled composites are in the nanometer range. There are several purposes for incorporating nanofillers in dental composites. First, the size of nanomeric particles is below that of visible light (400-800 nm), which provides the opportunity of creating highly translucent materials. In addition the surface area to volume ratio of the nanoparticles is quite large. The sizes of the smallest nanoparticles approach those of polymer molecules so they can form a molecular scale interaction with the host resin matrix.

Two types of nanoparticles have been synthesized and used for preparing this class of composite. The first type consists of nanomeric particles that are essentially monodisperse nonaggregates and nonagglomerated particles of silica or zirconia. The surface of the nanoparticles are treated with silane coupling agents that allow them to be bonded to the resin matrix when the composite is cured after placement. Nanomers are synthesized from sols, creating particles of the same size. Because of this, if nanomeric particles alone are used to make highly filled composites, the rheological properties are rather poor. To overcome this disadvantage, one manufacturer has designed a second type of nanofiller, which is called *nanocluster*. The nanoclusters are made by lightly sintering nanomeric oxides to form clusters of a controlled particle size distribution. Nanoclusters have been synthesized from silica sols alone as well as from mixed oxides of silica and zirconia. The primary particle size of the nanomers used to prepare the clusters range from 5 to 75 nm.

It is important to remember that in a nanocluster, the nanoparticles still maintain their individual form, much as in a cluster of grapes. The clusters can be made to have a wide size distribution ranging from 100 nm to submicron level and have an average size of 0.6 micrometers. Figure 9-3, *A*, shows a scanning electron microscopy (SEM)

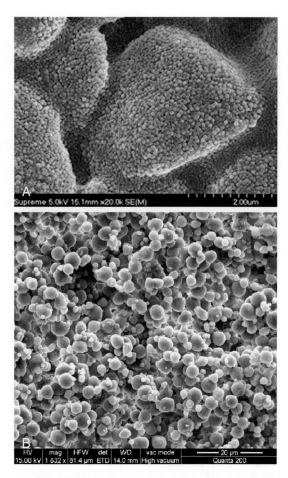

FIGURE 9.3 A, Scanning electron micrograph (SEM) image of a nanocluster of silica in a commercial composite 3M™ ESPE™ Filtek™ Supreme. **B,** Image of a nanocluster of zirconia-silica in Filtek Supreme Ultra. *(A, Courtesy of Dr. Jorge Perdigao, University of Minnesota; B, from SA Rodrigues Jr., SS Scherrer, JL Ferracane, A Della Bona Microstructural characterization and fracture behavior of a microhybrid and a nanofill composite. Dental Materials, Volume 24, Issue 9, September 2008, Pages 1281-1288.)*

image of a nanocluster of silica in a commercial composite after the resin matrix was removed by washing with acetone. In this material the surface of the nanoclusters are treated with a silane coupling agent to provide compatibility and chemical bonding with the resin system. Figure 9-3, *B*, shows the micrograph image of a nanocluster comprised of silica and zirconia. The differences in particle architecture of nanomers, nanoclusters, and conventional microhybrid fillers are readily apparent in transmission electron micrographs (TEMs) of composites prepared from these fillers. Figure 9-4, *A*, shows the TEM of a nanocomposite filled with 75-nm diameter nanoparticles only; Figure 9-4, *B*, is that of a nanocomposite filled with a mixture of

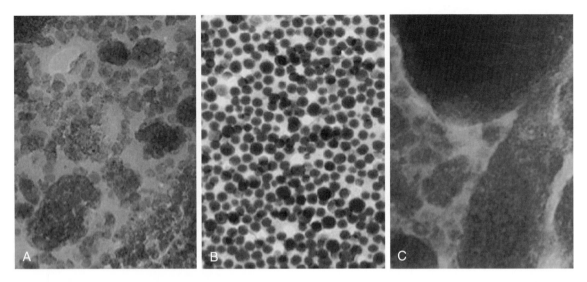

FIGURE 9.4 **A**, Transmission electron micrograph (TEM) image of composite with nanomeric particles (×60,000 magnification). **B**, TEM image of composite with nanocluster particles (×300,000 magnification). **C**, TEM image of composite with hybrid fillers (×300,000 magnification). *(A, B, and C from Mitra SB, Wu D, Holmes BN: J. Am. Dent. Assoc. 134, 1382, 2003.)*

nanoclusters alone, and Figure 9-4, *C*, is of a conventional microhybrid composite. To date there is only one true nanofilled dental composite available. In this manufactured composite, a combination of nanomeric particles and nanoclusters are used in optimum combinations. Figure 9-5, *A*, shows a schematic diagram of this nanocomposite containing a blend of nanocluster and nanomeric fillers and Figure 9-5, *B*, shows a TEM of the nanocomposite showing the presence of the two types of nanofillers.

The uniqueness of the nanofilled composite is that it has the mechanical strength of a microhybrid but at the same time retains smoothness during service like a microfill. The initial gloss of many restoratives is quite good, but in hybrid composites (microhybrids, nanohybrids) plucking of the larger fillers causes loss of gloss. In contrast, in the nanofilled composite, the nanoclusters shear at a rate similar to the surrounding matrix during abrasion. This allows the restoration to maintain a smoother surface for long-term polish retention. Optical analysis of the polish retention can be done using atomic force microscopy after extended toothbrush abrasion.

Nanofillers also offer advantages in optical properties. In general, it is desirable to provide low visual opacity in unpigmented dental composites. This allows for the creation of a wide range of shades and opacities so the clinician can design a highly esthetic restoration. In hybrid types of composites the filler particles are 0.4-3.0 μm in size. When particles and resin are mismatched in the refractive index, which measures the ability of the material

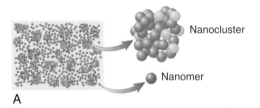

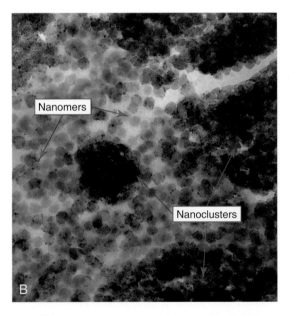

FIGURE 9.5 **A,** Schematic diagram of a nanofilled composite containing nanoclusters and nanomers. **B,** TEM image of a nanocomposite with nanocluster and nanomeric fillers. *(Courtesy of 3M ESPE Dental Products, St. Paul, MN.)*

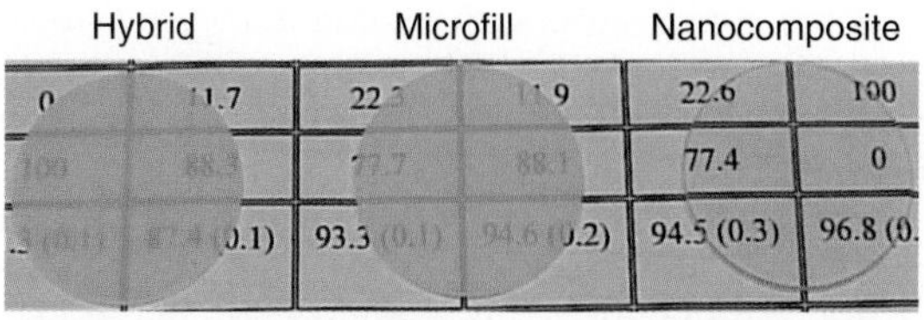

Hybrid		Microfill		Nanocomposite	
0	11.7	22.?	1.9	22.6	100
100	88.?	7.7	88.1	77.4	0
(0.1)	87.4 (0.1)	93.3 (0.1)	94.6 (0.2)	94.5 (0.3)	96.8 (0.

FIGURE 9.6 **Translucency of a hybrid composite, microfill composite, and a nanocomposite.** *(Courtesy of 3M ESPE Dental Products, St. Paul, MN.)*

to transmit light, the particles will scatter light and produce opaque materials. Nanomeric fillers particles are far smaller than the wavelength of light, making them unmeasurable by refractive index. When light enters, long wavelength light passes directly through and materials show high translucency. As shown by Figure 9-6, the discs made with hybrid and microfill fillers are rather opaque. The nanofill composite sample made predominantly with the nanomeric filler is quite clear; the background can be easily seen through the composite. In addition, when placed on a black background, the nanomeric and nanocluster particles preferentially scatter blue light, giving the composite an opalescent effect. This gives a more life-like appearance that matches natural enamel, which also exhibits the same effect.

The ability to create a nanocomposite with very low opacity provides the ability to formulate a vast range of shade and opacity options from the very translucent shades needed for the incisal edge and for the final layer in multilayered restorations to the more opaque shades desired in the enamel, body, and dentin shades. This allows the clinician the flexibility of choosing a single shade or a multi-shade layering technique depending on the esthetic needs. The wear resistance of this material after 3 and 5 years of clinical use was found to be similar to human enamel.

NANOHYBRID COMPOSITE

Several manufacturers have placed nano-sized particles in their microhybrids. These composites have been described as nanohybrids. Because the smoothness and wear of any composite is often determined by the size of its largest filler particles as with microhybrids, the surface of nanohybrids becomes gradually dull after a few years of clinical service.

Interfacial Phase and Coupling Agents

For a composite to have successful clinical performance, a good bond must form between the inorganic filler particles and the organic resin matrix during setting. This is achieved through the use of compounds called *coupling agents*, the most common of which are organic silicon compounds called *silane coupling agents*. The surface of the filler is treated with a coupling agent during the manufacture of the composite. A typical silane coupling agent is 3-methacryloxypropyltrimethoxysilane (MPTS), the chemical structure of which is shown below.

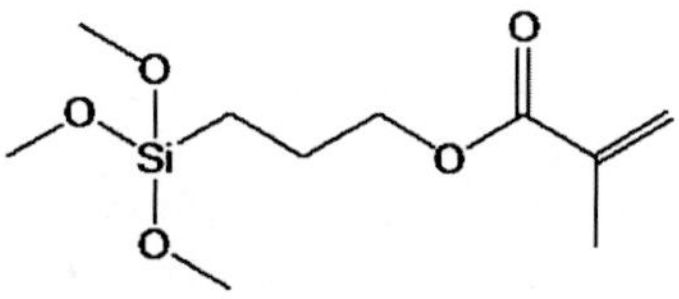

In the low-shrink silorane composite, an epoxy functionalized coupling agent, 3-glycidoxypropyltrimethoxysliane, is used to bond the filler to the oxirane matrix.

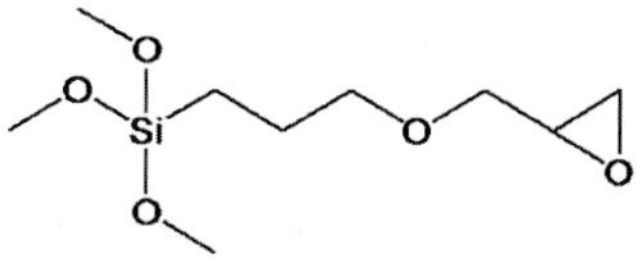

During the filler treatment process, the methoxy groups hydrolyze to generate hydroxyl groups through an acid or base catalyzed reaction. These hydroxyl groups then undergo condensation with the hydroxyl groups on the surface of the filler and become attached by covalent bonds (see the following schematic sketch). Condensation is also possible with the adjacent –OH groups of the hydrolyzed silanes or with water absorbed on the surface of the filler. This results in the formation of a very thin mono- or multilayer polymeric film on the surface of the filler with unreacted double bonds. During the curing of the composite, the double bonds of the methacryloxy groups of the treated surface co-reacts with the monomer resins. The coupling agent plays a critical role in the composite. Its functions are summarized below:

- It forms an interfacial bridge that strongly binds the filler to the resin matrix.
- It enhances the mechanical properties of the composite and minimizes the plucking of the fillers from the matrix during clinical wear.
- The resulting interfacial phase provides a medium for stress distribution between adjacent particles and the polymer matrix.
- It provides a hydrophobic environment that minimizes water absorption of the composite.

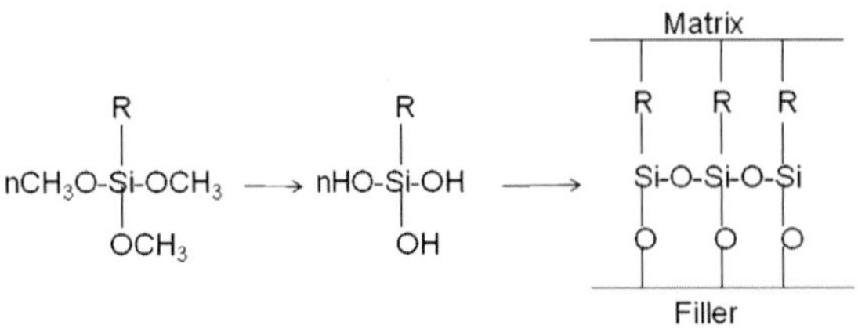

Initiators and Accelerators

The curing of composites is triggered by light or a chemical reaction, with the former being more common. Light activation is accomplished with blue light at a peak wavelength of about 465 nm, which is absorbed usually by a photo-sensitizer, such as camphorquinone, added to the monomer mixture during the manufacturing process in amounts varying from 0.1% to 1.0%.

In methacrylate composites, free radicals are generated upon activation. The reaction is accelerated by the presence of an organic amine. Various amines have been used, both aromatic and aliphatic. Examples of two such amines are shown below. The amine and the camphorquinone are stable in the presence of the oligomer at room temperature, as long as the composite is not exposed to light. Although camphorquinone is the most common photo-sensitizer, others are sometimes used to accommodate special esthetic considerations. Camphorquinone adds a slight yellow tint to the uncured composite paste. Although the color bleaches during cure, sometimes clinicians find shade matching difficult with the color shift.

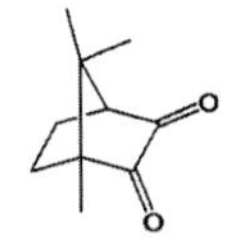

Camphorquinone 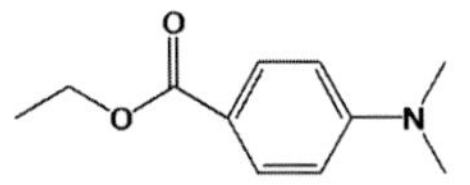   A typical amine

Chemical activation is accomplished at room temperature by an organic amine (catalyst paste) reacting with an organic peroxide (universal paste) to produce free radicals, which in turn attack the carbon double bonds, causing polymerization. Once the two pastes are mixed, the polymerization reaction proceeds rapidly.

Some composites, such as core and provisional products, are dual cured. These formulations contain initiators and accelerators that allow light activation followed by self-curing or self-curing alone.

In the silorane composite, the initiator system generates cations when irradiated with light. One of the components is the camphorquinone photosensitizer enabling the composite to be cured by a dental curing unit. Other components of the initiation system are iodonium salts and electron donors, which generate the reactive cationic species that start the ring opening polymerization process.

Pigments and Other Components

Inorganic oxides are usually added in small amounts to provide shades that match the majority of tooth shades. The most common pigments are oxides of iron. Numerous shades are supplied, ranging from very light shades to yellow to gray. Various color scales are used to characterize the shades of the composites. A UV absorber may be added to minimize color changes caused by oxidation. Darker and more opaque shades of composites cannot be cured to the same depth as the lighter translucent shades.

Fluorescent agents are sometimes added to enhance the optical vitality of the composite and mimic the appearance of natural teeth. These are dyes or pigments that absorb light in the ultraviolet and violet region (usually 340-370 nm) of the electromagnetic spectrum, and re-emit light in the blue region (typically 420-470 nm). These additives are often used to enhance the appearance of color causing a perceived "whitening" effect, making materials look less yellow by increasing the overall amount of blue light reflected.

Polymerization Reactions

Polymerization of Methacrylate Composites

Methacrylate composites form the workhorse of direct restorative materials. The polymer network of these composites are formed by a process called *free-radical addition polymerization of the corresponding methacrylate monomers*. The polymerization reaction takes place in three stages: initiation, propagation, and termination and is shown in the following scheme.

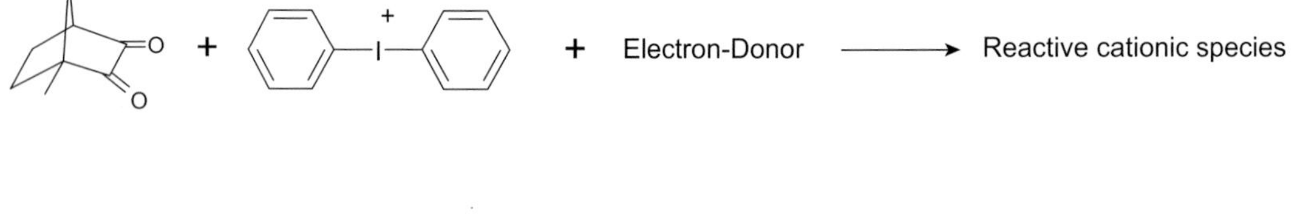

Initiation Stage

Initiator $\xrightarrow[\text{or chemical reaction}]{\text{light, heat}}$ Free radical $R^\bullet$

Example:

Benzoyl peroxide → 2 Free radical ($R^\bullet$)

Camphorquinone + Amine $\xrightarrow{\text{Light}}$ Free radical $R^\bullet$

Free radical + Monomer $\longrightarrow$ growing chain

Propagation Stage

Growing chain

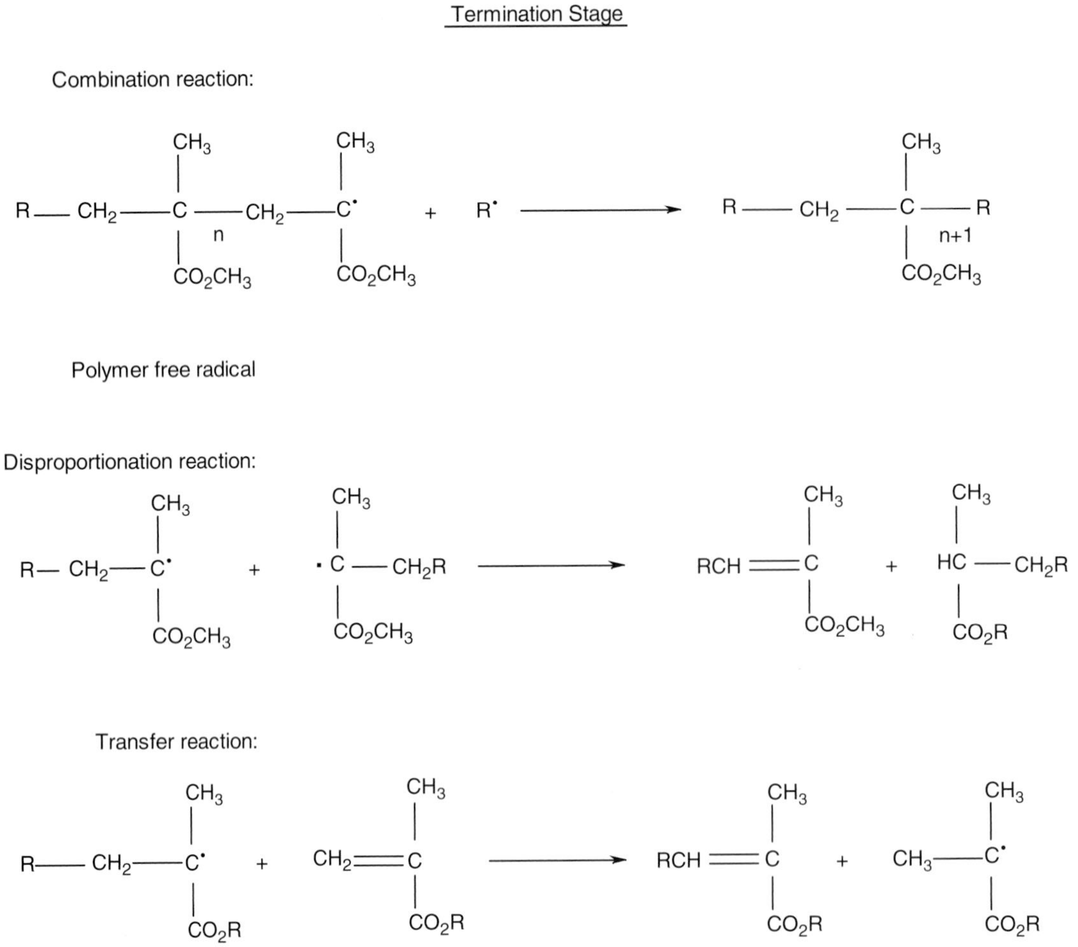

<u>Termination Stage</u>

Combination reaction:

$$R—CH_2—\underset{\underset{CO_2CH_3}{|}}{\overset{\overset{CH_3}{|}}{C}}—CH_2—\underset{\underset{CO_2CH_3}{|}}{\overset{\overset{CH_3}{|}}{\overset{\bullet}{C}}} \quad + \quad R^{\bullet} \quad \longrightarrow \quad R—CH_2—\underset{\underset{CO_2CH_3}{|}}{\overset{\overset{CH_3}{|}}{C}}—R$$

(subscript n on left structure, n+1 on right structure)

Polymer free radical

Disproportionation reaction:

$$R—CH_2—\underset{\underset{CO_2CH_3}{|}}{\overset{\overset{CH_3}{|}}{\overset{\bullet}{C}}} \quad + \quad \overset{\overset{CH_3}{|}}{\underset{\underset{CO_2CH_3}{|}}{\overset{\bullet}{C}}}—CH_2R \quad \longrightarrow \quad RCH=\underset{\underset{CO_2CH_3}{|}}{\overset{\overset{CH_3}{|}}{C}} \quad + \quad \overset{\overset{CH_3}{|}}{HC}—\underset{\underset{CO_2R}{|}}{CH_2R}$$

Transfer reaction:

$$R—CH_2—\underset{\underset{CO_2R}{|}}{\overset{\overset{CH_3}{|}}{\overset{\bullet}{C}}} \quad + \quad CH_2=\underset{\underset{CO_2R}{|}}{\overset{\overset{CH_3}{|}}{C}} \quad \longrightarrow \quad RCH=\underset{\underset{CO_2R}{|}}{\overset{\overset{CH_3}{|}}{C}} \quad + \quad CH_3—\underset{\underset{CO_2R}{|}}{\overset{\overset{CH_3}{|}}{\overset{\bullet}{C}}}$$

The polymerization reaction of self-cured composites is chemically initiated at room temperature with a peroxide initiator and an amine accelerator. Polymerization of light-cured composites is triggered by visible blue light. The photo-initiators used are described in the section on Initiators and Accelerators. Dual-cured products use a combination of chemical and light activation to carry out the polymerization reaction. At this stage, an active free radical species, designated as $R^{\bullet}$ in the foregoing scheme, is first formed as the initiating species. This free radical adds to a monomer species generating an active center monomer radical.

The initiation stage is followed by the propagation stage during which rapid addition of other monomers molecules to the active center occurs to provide the growing polymer chain. The propagation reaction continues to build molecular weight and cross-link density until the growing free radical is terminated. The termination stage may take place in several ways as indicated, where n represents the number of mer units.

The polymerized resin is highly cross-linked because of the presence of difunctional carbon double bonds. The degree of polymerization varies, depending on whether it is in the bulk or in the air-inhibited layer of the restoration. Polymerization of light-cured composites varies by the distance of the light from the restoration and the duration of light exposure. The percentage of double bonds that react may vary from 35% to 80%. The degree of polymerization is higher for laboratory composites that are post-cured at elevated temperatures and light intensities.

During polymerization, molecules have to approach their "neighbors" to form chemical bonds with them. Reduction of volume, or shrinkage, is generally observed during polymerization because two factors are reduced: the Van der Waals volume and the free volume. The Van der Waals volume is the volume of molecule itself derived from the atoms and bond lengths. Reduction in the Van der Waals volume takes place during polymerization because

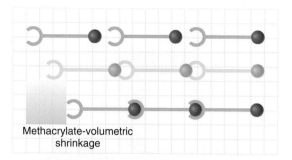

Methacrylate-volumetric shrinkage

FIGURE 9.7 **Schematic illustration of the polymerization of methacrylate resin and resulting volumetric shrinkage.**

of a change in the bond lengths (conversion of double bonds to single bonds). The free volume of a molecular species, whether a monomer or a polymer, is the volume occupied by it due to its random rotational and thermal movement. When monomers are converted to polymers, reduction of the free volume occurs because the rotation of the polymer chain is more restricted than in unpolymerized monomer

molecules. A schematic illustration of the polymerization of methacrylate resin resulting in shrinkage is shown in Figure 9-7.

Manufacturers have taken several steps to minimize the polymerization contraction in methacrylate composites by one or more of the following methods:

- Filling the monomer resins with prepolymerized resins
- Maximizing the amount of inorganic filler
- Using high molecular mass methacrylate monomers

In addition, incremental placement of methacrylate composites in the tooth cavity, necessitated by their limited depth of cure, controls shrinkage stress so that clinical success of the modern-day methacrylate composite is quite excellent.

Polymerization of Silorane Composites

Polymerization of the silorane molecule takes place through a cationic initiation process during which the oxirane segments undergo ring opening to form covalent single bonds with their neighbors. The chemistry of the polymerization is shown below:

Blue light

Cationic Photoinitiator ⟶ H^+

Proton Initiation   **Ring Opening Expansion**

Propagation   **Bond Forming Contraction**   **Expansion**

Contraction   **Expansion**   **Contraction....**

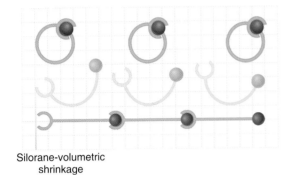

Silorane-volumetric
shrinkage

FIGURE 9.8 **Schematic illustration of the polymerization of silorane composite and resulting volumetric
shrinkage.**

The ring-opening chemistry of the siloranes starts with the cleavage and opening of the oxirane ring. This process gains space and counteracts some of the reduction in volume when chemical bonds are established to form the polymer. A schematic diagram to depict the polymerization is shown in Figure 9-8.

The silorane composites generate lower volume shrinkage and stress upon polymerization. It is still important to place these composites in increments because of limited depth of cure. In addition, special adhesives are needed.

Packaging of Composites

Composites as supplied from the manufacturer are in their pre-cured state and hence have to be packaged with adequate protection against inadvertent setting. The primary package is made from a plastic material that allows the diffusion of oxygen (which works as an inhibitor for methacrylate polymerization) and also prevents moisture absorption in humid environments.

Light-Cured Composites

Because the setting of light-cured composite is triggered by visible light, these materials have to be protected from premature curing when supplied from the manufacturer and stored in the dental office. Hence they are packaged in opaque, most often black, plastic syringes or unit-dose capsules, sometimes referred to as *compules*. In the latter case, a delivery gun for direct intra-oral placement is provided. An advantage of the capsule delivery is the lower risk of cross-infection. Composite packaging and delivery systems are shown in Figure 9-9. The composites are supplied in a variety of shades and opacities. Some manufacturers color code their capsule caps or syringe plungers for ease of identification of the shades and/or opacities.

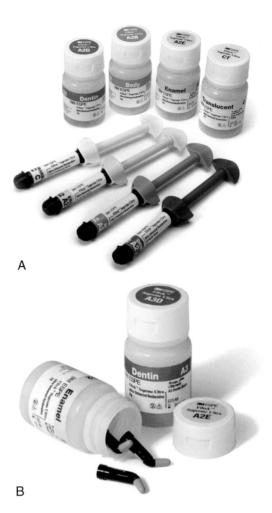

A

B

FIGURE 9.9 Single-paste, visible light-initiated composite in syringe (**A**) and capsules (**B**). *(Courtesy of 3M ESPE Dental Products, St. Paul, MN.)*

Self-Cured and Dual-Cured Composites

Self-cured and dual-cured materials are supplied in two syringes. Two pastes are mixed to initiate the chemical cure. An example of a two-paste core build-up composite is shown in Figure 9-10. It is advisable to store these materials in a cool temperature to prolong their shelf-life.

PROPERTIES OF COMPOSITES

Overview

In order to have good clinical service life, composites have to meet certain performance criteria. Important physical, mechanical, and clinical properties are described in this section. Selected properties of various types of composites are listed in Table 9-3. Values of properties for polymer-based filling and

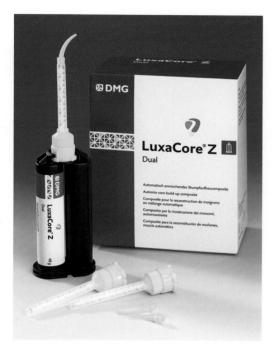

FIGURE 9.10 Dual-curing composite for core build-ups. *(Courtesy of DMG Chemisch-Pharmazeutische Fabrik GmbH, Hamburg, Germany)*

restorative materials based on ISO 4049 (ANSI/ADA No. 27) are summarized in Table 9-4.

Physical Properties

Working and Setting Times

For light-cured composites, curing is considered to be "on demand." Polymerization is initiated when the composite is first exposed to the curing light. Stiffening takes place within seconds after light exposure by a high-intensity curing light source. Although the composite restoration appears hard and fully cured after exposure to the curing light source, the setting reaction continues for a period of 24 hours. All of the available unsaturated carbon double bonds of methacrylate-based composites do not react; studies report that about 25% remain unreacted in the bulk of the restoration. A thin layer of air-inhibited, unpolymerized material remains on the surface of the polymerized layer, which is advantageous for subsequent incremental placement during layering. It is useful to protect the surface of the contoured restoration with a transparent matrix, to minimize the amount of unpolymerized resin in the final restoration. Although for some composites the final physical properties may not be reached until about 24 hours after the reaction is initiated, enough of the mechanical strength is attained immediately after curing so the restoration

can be finished and polished with abrasives and is functional.

For most composites that are initiated by visible light, bright operatory lights can initiate cure prematurely if the composite is left unprotected on a mixing pad. Within 60 to 90 seconds after exposure to ambient light, the surface of the composite may lose its capability to flow readily against the tooth, and further work with the material becomes difficult. The dispensed paste can be covered with an opaque or orange cover to prevent premature exposure to light.

The setting times for chemically activated composites range from 3 to 5 minutes. These short setting times have been accomplished by controlling the concentration of initiator and accelerator.

Polymerization Shrinkage and Stress

As explained in the section on Polymerization Reactions, all composites undergo volumetric shrinkage upon setting. Typical shrinkage values are listed in Table 9-3. Volumetric shrinkage results in the development of contraction stresses as high as 13 MPa between the composite and the tooth structure. These stresses severely strain the interfacial bond between the composite and the tooth, leading to a very small gap that can allow marginal leakage of saliva and microorganisms. Recurrent caries and marginal staining may result. This stress can exceed the tensile strength of enamel and result in stress cracking and enamel fractures along the interfaces. Because the development of shrinkage stress depends on the volumetric shrinkage strain and the stiffness of the composite at the time of shrinkage, low-shrinkage composites might exhibit high stress if the composite has a high elastic modulus. Adding the composite in 2-mm increments and polymerizing each increment independently can reduce the net effect of polymerization shrinkage. Net shrinkage stress is less because a smaller volume of composite is allowed to shrink before successive additions. A recent paper has reviewed the clinical and laboratory properties of several low-shrink/low-stress composites. Most of these products are universal composites, but two products are described as flowable composites. The shrinkage values are dependent on the method used. Volumetric polymerization shrinkage for low-shrink universal composites measured by a pycnometer vary from 0.9% to 1.8% whereas that of low-shrink flowables are 2.4% to 2.5%. When an ACTA linometer was used, the values were 1.0% to 1.4% and 2.6% to 2.9%, respectively. The polymerization stress was 1.2 to 1.6 MPa. In comparison, traditional universal composites have been reported to have polymerization stress of 0.8 to 2.4 MPa and flowables were reported to have stress values ranging from 1.3% to 3.2%.

TABLE 9-3   Properties of Various Types of Resin Composites, Compomers, Conventional Glass Ionomers and Resin-modified Glass Ionomers

Property	Nano-composite*	Multipurpose Composite	Microfill Composite	Packable Composite	Flowable Composite	Laboratory Composite	Core Composite	Conventional Glass Ionomer	Resin-modified Glass Ionomer
Flexural strength (MPa)	180	80-160	60-120	85-110	70-120	90-150[†]	—	7-15	50-60
Flexural modulus (GPa)	—	8.8-13	4.0-6.9	9.0-12	2.6-5.6	4.7-15[†]	—	—	—
Flexural fatigue limit (MPa)	—	60-110	—	—	—	—	—	—	—
Compressive strength (MPa)	460	240-290	240-300	220-300	210-300	210-280	210-250	10-15	200-250
Compressive modulus (GPa)	—	5.5-8.3	2.6-4.8	5.8-9.0	2.6-5.9	—	7.5-22	7.2-10.3	3.2-6.9
Diametral tensile strength (MPa)	81	30-55	25-40	—	33-48	—	40-50	7-15	30-40
Linear polymerization shrinkage (%)	—	0.7-1.4	2–3	0.6-0.9	—	—	—	—	—
Color stability, accelerated aging—450 kJ/m²(ΔE*)‡	—	1.5	—	—	15	1.1-2.3	—	—	—
Color stability, stained by juice/tea (ΔE*)‡	—	4.3	—	—	—	1.7-3.9	—	—	—

*Mitra SB, Wu D, Holmes BN: J Am Dent Assoc 134:1382, 2003.
#Mitra S, Glass ionomers and related filling materials. In Dhuru VB ed. Contemporary Dental Materials, Oxford, New Delhi, India: Oxford 2004:66-80.
†Without fiber reinforcement.
‡ΔE <3.3 is considered not clinically perceptible.

TABLE 9.4 Requirements for Polymer-Based Filling and Restorative Materials Based on ISO 4049

Property	Class 1	Class 2	Class 3
Working time (min, sec)	90	—	90
Setting time (max, min)	5	—	10
Depth of cure (min, mm)			
Opaque shades	—	1.0	—
Other shades	—	1.5	—
Water sorption (max, μg/mm^3)	40	40	40
Solubility (max, μg/mm^3)	7.5	7.5	7.5
Flexural strength (MPa)			
Type 1	80	80* 100†	80
Type 2	50	50*	50

*Group 1: cured intraorally.
†Group 2: cured extraorally.

Thermal Properties

The linear coefficient of thermal expansion (α) of composites ranges from 25 to 38 × 10^{-6}/° C for composites with fine particles to 55 to 68 × 10^{-6}/° C for composites with microfine particles. The α values for composites are less than the mean of its constituents added together; however, the values are higher than those for dentin (8.3 × 10^{-6}/° C) and enamel (11.4 × 10^{-6}/° C). The higher values for the microfilled composites are related mostly to the greater amount of polymer present. Certain glasses may be more effective in reducing the effect of thermal change than are others, and some resins have more than one type of filler to compensate for differential rates.

Thermal stresses place an additional strain on the bond to tooth structure, which adds to the detrimental effect of the polymerization shrinkage. Thermal changes are also cyclic in nature, and although the entire restoration may never reach thermal equilibrium during the application of either hot or cold stimuli, the cyclic effect can lead to material fatigue and early bond failure. If a gap forms, the difference between the thermal coefficient of expansion of composites and teeth could permit percolation of oral fluids.

The thermal conductivity of composites with fine particles (25 to 30 × 10^{-4} cal/sec/cm^2 [° C/cm]) is greater than that of composites with microfine particles (12 to 15 × 10^{-4} cal/sec/cm^2 [° C/cm]) because of the higher conductivity of the inorganic fillers compared with the polymer matrix. However, for highly transient temperatures, the composites do not change temperature as fast as tooth structure, and this difference does not present a clinical problem.

Water Sorption

The water sorption of composites with hybrid particles (5 to 17 μg/mm^3) is lower than that of composites with microfine particles (26 to 30 μg/mm^3) because of the lower volume fraction of polymer in the composites with fine particles. The quality and stability of the silane coupling agent are important in minimizing the deterioration of the bond between the filler and polymer and the amount of water sorption. Expansion associated with the uptake of water from oral fluids could relieve some polymerization stress, but water sorption is a slow process when compared to polymerization shrinkage and stress development. In the measurement of hygroscopic expansion starting 15 minutes after the initial polymerization, most resins required 7 days to reach equilibrium and about 4 days to show the majority of expansion. Because composites with fine particles have lower values of water sorption than composites with microfine particles, they exhibit less expansion when exposed to water.

Solubility

The water solubility of composites varies from 0.25 to 2.5 mg/mm^3. Inadequate light intensity and duration can result in insufficient polymerization, particularly at greater depths from the surface. Inadequately polymerized composites have greater water sorption and solubility, possibly manifested clinically with early color instability.

During the storage of microhybrid composites in water, the leaching of inorganic ions can be detected; such ions are associated with a breakdown in interfacial bonding. Silicon leaches in the greatest quantity (15 to 17 μg/mL) during the first 30 days of storage in water and decreases with time of exposure. Microfilled composites leach silicon more slowly and show a 100% increase in amount during the second 30-day period (14.2 μg/mL). Boron, barium, and strontium, which are present in glass fillers, are leached to various degrees (6 to 19 μg/mL) from the various resin-filler systems. Breakdown and leakage can be a contributing factor to the reduced resistance to wear and abrasion of composites.

Color and Color Stability

The color and blending of shades for the clinical match of esthetic restorations are important. The characteristics of color are discussed in Chapter 4, and these principles can be applied specifically to composites for determining appropriate shades for clinical use. Universal shades vary in color among currently marketed products. The modern day composites are often supplied by the manufacturer in multiple opacities. This allows for better esthetic outcome using multiple shades of different opacities to construct the restoration.

Change of color and loss of shade match with surrounding tooth structure are reasons for replacing restorations. Stress cracks within the polymer matrix and partial debonding of the filler to the resin as a result of hydrolysis tend to increase opacity and alter appearance. Discoloration can also occur by oxidation and result from water exchange within the polymer matrix and its interaction with unreacted polymer sites and unused initiator or accelerator.

Color stability of current composites has been studied by artificial aging in a weathering chamber (exposure to UV light and elevated temperatures of 70° C) and by immersion in various stains (coffee/tea, cranberry/grape juice, red wine, and sesame oil). As shown in Table 9-3, composites are resistant to color changes caused by oxidation but are susceptible to staining.

Mechanical Properties

Although composites take advantage of selected properties of each constituent material, the physical and mechanical properties of the composites are different from those of the separate phases.

Factors that affect the properties of composites include (1) the state of matter of the second (dispersed) phase; (2) the geometry of the second phase; (3) the orientation of the second phase; (4) the composition of the dispersed and continuous phases; (5) the ratio of the phases; and (6) bonding of the phases. Examples of properties that can be changed (improved if the composites are judiciously developed) are (1) modulus, (2) strength, (3) fracture toughness, (4) wear resistance, (5) thermal expansion, and (6) chemical and corrosion resistance.

Strength and Modulus

Values of compressive, tensile (tested by the diametral method) and flexural strengths and modulus for dental composites are listed in Table 9-3. Compressive strength is of importance because of the chewing forces. The flexural and compressive moduli of microfilled and flowable composites are about 50% lower than values for multipurpose hybrids and packable composites, which reflects the lower volume percent filler present in the microfilled and flowable composites (see Table 9-2). For comparison, the modulus of elasticity in compression is about 62 GPa for amalgam, 18-24 GPa for dentin, and 60-120 GPa for enamel.

Knoop Hardness

Knoop hardness for composites (22 to 80 kg/mm^2) is lower than enamel (343 kg/mm^2) or dental amalgam (110 kg/mm^2). The Knoop hardness of composites with fine particles is somewhat greater than values for composites with microfine particles

because of the hardness and volume fraction of the filler particles. These values indicate a moderate resistance to indentation under functional stresses for more highly filled composites, but this difference does not appear to be a major factor in resisting functional wear.

A microhardness measurement such as Knoop can be misleading on composites with large filler particles (>10 μm in diameter), in which the small indentation could be made solely on the organic or the inorganic phase. However, with most current products, filler particle sizes are much smaller (<1 μm), and the microhardness values appear more reliable.

Bond Strength to Dental Substrates

Bonding of composites to tooth structure and other dental substrates is discussed in detail in Chapter 13. A brief overview of bonding dental composites to various substrates is presented here.

Enamel and Dentin

The bond strength of composites to etched enamel and primed dentin is typically between 20 and 30 MPa. Bonding is principally a result of micromechanical retention of the bonding agent into the etched surfaces of enamel and primed dentin. In dentin, a hybrid layer of bonding resin and collagen is often formed, and the bonding adhesive penetrates the dentinal tubules (Figure 9-11).

Other Substrates

Composite can be bonded to existing composite restorations, ceramics, and alloys when the substrate is roughened and appropriately primed (see Chapter 13). In general, the surface to be bonded is sandblasted (microetched) with 50-μm alumina and then treated with a resin-silane primer for composite, a silane primer for silica-based ceramics, an acidic phosphate monomer for zirconia, or a special alloy primer. Bond strengths to treated surfaces are typically greater than 20 MPa.

Clinical Properties

Clinical requirements for composites accepted for unrestricted use, including cuspal replacement in posterior teeth, as defined by the American Dental Association (Proposed) Guidelines for Resin-based Composites for Posterior Restorations, are listed in Table 9-5.

Depth of Cure (Light-Cured Composites)

Light intensity decreases as the light source is moved away from the surface of an object. Furthermore, as the light travels through a scattering medium like a composite with filler particles, the

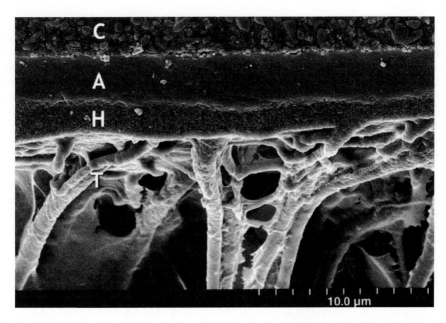

FIGURE 9-11 **Transverse section of composite bonded to dentin showing composite (C), adhesive layer (A), hybrid layer (H), and resin tags (T).**

TABLE 9.5 Clinical Requirements for Resin Composites Accepted for Unrestricted Use, Including Cuspal Replacement, in Posterior Teeth

Property	Criteria
Maintenance of color (18 mo)	No more than 5% failures
Marginal discoloration (18 mo)	No more than 5% failures
Marginal integrity (18 mo)	No more than 5% failures
Caries—recurrent or marginal (18 mo)	No more than 5%
Maintenance of interproximal contact (18 mo)	95% showing no observable broadening of contacts
Postoperative sensitivity	Thorough history of adverse sensitivity to hot, cold, and biting stimuli
Failure (18 mo)	No more than 5%
Wear between 6 and 18 mo	No more than 50 μm

From American Dental Association Acceptance Program guidelines for resin-based composites for posterior restorations, 2001.

light intensity is reduced. The depth of light penetration into a composite restoration depends on the wavelength of light, its irradiance, and the scattering that takes place within the restoration. A number of factors influence the degree of polymerization at given depths from the surface after light curing. The concentration of photo-initiator or light absorber in the composite must be such that it will react at the proper wavelength and be present in sufficient concentration. Both filler content and particle size are critical to dispersion of the light beam. For this reason, microfilled composites with smaller and more numerous particles scatter more light than microhybrid composites with larger and fewer glass particles. Longer exposure times are needed to obtain adequate polymerization of microfilled composites.

Another important consideration is the particular shade and opacity of the composite used. Many shades are intentionally opacified and have more pigments to mask discolored tooth after removal of carious tissue. These materials have higher concentration of opacifying agents and pigments that scatter more light and hence have lower depth of cure. In such cases, longer exposure times and smaller increments are essential for clinical success.

Light intensity at the surface is a critical factor in completeness of cure at the surface and within the material. The tip of the light source should be held within 1 mm of the surface to provide optimum exposure. More opaque shades reduce light transmission and cure only to minimal depths (1 mm). A standard exposure time using most dental curing lights is 20 seconds. In general, this is sufficient to cure a light shade of resin to a depth of 2 or 2.5 mm, assuming that the light guide is immediately adjacent to the restoration surface. The anatomy of the tooth often precludes the positioning of the light guide close to the restoration surface. A 40-second exposure improves the degree of cure at all depths, and is required to obtain sufficient cure with the darker shades. Because the light beam is partially collimated and does not spread sufficiently beyond the diameter of the tip at the emitting surface, it is necessary to "step" the light across the surface of large restorations so the entire surface receives a complete exposure. Larger tips have been manufactured for placement on most light-curing units. However, as the light beam is distributed over a larger surface area, the intensity at a given point is reduced. A longer exposure time of up to 60 seconds should be used when larger emitting tips are used.

Radiopacity

It is very difficult to locate enamel-composite margins radiographically because of the relatively low radiopacity of composites. Modern composites include glasses having atoms with high atomic numbers, such as barium, strontium, and zirconium. Some fillers, such as quartz, lithium-aluminum glasses, and silica, are not radiopaque and must be blended with other fillers to produce a radiopaque composite. Even at the highest volume fraction of filler, the amount of radiopacity is noticeably less than that exhibited by a metallic restorative like amalgam. Some microhybrid composites achieve some radiopacity by incorporating finely divided heavy-metal glass particles. Others use ceramic particles containing heavy metal oxides. In the nanofilled composite, radiopacity is achieved by using nanomeric zirconia (5-7 nm) or by incorporating the zirconia in the nanoclusters along with silica.

Wear Rates

Under clinical conditions, a composite restoration comes in contact with other surfaces such as the opposing tooth, food particles, and oral fluids, which can result in surface wear and degradation. The extent of wear is a complex phenomenon and depends on several intrinsic and extrinsic factors that are elaborated in Chapters 4 and 5. Many *in vitro* wear studies have been reported but because there are many different methodologies used, standardization and direct comparison of these results with actual clinical performance is not available. It is advisable to look at controlled clinical studies when choosing a composite, particularly for posterior restorations.

Clinical studies have shown that composites are ideal for anterior restorations in which esthetics is essential and occlusal forces are low. Wear rates are a larger concern in the posterior segments where occlusal forces and lateral excursive contacts are higher than in the anterior segment. Although earlier generations of composites exhibited attrition and abrasion wear, newer formulations minimize

the problem. Marginal degradation is still evident and is attributed to improper preparation design, inadequate adhesion, polymerization contraction of the composite, and marginal microcracks. Marginal degradation and stain are sometimes interpreted as recurrent caries, although this is not always the case. Currently accepted composites for posterior applications require clinical studies that demonstrate, over an 18-month period, a loss of surface contour less than 50 μm. Several clinical studies have been published showing that the newest generation of filled composite (nanocomposite) has excellent wear resistance. The nanofilled composite has been shown to exhibit wear resistance similar to that of natural human enamel in a 3-year and 5-year clinical study.

Biocompatibility

Details about the biocompatibility of composites are discussed in Chapter 6, but some of the central issues are discussed here. Nearly all of the major components of composites (Bis-GMA, TEGDMA, and UDMA, among others) are cytotoxic in vitro if tested as the bulk monomer, but the biological liability of a cured composite depends on the extent of release of these components from the composite. Although composites may release some low levels of components for weeks after curing, there is considerable controversy about the biological effects of these components. The amount of release depends on the type of composite and the method and efficiency of the cure of the composite. A dentin barrier markedly reduces the ability of components to reach pulpal tissues, but these components can traverse dentin barriers, albeit at reduced concentrations. The effects of low-dose, long-term exposures of cells to resin components are not generally known. On the other hand, the use of composite materials as direct pulp-capping agents poses a higher risk for adverse biological responses, because no dentin barrier exists to limit exposure of the pulp to the released components.

The effects of released components from composites on oral or other tissues are not known with certainty, although no studies have documented any adverse biological effects. The International Organization for Standardization (ISO) standard for testing of toxicity of dental materials requires the testing of composites after immersion in various aqueous and organic elution media followed by the testing of the eluants for adverse biological response. The tissue at highest risk from this type of release would appear to be the mucosa in close, long-term contact with composites. Components of composites are known allergens, and there has been some documentation of contact allergy to composites. Most of these reactions occur with dentists or dental personnel who regularly handle uncured composite and, therefore, have the greatest exposure. There are no good studies documenting the frequency of allergy to composites in the general population.

Finally, there has been some controversy about the ability of components of composites to act as xenoestrogens. Studies have proved that bisphenol A is estrogenic in vitro tests that measure this effect using breast cancer cell growth. Trace levels of these components have been identified in some commercial uncured composites; however, estrogenicity from cured commercial composites has not been demonstrated. Furthermore, there is considerable controversy about the accuracy and utility of in vitro tests using breast cancer cells to measure a true estrogenic effect. An early study in this area, which claimed that dental sealants and composites were estrogenic in children, has since been discredited.

Manipulation of composites can be found on the book's website at http://evolve.elsevier.com/sakaguchi/restorative ⊜

COMPOSITES FOR SPECIAL APPLICATIONS

Microfilled Composites

Microfilled composites are recommended for low stress bearing class 3 and class 5 restorations, in which a high polish and esthetics are most important. One product has been used successfully in posterior restorations. They are composed of light-activated, dimethacrylate resins with 0.04-μm colloidal silica fillers and prepolymerized resins, which are sometimes filled with colloidal silica. The total inorganic filler loading is 32% to 50% by volume (see Table 9-2).

Typical properties of microfilled composites are listed in Table 9-3. Because they are less highly filled, microfilled composites exhibit more water sorption, and thermal expansion than microhybrid composites or nanocomposites. Depending on the amount of prepolymerized resin, the shrinkage can be more than with microhybrids or nanocomposites.

Packable Composites

Packable is a term used for composite pastes that have very high viscosity and low surface tackiness. These materials are not condensable like amalgams, but can be compressed and forced to flow using flat-faced instruments. These composites (see Table 9-1) are recommended for use in classes 1 and 2 cavity preparations. They are composed of light-activated, dimethacrylate resins with fillers (porous or irregular particles) that have filler loading of 66% to 70% by volume (see Table 9-2). The interaction of the filler particles and modifications of the resin cause these composites to be packable.

Typical properties of packable composites are listed in Table 9-3. Important properties include greater depth of cure, lower polymerization shrinkage, radiopacity, and lower wear rate (3.5 μm/year). Several packable composites are packaged in unit-dose capsules. A bulk-fill technique is recommended by manufacturers but has not yet been demonstrated effective in clinical studies.

Flowable Composites

Flowable composites, which are light-activated, low-viscosity composites, are recommended for cervical lesions, restorations in deciduous teeth, and other small, low- or non-stress-bearing restorations (see Table 9-1). They contain dimethacrylate resin and inorganic fillers with a particle size of 0.4 to 3.0 μm and filler loading of 42% to 53% by volume (see Table 9-2). The newest generation of flowable composites contains nanofiller particles at a volume loading somewhat lower than universal or multipurpose composites. Recently, self-adhesive flowable composites have become available.

Typical properties of flowable composites are listed in Table 9-3. Flowable composites have a low modulus of elasticity, which may make them useful in cervical abrasion areas. Because of their lower filler content, they exhibit higher polymerization shrinkage and lower wear resistance than universal composites. The viscosity of these composites allows them to be dispensed by a syringe with a needle tip for easy handling. Gentle heating of higher viscosity composites can improve their flow and enable them to be placed as flowable composites.

Laboratory Composites

Crowns, inlays, and veneers bonded to metal copings can be prepared with composites processed in the laboratory (see Table 9-1), using various combinations of light, heat, pressure, and vacuum to increase the degree of polymerization, density, mechanical properties, and wear resistance.

Typical properties of laboratory composites are listed in Table 9-3. For increased strength and rigidity, laboratory composites can be combined with fiber reinforcement. Restorations are usually bonded with resin cements.

Core Build-Up Composites

If sufficient tooth structure remains to retain and support a full-coverage restoration, but extensive regions of dentin have been lost to disease, the core of

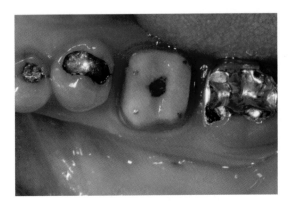

FIGURE 9.12 **A reconstructed composite resin pre-pared for a cast metal crown.** *(Courtesy of Dr. Charles Mark Malloy, Portland, OR.)*

the tooth can be restored before final preparation and impression. Composites are commonly used in this application. Core composites are available as self-cured (see Figure 9-4), light-cured, and dual-cured products. Core composites are usually tinted (blue, white, or opaque) to provide a contrasting color with the tooth structure. Some products release fluoride. An example of a composite core build-up is shown in Figure 9-12. Typical properties of core composites are listed in Table 9-3.

Composite cores have the following advantages as compared with amalgam: they can be bonded to dentin, can be finished immediately, are easy to contour, and can have a more natural color under ceramic restorations. Composite cores are bonded to remaining enamel and dentin using bonding agents. A bonding agent recommended by the manufacturer of the core material should be used because some self-cured composite core materials are incompatible with some light-cured bonding agents. Retention of the final restoration should not rely on the composite structure alone because adhesion of the composite core to remaining dentin alone is insufficient to resist rotation and dislodgement of the crown.

Provisional Composites

Provisional restorations maintain the position of the prepared tooth, seal and insulate the preparation and protect the margins, establish proper vertical dimension, aid in diagnosis and treatment planning, and help to evaluate candidates for esthetic replacements. Provisional inlays, crowns, and fixed partial dentures are usually fabricated from acrylic resins or composites. Provisional restorations fabricated from composites are generally harder, stiffer, and more color stable than those made from acrylics.

GLASS IONOMERS

Glass ionomers are water-based, self-adhesive restorative materials in which the filler is a reactive glass called *fluoroaluminosilicate glass* and the matrix is polymer or copolymer of carboxylic acids. The setting reaction of these materials involves an acid-base reaction. They are used as filling materials in clinical situations when isolation is a problem and fluoride release is desirable for the patient. There are two main types of glass ionomers:

- Conventional glass ionomer
- Resin-modified glass ionomer

Components and Setting Reaction of Conventional Glass Ionomer

Glass ionomers, invented in the 1970s, combine the technologies and chemistry of silicate and zinc polycarboxylate materials so as to incorporate the desirable characteristics of both. Thus they contain finely ground fluoroalumionosilicate glass filler that is ion-leachable but avoids the susceptibility to dissolution (a disadvantage in silicates) by substituting phosphoric acid with the polymeric carboxylic acids of zinc polycarboxylate materials. The materials are supplied as two-part powder-liquid systems that require mixing. The original systems have undergone several modifications, but all conventional glass ionomers have the following essential components:

- Polycarboxylic acid
- Fluoroaluminosilicate (FAS) glass
- Water
- Tartaric acid

The polymeric matrix of most glass ionomers is a copolymer of acrylic acid and itaconic acid or maleic acid. In most cases this is formulated as a concentrated aqueous liquid. Tartaric acid is added to control the working and setting characteristics of the material. The powder consists of an acid-reactive comminuted FAS glass and has ions such as calcium, strontium, and lanthanum. When heavy metal ions are used, the set material is radiopaque to x-rays. When the powder and liquid are mixed, an acid-base setting reaction begins between the FAS glass and the polycarboxylic acid. An initial set is achieved within 3 to 4 minutes of mixing, but the ionic reaction continues for at least 24 hours or more so that maturation is achieved much later. Maturation time has been improved in newer formulations to allow finishing after 15 minutes of placement of the mix. The actual process of ion extraction and complex formation is quite elaborate; however, the essential steps are described in the scheme shown.

All carboxylic acids have a common organic functional group denoted by COOH. In the presence of water, the COOH group undergoes partial ionization to yield a carboxylate anion COO^- and a hydrated proton, H_3O^+ (see scheme 1, reaction 1). The hydrated proton attacks the surface of the glass particles releasing calcium and aluminum ions. The carboxylate ions from the polymer react with these metallic ions to form a salt bridge, resulting in gelation and setting. During the initial setting, calcium ions are more rapidly bound to the polyacrylate chains; binding to the aluminum ions occurs at a later stage. The strength of the cement builds with time. Silicic acid is initially formed when the glass breaks down, but rapidly polymerizes to form silica hydrogel (reaction 4). A very important by-product of the setting reaction is the release of fluoride ions from the glass matrix. This fluoride release process is sustained and occurs over a long period of time. It is important to understand that this fluoride ion release is a result of the setting reaction and the ion exchange process in the cement. In this process the fluoride from the glass is being replaced by carboxylates and water. Hence, if properly formulated, there is little chance of the cement losing its strength with time. Considerable research has shown no loss of strength of the cement during years of storage in water.

Water plays several important roles in the overall setting. First, it provides for the ion transport needed for the acid base setting reaction and fluoride release. Second, a portion of the water is also chemically bound in the set complex and provides stability to the restorative material. Water also provides plasticity during the manipulative stages.

The set cement is constituted by a hydrogel of calcium, aluminum, and fluoroaluminum polyacrylates involving the unreacted glass particles sheathed by a weakly bonded siliceous hydrogel layer. About 20% to 30% of the glass is dissolved in the reaction. Smaller glass particles may be entirely dissolved and replaced by siliceous hydrogel particles containing fluorite crystallites. The stability of the matrix is given by an association of chain entanglement, weak ionic cross-linking, and hydrogen bonding.

Significant advances have been made in formulation of conventional glass ionomers in recent years to improve their manipulation and mechanical properties. Fast hardening has been achieved by

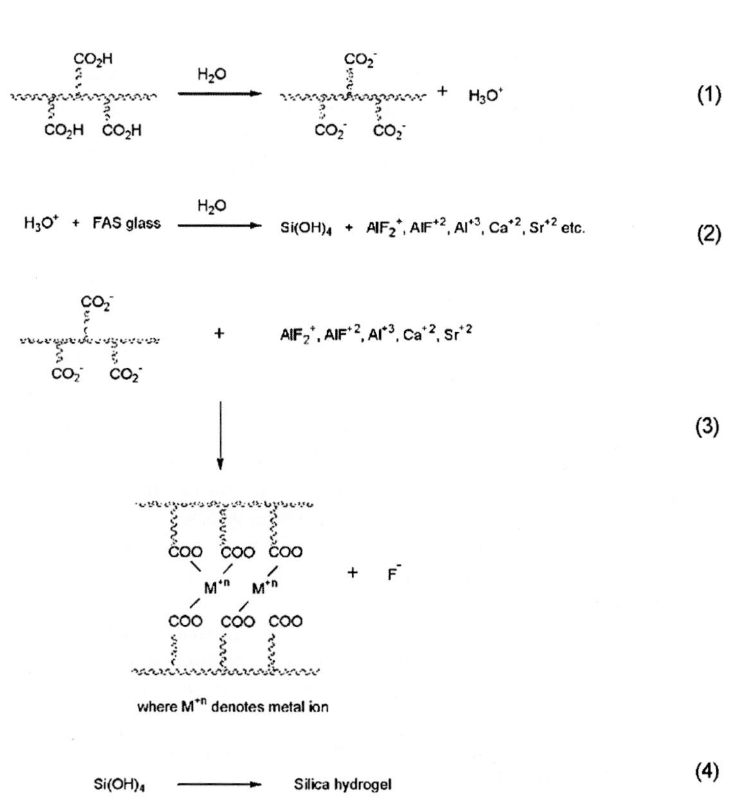

where M^{+n} denotes metal ion

Setting mechanism of conventional glass ionomers

altering the particle size and particle size distribution of the glass powder. One manufacturer coats the powder particles with a polymeric material for easy mixing.

Cermets

The early conventional glass ionomers were not very strong mechanically, so the glasses were fused with metals such as gold, silver, titanium, and silver to improve their strength. These materials are called *cermets*. The commercial systems are made from silver fused to the glass. Although the wear resistance is better than the conventional materials, the flexural strength and abrasion resistance are not significantly better, whereas the fluoride release is diminished. Because of the presence of metallic phase, the cermet cements are gray in color.

Components and Setting Reactions of Resin-Modified Glass Ionomers

To create a longer working time yet quick setting time so that immediate finishing can take place, the concept of resin-modified glass ionomer (RMGI) was introduced in the late 1980s. The essential components are similar to those in conventional GIs in which an aqueous polycarboxylic acid undergoes an acid-base setting reaction with fluoroalumionosilicate glass. To this methacrylate, components are added in limited amounts so a photo-initiated and/or redox curing reaction of the double bonds can also occur. Although commercial materials vary widely in composition, the essential components of true RMGIs are as follows:

- Polycarboxylic acid polymer—one manufacturer uses a polycarboxylic acid in which some pendent methacrylate groups are provided
- Fluoroaluminosilicate glass
- Water
- Hydrophilic methacrylate monomer
- Free radical initiators

The resin-modified glass ionomers contain some methacrylate components common in resin composites. There are two ways in which methacrylate components can be introduced. In the first type, the polycarboxylic acid polymer chain is modified to contain a pendent methacrylate group. A common way of doing this is to react some of the carboxylic acid groups of the polycarboxylic acid with isocyanatoethyl methacrylate to provide pendent methacrylate groups connected through the hydrolytically stable amide linkages. The first commercial

glass ionomer was introduced using this type of chemistry.

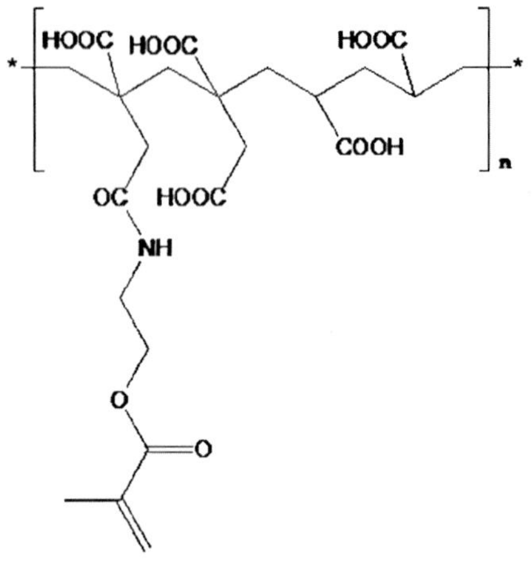

Polymeric component of some popular commercial resin-modified glass ionomers

In addition to the methacrylate-modified carboxylic acid, the liquid portion contains a water-miscible methacrylate monomer, for example, hydroxy ethylmethacrylate (HEMA) or glycerol dimethacrylate (GDMA). In another type of resin-modified glass ionomer system, the polymer is unmodified polycarboxylic acid. In this case the liquid is formulated with a mixture of hydrophilic methacrylate monomers and water. Generally, the water content of these materials is lower and the monomer content higher than for the first type. As a result, the coefficient of thermal expansion of these glass ionomers is high. Free radical initiators are added to trigger the curing of the methacrylate groups. Visible light initiators and/or self-cure redox initiators are employed to effect this curing and covalent cross-linking reaction.

The FAS glass of the resin-modified glass ionomer systems is similar in composition to the glasses described for conventional glass ionomers, although some variations are made in order to match the refractive index of the glass with that of the matrix. It is also common to treat the surface of the glass with an organic modifier.

Two distinct types of curing reactions take place in a true light-cure glass ionomer, the traditional acid-base glass ionomer cure and the free-radical methacrylate polymerization. In the laboratory the former can be followed by infrared spectroscopy through the appearance of carboxylate ion peaks. This is shown in the following reaction scheme. The methacrylate reaction, being a chain polymerization, proceeds at a rate that is several orders of magnitude higher than the acid-base reaction. In practice, the extent to which each of these two reactions occurs is very dependent on a particular system. If the system is low in water and high in the methacrylate components, the ionization of the polycarboxylic acid will be severely suppressed, resulting in little acid-base reaction. The extent of acid-base reaction is easily detected by chemical techniques such as Fourier transform infrared (FTIR) spectroscopy and electron spectroscopy for chemical analyses (ESCA).

Tri-Cure Glass Ionomer System

These are resin-modified glass ionomers with an additional curing mode. If only photo-initiators are used for cross-linking of the methacrylate groups, the resin-modified glass ionomer has to be cured in layers because penetration of visible light can occur only to a limited depth. This is not a disadvantage in applications where thin layers of materials are to be placed, for example, for lining or basing. However, for restorative and core build-up application, the need for incremental filling is a drawback. This problem has been overcome in the so-called *tri-cure glass ionomer system*. Here, in addition to the photo-initiators, self-cure redox imitators are added so that the methacrylate polymerization can proceed in the absence of light. The three curing reactions are as follows:

1. Acid-base glass ionomer reaction.
2. Light-activated polymerization
3. Chemically activated polymerization

Setting reaction of resin-modified glass ionomer (light-cure type)

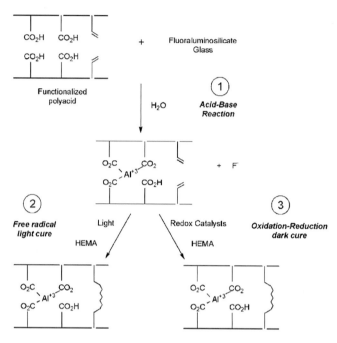

Setting reactions in tri-cure glass ionomer system.

Reactions 2 and 3 are chemically similar but differ in the mode of initiation. Reactions 1 and 3 take place spontaneously when the powder and liquid are mixed. Reaction 2 occurs only when initiated by light. The introduction of tri-cure technology has allowed resin-modified glass ionomers to be used as bulk-cured materials, thus saving time for the practitioner. In one commercial system, the redox initiators are microencapsulated separately in polymers and added to the powder. The spatulation and mixing of the powder and liquid trigger the release of the catalysts from the microcapsules resulting in the autocuring.

Although several commercial products claim to have the tri-cure chemistry, it is important to become familiar with the instructions for use and realize that there are very important differences between them. In a true tri-cure, the redox cure is quite rapid to allow the material to be placed in bulk, if desired.

Nanoionomer

The latest advancement in resin-modified glass ionomers is the nanoionomer available commercially since 2007. This material is a resin-modified glass ionomer in which some nanoparticles such as nanomers and nanoclusters (see section on Nanocomposites) are added to the FAS glass. Like all RMGIs, it has an aqueous component with a polycarboxylic acid and water-miscible methacrylate monomers. The addition of nanoparticles improves the polishability and the optical characteristics of the cured ionomer. The FAS of this material has very high surface area so that the fluoride release is not compromised. Infrared and ESCA analyses have confirmed the presence of significant acid-base reaction.

Packaging of Glass Ionomers

Glass ionomers are two-part systems. Until recently all glass ionomers consisted of a powder component and a liquid component. The powder is commonly provided in a jar and is dispensed with a measuring spoon and the liquid is provided in a vial with a dropper tip for use of dispensing. After dispensing the recommended ratio of powder and liquid according to the manufacturers' directions, the components are hand spatulated. In some cases, it is recommended that the mixed material be transferred to a syringe and injected into the tooth preparation.

To aid in the dispensing and mixing, the glass ionomers are also supplied in single-unit encapsulated version (see Figure 8-10). The powder and liquid are kept separated in the capsule for shelf-stability. Prior to clinical use the capsule is activated and then triturated in an amalgamator to mix the two components. An applicator is provided that pushes the mixed material through a narrow tip so that it can be directly placed in the oral preparation.

Recently, the RMGIs have been formulated in paste-liquid or two-paste systems. During manufacture the FAS powder component is mixed with a small amount of resin to provide a paste-like

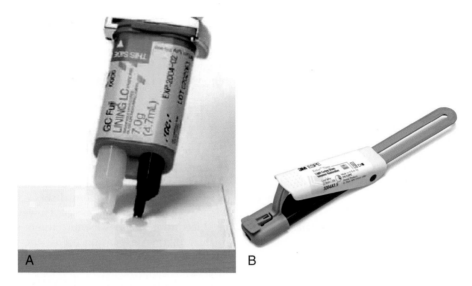

FIGURE 9-13 **Paste-liquid resin-modified glass ionomer dispensers (A & B).** *(A. Courtesy of GC America, Alsip, IL; B. Courtesy of 3M ESPE Dental Products, St. Paul, MN).*

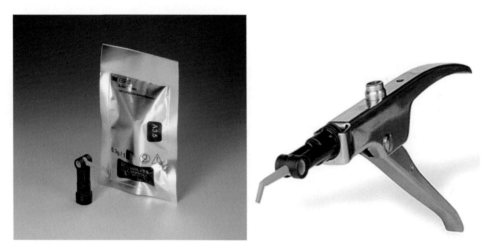

FIGURE 9.14 **Single-unit auto-mix dispensing capsule for a two-paste resin-modified glass ionomer.** The dispensing tip contains a mini static mixer for auto-mixing when expressed by a delivery gun device. *(Courtesy of 3M ESPE Dental Products, St. Paul, MN).*

consistency. The liquid may be left as such or alternatively formulated with a nonreactive glass and also provided as a paste. The manufacturer provides the two components in a dual-barrel syringe type of construction (Figure 9-13). During use, the two components are extruded by a lever in a predetermined ratio in the amount needed for the clinical preparation. The variability in dispensing is expected to be less in these types of dispensers. Furthermore, mixing by spatulation is more facile than with powder-liquid materials.

The latest advancement in dispensing of two paste systems is an auto-mixable, single-unit direct delivery device (Figure 9-14). In this device, the two

pastes are placed in two side-by-side compartments. The nozzle of the capsule contains a mini static mixer. In use the nozzle is lifted and positioned parallel to the barrels. An applicator then pushes out the two pastes into the nozzle where mechanical mixing occurs and the paste is extruded through the tip directly into the tooth preparation. The system is said to produce fewer microbubbles in the restoration, a condition that could potentially arise during trituration.

MANIPULATION OF GLASS IONOMERS can be found on the book's website at http://evolve. elsevier.com/sakaguchi/restorative ☉

Clinical Applications of Glass Ionomers

Clinically, both conventional and resin-modified glass ionomers are used for a variety of restorative applications, particularly in situations of high caries activity or where caries are likely to recur. The main clinical indications are for small lesions (long-term non-stress-bearing restorations in permanent teeth, interim restoration in permanent teeth, and in the atraumatic restoration technique [ART]) especially where one or more margins are on dentin. They make an excellent liner or base in all deep lesions where demineralized dentin remains on the cavity floor to be remineralized. They are also advocated for a technique known as *sandwiching*, *layering* or *stratification*, in which a resin composite is bonded over a base of the glass ionomer. Because of their low modulus, they are often advocated for class V restorations and abfraction lesions in which tooth flexure is more pronounced. Resin-modified glass ionomers are often the material of choice for pediatric restorations and preventive applications (direct filling as well as core build-up), because they are one-step procedures and require minimal isolation during placement. Some products are indicated for erupting permanent first and second molars with partially exposed grooves that are not yet able to be sealed with conventional resin sealant.

Properties of Glass Ionomers

Like many two part systems, the properties of glass ionomers, both conventional type and resin-modified, are quite dependent on the ratio of poly-carboxylic acid and fluoroaluminosilicate glass components dispensed. Particular care has to be exercised for powder-liquid hand-mixed systems to ensure accurate proportions. The ISO standard 9917 for water-based cements provides some requirements of glass ionomers as restorative materials and the ISO 9917-2 covers the properties of resin-modified glass ionomers. Comparative properties are shown in Table 9-3.

Physical, Mechanical Properties and Thermal Properties

The physical and mechanical properties of GIs are lower than that of composite resins and hence these materials are indicated for conservative restorations. The physical properties of the RMGIs, including wear resistance and dimensional stability, are improved over the conventional counterparts. The additional covalent cross-linking in the matrix due to the polymerization of the methacrylate groups contributes towards this improvement. The modulus of the resin modified glass ionomers is low during

the initial set by light activation but increases over time as the acid-base reaction completes. This unique characteristic makes the RMGI particularly attractive when used as liner or as the base in sandwich restorations under resin composites because it can relieve the stress associated with the polymerization shrinkage of the latter.

The thermal diffusivity and coefficient of thermal expansion (CTE) of several conventional and resin-modified glass ionomers have been shown to be closer to tooth structure (dentin) than are resin composites. Such materials should, therefore, serve as good insulation against thermal shock, particularly when used as liners and bases. However, because products from different manufacturers vary widely in their thermal expansion coefficient values, it is advisable to check the values of individual materials. In general, the products that have the smallest proportion of resin component exhibit the lowest CTE values.

Fluoride Ion Release and Uptake

A particularly beneficial characteristic of glass ionomers, conventional or resin modified, is that these materials act as a reservoir of fluoride ions. The fluoride is released by an ion-exchange mechanism from these materials. Research has shown that the released fluoride ions are taken up by the associated enamel and dentin, rendering those tooth structures less susceptible to acid challenge by a combination of decreased solubility and disruption of the activity of cariogenic bacteria. The release of fluoride ion is sustained over prolonged periods (Figure 9-15). These materials also have been shown to act as fluoride reservoirs in the oral environment by taking up salivary fluoride from dentifrices, mouthwashes, and topical fluoride solutions. Fluoride has been measured in plaque samples immediately adjacent to resin-modified glass ionomer restorations (see Figure 8-9). Fluoride ion dynamics is particularly advantageous for those with high susceptibility to dental caries. A vast amount of in vitro and in situ research and a limited number of clinical studies have been carried out to assess the clinical benefit of the fluoride. Most of these studies have shown the utility of these materials when medium to high caries activity is present.

Adhesion

Glass ionomer materials have good clinical adhesion to tooth structure. Unlike the resin-based composite materials, etching of the enamel or dentin surface by phosphoric acid is not needed. Hence these materials are sometimes referred to as being *self-adhesive*. Preconditioning of the tooth surface is recommended for some products, especially those with high powder-liquid ratio to ensure good

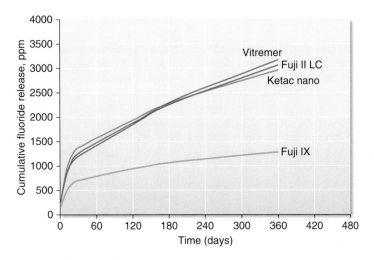

FIGURE 9.15 **Fluoride release from typical glass ionomers.**

wetting. One of the following procedures is used for the pretreatment:

- The cavity surface is conditioned using 10% to 20% polyacrylic acid for 10 seconds, washed well to remove the conditioner and surface debris, and dried.
- For some resin-modified glass ionomer restoratives (identified by manufacturers as primer or self-conditioner), a dilute polycarboxylic acid-based solution is applied on the cavity surface and set through light. This ensures good contact of the viscous mix of the glass ionomer with the tooth while not impeding ion exchange reactions.

The mechanism of adhesion to the tooth structure is mostly chemical in nature and proceeds through an exchange of ions arising from both the tooth and restoration. Calcium-polyacrylate bonds have been shown by some products by in vitro electron spectroscopy for chemical analysis (ESCA) studies. A small amount of micromechanical bonding has been exhibited by some resin-modified glass ionomers.

Laboratory measurements of bond strengths of conventional and resin-modified glass ionomers to tooth structure have generally yielded lower values than with the combination of resin adhesives and composites. The failure is usually cohesive in the glass ionomer; hence, it is doubtful whether these laboratory measurements reflect the actual interfacial adhesion. However, retrospective clinical analyses of in vivo studies have shown RMGIs to provide excellent retention and sealing of the tooth. One of the reasons for this is due to the relief of external stress provided by the dual-curing reactions of this class of materials.

Resin-modified glass ionomers have been recognized as one of the best treatments for minimizing

postoperative sensitivity in restored teeth. There are two reasons for this. First, because prior etching is not needed during placement, the collagen fibrils are not demineralized and collapse of the denuded layers cannot occur. Second, the dual-setting mechanism and gradual build-up of modulus allow the material to absorb a considerable amount of shrinkage stresses, thus minimizing the effect of contraction forces at the tooth-restoration interfaces.

COMPOMERS

Compomers or poly acid–modified composites are used for restorations in low stress–bearing areas, although a recent product is recommended by the manufacturer for class 1 and class 2 restorations in adults (see Table 9-1). Compomers are recommended for patients at medium risk of developing caries.

Composition and Setting Reaction

Compomers contain poly acid–modified monomers with fluoride-releasing silicate glasses and are formulated without water. Some compomers have modified monomers that provide additional fluoride release. The volume percent filler ranges from 42% to 67%, and the average filler particle size ranges from 0.8 to 5.0 μm. Compomers are packaged as single-paste formulations in compules and syringes.

Setting occurs primarily by light-cured polymerization, but an acid-base reaction also occurs as the compomer absorbs water after placement and upon contact with saliva. Water uptake is also important for fluoride transfer.

Properties

Typical properties of compomers are listed in Table 9-3. Compomers release fluoride by a mechanism similar to that of glass and hybrid ionomers. Because of the lower amount of glass ionomer present in compomers, the amount of fluoride release and its duration are lower than those of glass and hybrid ionomers. Also, compomers do not recharge from fluoride treatment or brushing with fluoride dentifrices as much as glass and hybrid ionomers.

Manipulation

Compomers are packaged in unit-dose compules. They require a bonding agent to bond to tooth structure. The material is to be cured by light in increments of 2 to 2.5 mm.

LIGHT-CURING UNITS

Overview

The most common light sources used in dentistry to photo-activate composites is quartz-tungsten-halogen and blue LED (light-emitting diode). Definitions of terms used to describe light sources used to activate dental resins are listed in Table 9-6.

Quartz-Tungsten-Halogen Light-Curing Units

An example of a quartz-tungsten-halogen (QTH) light-curing unit used to activate polymerization of composites is shown in Figure 9-16. The peak

wavelength varies among units from about 450 to 490 nm. Typically, the irradiance ranges from 400 to 800 mW/cm², but higher-intensity QTH units are available. Some units can be controlled to provide two or three different intensities (step cure) or at a continuously increasing (ramp cure) intensity. A typical 2-mm thick resin composite restoration requires a radiant exposure of 8 J/cm² (400 mW/cm² × 20 s = 8000 mW s/cm²) for proper polymerization.

A QTH light source consists of a broad-spectrum light bulb (typically 75 W), several filters, a reflector, a fan, a power supply, and a light guide. The broad-spectrum output of the QTH bulb is clipped by a blue bandpass filter that only allows a narrow band of wavelengths centered around 470 to 480 nm (blue wavelengths) to be transferred to the light guide. A UV filter blocks passage of UV wavelengths. A dichroic reflector focuses the light on the end of the light guide. The reflector also enables infrared wavelengths to dissipate as heat through the back of the housing. Because substantial heat is generated by the 75 W bulb, a fan is necessary to cool the bulb and assembly.

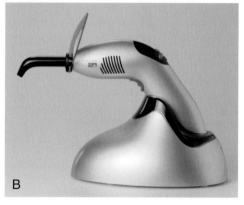

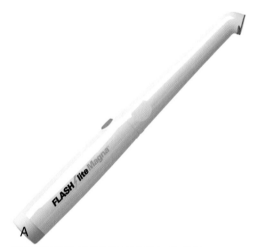

FIGURE 9.16 **Visible-light source for photo-initiation of light activated restorative materials.** *(A. Courtesy of Discus Dental, Culver City, CA; B. Courtesy of Ivoclar Vivadent, Amherst, NY.)*

TABLE 9.6   Definitions of Terms Used to Describe Light Sources for Polymerization of Dental Resins

Term	Unit	Definition
Spectral emission	nm	Effective bandwidth of wavelengths emitted by light source
Spectral requirement	nm	Bandwidth of wavelengths required to activate photo-initiator(s) of dental resin
Flux	mW	Number of photons per second emitted by light source
Irradiance or radiant exitance	mW/cm²	Number of photons per second emitted by light source per unit area of curing tip
Energy	J*	Flux × time
Energy density	J/cm²	Radiant exitance × time

*Joule (J) = 1000 mW × s.

A decrease in line voltage of 6% shows a corresponding reduction in output of about 25% in intensity in some lamps, but only 10% in lamps with voltage regulators in their circuitry. In general, the output from the various lamps decreases with continuous use and the intensity is not uniform for all areas of the light tip, being greatest at the center. Also, the intensity of the light decreases with distance from the source. Although the intensity is important with respect to the depth of cure, it has been shown for some products that a threefold difference in intensity had only a 15% difference in the depth of cure. Bulb life ranges from 50 to 75 hours.

Although there is minimal potential for radiation damage to surrounding soft tissue inadvertently exposed to visible light, caution should be used to prevent retinal damage to the eyes. Because of the high intensity of the light, the operator should not look directly at the tip or the reflected light from the teeth. A number of devices are marketed to filter the visible-light beam so the operator can directly observe the curing procedure and to protect the patient and staff. These orange-tinted devices are available as eyeglasses, flat shields that can be held over the field of vision, and curved shields that attach directly to the handpiece delivering the light beam.

Some lamps produce considerable heat at the curing tip, which can produce pulpal irritation. Too much heat is being generated if one cannot hold a finger 2 to 3 mm from the tip for 20 seconds. Maintenance of QTH lights must be provided on a regular basis, as summarized in Table 9-7.

TABLE 9.7 Factors Causing Decrease in Intensity of Light from Quartz-Tungsten-Halogen (QTH) Light-Curing Units and Maintenance Hints

Factors	Maintenance Hints
Dust or deterioration of reflector	Clean or replace reflector
Burn-out of bulb filament	Replace bulb
Darkening/frosting of bulb	Replace bulb
Age of components	Monitor intensity, replace unit
Chipping of light tip	Replace light tip
Resin deposit on light tip	Clean or replace light tip
Change in line voltage	Get built-in voltage regulator
Lack of uniformity across light tip	Overlap curing on larger surface
Increased distance of tip from material to be cured	Keep light tip close to material

Blue Light-Emitting Diodes

Solid-state light-emitting diodes (LEDs) use junctions of doped semiconductors (p-n junctions) based on gallium nitride to emit blue light. The spectral output of blue LEDs falls between 450 and 490 nm, so these units are effective for curing materials with camphorquinone photo-initiators. LED units do not require a filter, have a long life span, and do not produce as much heat as QTH devices. Heat becomes a concern even with LED sources, when large arrays are used. Because the output spectrum of blue LEDs matches the absorption spectrum of camphorquinone more closely than QTH sources, it is thought that blue LED sources are more efficient. For QTH sources, most of the light energy is discarded because QTH is a broad-spectrum source and only the wavelengths absorbed by camphorquinone are desired. For LED sources, the emission is not filtered. This, however, does not make LED sources more efficient in activating the camphorquinone photo-initiator than QTH. Creation of photons is dependent only on the energy applied in the absorbable wavelengths.

Composites cured with LED units have flexural properties similar to those cured with QTH units. Depth of cure with LED units appears to be higher.

PROSTHETIC APPLICATIONS OF POLYMERS

Acrylic polymers have a wide variety of applications in restorative dentistry as denture bases, artificial teeth, denture repair materials, impression trays, provisional restorations, and maxillofacial appliances for skeletal defects. The vast majority of dentures made today are fabricated from heat-cured poly(methyl methacrylate) and rubber-reinforced poly(methyl methacrylate). Fractures of dentures still occur, but are usually associated with carelessness or unreasonable use by the patient. Considering functional stresses, the oral environment, and expected service life, denture base materials perform remarkably well.

Physical Form and Composition

Denture base plastics are commonly supplied in a powder-liquid or a gel form. The powder-liquid type may contain the materials listed in Box 9-1.

Powder

Most commercial materials contain poly(methyl methacrylate), modified with small amounts of ethyl, butyl, or other alkyl methacrylates to produce a polymer somewhat more resistant to

---

BOX 9-1

PRINCIPAL INGREDIENTS OF ACRYLIC DENTURE BASE POWDER AND LIQUID

Powder

Acrylic polymer (or copolymer) beads
Initiator
Pigments
Dyes
Opacifier
Plasticizer
Dyed organic fibers
Inorganic particles

Liquid

Monomer
Inhibitor
Accelerator
Plasticizer
Cross-linking agent

---

fracture by impact. The powder also contains an initiator such as benzoyl peroxide or diisobutylazonitrile to initiate the polymerization of the monomer liquid after being added to the powder. The peroxide initiator may be added to the polymer or be present as a residual from the polymerization reaction and is present in amounts from 0.5% to 1.5%.

Pure polymers, such as poly(methyl methacrylate), are clear and are adaptable to a wide range of pigmentation. Colorants are added to obtain the various tissue-like shades, and zinc or titanium oxides are used as opacifiers. Dyed synthetic fibers made from nylon or acrylic are usually added to simulate the small capillaries of the oral mucosa.

Plasticizers such as dibutyl phthalate may be incorporated in the powder or the monomer. Adding glass fibers and alumina (sapphire) whiskers increases the stiffness, decreases the thermal coefficient of expansion, and increases thermal diffusivity. Polyethylene-woven yarn and polyaramid fabric have also been used to reinforce acrylic polymers.

Liquid

The liquid component of the powder-liquid type acrylic resin is methylmethacrylate, but it may be modified by the addition of other monomers. Because these monomers may be polymerized by heat, light, or traces of oxygen, inhibitors are added to give the liquid adequate shelf life. The inhibitor most commonly used to prevent premature polymerization is hydroquinone, which may be present in concentrations of 0.003% to 0.1%.

When a chemical accelerator rather than heat is used to speed up the peroxide decomposition and enable the polymerization of the monomer at room temperature, an accelerator is included in the liquid. Common accelerators are amines such as N,N-dimethyl-para-toluidine, and N,N-dihydroxyethyl-para-toluidine. These systems are referred to as *self-curing, cold-curing,* or *autopolymerizing resins*. The pour-type of denture resin is included in this category.

Plasticizers are sometimes added to produce a softer, more resilient polymer. They are generally relatively low-molecular-weight esters, such as dibutyl phthalate. Plasticizer molecules do not enter the polymerization reaction but do interfere with the interaction between polymer molecules, making the plasticized polymer softer than the pure polymer. One disadvantage in using plasticizers is that they gradually leach out of the plastic into oral fluids, resulting in hardening of the denture base. A polymer also may be plasticized by the addition of some higher ester such as butyl or octyl methacrylate to methylmethacrylate. The esters polymerize and form a more flexible plastic. This type of internal plasticizing does not leach out in the oral fluids, and the material remains flexible.

If a cross-linked polymer is desired, organic compounds such as glycol dimethacrylate are added to the monomer. Cross-linking compounds are characterized by reactive—CR–CH—groups at opposite ends of the molecules and serve to link long polymer molecules together. Using cross-linking agents provides greater resistance to minute surface cracking, termed *crazing,* and may decrease solubility and water sorption. Cross-linking materials may be present in amounts of 2% to 14%, but have little effect on the tensile strength, flexural properties, or hardness of acrylic plastics.

SELECTED PROBLEMS

PROBLEM 1

In selecting a composite for placing a large class 4 restoration, what advantages of a light-cured composite would you consider?

Solution

Contour can be more adequately achieved through incremental addition; fewer air voids should be incorporated, because mixing of two pastes is not necessary; shade development can more readily be accomplished through the increments of different-colored composites; and less excess material should exist after insertion and curing of the restoration; thus finishing should be facilitated.

PROBLEM 2

An extensive posterior core build-up is required on a lower molar. Why is a self-cured, core composite the material of choice?

Solution

Uniform curing takes place under a crown form, lower-viscosity resin adapts better to posts, and opaque, colored composites can be used to differentiate core from tooth structure during crown preparation.

PROBLEM 3

When small air voids appear on the surface of a self-cured composite restoration during finishing, what are the causative manipulative factors?

Solution

The problem may be caused by exposing the dispensed composite to operatory light before incremental insertion; extended working of each increment to the point that voids are incorporated between layers; mixing of increments of two different shades of pastes on a pad before insertion; or excessive use of alcohol as a lubricant on the insertion instrument.

PROBLEM 4

Is there reason to expect that the color of a large class 4 restoration will be more stable when a light-cured composite is used instead of a self-cured composite? Why?

Solution

Yes. A self-cured composite contains an aromatic amine accelerator that is more susceptible to breakdown by oxidation than the aliphatic amine in a light-cured system.

PROBLEM 5

When a thin composite anterior veneer is being placed to modify tooth color, what are the advantages of a microfilled composite?

Solution

The advantages are the following: greater translucency improves vitality in the final shade; smoother surface texture provides a glossy surface with light-reflective patterns similar to enamel; in a thin layer supported by the bond to enamel, high physical and mechanical properties are not as important as in a free-standing class 4 restoration.

PROBLEM 6

In polymerizing a large, light-cured, resin composite restoration, what manipulative variables can be controlled to improve the depth of cure?

Solution

The following variables can be controlled: the exposure time of the light can be increased for darker shades and thicker increments (beyond 2 mm); the light source can be maintained within 1 mm of the resin surface; and the light tip can be drawn across the composite surface in steps, with multiple exposures ensuring uniformity of cure.

PROBLEM 7

In selecting a composite for a large, class 4 anterior restoration with significant incisal function, what are the enhanced properties of microhybrid composite that make it the material of choice?

Solution

The beneficial properties are greater strength and elastic modulus, lower polymerization shrinkage, lower thermal coefficient of expansion, lower water sorption, and greater wear resistance.

PROBLEM 8

In the clinical evaluation of a 2-year-old composite restoration, penetrating marginal discoloration is noted. What factors contribute to this bond failure?

Solution

Contributing factors are residual stress from polymerization shrinkage; fatigue stresses on the bond from thermal cycling; contamination at the bond site during material insertion; deflection stress at the restoration margins caused by intermittent functional loading of the restoration; and hydrolytic breakdown of the bond at the tooth interface (particularly if it is dentin).

PROBLEM 9

When repairing an anterior veneer restoration with a small area of severe marginal leakage, the discolored composite is removed and the deficient area is rebonded with new material. What is the character of the bond between old cured composite and new?

Solution

The bond is primarily micromechanical and is formed against the roughened surface of the original composite. A weak chemical bond may be formed between exposed unreacted bonds in the old material and the new bonding agent/composite. The repaired

composite has less cohesive strength than the original composite and is more durable if an adjacent fresh enamel area can also be prepared by acid etching.

PROBLEM 10

In assessing the use of composites in posterior teeth, what are the factors that contribute to early wear and failure?

Solution

These factors are the loss of substance as a result of deterioration of the silane coupling agent that bonds the filler particles to the matrix; excessive polymerization shrinkage from the relatively large volume of such restorations; stress-crack propagation across filler-polymer interfaces; and the low abrasion resistance of a relatively large volume of polymer matrix.

Bibliography

History

British Dental Association Museum. http://www.bda.org/museum/

Fletcher T: British Patent 3028, 1878, Dental silicate cement.

Fletcher T: German Patent 8202, 1879, Dental silicate cement.

Wilson AD, Batchelor RF: Dental silicate cements. I. The chemistry of erosion, *J Dent Res* 46:1075, 1967.

Composites

Asmussen E: Clinical relevance of physical, chemical, and bonding properties of composite resins, *Oper Dent* 10:61, 1985.

Bayne SC, Thompson JY, Swift EJ Jr, et al: A characterization of first-generation flowable composites, *J Am Dent Assoc* 129:567, 1998.

Braem M, Davidson CL, Lambrechts P, et al: In vitro flexural fatigue limits of dental composites, *J Biomed Mater Res* 28:1397, 1994.

Braem M, Finger W, Van Doren VE, et al: Mechanical properties and filler fraction of dental composites, *Dent Mater* 5:346, 1989.

Braga RR, Ferracane JL: Alternatives in polymerization contraction stress management, *Crit Rev Oral Biol Med* 15:176, 2004.

Chantler PM, Hu X, Boyd NM: An extension of a phenomenological model for dental composites, *Dent Mater* 15:144, 1999.

Choi KK, Condon JR, Ferracane JL: The effects of adhesive thickness on polymerization contraction stress of composite, *J Dent Res* 79:812, 2000.

Condon JR, Ferracane JL: Factors affecting dental composite wear in vitro, *J Biomed Mater Res* 38:303, 1997.

Condon JR, Ferracane JL: In vitro wear of composite with varied cure, filler level, and filler treatment, *J Dent Res* 76:1405, 1997.

Condon JR, Ferracane JL: Reduction of composite contraction stress through non-bonded microfiller particles, *Dent Mater* 14:256, 1998.

Council on Scientific Affairs: Posterior resin-based composites, *J Am Dent Assoc* 129:1627, 1998.

Council on Scientific Affairs: *American Dental Association acceptance program guidelines for resin-based composites for posterior restorations, Council on Scientific Affairs*, Chicago, 2001, American Dental Association.

Cross M, Douglas WH, Fields RP: The relationship between filler loading and particle-size distribution in composite resin technology, *J Dent Res* 62:850, 1983.

Dauvillier BS, Feilzer AJ, de Gee AJ, et al: Visco-elastic parameters of dental restorative materials during setting, *J Dent Res* 79:818, 2000.

DeWald J, Ferracane JL: A comparison of four modes of evaluating depth of cure of light-activated composites, *J Dent Res* 66:727, 1987.

Dietschi D, Holy J: A clinical trial of four light-curing posterior composite resins: two-year report, *Quint Int* 21:965, 1990.

Doray PG, Wang X, Powers JM, et al: Accelerated aging affects color stability of provisional restorative materials, *J Prosthodont* 6:183, 1997.

El Hejazi AA, Watts DC: Creep and visco-elastic recovery of cured and secondary-cured composites and resin-modified glass-ionomers, *Dent Mater* 15:138, 1999.

Eldiwany M, Friedl K-H, Powers JM: Color stability of light-cured and post-cured composites, *Am J Dent* 8:179, 1995.

Eldiwany M, Powers JM, George LA: Mechanical properties of direct and post-cured composites, *Am J Dent* 6:222, 1993.

Farah JW, Powers JM: Composite update, *Dent Advis* 26(8):1, 2009.

Farah JW, Powers JM, editors: Finishing and polishing of composites, *Dent Advis* 24(7):1, 2007.

Farah JW, Powers JM, editors: Focus on composite cores, *Dent Advis* 26(4):1, 2009.

Farah JW, Powers JM, editors: Laboratory composites, *Dent Advis* 22(3):1, 2005.

Farah JW, Powers JM, editors: Layered resin composites, *Dent Advis* 20(7):1, 2003.

Farah JW, Powers JM, editors: Update: flowable composites, *Dent Advis* 22(4):1, 2005.

Fay R-M, Servos T, Powers JM: Color of restorative materials after staining and bleaching, *Oper Dent* 24:292, 1999.

Feilzer AJ, de Gee AJ, Davidson CL: Setting stress in composite resin in relation to configuration of the restoratives, *J Dent Res* 66:1636, 1987.

Feilzer AJ, de Gee AJ, Davidson CL: Quantitative determination of stress reduction by flow in composite restorations, *Dent Mater* 6:167, 1990.

Ferracane JL: Elution of leachable components from composites, *J Oral Rehabil* 21:441, 1994.

Ferracane JL: Current trends in dental composites, *Crit Rev Oral Biol Med* 6:302, 1995.

Ferracane JL, Mitchem JC, Condon JR, et al: Wear and marginal breakdown of composites with various degrees of cure, *J Dent Res* 76:1508, 1997.

Ferracane JL, Moser JB, Greener EH: Rheology of composite restoratives, *J Dent Res* 60:1678, 1981.

Ferracane JL: Developing a more complete understanding of stresses produced in dental composites during polymerization, *Dent Mater* 21:36, 2005.

Filho HN, D'Azevedo MT, Nagem HD, Marsola FP: Surface roughness of composite resins after finishing and polishing, *Braz Dent J* 14:37, 2003.

Gerzina TM, Hume WR: Effect of dentine on release of TEGDMA from resin composite *in vitro, J Oral Rehabil* 21:463, 1994.

Geurtsen W: Biocompatibility of resin-modified filling materials, *Crit Rev Oral Biol Med* 11:333, 2000.

Hanks CT, Strawn SE, Wataha JC, et al: Cytotoxic effects of composite resin components on cultured mammalian fibroblasts, *J Dent Res* 70:1450, 1991.

Hanks CT, Wataha JC, Parsell RR, et al: Permeability of biological and synthetic molecules through dentine, *J Oral Rehabil* 21:475, 1994.

Hu X, Harrington E, Marquis PM, et al: The influence of cyclic loading on the wear of a dental composite, *Biomaterials* 20:907, 1999.

Hu X, Marquis PM, Shortall AC: Two-body in vitro wear study of some current dental composites and amalgams, *J Prosthet Dent* 82:214, 1999.

Kalachandra S: Influence of fillers on the water sorption of composites, *Dent Mater* 5:283, 1989.

Kim K-H, Park J-H, Imai Y, et al: Fracture toughness and acoustic emission behavior of dental composite resins, *Engin Fract Mech* 40:811, 1991.

Labella R, Lambrechts P, Van Meerbeek B, et al: Polymerization shrinkage and elasticity of flowable composites and filled adhesives, *Dent Mater* 15:128, 1999.

Lee Y-K, Powers JM: Calculation of colour resulting from composite/compomer layering techniques, *J Oral Rehabil* 31:1102, 2004.

Lee Y-K, El Zawahry M, Noaman KM, et al: Effect of mouthwash and accelerated aging on the color stability of esthetic restorative materials, *Am J Dent* 13:159, 2000.

Leinfelder KF: Posterior composite resins: the materials and their clinical performance, *J Am Dent Assoc* 126:663, 1995.

Letzel H: Survival rates and reasons for failure of posterior composite restorations in multicentre clinical trial, *J Dent* 17:S10, 1989.

Lu H, Roeder LB, Powers JM: Effect of polishing systems on the surface roughness of microhybrid composites, *J Esthet Restor Dent* 15:297, 2003.

Manhart J, Kunzelmann K-H, Chen HY, et al: Mechanical properties and wear behavior of light-cured packable composite resins, *Dent Mater* 16:33, 2000.

Mitchem JC, Gronas DG: The continued in vivo evaluation of the wear of restorative resins, *J Am Dent Assoc* 111:961, 1985.

Mitra SB, Wu D, Holmes BN: An application of nanotechnology in advanced dental materials, *J Am Dent Assoc* 134:1382, 2003.

Ortengren U, Wellendorf H, Karlsson S, et al: Water sorption and solubility of dental composites and identification of monomers released in an aqueous environment, *J Oral Rehabil* 28:1106, 2001.

Oysaed H, Ruyter IE: Water sorption and filler characteristics of composites for use in posterior teeth, *J Dent Res* 65:1315, 1986.

Paravina RD, Ontiveros JC, Powers JM: Accelerated aging effects on color and translucency of bleaching-shade composites, *J Esthet Restor Dent* 16:117, 2004.

Paravina RD, Ontiveros JC, Powers JM: Curing-dependent changes in color and translucency parameter of composite bleach shades, *J Esthet Restor Dent* 14:158, 2002.

Paravina RD, Roeder L, Lu H, et al: Effect of finishing and polishing procedures on surface roughness, gloss and color of resin-based composites, *Am J Dent* 17:262, 2004.

Park Y-J, Chae K-H, Rawls HR: Development of a new photoinitiation system for dental light-cure composite resins, *Dent Mater* 15:120, 1999.

Perry R, Kugel G, Kunzelmann K-H, et al: Composite restoration wear analysis: conventional methods vs. three-dimensional laser digitizer, *J Am Dent Assoc* 131:1472, 2000.

Powers JM: Lifetime prediction of dental materials: an engineering approach, *J Oral Rehabil* 22:491, 1995.

Powers JM, Burgess JO: Performance standards for competitive dental restorative materials, *Trans Acad Dent Mater* 9:68, 1996.

Powers JM, Dennison JB, Lepeak PJ: Parameters that affect the color of direct restorative resins, *J Dent Res* 57:876, 1978.

Powers JM, Hostetler RW, Dennison JB: Thermal expansion of composite resins and sealants, *J Dent Res* 58:584, 1979.

Powers JM, Smith LT, Eldiwany M, et al: Effects of postcuring on mechanical properties of a composite, *Am J Dent* 6:232, 1993.

Price RB, Felix CA, Andreou P: Knoop hardness of ten resin composites irradiated with high-power LED and quartz-tungsten-halogen lights, *Biomaterials* 26:2631, 2005.

Price RB, Derand T, Loney RW, et al: Effect of light source and specimen thickness on the surface hardness of resin composite, *Am J Dent* 15:47, 2002.

Pratten DH, Johnson GH: An evaluation of finishing instruments for an anterior and a posterior composite, *J Prosthet Dent* 60:154, 1988.

Rathbun MA, Craig RG, Hanks CT, et al: Cytotoxicity of a Bis-GMA dental composite before and after leaching in organic solvents, *J Biomed Mater Res* 25:443, 1991.

Roeder LB, Powers JM: Surface roughness of resin composite prepared by single-use and multi-use diamonds, *Am J Dent* 17:109, 2004.

Roeder LB, Tate WH, Powers JM: Effect of finishing and polishing procedures on the surface roughness of packable composites, *Oper Dent* 25:534, 2000.

Sakaguchi RL, Berge HX: Reduced light energy density decreases post-gel contraction while maintaining degree of conversion in composites, *J Dent* 26:695, 1998.

Sakaguchi RL, Peters MCRB, Nelson SR, et al: Effects of polymerization contraction in composite restorations, *J Dent* 20:178, 1992.

Sakaguchi RL, Wiltbank BD, Murchison CF: Prediction of composite elastic modulus and polymerization shrinkage by computational micromechanics, *Dent Mater* 20:397, 2004.

Sakaguchi RL, Wiltbank BD, Shah NC: Critical configuration analysis of four methods for measuring polymerization shrinkage strain of composites, *Dent Mater* 20:388, 2004.

Sakaguchi RL, Wiltbank BD, Murchison CF: Cure induced stresses and damage in particulate reinforced polymer matrix composites: a review of the scientific literature, *Dent Mater* 21:43, 2005.

Sarrett DC: Clinical challenges and the relevance of materials testing for posterior composite restorations, *Dent Mater* 21:9, 2005.

Sideridou I, Tserki V, Papanastasiou G: Study of water sorption, solubility and modulus of elasticity of light-cured dimethacrylate-based dental resins, *Biomaterials* 24:655, 2003.

Soderholm K-JM: Leaking of fillers in dental composites, *J Dent Res* 62:126, 1983.

Soderholm K-J, Zigan M, Ragan M, et al: Hydrolytic degradation of dental composites, *J Dent Res* 63:1248, 1984.

Stanford CM, Fan PL, Schoenfeld CM, et al: Radiopacity of light-cured posterior composite resins, *J Am Dent Assoc* 115:722, 1987.

Stansbury JW, Trujillo-Lemon M, Lu H, et al: Conversion-dependent shrinkage stress and strain in dental resins and composites, *Dent Mater* 21:56, 2005.

Suh BI, Ferber C, Baez R: Optimization of hybrid composite properties, *J Esthetic Dent* 2:44, 1990.

Tate WH, Friedl K-H, Powers JM: Bond strength of composites to hybrid ionomers, *Oper Dent* 21:147, 1996.

Tate WH, Powers JM: Surface roughness of composites and hybrid ionomers, *Oper Dent* 21:53, 1996.

Tirtha R, Fan PL, Dennison JB, et al: In vitro depth of cure of photo-activated composites, *J Dent Res* 61:1184, 1982.

Trajtenberg CP, Powers JM: Bond strengths of repaired laboratory composites using three surface treatments and three primers, *Am J Dent* 17:123, 2004.

Trajtenberg CP, Powers JM: Effect of hydrofluoric acid on repair bond strength of a laboratory composite, *Am J Dent* 17:173, 2004.

Van Dijken JWV: A clinical evaluation of anterior conventional, microfiller, and hybrid composite resin fillings: a 6-year follow-up study, *Acta Odontol Scand* 44:357, 1986.

Vandewalle KS, Ferracane JL, Hilton TJ, et al: Effect of energy density on properties and marginal integrity of posterior resin composite restorations, *Dent Mater* 20:96, 2004.

Wataha JC, Hanks CT, Strawn SE, et al: Cytotoxicity of components of resin and other dental restorative materials, *J Oral Rehabil* 21:453, 1994.

Weinmann W, Thalacker C, Guggenberger R: Siloranes in dental composites, *Dent Mater* 21:68, 2005.

Wendt SL Jr: The effect of heat used as a secondary cure upon the physical properties of three composite resins. I. Diametral tensile strength, compressive strength, and a marginal dimensional stability, *Quint Int* 18:265, 1987.

Wendt SL Jr, Leinfilder KF: The clinical evaluation of heat-treated composite resin inlays, *J Am Dent Assoc* 120:177, 1990.

Xu HH: Whisker-reinforced heat-cured dental resin composites: effects of filler level and heat-cure temperature and time, *J Dent Res* 79:1392, 2000.

Nanocomposites

Curtis AR, Palin WM, Fleming GJ, et al: The mechanical properties of nanofilled resin-based composites: the impact of dry and wet cyclic pre-loading on bi-axial flexural strength, *Dent Mater* 25:188–197, 2009.

Ernst CP, Brandenbusch M, Meyer G, et al: Two-year clinical performance of a nanofiller vs a fine-particle hybrid resin composite, *Clin Oral Investig* 10:1125–1191, 2006.

Endo T, Finger WJ, Kanehira M, et al: Surface texture and roughness of polished nanofill and nanohybrid resin composites, *Dent Mater J* 29:213–223, 2010.

Farah JW, Powers JM: Composite update, *Dent Advis* 26(8):1, 2009.

Mahmoud SH, El-Embaby AE, Abdallah AM, Hamama HH: "Two-year clinical evaluation of ormocer, nanohybrid and nanofilled composite restorative systems in posterior teeth", *Adhes Dent* 19(4): 315–322, 2008.

Mitra SB, Wu D, Holmes BN: An application of nanotechnology in advanced dental materials, *J Am Dent Assoc* 134:1382–1390, 2003.

Palaniappan S, Peumans M, Van Meerbeek B, Lambrechts P: "Clinical and in-vitro evaluation of posterior composite Wear: Five-year RCT", *J Dent Res* 87, 2008:Special issue B, Abstract 0240.

Palaniappan S, Bharadwaj D, Mattar DL, et al: Three-year randomized clinical trial to evaluate the clinical performance and wear of a nanocomposite versus a hybrid composite, *Dent Mater* 25:1302–1314, 2009.

Senawongse P, Pongpreuksa P: Surface roughness of nanofill and nanohybrid resin composites after polishing and brushing, *J Esthet Restor Dent* 19:265–273, 2007.

Ure D, Harris J: Nanotechnology in dentistry: reduction to practice, *Dent Update* 30:10–15, 2003.

Yamazaki PC, Bedran-Russo AK, Pereira PN, Wsift EJ Jr: Microleakage evaluation of a new low-shrinkage composite restorative material, *Oper Dent* 31:670–676, 2006.

Yap SH, Yap AU, Teo CK, Ng JJ: Polish retention of new aesthetic restorative materials over time, *Singapore Dent J* 26:39–43, 2004.

Yazici AR, Celik C, Ozgunaltay G, Dayanagac B: The effect of different light-curing units on the clinical performance of nanofilled composite resin restorations in noncarious cervical lesions: 3-year follow-up, *J Adhes Dent* 12:231–236, 2010.

Low-Shrink Composites

Ilie N, Jelen E, Clementino-Ludeemann T, Hickel R: Low-shrinkage composite for dental application, *Dent Mater J* 26:149–155, 2007.

Lien W, Vandewalle KS: Physical preperties of a new silorane-based restorative system, *Dent Mater* 26:337–344, 2010.

Mozner N, Salz U: Recent Developments of New Components for Dental Adhesives and Composites, *Macromol Mater Eng* 292:245–271, 2007.

Schmidt M, Kirkevang LL, Horsted-Bindslev P, Poulsen S: Marginal adaptation of a low-shrink silorane-based composite: 1-year randomized clinical trial, *Clin Oral Investig* 15(2):291–295, 2011.

Weinmann W, Thalacker C, Guggenberger R: Siloranes in dental composites, *Dent Mater* 21:68–74, 2005.

Yamazaki PC, Bedran-Russo AK, Periera PN, Swift EJ Jr: Microleakage evaluation of a new low-shrinkage composite restorative material, *Oper Dent* 31:670–676, 2006.

Glass Ionomers and Resin-Modified Glass Ionomers

Billington RW, Williams JA, Pearson GJ: Ion processes in glass ionomer cements, *J Dent* 34:544–555, 2006.

Bui HT, Falsafi A, Mitra S: Fluoride release of a new nanoionomer restorative material, *J Dent Res* 87(Spec Iss A), 2008:[Abst. No 987].

Burke FJT, Wilson NH: Glass-ionomer restorations in stress bearing and difficult to access cavities. In Davidson CL, Mjor IA, editors: *Advances in Glass Ionomer Cements*, Illinois, USA, 1999, Quintessence, pp 253–268.

Croll TP, Nicholson JW: Glass-ionomer cements: history and current status, *Inside Dentistry* 4:76–84, 2008.

Croll TP, Bar-Zion Y, Segura A, Donly KJ: Clinical performance and caries inhibition of resin-modified glass ionomer restorations in primary teeth. A retrospective evaluation, *J Amer Dent Assoc* 132:1110–1116, 2001.

Croll TP, Berg JH: Resin-modifed glass-ionomer restoration of primary molars with proximating class II caries lesions, *Compend Contin Educ Dent* 28:372–376, 2007.

Croll TP, Berg JH: Nano-ionomer restorative cement: observations after 2 years of use, *Inside Dentistry* 5:60–67, 2009.

Croll TP, Cavanaugh RR: Tissue-specific, direct application class II tooth repair: a case report, *Compend Contin Educ Dent* 30:2–6, 2009.

Donly KJ, Segura A, Kanellis M, Erickson RC: Clinical performance and caries inhibition of resin-modified glass ionomer cement and amalgam restorations, *J Amer Dent Assoc* 13:1459–1466, 1999.

Farah JW, Powers JM, editors: Fluoride-releasing restorative materials, *Dent Advis* 15:2, 1998.

Wilson AD, McLean JW: *Glass-ionomer cements*, London, 1988, Quintessence.

Forsten L: Fluoride release and uptake by glass ionomers and related materials and its effect, *Biomaterials* 19:503–508, 1998.

Haveman CW, Summit JB, Burgess JO, Carlson K: Three restorative materials and topical fluoride gel used in xerostomic patients: a clinical comparison, *J Am Dent Assoc* 134:177–184, 2003.

McComb D, Erickson RL, Maxymiw WG, Wood RE: A clinical comparison of glass ionomer, resin-modofied glass ionomer and resin composite restorations in the treatment of cervical caries in xerostomic head and neck cancer patients, *Oper Dent* 27:430–437, 2002.

Mickenautsch S, Yengopal V, Banerjee A: Pulp response to resin-modified glass ionomer and calcium hydroxide cements in deep cavities: a quantitative systematic review, *Dent Mater* 26:761–770, 2010.

Mitra SB, Curing reactions of glass ionomer materials, Glass Ionomers: *The Next Generation (Proceedingsof the 2nd International Conference on Glass Ionomers)*, Hunt PR ed., Philadelphia, USA, 1994, pp 13–22.

Mitra SB, Kedrowski BL: Long-term mechanical properties of glass ionomers, *Dent Mater* 10:78–82, 1994.

Mitra S: Glass ionomers and related filling materials. In Dhuru VB, editor: *Contemporary Dental Materials*, New Delhi, India, 2004, Oxford, pp 66–80.

Mitra S, Falsafi A, Oxman J, Ton T: Fluoride release of nanoionomer and compomer materials with adhesive coatings, *J Dent Res* 87(Spec Issue B):243, 2008.

Mitra SB, Lee C-Y, Bui HT, et al: Long-term adhesion and mechanism of bonding of a paste-liquid resin-modified glass-ionomer, *Dent Mater* 25:459–466, 2009.

Mount GJ: Description of glass ionomers. In *An atlas of glass ionomer cements a clinician's guide*, ed 3, London, UK, 2002, Martin Dunitz Ltd, pp 1-42.

Mount GJ, Tyas MJ, Ferracane JI, et al: A revised classification for direct tooth-colored restorative materials, *Quintessence Int* 40:691–697, 2009.

Peumans M, Kanumilli P, De Munck J, van Landuyt K, Lambrechts P, Van Meerbeek B: Clinical effectiveness of contemporary adhesives: a systematic review of current clinical trials, *Dent Mater* 21:864–881, 2005.

Ruiz JL, Mitra S: Using cavity liners with direct posterior composite restorations, *Compend Contin Educ Dent* 27:347–351, 2006.

Tantbirojn D, Rusin RP, Mitra SB: Inhibition of dentin demineralization adjacent to a glass ionomer/composite sandwich restoration, *Quintessence Int* 40:287–294, 2009.

Van Meerbeek B, Peumans M, Poitevin A, et al: Relationship between bond-strength test and clinical outcomes, *Dent Mater* 26:100–121, 2010.

Xie D, Brantley WA, Culbertson BM, Wang G: Mechanical properties and microstructure of glass-ionomer cements, *Dent Mater* 16:129–138, 2000.

Xu X, Burgess JO: Compressive strength, fluoride release and recharge of fluoride-releasing materials, *Biomaterials* 24:2451–2461, 2003.

Compomers

Cattani-Lorente MA, Dupuis V, Moya F, et al: Comparative study of the physical properties of a polyacid-modified composite resin and a resin-modified glass ionomer cement, *Dent Mater* 15:21, 1999.

Farah JW, Powers JM: Compomers, *Dent Advis* 15(8):1, 1998.

Nicholson JW: Polyacid-modified composite resins ("compomers") and their use in clinical dentistry, *Dent Mater* 23:615–622, 2007.

Light-Curing Units

Albers HF: Resin polymerization, *Adept Report* 6:1, 2000.

Farah JW, Powers JM: Update on LED curing lights, *Dent Advis* 26(9):1, 2009.

Ferracane JL, Ferracane LL, Musanje L: Effect of light activation method on flexural properties of dental composites, *Am J Dent* 16:318, 2003.

Harrington E, Wilson HJ: Determination of radiation energy emitted by light activation, *J Oral Rehabil* 22:377, 1995.

Jandt KD, Mills RW, Blackwell GB, et al: Depth of cure and compressive strength of dental composites cured with blue light emitting diodes (LEDs), *Dent Mater* 16:41, 2000.

Kirkpatrick SJ: A primer on radiometry, *Dent Mater* 21:21, 2005.

Mills RW, Jandt KD, Ashworth SH: Dental composite depth of cure with halogen and blue light emitting diode technology, *Br Dent J* 186:388, 1999.

Peutzfeldt A, Sahafi A, Asmussen E: Characterization of resin composites polymerized with plasma arc curing units, *Dent Mater* 16:330, 2000.

Price RB, Felix CA, Andreou P: Effects of resin composite composition and irradiation distance on the performance of curing lights, *Biomaterials* 25:4465, 2004.

Price RB, Ehrnford L, Andreou P, et al: Comparison of quartz-tungsten-halogen, light-emitting diode, and plasma arc curing lights, *J Adhes Dent* 5:193, 2003.

Sakaguchi RL, Berge HX: Reduced light energy density decreases postgel contraction while maintaining degree of conversion in composites, *J Dent* 26:695, 1998.

Sakaguchi RL, Wiltbank BD, Murchison CF: Contraction force rate of polymer composites is linearly correlated with irradiance, *Dent Mater* 20:402, 2004.

Satrom KD, Morris MA, Crigger LP: Potential retinal hazards of visible light photopolymerization units, *J Dent Res* 66:731, 1987.

Stahl F, Ashworth SH, Jandt KD, et al: Light emitting diodes (LED) polymerisation of dental composites: flexural properties and polymerisation potential, *Biomaterials* 21:1379, 2000.

Watts DC: Al Hindi A: Intrinsic "soft-start" polymerisation shrinkage-kinetics in an acrylic-based resin-composite, *Dent Mater* 15:39, 1999.

Wataha JC, Lockwood PE, Lewis JB, et al: Biological effects of blue light from dental curing units, *Dent Mater* 20:150, 2004.

Provisional Materials

Chung K, Lin T, Wang F: Flexural strength of a provisional resin material with fibre addition, *J Oral Rehabil* 25:214, 1998.

Doray PG, Eldiwany MS, Powers JM: Effect of resin surface sealers on improvement of stain resistance for a composite provisional material, *J Esthet Restor Dent* 15:244, 2003.

Doray PG, Li D, Powers JM: Color stability of provisional restorative materials after accelerated aging, *J Prosthodont* 10:212, 2001.

Farah JW, Powers JM: Provisional composites and liquid polishes, *Dent Advis* 27(4):1, 2010.

Grajower R, Shaharbani S, Kaufman E: Temperature rise in pulp chamber during fabrication of temporary self-curing resin crowns, *J Prosthet Dent* 41:535, 1979.

Ireland MF, Dixon DL, Breeding LC, et al: In vitro mechanical property comparison of four resins used for fabrication of provisional fixed restorations, *J Prosthet Dent* 80:158, 1998.

Lepe X, Bales DJ, Johnson GH: Retention of provisional crowns fabricated from two materials with the use of four temporary cements, *J Prosthet Dent* 81:469, 1999.

Lui JL: Hypersensitivity to a temporary crown and bridge material, *J Dent* 7:22, 1979.

Robinson FB, Hovijitra S: Marginal fit of direct temporary crowns, *J Prosthet Dent* 47:390, 1982.

Restorative Materials—Metals

AMALGAM

An amalgam is an alloy of mercury and one or more other metals. Dental amalgam is produced by mixing liquid mercury with solid particles of an alloy containing predominantly silver, tin, and copper. Zinc and palladium may also be present in small amounts. This combination of solid metals is known as *amalgam alloy*. It is important to differentiate between dental amalgam and the amalgam alloy that is commercially produced and marketed as small filings, spheroid particles, or a combination of these, suitable for mixing with liquid mercury to produce the dental amalgam.

Once amalgam alloy is freshly mixed with liquid mercury, it has the plasticity that permits it to be conveniently packed or condensed into a prepared tooth cavity. After condensing, the dental amalgam is carved to generate the required anatomical features and then hardens with time. Amalgam is used most commonly for direct, permanent, posterior restorations and for large foundation restorations, or cores, which are precursors to placing crowns. Dental amalgam restorations are reasonably easy to insert, are not overly technique sensitive, maintain anatomical form, have reasonably adequate resistance to fracture, prevent marginal leakage after a period of time in the mouth, can be used in stress-bearing areas, and have a relatively long service life.

The principal disadvantage of dental amalgam is that its silver color does not match tooth structure. In addition, amalgam restorations are somewhat brittle, are subject to corrosion and galvanic action, may demonstrate a degree of breakdown at the margins of tooth and amalgam, and do not help retain weakened tooth structure. Finally, there are regulatory concerns about amalgam being disposed of in the wastewater. Despite these shortcomings, dental amalgam is a highly successful restorative material and is cost effective. However, alternatives such as cast gold, ceramics, and resin composite restorative materials are now competitive in terms of frequency of use. Many argue, however, that the use of amalgam must be strongly supported given its large public health benefit in the United States and many other countries.

In this chapter, the composition and morphology of the different dental amalgams are presented, followed by a discussion of low- and high-copper amalgams, the chemical reactions that occur during amalgamation, and the resultant microstructures. Various physical and mechanical properties are covered in the next section, as well as factors related to the manipulation of amalgam.

Dental Amalgam Alloys

History

Amalgam has been used for many years as a dental restorative material. Prior to 1900 many compositions were tried but few were successful when placed in the oral environment. Around 1900 scientific testing was applied to the problem, which led to a so-called *balanced composition* of silver and tin in the form of Ag_3Sn with small amounts of copper and occasionally zinc added. Amalgam restorations made from this balanced formula were reasonably successful, and it was not uncommon to see 10- to 20-year-old amalgam restorations still in service. However, one disadvantage that remained was a propensity for fracture at the edge or margin of the amalgam restoration next to tooth structure, commonly called *marginal fracture*. Such fractures were considered to be exacerbated by the presence of the tin-mercury phase ($Sn_{7-8}Hg$), which results when Ag_3Sn reacts with mercury. This phase has been shown to be the weakest phase in the hardened amalgam and is subject to corrosive breakdown, particularly at the restoration/tooth margin where a most active form of corrosion known as *crevice corrosion* is likely to occur. Although a significant amount of *marginal fracture* was exhibited among the commercial alloys at the time, this type of fracture was accepted as an indigenous characteristic of dental amalgam restorations.

In 1962 a new amalgam alloy, called *Dispersalloy*, was introduced that consisted of the addition of a spherical silver-copper eutectic particle to the traditional lathe-cut Ag_3Sn particle in a ratio of 1:2. The mixing of these two types of particles led to the term *admix alloy*. Although the rationale for this admix alloy was to strengthen the amalgam, an unanticipated but highly significant benefit proved to be the elimination of the tin-mercury phase ($Sn_{7-8}Hg$). This elimination occurred because the increased copper in the silver-copper eutectic reacted preferentially with tin so that $Sn_{7-8}Hg$ could not form. Early results from the clinical use of this new amalgam showed what appeared to be improved marginal integrity. However, it took carefully designed clinical studies to show, unequivocally, that the extent of marginal fracture was either eliminated or reduced significantly in restorations made from Dispersalloy.

About 10 years later, another alloy, called *Tytin*, was introduced using the same principle of adding increased copper to eliminate the tin-mercury phase. However, in this case, this was done by combining a significant amount of Cu_3Sn together with Ag_3Sn in the form of a unicompositional spherical particle.

Both of these relatively new alloys raised the copper content from 5%, present in the older balanced composition alloy, to about 13% for the newer alloys. Thus, the term *low-copper alloys* refers to alloys that do not contain sufficient copper to prevent the formation of $Sn_{7-8}Hg$, whereas the term *high-copper alloys* refers to alloys that do have sufficient copper to prevent the formation of $Sn_{7-8}Hg$.

In Figure 10-1, two restorations are shown, after 3 years of clinical service, that were placed at the same time in the same patient. The restoration on the left was made from a low-copper alloy, whereas the restoration on the right was made from a high-copper alloy. The higher extent of marginal fracture for the low-copper alloy is clearly shown.

Notice also that in the low-copper restoration, deep indentations were produced by occlusal forces acting through the cusps of opposing teeth that is not shown in the high-copper restoration. This observation suggests that the viscoelastic behavior or creep of dental amalgam has clinical implications.

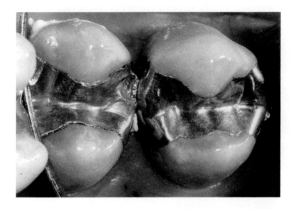

FIGURE 10.1 **Amalgam restorations from a low-copper lathe cut alloy (left) and a high-copper admix alloy (right) after 3 years of clinical service.** *(Courtesy of D.B. Mahler, OHSU School of Dentistry, Portland, Oregon.)*

Composition and Morphology

ANSI/ADA (American National Standards Institute/American Dental Association) specification No. 1 (ISO 24234) for amalgam alloy includes a requirement for composition. This specification does not state precisely what the composition of alloys shall be; rather, it permits some variation in composition. Specifically, it states that the chemical composition shall consist primarily of silver, tin, and copper. Indium, palladium, platinum, zinc, or mercury may also be included in lesser amounts.

The ANSI/ADA specification also includes a notation about the presence of zinc in amalgam alloys, with more than 0.01% zinc classified as zinc containing and those with less than 0.01% as nonzinc alloys. Zinc has been included in amalgam alloys as an aid in manufacturing; it helps produce clean, sound castings of the ingots used for producing cut-particle alloys. However, the presence of zinc has been shown to produce a delayed expansion if water-based fluids such as blood or saliva are present within the amalgam during condensation. Therefore, practitioners are informed of this possible problem. Possible remedies are the use of zinc-free alloys and careful attention given to rubber dam isolation of the prepared tooth. The presence of contamination within the amalgam must be avoided because it can degrade the integrity of the restoration. The approximate composition of commercial amalgam alloys are shown in Table 10-1.

The alloys are broadly classified as low-copper (5% or less copper) and high-copper alloys (13% to 30% copper). Particles are irregularly shaped microspheres of various sizes or a combination of the two. Scanning electron micrographs of the particles are shown in Figure 10-2. The low-copper alloys have either irregular or spherical particles. Both morphologic types contain silver and tin in a ratio approximating the intermetallic compound Ag_3Sn.

TABLE 10.1 Approximate Composition of Low- and High-Copper Amalgam Alloys

Alloy	Particle Shape	Element (wt%)					
		Ag	Sn	Cu	Zn	In	Pd
Low copper	Irregular or spherical	63-70	26-28	2-5	0-2	0	0
High copper							
Admixed regular	Irregular	40-70	26-30	2-30	0-2	0	0
	Spherical	40-65	0-30	20-40	0-1	0	0-1
Admixed unicomposition	Irregular	52-53	17-18	29-30	0	0	0.3
	Spherical	52-53	17-18	29-30	0	0	0.3
Unicompositional	Spherical	40-60	22-30	13-30	0	0-5	0-1

Ag, *Silver;* Cu, *copper;* In, *indium;* Pd, *palladium;* Sn, *tin;* Zn, *zinc.*

High-copper alloys contain either spherical particles of the same composition (unicompositional) or a mixture of irregular and spherical particles of different or the same composition (admixed).

When the particles have different compositions, the admixed alloys are made by mixing particles of silver and tin with particles of silver and copper. The silver-tin particle is usually irregular in shape, whereas the silver-copper particle is usually spherical. The composition of the silver-tin particles in most commercial alloys is the same as that of the low-copper alloys. Different manufacturers, however, have somewhat different compositions for the silver-copper particle. The compositional ranges of the spherical silver-copper particles are shown in Table 10-1. The admixed regular alloy contains 33% to 60% spherical particles that have a composition close to the eutectic composition of Ag_3Cu_2 (see Figure 10-2); the balance is irregular particles.

Like the admixed alloy, the unicompositional alloys have higher copper contents than the traditional lathe-cut or spherical low-copper alloys, but all the particles are spherical, as seen in Figure 10-2. The silver content of the unicompositional alloys varies from 40% to 60%, copper content varies from 13% to 30%, and tin content varies only slightly.

A high-copper admixed alloy is also available, in which both spherical and irregular particles have the same composition and the copper content is between 29% and 30%. High-copper alloys are less commonly supplied as unicompositional and irregular particles. The lathe-cut, high-copper alloys contain more than 23% copper.

It is estimated that more than 90% of the dental amalgams currently placed are high-copper alloys. Of the high-copper alloys, admixed alloys are used more often than spherical types, and fewer irregularly shaped or lathe-cut types are selected. A high-copper alloy is selected to obtain a restoration with high early strength, low creep, good corrosion resistance, and good resistance to marginal fracture.

In general, alloy composition—particle size, shape, and distribution—and heat treatment control the characteristic properties of the amalgam.

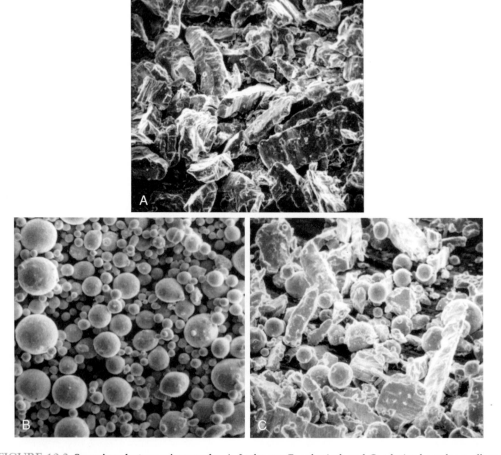

FIGURE 10.2 **Scanning electron micrographs. A**, Lathe-cut; **B**, spherical; and **C**, admixed amalgam alloys.

Production

IRREGULAR PARTICLES

To produce lathe-cut alloys, the metal ingredients are heated and protected from oxidation until melted, then poured into a mold to form an ingot. The ingot is cooled relatively slowly, leading to the formation of mainly Ag_3Sn (γ) and some Cu_3Sn (ε), Cu_6Sn_5 (η'), and Ag_4Sn (β). After the ingot is completely cooled, it is heated for various periods of time (often 6 to 8 hours) at 400° C to produce a more homogeneous distribution of Ag_3Sn. The ingot is then reduced to filings by being cut on a lathe and ball milled. The particles are passed through a fine sieve and then ball milled to form the proper particle size. The particles are typically 60 to 120 μm in length, 10 to 70 μm in width, and 10 to 35 μm in thickness. Most products are labeled as fine-cut. The particle size and shape of lathe-cut amalgam alloys are shown in Figure 10-2, A.

In general, freshly cut alloys amalgamate and set more promptly than aged particles, but some aging of the alloy is desirable to improve the shelf life of the product. The aging is related to relief of stress in the particles produced during the cutting of the ingot. The alloy particles are aged by subjecting them to a controlled temperature of 60° to 100° C for 1 to 6 hours. Irregularly shaped high-copper particles are made by spraying the molten alloy into water under high pressure.

SPHERICAL PARTICLES

Spherical particles of low- or high-copper alloys are produced when all the desired elements are melted together. In the molten stage the metallic ingredients form the desired alloy. The liquid alloy is then sprayed, under high pressure of an inert gas, through a fine crack in a crucible into a large chamber. Depending on the difference in surface energy of the molten alloy and the gas used in the spraying process, the shape of the sprayed particles may be spherical or somewhat irregular, as shown in Figure 10-2, B. The diameter of the spheres varies from 2 to 43 μm.

Silver-Tin Alloy

Because two of the principal ingredients in the amalgam alloy are silver and tin, it is appropriate to consider the equilibrium phase diagram for these two metals, as shown in Figure 10-3.

The most important feature in this diagram concerning the silver-tin alloy is that when an alloy containing approximately 27% tin is slowly cooled below a temperature of 480° C, an intermetallic compound (Ag_3Sn) known also as the *gamma* (γ) *phase*

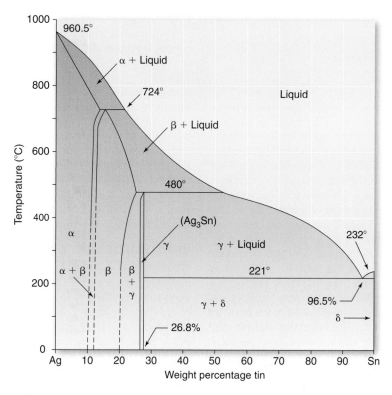

FIGURE 10.3 **Equilibrium phase diagram for silver and tin.** *Ag,* Silver; *Sn,* tin. *(Modified from Murphy AJ, Inst. Metals. J. 35, 107, 1926.)*

is produced. This Ag_3Sn compound is an essential ingredient in the silver amalgam alloy and combines with mercury to produce a dental amalgam of desired mechanical properties and handling characteristics. This silver-tin compound is formed over only a narrow composition range. The silver content for such an alloy would be approximately 73%. Practically, the tin content is held between 26% and 30%, and the remainder of the alloy consists of copper, and in some cases, zinc. If the concentration of tin is less than 26%, the beta (β) phase, which is a solid solution of silver and tin, forms. The replacement of silver by an equal amount of copper produces a copper-tin compound (Cu_3Sn).

In general, larger (greater than 30%) or smaller (less than 26%) quantities of tin in the alloy are detrimental to the final properties of the amalgam. The reason for this unfavorable shift in properties is generally considered to be a reduction in the amount of Ag_3Sn as the percentage of tin is altered beyond the indicated limits. This is the basis for the rather narrow limits of the alloy compositions of current products with acceptable properties.

Silver-tin amalgam alloys compounded to produce largely Ag_3Sn react favorably with mercury to produce only slight dimensional setting changes when properly manipulated. In addition, setting time is shortened by increasing silver content, and mechanical properties are superior when an alloy of Ag_3Sn is used rather than one with higher tin content.

Amalgamation Processes
Low-Copper Alloys

All dental amalgam alloys, including both low- and high-copper types, have Ag_3Sn as their primary component, which reacts with mercury to form Ag_2Hg_3, the major matrix phase of the set amalgam. Because of this basic similarity, an initial discussion of the amalgamation of the low-copper alloys is a significant preliminary to that of the high-copper alloys.

The amalgam alloy is intimately mixed with liquid mercury to wet the surface of the particles so that the reaction between liquid mercury and alloy can proceed at a reasonable rate. This mixing is called *trituration*, which has the dual function of mixing the ingredients and removing surface oxide layers that have formed on the alloy particles. During this process, mercury diffuses into the alloy particles and reacts with the silver and tin portions of the particles to form predominantly silver-mercury and tin-mercury compounds. The silver-mercury compound is Ag_2Hg_3 and is known as the *gamma one* (γ_1) phase, and the tin-mercury compound is $Sn_{7-8}Hg$, known as the *gamma two* (γ_2) phase. However, the silver-tin, silver-mercury, and tin-mercury phases are not pure. For example, the alloy particles usually contain small

amounts of copper in the form of Cu_3Sn and occasionally small amounts of zinc. Ag_2Hg_3 contains 1% to 2% of tin.

While crystals of the γ_1 and γ_2 phases are being formed, the amalgam is relatively soft and easily condensable and carvable. As time progresses, more crystals of γ_1 and γ_2 are formed; the amalgam becomes harder and stronger and is no longer condensable or carvable. The lapse of time between the end of the trituration and when the amalgam hardens and is no longer workable is called *working time*.

The amount of liquid mercury used to amalgamate the alloy particles is not sufficient to react with the particles completely. Therefore, the set mass of amalgam contains about 27% unreacted particles. A simplified reaction of a low-copper amalgam alloy with mercury can be summarized in the following manner:

$$\gamma \, (Ag_3Sn) + Hg \rightarrow$$
$$\gamma_1 \, (Ag_2Hg_3) + \gamma_2 \, (Sn_{7-8}Hg) + \text{unreacted } \gamma \, (Ag_3Sn)$$

The dominant phase in a well-condensed, low-copper dental amalgam is the Ag_2Hg_3 (γ_1) phase, which is about 54% to 56% by volume. The percentages of the γ and γ_2 phases are 27% to 35% and 11% to 13%, respectively. The Ag_2Hg_3 phase serves as the matrix phase surrounding the unreacted alloy particles, whereas the $Sn_{7-8}Hg$ (γ_2) phase pervades the structure in a continuous skeleton type form.

High-Copper Alloys

The main difference between the low- and high-copper amalgam alloys is not merely the percentage of copper but also the effect that the higher copper content has on the amalgam reaction. The higher copper content in these alloys is supplied by either the silver-copper eutectic or the Cu_3Sn (ϵ) phase. This proper amount of copper results in the elimination of the $Sn_{7-8}Hg$ (γ_2) phase, which is the weakest phase and most susceptible to corrosion in a low-copper amalgam. Therefore, restorations using amalgam made with sufficient copper tend to have superior physical and mechanical properties and a longer period of clinical serviceability than restorations made from the low-copper amalgams.

REACTION OF MERCURY IN AN ADMIXED HIGH-COPPER AMALGAM ALLOY

In high-copper admix alloys, additional copper is supplied by adding spherical particles of the silver-copper eutectic alloy to a low-copper lathe-cut alloy in a ratio of 1:2. The solubility of silver, tin, and copper in mercury differs considerably. One mg of copper, 10 mg of silver, and 170 mg of tin can dissolve in mercury, all at the same temperature. Therefore, mercury dissolves mainly the silver and tin in Ag_3Sn, whereas very little of the silver-copper eutectic particles are dissolved. During trituration, the dissolved silver from the silver-tin particles reacts, as in low-copper alloys, to form the γ_1 phase while the dissolved tin migrates to the outside of the silver-copper particles to form Cu_6Sn_5, the eta prime (η') phase of the copper-tin system. Thus the tin is tied up by sufficient copper to prevent the formation of γ_2. The amalgamation reaction may be simplified as follows

$$\gamma(Ag_3Sn) + Ag\text{-}Cu \text{ (eutectic)} + Hg \rightarrow$$
$$\gamma_1(Ag_2Hg_3) + \eta'(Cu_6Sn_5) + \text{unreacted } \gamma (Ag_3Sn)$$
$$+ \text{unreacted Ag-Cu (eutectic)}$$

REACTION OF MERCURY IN A UNICOMPOSITIONAL ALLOY

In high-copper unicompositional alloys, the alloy particles contain both $Ag_3Sn(\gamma)$ and $Cu_3Sn(\varepsilon)$, similar to the low-copper lathe-cut alloys, but the amount of the $Cu_3Sn(\varepsilon)$ phase is much greater to accommodate additional copper. These alloys are usually spherical in nature, and because spherical particles cool very rapidly, the Cu_3Sn phase is finely dispersed throughout the Ag_3Sn phase. When liquid mercury is mixed with these alloys, it diffuses into the surface of these particles and Ag_2Hg_3 as well as Cu_6Sn_5 are formed. The reaction occurs in a ring around the spherical particles and consists of γ_1 and η' with no remaining γ or ε in this ring. The reaction can be summarized as follows:

$$[\gamma(Ag_3Sn) + \varepsilon(Cu_3Sn)] + Hg \rightarrow$$
$$\gamma_1 (Ag_3Hg_3) \text{ and } \eta'(Cu_6Sn_5)$$
$$+ \text{unreacted } [\gamma (Ag_3Sn) + \varepsilon (Cu_3Sn)]$$

Thus the reaction of mercury with either the high-copper admixed or the unicompositional alloys results in a final reaction with Cu_6Sn_5 (η') being produced rather than $Sn_{7-8}Hg$ (γ_2).

Microstructure of Amalgam

In dental applications the amount of liquid mercury used to amalgamate with the alloy particles is less than that required to complete the reaction. Thus the set amalgam mass consists of unreacted particles surrounded by a matrix of the reaction products. The reaction is principally a surface reaction, and the matrix bonds the unreacted particles together. The initial diffusion and reaction of mercury and alloy are relatively rapid, and the mass changes rapidly from a plastic consistency to a hard mass. Completion of the reaction may take several days to several weeks, which is reflected by the change in mechanical properties over this time.

The microstructures of the set amalgams of the low-copper, lathe-cut, the high-copper admix, and the high-copper, unicompositional types are shown in Figure 10-4. These photographs were made by superimposing microprobe x-ray scans of the elements through colored filters; blue for silver, red for copper, and green for tin. The blue/black matrix phase

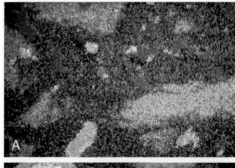

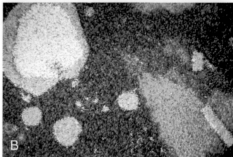

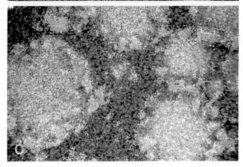

FIGURE 10.4 Microstructures of the set amalgams of the (A) low-copper, lathe-cut, (B) the high-copper, admix and (C) the high-copper, unicompositional types. These photographs were made by superimposing microprobe X-ray scans of the elements through colored filters; blue for silver, red for copper, and green for tin. The blue/black matrix phase is A_2Hg_3 (γ_1) for all amalgams. The green colored $Sn_{7-8}Hg$ (γ_2) phase is only present in the low-copper alloy **A**. The tangerine colored Cu_6Sn_5 (η') phase is minimal in alloy **A** but substantial in alloys **B** and **C**. In alloy **B**, the source of the increased copper is in the spherical silver-copper eutectic phase where the η' surrounds this spherical particle. In alloy **C**, the source of the increased copper is in the additional Cu_3Sn added to the spherical Ag_3Sn particle and Cu_6Sn_5 (η') phases are present around this spherical particle. *(Courtesy of Mahler DB, OHSU School of Dentistry, Portland, Oregon.)*

is A_2Hg_3 (γ_1) for all amalgams. The green colored $Sn_{7-8}Hg$ (γ_2) phase is only present in the low-copper alloy *A*. The tangerine colored Cu_6Sn_5 (η') phase is minimal in alloy *A* but substantial in alloys *B* and *C*. In alloy *B*, the source of the increased copper is in the spherical silver-copper eutectic phase where the η' surrounds this spherical particle. In alloy *C*, the source of the increased copper is in the additional Cu_3Sn added to the spherical Ag_3Sn particle, and the Cu_6Sn_5 (η') phase is present around this spherical particle.

STRENGTH OF VARIOUS PHASES

The relative strengths of the different amalgam phases are important. By studying the initiation and propagation of a crack in a set amalgam, the relative strength of the different phases can be observed. Figure 10-5 shows the propagation of a crack in a dental amalgam specimen. It is possible to view the crack initiation and propagation of an amalgam specimen under a conventional metallographic microscope with a strain viewer. The propagation of the crack can be halted and the specimen etched to identify the various phases. Results of such studies have led to the following ranking of the different phases of a set low-copper amalgam from strongest to weakest: Ag_3Sn (γ), the silver-mercury phase (γ_1), the tin-mercury phase (γ_2), and the voids.

Silver-mercury and tin-mercury act as a matrix to hold the unreacted amalgam alloy together. When relatively smaller amounts of silver-mercury and tin-mercury phases form, up to a certain minimum required for bonding the unreacted particles, a set amalgam is stronger. When a higher percentage of mercury is left in the final mass, it reacts with more of the amalgam alloy, producing larger amounts of silver-mercury and tin-mercury phases and leaving relatively smaller amounts of unreacted particles. The result is a weaker mass. In high-copper amalgams, there is preferential crack propagation through the γ_1 phase and around copper-containing particles.

Physical and Mechanical Properties

ANSI/ADA Specification for Amalgam Alloy

ANSI/ADA specification No. 1 (ISO 24234) for amalgam alloy contains requirements that help control the qualities of dental amalgam. The specification lists three physical properties as a measure of amalgam quality: compressive strength, creep, and dimensional change. The minimum allowable compressive strength is 80 MPa for 1 hour after setting and 300 MPa for 24 hours after setting, the maximum allowable creep is 1%, and the dimensional change between 5 minutes and 24 hours must fall within the range of −15 to +20 μm/cm. The physical properties for several amalgams are shown in Table 10-2.

Mercury in Mix

In general, irregular particles have higher surface areas than spherical particles and, therefore, require more mercury to wet their surfaces. In turn, higher percentages of mercury in the mix will result in higher mercury contents and lower strengths of the hardened amalgams. This effect is clearly shown in Table 10-2.

Compressive Strength

Resistance to compression forces is an important strength characteristic of amalgam. Because amalgam is strongest in compression and much weaker in tension and shear, the prepared cavity design should maximize compressive stresses in service and minimize tension or shear stresses. When subjected to a rapid application of stress either in tension or in compression, a dental amalgam does not exhibit significant deformation or elongation and, as a result, functions as a brittle material. Therefore, a sudden application of excessive force to amalgam may lead to fracture of the amalgam restoration.

The early compressive strengths after 1 hour of setting for several low- and high-copper alloys are listed in Table 10-2. The high-copper unicompositional materials have the highest early compressive strengths of more than 250 MPa. The compressive strength at 1 hour is lowest for the low-copper lathe-cut alloy (45 MPa). These data indicate that only some of the older lathe-cut alloys would meet the

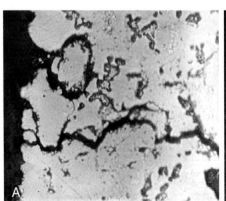 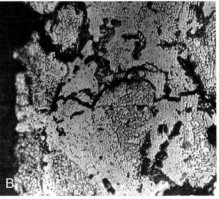

FIGURE 10.5 **Propagation of a crack in a dental amalgam. A,** Unetched. **B,** After etching. *(From Asgar K, Sutfin L: J. Dent. Res. 44,985, 1965.)*

requirement for compressive strength at the 1-hour limit of ANSI/ADA specification No. 1. High values for early compressive strength are an advantage for an amalgam, because they reduce the possibility of fracture by the application of prematurely high occlusal forces by the patient before the final strength is reached. The compressive strengths at 7 days are again highest for the high-copper unicompositional alloys, with only modest differences in the other alloys.

Tensile Strength

The tensile strengths of various amalgams after 15 minutes and 7 days are also listed in Table 10-2. The tensile strengths at 7 days for both non-γ_2 and γ_2-containing alloys are about the same. The tensile strengths are only a fraction of their compressive strengths; therefore, cavity designs should be constructed to reduce tensile stresses resulting from biting forces. The tensile strengths at 15 minutes for the high-copper unicompositional alloys are significantly higher than for the other alloys.

Flexural Strength

Flexural strength (also called *transverse strength*) is determined by the application of load to cause bending in a rectangular specimen of amalgam. In this test, the top layer of the specimen is under compressive stress while the bottom layer is under tensile stress. The results of this test correlate to tensile strength and the test is much easier to conduct.

Elastic Modulus

When the elastic modulus is determined for dental amalgam, values in the range of 40 to 60 GPa are obtained. As a comparison, the elastic modulus of resin composites is only 5 to 20 GPa, which can be of significance when considering amalgam versus composites in certain clinical applications. High-copper alloys tend to be stiffer that low-copper alloys.

Creep

Creep is the time-dependent inelastic deformation of materials that are used at temperatures that are close to their melting points. Expressed in absolute temperatures, the melting point of the major matrix phase (γ_1) in dental amalgam is 400 K, whereas it is used at the mouth temperature of 310 K for a ratio of 0.8. In metals, ratios that exceed 0.5 are considered to be a forerunner for examining creep behavior. Therefore, dental amalgam is an appropriate candidate for this examination.

A number of amalgam alloys, which included the newly introduced high-copper alloy Dispersalloy, were subjected to creep testing. The results were surprising in that the creep of Dispersalloy was an order of magnitude lower than the other alloys tested, which were all traditional low-copper alloys.

TABLE 10-2 Mercury in Mix, Compressive Strength, Tensile Strength, Creep and Dimensional Change

| | Mercury In Mix (%) | Compressive Strength (MPa) | | Tensile Strength (MPa) | | Creep (%) | Dimensional Change (mm/cm) |
		1 hr	7 days	15 min	7 days		
LOW-COPPER							
Alloys							
Lathe-cut							
Caulk 20th Cent	53.7	45	302	3.2	51	6.3	-19.7
Spherical							
Caulk Spherical	46.2	141	366	4.7	55	1.5	-10.6
HIGH-COPPER							
Alloys							
Admixed							
Dispersalloy	50.0	118	387	3.8	43	0.45	-1.9
Unicompositional							
Sybraloy	46.0	252	455	8.5	49	0.05	-8.8
Tytin	43.0	292	516	8.1	56	0.09	-8.1

Adapted from Malhotra ML, Asgar K: J Amer Dent Assoc 96:446, 1978.

Dispersalloy was then subjected to electron microprobe analysis, and the next surprising event was the observation that there was no $Sn_{7-8}Hg$ (γ_2) present in the Dispersalloy amalgam. Furthermore, objective clinical studies that followed showed that clinical restorations made from Dispersalloy exhibited a significant reduction in the marginal fracture normally exhibited by the traditional low-copper amalgams. Further testing of other high-copper alloys, as they became available, verified this difference. The value of 1.0% creep was determined to be a limiting value. Amalgams exhibiting values higher that 1.0% were found to contain γ_2 whereas amalgams having creep values less than 1.0% were free of γ_2. Thus creep became a valuable test for predicting both the presence and absence of $Sn_{7-8}Hg$ (γ_2) and the clinical performance of amalgam restorations and was subsequently adopted as one of the prime tests in both the American Dental Association (ADA) and the FDI World Dental Federation (FDI) specifications.

The mechanism of creep in dental amalgam is the sliding of γ_1 grains. In the low-copper amalgams, the γ_2 phase pervades the γ_1 grain boundaries, thereby exasperating the sliding action, which gives rise to higher creep values. In the high-copper amalgams, lower creep values prevail because the γ_2 phase has been eliminated.

The creep test in the specifications is conducted by applying a compressive stress of 36 MPa on a 7-day-old cylindrical specimen in a 37° C environment. Creep is measured by the shortening of the test specimen between 1 and 4 hours of testing, and the specification sets the acceptable limit for creep of 1.0%.

However, amalgams whose creep values vary within the range of less than 1.0% do not show differences in clinical performance. For example, referring to Table 10-2, unicompositional alloys with creep values of 0.05 and 0.09 do not show superior clinical performance compared to the admix alloy with a creep value of 0.45. Therefore, physical properties are helpful in predicting clinical performance but care should be exercised in the limits of their interpretation.

The ability of creep to demonstrate the inelastic properties of dental amalgam in the clinical environment is shown to be of significance in Figure 10-1. However, the primary importance of creep is to determine the presence or absence of the tin-mercury phase (γ_2), which has the most important role of predicting the extent of marginal fracture in clinical service.

Dimensional Change

The dimensional change during the setting of amalgam is one of its most significant properties. Modern amalgams mixed with mechanical amalgamators usually have negative dimensional changes. The initial contraction after a short time (the first 20 minutes) is believed to be associated with the solution of the alloy particles in mercury. After this period, an expansion occurs that is believed to be a result of the reaction of mercury with silver and tin and the formation of the intermetallic compounds. The dimensions become nearly constant after 6 to 8 hours, and thus the values after 24 hours are final values. The only exception to this statement is the excessive delayed dimensional change resulting from contamination of a zinc-containing alloy with water-based fluids during trituration or condensation.

Dimensional change is measured by the change in length of an 8-mm cylindrical specimen between 5 minutes and 24 hours after trituration. The change in length can be determined continuously, although ANSI/ADA specification No. 1 requires only the value at 24 hours.

The dimensional changes in micrometers per centimeter for various alloys are listed in Table 10-2. The largest dimensional change of -19.7 $\mu m/cm$ occurred with the low-copper, lathe-cut alloy, and the lowest change of -1.9 $\mu m/cm$ was for the high-copper admixed alloy. All the amalgams meet the requirements of ANSI/ADA specification No. 1 of -15 to $+20$ $\mu m/cm$ but are susceptible to influence from various manipulative factors.

An additional clinical significance of dimensional change is related to the occasional occurrence of postoperative sensitivity associated with newly placed amalgam restorations. Amalgam does not adhere to tooth structure; therefore, a negative dimensional change would result in the presence of an interfacial gap between the amalgam restoration and tooth structure. When a cavity is prepared that cuts through dentin in a tooth requiring restoration, pulpal fluid in the tubules can flow outward into the interfacial gap. Changes in pressure of this fluid are considered to be one of the major causes of postoperative sensitivity. Apparently, the size of the interfacial gap is a key factor in determining whether sensitivity will occur, with larger gaps being particularly prone in this regard.

Although most alloys that pass ANSI/ADA specification No. 1 for negative dimensional changes of -15 $\mu m/cm$ or less have not been shown to have an uncommon amount of postoperative sensitivity, some of the newer high-copper amalgams consisting of only spherical particles have been reported to show a propensity for this sensitivity. The reason for this anomaly was found by in vitro microleakage studies using air pressure through the marginal gaps of simulated class I restorations. These studies showed that spherical particle alloys leaked more than lathe-cut particle alloys, even though their respective dimensional changes were not significantly different. Examination showed that the surfaces of these amalgams next to the cavity walls exhibited a relatively uneven texture for the spherical particle alloys compared to a smoother texture for the lathe-cut alloys. Thus the interfacial space filled by pulpal fluid was greater for the spherical particle alloys but was not measured by the dimensional change test. In Figure 10-6, the microleakage of a number of dental amalgams are shown where spherical particle alloys are marked with a capital S. It is clear that the presence of higher microleakage values are associated with the spherical alloys. Bars that are shaded refer to alloys in which data were available to indicate an unusual propensity for postoperative sensitivity.

The use of film-forming agents such as dentin bonding agents to seal the dentinal tubules before placement of an amalgam restoration has proven to be an effective solution to the problem of postoperative sensitivity of spherical particle amalgams.

Corrosion

In general, corrosion is the progressive destruction of a metal by chemical or electrochemical reaction with its environment. Excessive corrosion can lead to increased porosity, reduced marginal integrity, loss of strength, and the release of metallic products into the oral environment.

The following compounds have been identified on dental amalgams in patients: SnO, SnO_2, $Sn_4(OH)_6Cl_2$, Cu_2O, $CuCl_2 \cdot 3Cu(OH)_2$, $CuCl$, $CuSCN$, and $AgSCN$.

Because of their different chemical compositions, the different phases of an amalgam have different corrosion potentials. Electrochemical measurements on pure phases have shown that the Ag_2Hg_3 (γ_1) phase has the highest corrosion resistance, followed by Ag_3Sn (γ), Ag_3Cu_2, Cu_3Sn (ϵ), Cu_6Sn_5 (η'), and $Sn_{7-8}Hg$ (γ_2). However, the order of corrosion resistance assigned is true only if these phases are pure, and they are not in the pure state in dental amalgam.

The presence of small amounts of tin, silver, and copper that may dissolve in various amalgam phases has a great influence on their corrosion resistance. The γ_1 phase has a composition close to Ag_2Hg_3 with 1% to 3% of dissolved tin. The higher the tin concentration in Ag_2Hg_3 (γ_1), the lower its corrosion resistance. In general, the tin content of the γ_1 phase is higher for low-copper alloys than for high-copper alloys. The average depth of corrosion for most amalgam alloys is 100 to 500 µm, measured from the amalgam/tooth margin.

In the low-copper amalgam system, the most corrodible phase is the $Sn_{7-8}Hg$ or γ_2 phase. Although a relatively small portion (11% to 13%) of the amalgam mass consists of the γ_2 phase, in time and in the oral environment the structure of such an amalgam will contain a higher percentage of corroded phase. On the other hand, neither the γ nor the γ_1 phase is corroded as easily. Studies have shown that corrosion of the γ_2 phase occurs throughout the restoration, because it is a network structure. Corrosion results in the formation of tin oxychloride from the tin in the γ_2,

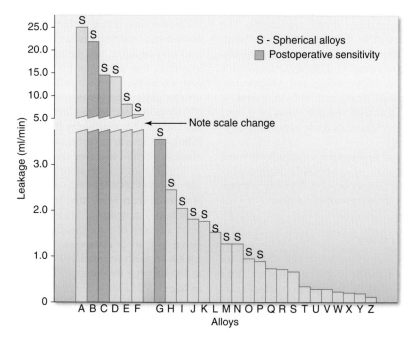

FIGURE 10.6 **In vitro microleakage of various commercial amalgams.** *(From Mahler DB, Nelson LW: J. Am. Dent. Assoc. 125, 282, 1994.)*

and also liberates mercury, as shown in the following equation:

$$Sn_{7-8}Hg + \frac{1}{2}O_2 + H_2O + Cl \rightarrow Sn_4(OH)_6Cl_2 + Hg$$

The reaction of the liberated mercury with unreacted γ can produce additional γ_1 and γ_2. It has been proposed that the dissolution of the tin oxide or tin chloride and the production of additional γ_1 and γ_2 result in porosity and lower strength.

The high-copper admixed and unicompositional alloys do not have any γ_2 phase in the final set mass, but they do have a significant amount of the Cu_6Sn_5 phase or η'. The η' phase is the least corrosion resistant phase in the high-copper amalgams, but it is not an interconnected phase like the γ_2 phase in the low-copper amalgams and therefore does not significantly contribute to corrosion throughout the amalgam. The corrosion product, $CuCl_3Cu(OH)_2$, has been associated with storage of amalgams in synthetic saliva, as shown here:

$$Cu_6Sn_5 + \frac{1}{2}O_2 + H_2O + Cl^- \rightarrow$$
$$CuCl_2 \cdot 3Cu(OH)_2 + SnO$$

Phosphate buffer solutions inhibit the corrosion process; thus saliva may provide some protection of dental amalgams from corrosion.

A study of amalgams that had been in service for 2 to 25 years revealed that the bulk elemental compositions were similar to newly prepared amalgams, except for the presence of a small amount of chloride and other contaminants. The compositions of the phases were also similar to new amalgams, except for internal amalgamation of the γ particles. The distribution of phases in the clinically aged amalgams, however, differed from that of new amalgams. The low-copper amalgams had decreased amounts of γ, γ_1, and γ_2 and increased β_1 and tin-chloride. High-copper admixed amalgams had decreased γ_1, increased β_1, and enlarged reaction rings of γ_1 and η'. There was also evidence of a conversion of γ_1 to β_1 and γ_2 to η'.

Surface tarnish of low-copper amalgams is more associated with γ than γ_1, whereas in high-copper amalgams, surface tarnish is related to the copper-rich phases, η' and the silver-copper eutectic.

Properties of Mercury

ANSI/ADA specification No. 6 (ISO 24234) for dental mercury requires that mercury have a clean reflecting surface that is free from surface film when agitated in air. It should have no visible evidence of surface contamination and contain less than 0.02% nonvolatile residue. Mercury that complies with the requirements of the United States Pharmacopoeia also meets requirements for purity in ISO 24234.

Mercury, which has a freezing point of $-38.87°$ C, is the only metal that remains in the liquid state at room temperatures. It combines readily to form an amalgam with several metals such as gold, silver, copper, tin, and zinc.

Mercury with a very high degree of purity exhibits a slight tarnish after a short time because impurities contaminate the metal and produce a dull surface appearance. Impurities in mercury can reduce the rate at which it combines with the silver alloy.

Bonding of Amalgam

Although amalgam has been a highly successful restorative material when used as an intercoronal restoration, it does not bond to tooth structure and therefore does not restore the original strength of the clinical crown. For large restorations, features such as pins, slots, holes, and grooves must be supplied to provide retention for large restorations, but they do not reinforce the amalgam or increase its strength.

With the development of adhesive systems for dental composites came the opportunity to attempt to bond amalgams to tooth structure. Bonding agents containing 4-META, an acronym for 4-methacryloxyethyl trimellitic anhydride (see Chapter 13), have been the most successful products. Shear bond strengths of amalgam to dentin as high as 10 MPa have been reported using these adhesives whereas comparable values for the shear bond strength of microfilled composites to dentin using these same adhesives have been 20 to 22 MPa.

There is no true adhesion between amalgam and tooth structure. Bonding that has been shown by shear bond tests is strictly produced by the commingling of the bonding agent and the amalgam at their common interface. The technique for placing a bonded amalgam consists of initially placing the bonding agent into the cavity and before the bonding agent has completely polymerized, the amalgam is condensed into the cavity. This represents the technical challenge of filling the retentive features of the preparation with amalgam mixed together with the bonding agent.

The fracture resistance of teeth restored with amalgam-bonded MOD (mesio-occlusal-distal) restorations was more than twice that of restorations containing unbonded amalgams. Also, in spite of the lower shear-bond strength of amalgam bonded to dentin as compared to that for composites, the fracture strength of MODs in teeth restored with bonded amalgams was as high as that for composites, although neither were as high (45% to 80%) as values for the intact tooth. As expected, amalgam-bonded MODs with narrow preparations had higher strengths than those with wide preparations. Other studies showed the retention of amalgam-bonded MODs with proximal boxes was as great as pin-retained amalgams. In addition, amalgam-bonded restorations decreased marginal leakage in class 5 restorations compared with unbonded amalgams. Finally, the bonding agents for amalgam have not been successful in increasing the amalgam-to-amalgam bond strength for the repair of amalgam restorations.

Manipulation of dental amalgam can be found on the website http://evolve.elsevier.com/sakaguchi/restorative ⊖

DENTAL CASTING ALLOYS

This section is divided into noble alloys and base-metal alloys. Fluctuations in the price of gold, platinum, and palladium influence the selection of alloys for cast restorations. Each alloy has specific physical and mechanical properties that affect its manipulation and application. Tooth preparation and restoration design will determine the required physical and mechanical properties of the alloy, so all factors should be kept in mind during the process of treatment planning.

Types and Composition

The ADA specification for dental casting alloys classifies alloys by composition, dividing alloys into three groups: (1) *high-noble,* with a noble metal

content of at least 60 wt% and a gold content of at least 40%; (2) *noble,* with a noble metal content at least 25% (no stipulation for gold); and (3) *predominately base metal,* with a noble metal content less than 25% (Table 10-3). It is important to keep in mind that the percentages used as boundaries in the specification are somewhat arbitrary.

ANSI/ADA specification No. 5 (ISO 1562) uses a type I through IV classification system with each alloy type recommended for specific applications, in addition to the compositional classification previously described (Table 10-4). Thus a high-noble alloy might be type I or type IV, depending on its mechanical properties. This situation is somewhat confusing, because in the old specification the alloy type was tied to its composition and virtually all alloys were gold based. In the current system, each type of alloy is recommended for intraoral use based on the amount of stress the restoration is likely to receive. Alloy types I and II have high elongation and are therefore easily burnished, but are appropriate only in low-stress environments, such as inlays that experience no occlusal forces. Type IV alloys are to be used in clinical situations where very high stresses are involved, such as long-span, fixed dental prostheses. Type III alloys are the most commonly used in dental practices.

Although the number of casting alloys is immense, it is possible to subdivide each ADA compositional group into several classes (Table 10-5). These classes are simply a convenient way of organizing the diverse strategies that have been used to formulate casting alloys. For each class of alloy shown in Table 10-5, there are many variations; the compositions shown are meant only to be representative. Note that both the wt% (weight percent) and at% (atomic percent) compositions of the alloys are shown in Table 10-5. For the sake of simplicity, the following discussion will be in terms of wt% composition. Most of the alloys contain some zinc as a deoxidizer and either iridium (Ir) or ruthenium (Ru) as grain refiners. Some of these compositions are used for both full metal castings and ceramic-metal restorations.

TABLE 10.3 Revised American Dental Association Classification of Prosthodontic Alloys

Class	Required Noble Content (%)	Required Gold Content (%)	Required Titanium Content (%)
High noble alloys	≥60	≥40	
Titanium and titanium alloys			≥85
Noble alloys	≥25		
Predominantly base materials	≥25		

From Givan DA: Dent. Clin. N. Am. 51, 591-601, 2007.

TABLE 10.4 ANSI/ADA Specification No. 5, Mechanical Properties of Dental Casting Alloys

Alloy Type	Description	Use	Yield Strength (annealed, MPa)	Elongated (annealed, %)
I	Soft	Restorations subjected to low stress: some inlays	<140	18
II	Medium	Restorations subjected to moderate stress: inlays and onlays	140-200	18
III	Hard	Restorations subjected to high stress: crowns, thick-veneer crowns, short-span fixed dental prostheses	201-340	12
IV	Extra-hard	Restorations subjected to very high stress: thin-veneer crowns, long-span fixed dental prostheses, removable dental prostheses	>340	10

TABLE 10.5   Typical Compositions (wt%/at%) of Noble Dental Casting Alloys

Alloy Type	Ag	Au	Cu	Pd	Pt	Zn	Other
HIGH-NOBLE							
Au-Ag-Pt	11.5/19.3	78.1/71.4	—	—	9.9/9.2	—	Ir (trace)
Au-Cu-Ag-Pd-*I*	10.0/13.6	76.0/56.5	10.5/24.2	2.4/3.4	0.1/0.1	1.0/2.0	Ru (trace)
Au-Cu-Ag-Pd-*II*	25.0/30.0	56.0/36.6	11.8/23.9	5.0/6.1	0.4/0.3	1.7/3.4	Ir (trace)
NOBLE							
Au-Cu-Ag-Pd-*III*	47.0/53.3	40.0/24.8	7.5/14.4	4.0/4.7	—	1.5/2.8	Ir (trace)
Au-Ag-Pd-In	38.7/36.1	20.0/10.3	—	21.0/33.3	—	3.8/5.8	In 16.5
Pd-Cu-Ga	—	2.0/1.0	10.0/15.8	77.0/73.1	—	—	Ga 7.0/10.1
Ag-Pd	70.0/69.0	—	—	25.0/25.0	—	2.0/3.3	In 3/2.3

Note: *Percentages may not add to exactly 100.0 because of rounding error in calculation of the atomic percentages (at%).*
Ag, *Silver;* Au, *gold;* Cu, *copper;* Ga, *gallium;* In, *indium;* Ir, *iridium;* Pd, *palladium;* Pt, *platinum;* Ru, *ruthenium;* Zn, *zinc.*

There are three classes of high-noble alloys: the Au-Ag-Pt alloys; the Au-Cu-Ag-Pd alloys with a gold content greater than 70 wt% (Au-Cu-Ag-Pd-*I* in Table 10-5); and the Au-Cu-Ag-Pd alloys with a gold content of about 50% to 65% (Au-Cu-Ag-Pd-*II*). The Au-Ag-Pt alloys typically consist of 78 wt% gold with roughly equal amounts of silver and platinum. These alloys have been used as casting alloys and porcelain-metal alloys. The Au-Cu-Ag-Pd-*I* alloys are typically 75 wt% gold with approximately 10 wt% each of silver and copper and 2 to 3 wt% palladium. The Au-Cu-Ag-Pd-*II* alloys typically have less than 60 wt% gold, with the silver content increased to accommodate the reduced gold content. Occasionally, these alloys will have slightly higher palladium and lower silver percentages.

There are four classes of noble alloys: the Au-Cu-Ag-Pd alloys (Au-Cu-Ag-Pd-*III* in Table 10-5); Au-Ag-Pd-In alloys; Pd-Cu-Ga alloys; and Ag-Pd alloys. The Au-Cu-Ag-Pd-*III* alloys typically have a gold content of 40 wt%. The reduced gold is compensated primarily with silver, thus the copper and palladium contents are not changed much from the Au-Cu-Ag-Pd-*II* alloys. The Au-Ag-Pd-In alloys have a gold content of only 20 wt% and have about 40 wt% silver, 20 wt% palladium, and 15 wt% indium. The Pd-Cu-Ga alloys have little or no gold, with about 75 wt% palladium and roughly equal amounts of copper and gallium. Finally, the Ag-Pd alloys have no gold, but have 70 wt% silver and 25 wt% palladium. By the ADA specification, these alloys are considered noble because of their palladium content.

As Table 10-5 shows, the wt% and at% of dental casting alloys can differ considerably. For example, by weight, the Au-Cu-Ag-Pd-*I* alloys have 76% gold. However, only 57% of the atoms in these alloys are gold. Other elements that have less mass than gold increase in atomic percentage. For these same alloys, the copper content by weight is 10%, but by atoms is 24%. For other alloys whose elements have similar mass, the differences between wt% and at% are less pronounced. For example, in the Ag-Pd alloys, the weight and atomic percentages are similar. Weight percentages of the alloys are most commonly used by manufacturers in the production and sales of the alloys. However, the physical, chemical, and biological properties are best understood in terms of atomic percentages.

The compositions of casting alloys determine their color. In general, if the palladium content is over 10 wt%, the alloy will be white. Thus the Pd-Cu-Ga and Ag-Pd alloys in Table 10-5 are white, whereas the other alloys are yellow. The Au-Ag-Pd-In alloys are an exception because they have palladium content over 20% and retain a light yellow color. The color of this alloy results from interactions of the indium with the palladium in the alloy. Among the yellow alloys, the composition will modify the shade of yellow. Generally, copper adds a reddish color and silver lightens either the red or yellow color of the alloys.

Metallic Elements Used in Dental Alloys

For dental restorations, various elements are combined to produce alloys with adequate properties for dental applications because none of the elements by themselves have properties that are suitable. These alloys may be used for dental restorations as cast alloys or may be manipulated into wire or other wrought forms. The metallic elements that make up dental alloys can be divided into two major groups, the noble metals and the base metals.

Noble Metals

Noble metals are elements with a good metallic surface that retain their surface in dry air. They react easily with sulfur to form sulfides, but their

TABLE 10.6   Properties of Elements in Dental Casting Alloys

Element	Symbol	Atomic Number	Atomic Mass	Density (g/cm³)	Melting Temp. (° C)	Color	Comments
NOBLE							
Ruthenium	Ru	44	101.07	12.48	2310.0	White	Grain refiner, hard
Rhodium	Rh	45	102.91	12.41	1966.0	Silver-white	Grain refiner, soft, ductile
Palladium	Pd	46	106.42	12.02	1554.0	White	Hard, malleable, ductile
Osmium	Os	76	190.20	22.61	3045.0	Bluish-white	Not used in dentistry
Iridium	Ir	77	192.22	22.65	2410.0	Silver-white	Grain refiner, very hard
Platinum	Pt	78	195.08	21.45	1772.0	Bluish-white	Tough, ductile, malleable
Gold	Au	79	196.97	19.32	1064.4	Yellow	Ductile, malleable, soft, conductive
BASE							
Nickel	Ni	28	58.69	8.91	1453.0	White	Hard
Copper	Cu	29	63.55	8.92	1083.4	Reddish	Malleable, ductile, conductive
Zinc	Zn	30	65.39	7.14	419.6	Bluish-white	Soft, brittle, oxidizes
Gallium	Ga	31	69.72	5.91	29.8	Grayish-white	Low-melting
Silver	Ag	47	107.87	10.49	961.9		Soft, malleable, ductile, conductive
Tin	Sn	50	118.71	7.29	232.0	White	Soft
Indium	In	49	114.82	7.31	156.6	Gray-white	Soft

resistance to oxidation, tarnish, and corrosion during heating, casting, soldering, and use in the mouth is very good. The noble metals are gold, platinum, palladium, iridium, rhodium, osmium, and ruthenium (Table 10-6). These metals can be subdivided into two groups. The metals of the first group, consisting of ruthenium, rhodium, and palladium, have atomic weights of approximately 100 and densities of 12 to 13 g/cm³. The metals of the second group, consisting of osmium, iridium, platinum, and gold, have atomic weights of about 190 and densities of 19 to 23 g/cm³. The melting points of members of each group decrease with increasing atomic weight. Thus ruthenium melts at 2310° C, rhodium at 1966° C, and palladium at 1554° C. In the second group the melting points range from 3045° C for osmium to 1064° C for gold. The noble metals, together with silver, are sometimes called *precious metals*. The term *precious* comes from the relatively high cost of these metals and their trading on the commodities market. Some metallurgists consider silver a noble metal, but it is not considered a noble metal in dentistry because it corrodes considerably in the oral cavity. Thus the terms *noble* and *precious* are not synonymous in dentistry.

GOLD (AU)

Pure gold is a soft, malleable, ductile metal that has a rich yellow color with a strong metallic luster. Although pure gold is the most ductile and malleable of all metals, it is relatively low in strength. The density of gold depends somewhat on the condition of the metal, whether it is cast, rolled, or drawn into wire. Small amounts of impurities have a pronounced effect on the mechanical properties of gold and its alloys. The presence of less than 0.2% lead causes gold to be extremely brittle. Mercury in small quantities also has a harmful effect. Therefore, scrap of other dental alloys, such as technique alloy or other base-metal alloys, including amalgam, should not be mixed with gold used for dental restorations.

Air or water at any temperature does not affect or tarnish gold. Gold is not soluble in sulfuric, nitric, or hydrochloric acids. However, it readily dissolves in combinations of nitric and hydrochloric acids (aqua regia, 18 vol% nitric and 82 vol% hydrochloric acids) to form the trichloride of gold ($AuCl_3$). It is also dissolved by a few other chemicals, such as potassium cyanide and solutions of bromine or chlorine.

Because gold is nearly as soft as lead, it must be alloyed with copper, silver, platinum, and other metals to develop the hardness, durability, and elasticity necessary in dental alloys, coins, and jewelry (Table 10-7). Through appropriate refining and purification, gold with an extremely high degree of purity may be produced. Gold can be work hardened to improve its physical properties. Without the improvement, cast gold would lack sufficient strength and hardness.

CARAT AND FINENESS OF GOLD-BASED ALLOYS. For many years the gold content of gold-containing alloys has been described on the basis of the carat, or in terms of fineness, rather than by weight percentage. The term *carat* refers only to the gold content of the alloy; a carat represents a $\frac{1}{24}$ part of the whole. Thus 24 carat indicates pure gold. The carat of an alloy is designated by a small letter *k*, for example, 18k or 22k gold.

The use of the term *carat* to designate the gold content of dental alloy is less common now. It is not unusual to find the weight percentage of gold listed or to have the alloy described in terms of fineness. *Fineness* also refers only to the gold content, and represents the number of parts of gold in each 1000 parts of alloy. Thus 24k gold is the same as 100% gold or 1000 fineness (i.e., 1000 fine). The fineness represents a precise measure of the gold content of the alloy and is often the preferred measurement when an exact value is to be listed. An 18k gold would be designated as 750 fine, or, when the decimal system is used, it would be 0.750 fine; this indicates that 750/1000 of the total is gold. A comparison of the carat, fineness, and weight percentage of gold is given in Table 10-8. Both the whole number and the decimal system are in common use, especially for noble dental solders. The fineness system is somewhat less relevant today because of the introduction of alloys that are not gold-based. It is important to emphasize that the terms *carat* and *fineness* refer only to gold content, not noble-metal content.

PLATINUM (Pt)

Platinum is a bluish white metal; is tough, ductile, and malleable; and can be produced as foil or fine-drawn wire. Platinum has hardness similar to that of copper. Pure platinum has numerous applications in dentistry because of its high fusing point and resistance to oral conditions and elevated temperatures.

Platinum increases the hardness and elastic qualities of gold, and some dental casting alloys and wires contain quantities of platinum up to 8% combined

TABLE 10.7 Physical and Mechanical Properties of Cast Pure Gold, Gold Alloys, and Condensed Gold Foil

Material	Density (g/cm³)	Hardness (VHN/BHN) (kg/mm²)	Tensile Strength (MPa)	Elongation (%)
Cast 24k gold	19.3	28 (VHN)	105	30
Cast 22k gold	—	60 (VHN)	240	22
Coin gold	—	85 (BHN)	395	30
Typical Au-based casting alloy (70 wt% Au)*	15.6	135/195 (VHN)	425/525	30/12
Condensed gold foil†	19.1	60 (VHN)	250	12.8

Values are for softened/hardened condition.
†Modified from Rule, R.W., 1937. J. Am. Dent. Assoc. 24, 583.
VHN/BHN, Vickers hardness number/Brinell hardness number.

TABLE 10.8 Comparison of Carat, Fineness, and Weight Percentage of Gold in Gold Alloys

Carat	Amount of Gold by Carats	Weight (%) of Gold	Fineness Parts/1000	Fineness Decimal
24	$^{24}/_{24}$	100.0	1000.00	1.000
22	$^{22}/_{24}$	91.7	916.66	0.916
20	$^{20}/_{24}$	83.3	833.33	0.833
18	$^{18}/_{24}$	75.0	750.00	0.750
16	$^{16}/_{24}$	66.7	666.66	0.666
14	$^{14}/_{24}$	58.3	583.33	0.583
9	$^{9}/_{24}$	37.5	374.99	0.375

with other metals. Platinum tends to lighten the color of yellow gold-based alloys.

PALLADIUM (Pd)

Palladium is a white metal somewhat darker than platinum. Its density is a little more than half that of platinum and gold. Palladium has the quality of absorbing or occluding large quantities of hydrogen gas when heated. This can be an undesirable quality when alloys containing palladium are heated with an improperly adjusted gas-air torch.

Palladium is not used in the pure state in dentistry, but is used extensively in dental alloys. Palladium can be combined with gold, silver, copper, cobalt, tin, indium, or gallium for dental alloys. Alloys are readily formed between gold and palladium, and palladium quantities of as low as 5% by weight have a pronounced effect on whitening yellow gold-based alloys. Palladium-gold alloys with a palladium content of 10% or more by weight are white. Alloys of palladium and the other elements previously mentioned are available as substitutes for yellow-gold alloys, and the mechanical properties of the palladium-based alloys may be as good as or better than many traditional gold-based alloys. Although many of the palladium-based alloys are white, some, such as palladium-indium-silver alloys, are yellow.

IRIDIUM (Ir), RUTHENIUM (Ru), AND RHODIUM (Rh)

Iridium and ruthenium are used in small amounts in dental alloys as grain refiners to keep the grain size small. A small grain size is desirable because it improves the mechanical properties and uniformity of properties within an alloy. As little as 0.005% (50 ppm) of iridium is effective in reducing the grain size. Ruthenium has a similar effect. The grain-refining properties of these elements are largely due to their extremely high melting points. Iridium melts at 2410° C and ruthenium at 2310° C. Thus these elements do not melt during the casting of the alloy and serve as nucleating centers for the melt as it cools, resulting in a fine-grained alloy.

Rhodium also has a high melting point (1966° C) and has been used in alloys with platinum to form wire for thermocouples. These thermocouples help measure the temperature in porcelain furnaces used to make dental restorations.

Base Metals

Several base metals are combined with noble metals to develop alloys with properties suitable for dental restorations. Base metals used in dental alloys include silver, copper, zinc, indium, tin, gallium, and nickel (see Table 10-6).

SILVER (Ag)

Silver is a malleable, ductile white metal. It is the best-known conductor of heat and electricity and is stronger and harder than gold but softer than copper. At 961.9° C, the melting point of silver is below the melting points of both copper and gold. It is unaltered in clean, dry air at any temperature, but combines with sulfur, chlorine, phosphorus, and vapors containing these elements or their compounds. Foods containing sulfur compounds cause severe tarnish on silver, and for this reason silver is not considered a noble metal in dentistry.

Pure silver is not used in dental restorations because of the black sulfide that forms on the metal in the mouth. Adding small amounts of palladium to silver-containing alloys prevents the rapid corrosion of such alloys in the oral environment.

Silver forms a series of solid solutions with palladium (Figure 10-7, *D*) and gold (Figure 10-7, *C*), and is therefore common in gold- and palladium-based dental alloys. In gold-based alloys, silver is effective in neutralizing the reddish color of alloys containing appreciable quantities of copper. Silver also hardens the gold-based alloys via a solid-solution hardening mechanism. In palladium-based alloys, silver is important in developing the white color of the alloy. Although silver is soluble in palladium, the addition of other elements to these alloys, such as copper or indium, may cause the formation of multiple phases and increased corrosion.

COPPER (Cu)

Copper is a malleable and ductile metal with high thermal and electrical conductivity and a characteristic red color. Copper forms a series of solid solutions with both gold (Figure 10-7, *A*) and palladium (Figure 10-7, *B*) and is therefore an important component of noble dental alloys. When added to gold-based alloys, copper imparts a reddish color to the gold and hardens the alloy via a solid-solution or ordered-solution mechanism. The presence of copper in gold-based alloys in quantities between approximately 40% and 88% by weight allows the formation of an ordered phase. Copper is also commonly used in palladium-based alloys, where it can be used to reduce the melting point and strengthen the alloy through solid-solution hardening and formation of ordered phases when Cu is between 15 and 55 wt%. The ratio of silver and copper must be carefully balanced in gold- and palladium-based alloys, because silver and copper are not miscible. Copper is also a common component of most hard dental solders.

ZINC (Zn)

Zinc is a blue-white metal with a tendency to tarnish in moist air. In its pure form, it is a soft, brittle metal with low strength. When heated in air, zinc

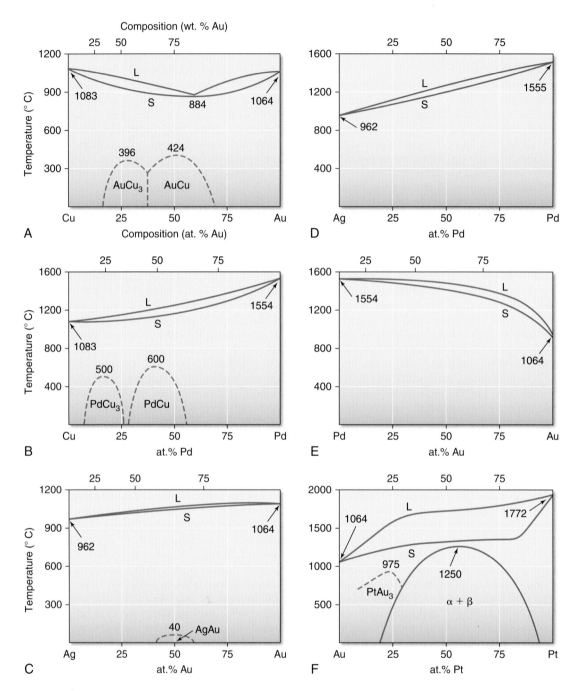

FIGURE 10.7 **Phase diagrams for binary combinations. A,** Copper (*Cu*) and gold (*Au*); **B,** copper and palladium (*Pd*); **C,** silver and gold; **D,** silver and palladium; **E,** palladium and gold; and **F,** gold and platinum (*Pt*). Atomic percentages are shown along the bottom of each graph; weight percentages are shown along the top. *L,* liquidus; *S,* solidus. (*Modified from Hansen M: Constitution of binary alloys. McGraw Hill, New York, 1958.*)

oxidizes readily to form a white oxide of relatively low density. This oxidizing property is exploited in dental alloys. Although zinc may be present in quantities of only 1% to 2% by weight, it acts as a scavenger of oxygen when the alloy is melted. Thus zinc is referred to as a *deoxidizing agent.* Because of its low density, the resulting zinc oxide lags behind the denser molten mass during casting and is therefore excluded from the casting. If too much zinc is present, it will markedly increase the brittleness of the alloy.

INDIUM (In)

Indium is a soft, gray-white metal with a low melting point of 156.6° C. Indium is not tarnished by air or water. It is used in some gold-based alloys as a replacement for zinc and is a common minor component of some noble ceramic dental alloys. Recently, indium has been used in greater amounts (up to 30% by weight) to impart a yellow color to palladium-silver alloys.

TIN (Sn)

Tin is a lustrous, soft, white metal that is not subject to tarnish in normal air. Some gold-based alloys contain limited quantities of tin, usually less than 5% by weight. Tin is also an ingredient in gold-based dental solders. It combines with platinum and palladium to produce a hardening effect, but also increases brittleness.

GALLIUM (Ga)

Gallium is a grayish metal that is stable in dry air but tarnishes in moist air. It has a very low melting point of 29.8° C and a density of only 5.91 g/cm³. Gallium is not used in its pure form in dentistry, but is used as a component of some gold- and palladium-based dental alloys, especially ceramic alloys. The oxides of gallium are important to the bonding of the ceramic to the metal.

NICKEL (Ni)

Nickel has limited application in gold- and palladium-based dental alloys, but is a common component in nonnoble dental alloys. Nickel has a melting point of 1453° C and a density of 8.91 g/cm³. When used in small quantities in gold-based alloys, nickel whitens the alloy and increases its strength and hardness.

Binary Combinations of Noble Metals

Although most noble casting alloys have three or more elements, the properties of certain binary alloys are important because these binary combinations constitute the majority of the mass of many noble alloys. An understanding of the physical and manipulative properties of these binary alloys is therefore useful in understanding the behavior of the more complex alloys. Among the noble alloys, six binary combinations of elements are important: Au-Cu, Pd-Cu, Au-Ag, Pd-Ag, Au-Pd, and Au-Pt. Phase diagrams for these binary systems are shown in Figure 10-7. Phase diagrams are powerful tools for understanding the physical and manipulative properties of binary alloys.

ALLOY COMPOSITION AND TEMPERATURE

In each phase diagram in Figure 10-7, the horizontal axis represents the composition of the binary alloy. For example, in Figure 10-7, *A*, the horizontal axis represents a series of binary alloys of gold and copper ranging in composition from 0% gold (or 100% copper) to 100% gold. The composition can be given in atomic percent (at%) or weight percent (wt%). Weight percent compositions give the relative mass of each element in the alloy, whereas atomic percentages give the relative numbers of atoms in the alloys. It is a simple calculation to convert weight percentages to atomic percentages, and vice versa. Note that for the binary alloys shown in Figure 10-7, the atomic percent composition is shown along the bottom of the phase diagram, whereas the weight percent composition is shown along the top.

The atomic and weight percent compositions of the binary alloys can differ considerably. For example, for the Au-Cu system shown in Figure 10-7, *A*, an alloy that is 50% gold by weight is only 25% gold by atoms. For other systems, like the Au-Pt system in Figure 10-7, *F*, there is little difference between atomic and weight percentages. The difference between atomic and weight percentages depends on the differences in the atomic masses of the elements involved. The bigger the difference in atomic mass, the bigger the difference between the atomic and weight percentages in the binary phase diagram.

Because it is more convenient to use masses in the manufacture of alloys, the most common method for reporting composition is by weight percentages. However, the physical and biological properties of alloys relate best to atomic percentages. It is therefore important to keep the difference between atomic and weight percent in mind when selecting and using noble dental casting alloys. Alloys that appear high in gold by weight percentage may in reality contain far fewer gold atoms than might be thought.

Other aspects of the phase diagrams that deserve attention are the liquidus and solidus lines. The y-axes in Figure 10-7 show temperature. If the temperature is above the liquidus line (marked *L*), the alloy will be completely molten. If the temperature is below the solidus line (marked *S*), the alloy will be solid. If the temperature lies between the liquidus and solidus lines, the alloy will be partially molten. Note that the distance between the liquidus and solidus lines varies among systems in Figure 10-7. For example, the temperature difference between these lines is small for the Ag-Au system (see Figure 10-7, *C*), is much larger for the Au-Pt system (see Figure 10-7, *F*), and varies considerably with composition for the Au-Cu system (see Figure 10-7, *A*).

From a manipulative standpoint, it is desirable to have a narrow liquidus-solidus range, because one would like to keep the alloy in the liquid state for as short a time as possible before casting. While in the liquid state, the alloy is susceptible to significant oxidation and contamination. If the liquidus-solidus range is broad, the alloy will remain at least partially molten for a longer period after it is cast.

The temperature of the liquidus line is also important, and varies considerably among alloys and with composition. For example the liquidus line of the Au-Ag system ranges from 962° to 1064° C (see Figure 10-7, C) but the liquidus line of the Au-Pd system ranges from 1064° to 1554° C (see Figure 10-7, E). It is often desirable to have an alloy with a liquidus line at lower temperatures; the method of heating is easier, fewer side reactions occur, and shrinkage is generally less of a problem.

PHASE STRUCTURE OF NOBLE ALLOYS

The area below the solidus lines in Figure 10-7 is also important to the behavior of the alloy. If this area contains no boundaries, then the binary system is a series of *solid solutions*. This means that the two elements are completely soluble in one another at all temperatures and compositions. The Ag-Pd system (see Figure 10-7, D) and Pd-Au system (see Figure 10-7, E) are examples of solid-solution systems. If the area below the solidus line contains dashed lines, then an ordered solution is present within the dashed lines.

An *ordered solution* occurs when the two elements in the alloy assume specific and regular positions in the crystal lattice of the alloy. This situation differs from a solid solution in which the positions of the elements in the crystal lattice are random. Examples of systems containing ordered solutions are the Au-Cu system (see Figure 10-7, A) the Pd-Cu system (see Figure 10-7, B), and the Au-Ag system (see Figure 10-7, C). Note that the ordered solutions occur over a limited range of compositions because the ratios between the elements must be correct to support the regular positions in the crystal lattices.

If the area below the solidus line contains a solid line, it indicates the existence of a second phase. A *second phase* is an area with a composition distinctly different from the first phase. In the Au-Pt system (see Figure 10-7, F) a second phase forms between 20 and 90 at% platinum. If the temperature is below the phase boundary line within these compositions, two phases exist in the alloy.

The presence of a second phase is important because it significantly changes the corrosion properties of an alloy. Figure 10-8 shows electron micrographs of single- and multiple-phase alloys. The single-phase alloy has little visible microstructure because its composition is more or less homogeneous. In the multiple-phase alloy, areas that have distinct compositions are clearly visible. These areas correspond to the different phases under the solidus in a phase diagram. Because the different phases may interact electrochemically, the corrosion of multiple-phase alloys may be higher than for a single-phase alloy.

HARDENING OF NOBLE ALLOYS

The use of pure cast gold is not practical for dental restorations because cast gold lacks sufficient strength and hardness. Solid-solution and ordered-solution hardening are two common ways of strengthening noble dental alloys sufficiently for use in the mouth. By mixing two elements in the crystal lattice randomly (forming a solid solution), the force needed to distort the lattice may be significantly increased. For example, adding just 10% by weight of copper to gold, the tensile strength increases from 105 to 395 MPa and the Brinell hardness increases from 28 to 85 (see Table 10-7). If the positions of the two elements become ordered (forming an ordered solution), the properties of the alloy are improved further

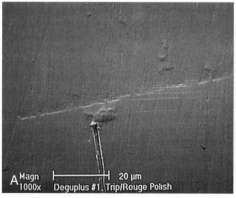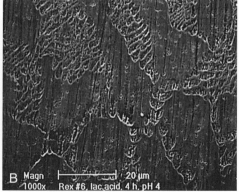

FIGURE 10.8 **Electron micrographs of single-phase (A) and multiple-phase (B) alloys. A,** Few distinguishing microstructure characteristics are seen because the alloy is nearly homogeneous. Only a few scratches from polishing and some debris on the surface are visible. **B,** A rich microstructure is evident, reflecting the several phases present. Each phase has a different composition.

(see Table 10-7). For a typical gold-based casting alloy, the formation of an ordered solution may increase yield strength by 50%, tensile strength by 25%, and hardness by at least 10%. It is important to note that the elongation of an alloy is reduced by the formation of the ordered solution. For the typical gold-based alloy, the percentage elongation will decrease from 30% to about 12%.

The formation of ordered solutions has been commonly used to strengthen cast dental restorations, particularly in gold-based alloys. As shown in Figure 10-7, *A*, the Au-Cu system supports ordered solutions between about 20 and 70 at% gold. However, the manipulation of the alloy during casting will determine whether the ordered solution will form. If Au-Cu containing about 50 at% gold is heated to the molten state and then cooled slowly, the mass will solidify at about 880° C as a solid solution. As the mass cools slowly to 424° C, the ordered solution will then form and will remain present at room temperature. However, if the mass is cooled rapidly to room temperature after the initial solidification, the ordered solution will not form because there is insufficient time for the mass to reorganize. Thus the alloy will be trapped in a nonequilibrium state of a solid solution and will be softer, weaker, and have greater elongation.

The conversion between the ordered solution and solid solution is reversible in the solid state. By heating an alloy in either condition above 424° C (but below the solidus), the state of the alloy can be selected by picking the cooling rate. Rapid cooling will preserve the solid solution and the soft condition, whereas slow cooling will allow the formation of the ordered solution and the hardened condition. In alloys of gold and copper with other elements, Au-Cu ordered solutions are still possible as long as the ratio of copper to gold is greater than 30:70 (at%). As shown in Figure 10-8, the formation of ordered solutions is possible in other noble alloy systems, such as Pd-Cu and Au-Pt. The ordered solution of the Ag-Au system exists but cannot be used in practice because the transition temperature is too low (almost body temperature).

The formation of a second phase has also been used to harden dental alloys, but this method is not commonly used for noble dental alloys. The dispersion of the second phase is very important to the effectiveness of the hardening. Recent evidence indicates that some Au-based alloys may contain Ag-rich coherent precipitates that, along with ordered solutions, contribute to alloy hardening. The advantages of the hardening must be balanced against the liabilities of the increased corrosion often seen with multiple-phase systems. It should be noted that, unlike the ordered solutions, the formation of second phases are not usually easily controlled by heat treatments

and may not be reversible in the solid state. In fact, heat treatment commonly causes a deterioration of properties with these systems.

FORMULATION OF NOBLE ALLOYS

The desired qualities of noble dental casting alloys determine the selection of elements that will be used to formulate the alloys. The ideal noble casting alloy should have (1) a low melting range and narrow solidus-liquidus temperature range, (2) adequate strength, hardness, and elongation, (3) a low tendency to corrode in the oral environment, and (4) low cost, among other properties. Traditionally, the noble elements gold and palladium have generally been the foundation to which other elements are added to formulate dental casting alloys. Gold and palladium are preferable to other noble elements because they have relatively low melting points, low corrosion, and form solid solutions with other alloy elements, such as copper or silver (see Figure 10-7). Solid-solution systems are desirable for the formulation of alloys because they are generally easier to manufacture and manipulate, have a lower tendency to corrode than multiple phase systems, and provide increased strength through solid-solution or ordered-solution hardening. Furthermore, the systems shown in Figure 10-7 generally have narrow liquidus-solidus ranges. Thus it is not surprising that combinations of these elements have been extensively used in the formulation of noble dental casting alloys.

Grain Size

Studies have shown that minute quantities of various elements can influence the grain size of dental casting alloys. With the addition of small amounts (0.005% or 50 ppm) of elements such as iridium and ruthenium, fine-grained castings are produced. Adding one of these elements to the alloy is believed to develop centers for nucleating grains throughout the alloy. Most alloy manufacturers use grain refinement in present-day products. The mechanical properties of tensile strength and elongation are improved significantly (30%) by the fine grain structure in castings, which contributes to uniformity of properties from one casting to another. Other properties, however, such as hardness and yield strength, show less effect from the grain refinement.

Properties
MELTING RANGE

Dental casting alloys do not have melting points, but rather melting ranges, because they are combinations of elements rather than pure elements. The magnitude of the solidus-liquidus melting range is important to the manipulation of the alloys (see Figure 10-7 and Table 10-9). The solidus-liquidus range should be narrow to avoid having the alloy

TABLE 10.9   Physical and Mechanical Properties of Several Types of Noble Dental Casting Alloys

Alloy	Solidus (° C)	Liquidus (° C)	Color	Density (g/cm³)	Yield Strength at 0.2% Offset (Soft/Hard) (MPa)	Elongation (Soft/Hard) (%)	Vickers Hardness (Soft/Hard) (kg/mm²)
Property							
HIGH-NOBLE							
Au-Ag-Pt	1045	1140	Yellow	18.4	420/470	15/9	175/195
Au-Cu-Ag-Pd-*I*	910	965	Yellow	15.6	270/400	30/12	135/195
Au-Cu-Ag-Pd-*II*	870	920	Yellow	13.8	350/600	30/10	175/260
NOBLE							
Au-Cu-Ag-Pd-*III*	865	925	Yellow	12.4	325/520	27.5/10	125/215
Au-Ag-Pd-In	875	1035	Light yellow	11.4	300/370	12/8	135/190
Pd-Cu-Ga	1100	1190	White	10.6	1145	8	425
Ag-Pd	1020	1100	White	10.6	260/320	10/8	140/155

Ag, *Silver;* Au, *gold;* Cu, *copper;* Ga, *gallium;* In, *indium;* Pd, *palladium;* Pt, *platinum.*

in a molten state for extended times during casting. If the alloy spends a long time in the partially molten state during casting, there is increased opportunity for the formation of oxides and contamination. Most of the alloys in Table 10-9 have solidus-liquidus ranges of 70° C or less. The Au-Ag-Pt, Pd-Cu-Ga, and Ag-Pd alloys have wider ranges, which makes them more difficult to cast without problems.

The liquidus temperature of the alloys determines the burnout temperature, type of investment, and type of heat source that must be used during casting. In general, the burnout temperature must be about 500° C below the liquidus temperature. For the Au-Cu-Ag-Pd-*I* alloys, therefore, a burnout temperature of about 450° to 475° C should be used. If the burnout temperature approaches 700° C, a gypsum-bonded investment cannot be used because the calcium sulfate will decompose and embrittle the alloys. At temperatures near 700° C or greater, a phosphate-bonded investment is used. As shown in Table 10-9, a gypsum-bonded investment may be used with the Au-Cu-Ag-Pd-*I, II,* and *III* and the Au-Ag-Pd-In alloys, but a phosphate-bonded investment is advisable for the other alloys. The gas-air torch will adequately heat alloys with liquidus temperatures below 1100° C. Above this temperature, a gas-oxygen torch or electrical induction method must be used. Again from Table 10-9, a gas-air torch would be acceptable only for the Au-Cu-Ag-Pd-*I, II,* and *III* and the Au-Ag-Pd-In alloys.

The composition of the alloys determines the liquidus temperatures. If the alloy contains a significant amount of an element that has a high melting point, it is likely to have a high liquidus. Thus alloys that contain significant amounts of palladium or platinum, both of which have high melting points (see Table 10-6), will have high liquidus temperatures. In Table 10-9, these alloys include the Pd-Cu-Ga, Ag-Pd, and Au-Ag-Pt alloys.

The solidus temperature is important to soldering and formation of ordered phases, because during both of these operations, the shape of the alloys is to be retained. Therefore during soldering or hardening-softening, the alloy may be heated only to the solidus before melting occurs. In practice, it is desirable to limit heating to 50° C below the solidus to avoid local melting or distortion of the casting.

DENSITY

Density is important during the acceleration of the molten alloy into the mold during casting. Alloys with high densities will generally accelerate faster and tend to form complete castings more easily. Among the alloys shown in Table 10-9, all have densities sufficient for convenient casting. Lower densities (7 to 8 g/cm³) seen in the predominantly base-metal alloys sometimes present problems in this regard. Alloys in Table 10-6 with high densities generally contain higher amounts of denser elements such as gold or platinum. Thus the Au-Ag-Pt alloys and Au-Cu-Ag-Pd-*I* alloys are among the densest of the casting alloys.

STRENGTH

Strength of alloys can be measured by either the yield strength or tensile strength. Although tensile strength represents the maximum strength of the alloy, the yield strength is more useful in dental applications because it is the stress at which permanent deformation of the alloys occurs (see Chapter 4). Because permanent deformation of dental castings is generally undesirable, the yield strength is a reasonable practical maximum strength for dental applications. The yield strengths for the different classes of alloys are shown in Table 10-6. Where applicable, the hard and soft conditions, resulting from the formation of ordered solutions, are shown. For several alloys, such as Au-Cu-Ag-Pd-*I*, *II*, and *III*, the formation of the ordered phase increases the yield strength significantly. For example, the yield strength of the Au-Cu-Ag-Pd-*II* alloys increases from 350 to 600 MPa with the formation of an ordered phase. For other alloys, such as the Au-Ag-Pt and Ag-Pd alloys, the increase in yield strength is more modest in the hardened condition. The Pd-Cu-Ga alloys do not support the formation of ordered phase because the ratio of palladium and copper are not in the correct range for ordered phase formation (see Table 10-9 and Figure 10-7, *B*).

The yield strengths of these alloys range from 320 to 1145 MPa (hard condition). The strongest alloy is Pd-Cu-Ga, with a yield strength of 1145 MPa. The other alloys range in strength from 320 to 600 MPa. These latter yield strengths are adequate for dental applications and are generally in the same range as those for the base-metal alloys, which range from 495 to 600 MPa. The effect of solid-solution hardening by the addition of copper and silver to the gold or palladium base is significant for these alloys. Pure cast gold has a tensile strength of 105 MPa (see Table 10-7). With the addition of 10 wt% copper (coin gold), solid-solution hardening increases the tensile strength to 395 MPa. With the further addition of 10 wt% silver and 3 wt% palladium (Au-Cu-Ag-Pd-*I*), the tensile strength increases to about 450 MPa and 550 MPa in the hard condition.

HARDNESS

Hardness is a good indicator of the ability of an alloy to resist local permanent deformation under occlusal load. Although the relationships are complex, hardness is related to yield strength and gives some indication of the difficulty in polishing the alloy. Alloys with high hardness will usually have high yield strengths and are more difficult to polish. As Table 10-9 shows, the values for hardness generally parallel those for yield strength. In the hard condition, the hardness of these alloys ranges from 155 kg/mm^2 for the Ag-Pd alloys to 425 kg/mm^2 for the Pd-Cu-Ga alloys. More typically, the hardness of the noble casting alloys is around 200 kg/mm^2. The Ag-Pd alloys are particularly soft because of the high concentration of silver, which is a soft metal. The Pd-Cu-Ga alloys are particularly hard because of the high concentration of Pd, which is a hard metal.

The hardness of most noble casting alloys is less than that of enamel (343 kg/mm^2), and typically less than that of base-metal alloys. If the hardness of an alloy is greater than enamel, it may wear the enamel of the teeth opposing the restoration.

ELONGATION

Elongation is a measure of the ductility of the alloy. For crown and bridge applications, a low value of elongation for an alloy is generally not a big concern, because permanent deformation of the alloys is generally not desirable. However, the elongation will indicate whether the alloy can be burnished. Alloys with high elongation can be burnished without fracture. Elongation is sensitive to the presence or absence of an ordered phase, as shown in Table 10-9. In the hardened condition, the elongation will drop significantly. For example, for the Au-Cu-Ag-Pd-*II* alloys, the elongation is 30% in the soft condition versus only 10% in the hard condition. In the soft condition, the elongation of noble dental casting alloys ranges from 8% to 30%. These alloys are substantially more ductile than the base-metal alloys, which have elongation on the order of 1% to 2%.

BIOCOMPATIBILITY

The *biocompatibility* of noble dental alloys is equally important as other physical or chemical properties. A detailed discussion about the principles of biocompatibility can be found in Chapter 6, but a few general principles are mentioned here. The biocompatibility of noble dental alloys is primarily related to elemental release from these alloys (i.e., their corrosion). Thus any toxic, allergic, or other adverse biological response is primarily influenced by elements released from these alloys into the oral cavity. The biological response is also influenced significantly by exactly which elements are released, their concentrations, and duration of exposure to oral tissues. For example, the short-term (more than 1 to 2 days) release of zinc may not be significant biologically, but longer-term (more than 2 to 3 years) release might have more significant effects. Similarly, equivalent amounts (in moles) of zinc, copper, or silver will have quite different biological effects, because each of the elements is unique in its interactions with tissues.

Unfortunately, there is currently no way of completely assessing the biocompatibility of noble alloys (or any other material), because the effects of elemental release on tissues are not completely understood. However, in general, several principles apply to alloy biocompatibility. The elemental release from noble alloys is not proportional to alloy composition, but rather is influenced by the numbers and types of phases in the alloy microstructure and the composition of the phases. In general, multiple-phase alloys release more mass than single-phase alloys. Some elements, such as copper, zinc, silver, cadmium, and nickel, are inherently more prone to be released from dental alloys than others, such as gold, palladium, platinum, and indium. Alloys with high noble metal content generally release less mass than alloys with little or no noble metal content. However, the only reliable way to assess elemental release is by direct measurement, because there are exceptions to each of the generalizations just mentioned. Similarly, it is difficult to predict, even knowing the elemental release from an alloy, what the biological response to the alloy will be. Thus the only reliable way is to measure the biological response directly, either in vitro, in animals, or in humans (see Chapter 6). It is important to also remember that combinations of alloys used in the mouth may alter their corrosion and biocompatibility.

The Identalloy program was developed in an effort to make dentists and patients more aware of the composition of dental alloys that are used. Under this program, each alloy has a certificate (Figure 10-9) that lists the complete composition of the alloy, its manufacturer, name, and the ADA compositional classification (high-noble, noble, or predominantly base metal). When the dental prosthesis is delivered by the laboratory to the dental office, a certificate is placed in the patient's chart. In this manner, all parties know the exact composition of the material used. This information can be invaluable later if there are problems with the restoration; for example, if the patient develops an allergic reaction. This information is also useful when planning additional restorations that may contact the existing restoration, or if some modification (such as occlusal adjustment or contouring) becomes necessary.

Composition and Properties of Noble-Metal Alloys for Ceramic-Metal Restorations

Ceramic-metal restorations consist of a cast metallic framework (or core) on which at least two layers of ceramic are baked. It is essential that the coefficient of thermal expansion of the alloy be slightly higher than that of the veneering ceramic to ensure that the ceramic is in slight compression after cooling. This will establish a better resistance to crack propagation of the ceramic-metal restoration. There are several requirements for the alloy in a ceramic-metal system (a complete list of requirements for both the alloy and ceramic can be found in Chapter 11).

1. The alloy must have a high melting temperature. The melting range must be substantially higher (greater than 100° C) than the firing temperature of the ceramic and solders used to join segments of a bridge.
2. A good bond between the ceramic and metal is essential and is achieved by the interactions of the ceramic with metal oxides on the surface of metal (Figure 10-10) and by the roughness of the metal coping.
3. Coefficients of thermal expansion of the ceramic and metal must be compatible so that the ceramic does not crack during fabrication. The system is designed so the value for the metal is slightly higher than for the ceramic, thus putting the ceramic in compression (where it is stronger) following cooling (Figure 10-11).
4. Adequate stiffness and strength of the alloy core are especially important for fixed bridges and posterior crowns. High stiffness in the alloy reduces stresses in the ceramic by reducing

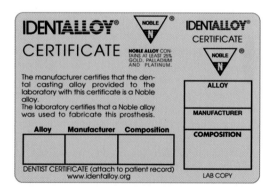

FIGURE 10-9 **An example of an Identalloy certificate showing the alloy name, manufacturer, composition, and American Dental Association (ADA) classification.** This section of the certificate is for the dentist's records. A duplicate retained by the laboratory is not shown here. Many dentists will give this information to the patient upon delivery of the prosthesis.

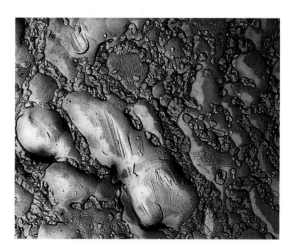

FIGURE 10.10 **Electron micrograph of replicated oxidized surface of a Au-Pt-Pd (gold-platinum-palladium) alloy (×8000).** *(From Kelly M, Asgar K, O'Brien WJ: J. Biomed. Mater. Res. 3, 403, 1969.)*

deflection and strain. High strength is essential in the interproximal regions in fixed bridges.

5. High sag resistance is essential. The alloy copings are relatively thin; no distortion should occur during firing of the ceramic, or the fit of the restoration will be compromised.

6. An accurate casting of the metal coping is required even with the higher melting range of the alloy.

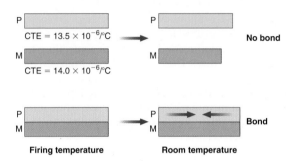

FIGURE 10.11 Diagram of the ceramic-metal bond. Shown at the firing temperature and at room temperature, when the thermal coefficient of expansion of the metal is $0.5 \times 10^{-6}/°$ C greater than the ceramic, thus placing the ceramic in compression at room temperature. *CTE*, Coefficient of thermal expansion; *M*, *metal*; *P*, *porcelain*. (*From Craig RG, Powers JM, Wataha JC: Dental materials: properties and manipulation,* 9th *ed. Mosby, St Louis, 2008.*)

7. Adequate design of the restoration is critical. The preparation should provide for adequate thickness of alloy as well as enough space for an adequate thickness of ceramic to yield an esthetic restoration.

The composition ranges and colors of five types of noble alloys for ceramic-metal restorations are listed in Table 10-10. The properties of these alloys are given in Table 10-11.

Au-Pt-Pd ALLOYS

The Au-Pt-Pd alloys contain very high noble-metal content, mainly gold with platinum and palladium to increase the melting range. The high-noble content provides good corrosion resistance. Indium, tin, and iron (Fe) are present and form oxides to produce a ceramic-metal bond. Rhenium (Re) is added as a grain refiner. Hardening of Au-Pt-Pd alloys results from solid-solution hardening and the formation of a $FePt_3$ precipitate. Optimum heat treatment for hardening is 30 minutes at 550° C, but practically the hardening occurs during firing of the ceramic. During the casting of these alloys, some of these base elements are lost; it is therefore recommended that 50% new alloy be used with a sprue button if it is used to make a second casting. The new alloy will provide enough of the base elements so that adequate oxides and hardening result.

TABLE 10.10   Composition Ranges and Color of Noble Alloys for Ceramic-Metal Restorations (wt%)

Type	Au (%)	Pt (%)	Pd (%)	Ag (%)	Cu (%)	Other (%)	Total Noble-Metal Content (%)	Color
Au-Pt-Pd	84-86	4-10	5-7	0-2	—	Fe, In, Re, Sn 2-5	96-98	Yellow
Au-Pd	45-52	—	38-45	0	—	Ru, Re, In 8.5, Ga 1.5	89-90	White
Au-Pd-Ag	51-52	—	26-31	14-16	—	Ru, Re, In 1.5, Sn 3-7	78-83	White
Pd-Ag	—	—	53-88	30-37	—	Ru, In 1-5, Sn 4-8	49-62	White
Pd-Cu	0–2	—	74-79	—	10-15	In, Ga 9	76-81	White

Ag, *Silver*; Au, *gold*; Cu, *copper*; Fe, *iron*; Ga, *gallium*; In, *indium*; Pd, *palladium*; Pt, *platinum*; Re, *rhenium*; Ru, *ruthenium*; Sn, *tin*.

TABLE 10.11   Properties and Casting Temperatures of Noble Alloys Used in Ceramic-Metal Restorations

Type	Ultimate Tensile Strength (MPa)	Yield Strength at 0.2% Offset (MPa)	Elastic Modulus (GPa)	Elongation (%)	VHN (kg/mm^2)	Density (g/cm^3)	Casting Temperature (° C)
Au-Pt-Pd	480-500	400-420	81-96	3-10	175-180	17.4-18.6	1150
Au-Pd	700-730	550-575	100-117	8-16	210-230	13.5-13.7	1320-1330
Au-Pd-Ag	650-680	475-525	100-113	8-18	210-230	13.6-13.8	1320-1350
Pd-Ag	550-730	400-525	95-117	10-14	185-235	10.7-11.1	1310-1350
Pd-Cu	690-1300	550-1100	94-97	8-15	350-400	10.6-10.7	1170-1190

Ag, *Silver*; Au, *gold*; Cu, *copper*; Pd, *palladium*; Pt, *platinum*; VHN, *Vickers hardness number.*

From Table 10-11 it is seen that these alloys have high stiffness (elastic modulus), strength, and hardness and reasonable elongation; however, they have somewhat low sag resistance. The alloys are very costly because of their high noble-metal content and high density; they are sold on a weight basis but used on a volume basis. The casting temperature is reasonably high, and although reasonably easy to solder, care must be taken because the soldering temperature is only about 50° C below the melting range of the alloys. Finally, although considerable platinum and palladium are present, these alloys are still yellow, which makes producing pleasing esthetics with the ceramic easier than with white alloys.

Au-Pd ALLOYS

The Au-Pd high-noble alloys with good corrosion resistance have decreased gold but increased palladium content. These alloys contain no platinum or iron and thus are solution- rather than precipitation-hardened. They contain indium for bonding, gallium (Ga) to decrease the fusion temperature, rhenium for grain refining, and ruthenium (Ru) for castability. Because of their high palladium content, the alloys are white (some call it gray) rather than yellow, even though they contain about 50% gold. This color causes increased difficulty in producing esthetic restorations.

These alloys are stronger, stiffer, and harder than the Au-Pt-Pd alloys and have higher elongation (more ductile) and casting temperatures (easier to solder). They have lower densities, and when introduced they were less costly than the Au-Pt-Pd alloys, because palladium was cheaper than gold. With palladium now being more costly than gold, there is no longer a cost advantage. The decrease in density indicates more care should be taken during casting because of the decrease in the force with which the alloy enters the casting ring. However, these alloys are easy to cast, and soldering is easy because of the higher casting temperature.

Au-Pd-Ag ALLOYS

The Au-Pd-Ag alloys contain less palladium than the Au-Pd alloys; the decrease is made up by adding silver. However, they still have good corrosion resistance. Again, indium and tin are added for bonding with the ceramics, ruthenium for castability, and rhenium for grain refining. Hardening results from solution hardening. As seen in Table 10-11, the properties of the Au-Pd-Ag alloys are similar to those of the Au-Pd alloys.

Pd-Ag ALLOYS

The Pd-Ag alloys, which contain no gold and have a moderately high silver content, have the lowest noble-metal content of the five noble alloys. They contain indium and tin for bonding and ruthenium for castability. Their properties are similar to those of the Au-Pd-Ag alloys, except they are less dense ($\approx$11 g/cm^3 versus 14 g/cm^3). Some ceramics used with these high-gold alloys resulted in what was called "greening" really a color shift toward yellow. Contamination and technique were blamed to some extent for this problem.

Pd-Cu ALLOYS

The Pd-Cu alloys contain very high palladium content with 10% to 15% copper. They contain indium for bonding and gallium for controlling casting temperature. These alloys have high strength and hardness, moderate stiffness and elongation, and low density. However, they have low sag resistance and form dark oxides. They are white alloys, like all the other metals except the yellow Au-Pt-Pd alloys.

BASE-METAL ALLOYS

Base-metal alloys are used extensively in dentistry for a variety of restorations and instruments, as shown in Box 10-1. Cast cobalt-chromium alloys have been used for many years for fabricating removable dental prosthesis frameworks and have replaced type IV gold alloys almost completely for this application. Nickel-chromium and cobalt-chromium alloys are used in ceramic-metal restorations.

The addition of beryllium to base metal alloys improves its castability by lowering the alloy's melting temperature and surface tension and increasing the strength of the porcelain-metal bond. However, beryllium, in vapor or particulate form, is associated with several diseases, including contact dermatitis, chronic lung disease, lung carcinoma, and osteosarcoma. Laboratory personnel are at greatest risk for beryllium exposure when performing melting, grinding, polishing, and finishing procedures. The safety standard for pure beryllium dust is 2 μg/m^3 of air for a time-weighted, 8-hour day. A higher limit of 25 μg/m^3 is allowed for a minimum exposure time of less than 30 minutes. Efficient local exhaust and filtration systems as well as adequate general ventilation should be used when casting, finishing, and polishing these beryllium-containing alloys. The ADA Council on Scientific Affairs recommends that, where possible, beryllium-containing alloys should not be used in the fabrication of dental restorations. If alloys containing beryllium must be used, the OSHA (Occupational Safety and Health Administration) guideline (OSHA Hazard Information Bulletin 02-04-19) must be followed. Several manufacturers

---

BOX 10.1

Dental Applications of Cast and Wrought Base–Metal Alloys

Cast cobalt-chromium alloys
    Removable dental prosthesis framework
    Ceramic-metal restorations
Cast nickel-chromium alloys
    Ceramic-metal restorations
Cast titanium and titanium alloys
    Crowns
    Fixed partial prosthesis
    Removable dental prosthesis framework
    Implants
Wrought titanium and titanium alloys
    Implants
    Crowns
    Fixed partial prosthesis

Wrought stainless steel alloys
    Endodontic instruments
    Orthodontic wires and brackets
    Preformed crowns
Wrought cobalt-chromium-nickel alloys—
    orthodontic wires and endodontic files
Wrought nickel-titanium alloys—orthodontic wires
    and endodontic files

---

have eliminated beryllium content in their alloys. The ISO standard limits beryllium content to 0.02 wt%. The Food and Drug Administration (FDA) has accepted the ISO standard but has grandfathered beryllium-containing alloys on the market before 1976. Beryllium-containing alloys are not emphasized in this chapter.

The presence of nickel in nickel-chromium alloys and stainless steel is of significant importance because it is a known allergen. The incidence of allergic sensitivity to nickel has been reported to be from 5 to 10 times higher for females than for males, with 5% to 8% of females showing sensitivity. However, no correlation has been found between the presence of intraoral nickel-based restorations and sensitivity. A cobalt-chromium alloy without nickel or other non-nickel-containing alloy should be used on patients with a medical history indicating an allergic response to nickel. The safety standard for pure nickel is 15 $\mu g/m^3$ of air for a 40-hour week. The amount of nickel in base metal alloys used in direct soft tissue contact, such as in removable dental prosthesis frameworks is diminishing. Nickel is mostly found in alloys for ceramic-metal restorations and for wrought applications such as wires. To minimize exposure of patients to metallic dust containing nickel or beryllium, intraoral finishing should be done with a high-speed evacuation system and preferably in a wet environment.

The use of titanium and titanium alloys is rapidly increasing for implants, orthodontic wires, and endodontic files. Stainless steel alloys are used principally for orthodontic wires, in fabricating endodontic instruments, and for preformed crowns.

General Requirements of a Dental Base-Metal Alloy

The metals and alloys used as substitutes for noble alloys in dental restorations must possess certain minimal fundamental characteristics:

1. The alloy's chemical nature should not produce harmful toxicologic or allergic effects in the patient or the operator.
2. The chemical properties of the prosthesis should provide resistance to corrosion and physical changes when in the oral fluids.
3. The physical and mechanical properties, such as thermal conductivity, melting temperature, coefficient of thermal expansion, and strength, should all be satisfactory, meeting certain minimum values and being variable for various prostheses.
4. The technical expertise needed for fabrication and use should be feasible for the average dentist and skilled technician.
5. The metals, alloys, and companion materials for fabrication should be plentiful, relatively inexpensive, and readily available, even in periods of emergency.

When base-metal alloys are used in ceramic-metal systems, the same requirements as listed for noble alloys apply.

This list of requirements for the ideal substitute for noble alloys calls attention to the fact that a combination of chemical, physical, mechanical, and biological qualities is involved in the evaluation of each alloy. Properties depend on material, compositional, and processing factors.

Cast and wrought base-metal alloys, including cobalt-chromium-nickel, nickel-chromium-iron, commercially pure titanium, titanium-aluminum-vanadium, stainless steel, nickel-titanium, and titanium-molybdenum (beta-titanium) alloys are discussed in this section. The discussion is based on the synergistic relationship between processing, composition, structure, and properties of the materials.

Cobalt-Chromium and Nickel-Chromium Casting Alloys for Removable Dental Prostheses

Almost all metal frameworks of removable dental prostheses are made from cobalt-chromium alloys.

ANSI/ADA Specification No. 14 (ISO 6871)

According to ANSI/ADA specification No. 14, the weight of chromium should be no less than 20%, and the total weight of chromium, cobalt, and nickel should be no less than 85%. Alloys having other compositions may also be accepted by the ADA, provided the alloys comply satisfactorily with requirements on toxicity, hypersensitivity, and corrosion. Elemental composition to the nearest 0.5% must be marked on the package, along with the presence and percentage of hazardous elements and

recommendations for processing the materials. The specification also requires minimum values for elongation (1.5%), yield strength (500 MPa), and elastic modulus (170 GPa).

An important feature of this specification is that it made available a standardized method of testing, which has, in turn, made it possible to compare results from one investigation with those of another.

Composition
PRINCIPAL ELEMENTS

The principal elements present in cast base metals for removable dental prostheses are chromium, cobalt, and nickel, which together account for 82 to 92 wt% of most alloys used for dental restorations. Representative compositions of five commercial dental casting alloys, including three that are used for ceramic-metal restorations, are listed in Table 10-12. Chromium, cobalt, and nickel compose about 85% of the total weight of these alloys, yet their effect on the physical properties is rather limited. As discussed in this chapter, the physical properties of these alloys are controlled by the presence of minor alloying elements such as carbon, molybdenum, tungsten, manganese, nitrogen, tantalum, gallium, and aluminum.

TABLE 10.12   Composition of Major Cast Base-Metal Alloys Used in Dentistry

Elements	Alloy (% weight)					
	Vitallium*	Ticonium*	Ni-Cr Alloy with Be[†]	Ni-Cr Alloy without Be[†]	Co-Cr Alloy[†]	Co-Cr with Some Noble Metals[‡]
Chromium (Cr)	30	17	13	22	26	20
Cobalt (Co)	Balance	—	—	—	Balance	Balance
Nickel (Ni)	—	Balance	Balance	Balance	—	—
Molybdenum (Mo)	5	5	5.5	9	6	4
Tungsten (W)	—	—	—	—	5	—
Niobium (Nb)	—	—	—	3.5	—	—
Aluminum (Al)	—	5	2.5	0.25	—	2
Iron (Fe)	1	0.5	—	1.75	0.5	—
Carbon (C)	0.5	0.1	<0.1	<0.1	<0.1	<0.1
Beryllium (Be)	—	1.0	1.9	—	—	—
Silicon (Si)	0.6	0.5	—	0.6	1	—
Manganese (Mn)	0.5	5	—	0.3	—	4
Gold (Au)	—	—	—	—	—	2
Gallium (Ga)	—	—	—	—	—	6
Rare earth	—	—	—	—	0.5	<0.25

*Data from Asgar K: An overall study of partial dentures, USPHS Research Grant DE-02017. National Institute of Health (NIH): Washington, DC; Baran G: J. Prosthet. Dent. 50, 539, 1983.
[†]Typical alloy compositions for ceramic-metal restorations with conventional porcelains.
[‡]Alloy suitable for high-expansion porcelain.

FUNCTION OF VARIOUS ALLOYING ELEMENTS

Chromium is responsible for the tarnish and corrosion resistance of these alloys. When the chromium content of an alloy is higher than 30%, the alloy is more difficult to cast. With this percentage of chromium, the alloy also forms a brittle phase, known as the *sigma* (σ) *phase*. Therefore, cast base-metal dental alloys should not contain more than 28% or 29% chromium. In general, cobalt and nickel, up to a certain percentage, are interchangeable elements. Cobalt increases the elastic modulus, strength, and hardness of the alloy more than does nickel.

The effect of other alloying elements on the properties of these alloys is much more pronounced. One of the most effective ways of increasing the hardness of cobalt-based alloys is by increasing their carbon content. A change in the carbon content of approximately 0.2% changes the properties to such an extent that the alloy would no longer be usable in dentistry. For example, if the carbon content is increased by 0.2% over the desired amount, the alloy becomes too hard and brittle and should not be used for making any dental prostheses. Conversely, a reduction of 0.2% in the carbon content would reduce the alloy's yield and ultimate tensile strengths to such low values that, once again, the alloy would not be usable in dentistry. Furthermore, almost all elements in these alloys, such as chromium, silicon, molybdenum, cobalt, and nickel, react with carbon to form carbides, which change the properties of the alloys. Note that, as shown in Table 10-12, the nickel-chromium alloys used with ceramic contain significantly less carbon than the alloys used for removable dental prostheses. The presence of 3% to 6% molybdenum contributes to the strength of the alloys.

Microstructure of Cast Base-Metal Alloys

The microstructure of any substance is the basic factor that controls properties. In other words, a change in the physical properties of a material is a strong indication that there must have been some alteration in its microstructure. Sometimes this variation in microstructure cannot be distinguished by ordinary means. Neither cobalt-chromium nor nickel-chromium alloys have simple microstructures, and their microstructures change with slight alterations of manipulative conditions.

The microstructure of cobalt-chromium alloys in the cast condition is inhomogeneous, consisting of an austenitic matrix composed of a solid solution of cobalt and chromium in a cored dendritic structure. The dendritic regions are cobalt-rich, whereas the interdendritic regions can be a quaternary mixture consisting of a cobalt-rich γ-phase; a chromium-rich $M_{23}C_6$ phase, where M is Co, Cr, or Mo; an M_7C_3 carbide phase; and a chromium- and molybdenum-rich

σ-phase. Interdendritic casting porosity is also associated with this structure.

Many elements present in cast base-metal alloys, such as chromium, cobalt, and molybdenum, are carbide-forming elements. Depending on the composition of a cast base-metal alloy and its manipulative condition, it may form many types of carbide. Furthermore, the arrangement of these carbides may also vary depending on the manipulative condition.

The microstructure of a commercial cobalt-chromium alloy is illustrated in Figure 10-12. In Figure 10-12, *A*, the carbides are continuous along the grain boundaries. Such a structure is obtained when the metal is cast as soon as it is completely melted. In this condition, the cast alloy possesses low elongation values with a good and clean surface. Carbides that are spherical and discontinuous, like islands, are shown in Figure 10-12, *B*. Such a structure can be obtained if the alloy is heated about 100° C above its normal melting temperature; this results in a casting with good elongation values but with a very poor surface because of an increased reaction with the investment. The surface is so poor that the casting cannot be used in dentistry.

Dark eutectoid areas, which are lamellar in nature, are shown in Figure 10-12, *C*. Such a structure is responsible for very low elongation values but a good and clean casting. From these three examples, it is clear that microstructure can strongly affect physical and mechanical properties. The microstructure of Ni-Cr alloys is strongly dependent on alloy composition.

Alloys not containing Be have complicated, multiphase microstructures such as that shown in Figure 10-12, *E*. The precipitates dispersed within the matrix include complex carbides, and, in alloys where niobium (Nb) is present, Mo-Nb-Si compounds. All these precipitates are relatively unaffected by the short heat-treatment cycles that the alloys are subjected to during the ceramic firing procedures.

Heat Treatment of Base-Metal Alloys

The early base-metal alloys used in removable dental prostheses were primarily cobalt-chromium and were relatively simple. Heat-treating these alloys up to 1 hour at 1000° C did not change their mechanical properties appreciably. Base-metal alloys available today for removable dental prostheses, however, are more complex. Presently, complex cobalt-chromium alloys, nickel-chromium, and iron-chromium alloys are used for this purpose.

Studies have shown that many heat treatments of cobalt-based alloys reduce both the yield strength and elongation. If for any reason some soldering or welding must be performed on these removable dental prostheses, the lowest possible temperature should be used with the shortest possible time of heating to the elevated temperature.

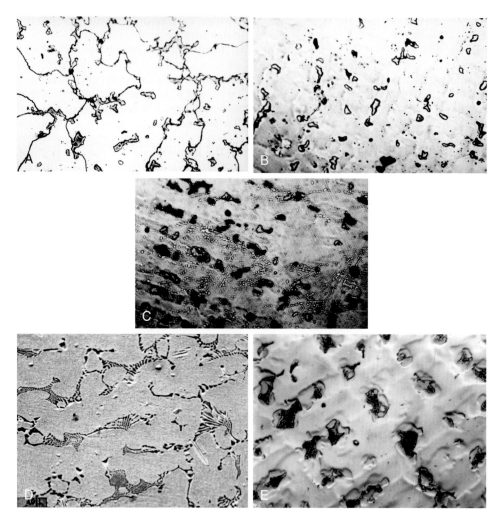

FIGURE 10.12 **Microstructure of alloys. A,** Cast cobalt-chromium alloy, where the carbides are continuous around the grain boundaries. **B,** The island-like structures are carbides, which are dispersed throughout the entire area. **C,** The dark areas are eutectoid, which are lamellar in nature. **D,** The microstructure of a beryllium-containing nickel-chromium alloy. **E,** The microstructure of a boron- and silicon-containing nickel-chromium alloy. (*A, B, and C from Asgar K, Peyton FA: J. Dent. Res. 40, 68, 1961; **D** and **E,** Courtesy of G. Baran, Temple University.*)

Physical Properties
MELTING TEMPERATURE

The melting temperature of base-metal alloys differs significantly from that of dental gold casting alloys. Most base-metal alloys melt at temperatures of 1150° to 1500° C, as compared with cast gold alloy types I to IV, which have a melting range of 800° to 1050° C.

DENSITY

The average density of cast base-metal alloys is between 7 and 8 g/cm^3, which is about half the density of most dental gold alloys. Density is of some importance in bulky maxillary prostheses, in which the force of gravity causes the relative weight of the casting to place additional forces on the supporting teeth. With certain prostheses, therefore, the reduction of weight resulting from the lower density of the cast base-metal alloys can be considered an advantage.

Mechanical Properties

Typical mechanical properties of the removable dental prothesis alloys listed in Table 10-12 have been assembled in Table 10-13, together with a representative range of values for type IV casting gold alloys subjected to a hardening heat treatment.

YIELD STRENGTH

The yield strength gives an indication of when a permanent deformation of a device or part of a device, such as a clasp, will occur. As such, it is one

TABLE 10.13   Mechanical Properties of Alloys Used in Removable Dental Prostheses

	Yield Strength at 0.2% Offset (MPa)	Tensile Strength (MPa)	Elongation (%)	Elastic Modulus (GPa)	Vickers Hardness Number (kg/mm²)
Cast base-metal alloys*					
Vitallium	644	870	1.5	218	380
Ticonium	710	807	2.4	186	340
Hardened removable dental prosthesis gold alloys†	480-510	700-760	5-7	90-100	220-250

*Data from Asgar K, Techow BO, Jacobson JM: J. Prosthet. Dent. 23, 36, 1970; Morris HF, Asgar K: J. Prosthet. Dent. 33, 36, 1975; Moffa JP, Lugassy AA, Guckes AD, et al: J. Prosthet. Dent. 30, 424, 1973.
†Data from Oilo G, Gjerdet NR: Acta. Odontal. Scand. 41, 111, 1983.

of the important properties of alloys intended for removable dental prostheses. It is believed that dental alloys should have yield strengths of at least 415 MPa to withstand permanent deformation when used as removable prosthesis clasps. It may be seen from Table 10-13 that base-metal dental alloys have yield strengths greater than 600 MPa.

TENSILE STRENGTH

The ultimate tensile strength of cast base-metal alloys is less influenced by variations in specimen preparation and test conditions than are some other properties, such as elongation. Table 10-13 shows that the ultimate tensile strength of cast base-metal dental alloys is greater than 800 MPa. Table 10-13 also demonstrates that hardened removable dental prosthesis gold alloys can have ultimate tensile strengths almost equal to those of cast base-metal alloys.

ELONGATION

The percent elongation of an alloy is important as an indication of the relative brittleness or ductility a restoration will exhibit. There are many occasions, therefore, when elongation is an important property for comparison of alloys for removable dental prostheses. For example, as described in Chapter 4, the combined effect of elongation and ultimate tensile strength is an indication of toughness of a material. Because of their toughness, removable dental prosthesis clasps cast of alloys with a high elongation and tensile strength do not fracture in service as often as do those with low elongation.

The percent elongation is one of the properties critical to accurate testing and to proper control during test preparation. For example, a small amount of microporosity in the test specimen will decrease the elongation considerably, whereas its effect on yield strength, elastic modulus, and tensile strength is rather limited. One can therefore assume that practical castings may exhibit similar variations in elongation from one casting to another. To some degree this

is borne out in practice, with some castings from the same product showing a greater tendency toward brittleness than others. This observation indicates that control of the melting and casting variables is of extreme importance if reproducible results are to be obtained.

Although nickel and cobalt are interchangeable in cobalt-nickel-chromium alloys, increasing the nickel content with a corresponding reduction in cobalt generally increases the ductility and elongation. High values of elongation are obtained by casting at the normal melting temperature and by not heating the alloy 100° C above its normal casting temperature. High elongation is achieved without sacrificing strength and is the result of the precise and proper combination of carbon, nitrogen, silicon, manganese, and molybdenum content.

ELASTIC MODULUS

The higher the elastic modulus, the more rigid a structure can be expected, provided the dimensions of the casting are the same in both instances. Some dental professionals recommend the use of a well-designed, rigid prosthesis because it properly distributes forces on the supporting tissues when in service. With a greater elastic modulus, one can design the restoration with slightly reduced dimensions. From Table 10-13, it can be seen that the elastic modulus of base-metal alloys is approximately double the modulus of type IV cast dental gold alloys.

HARDNESS

Differences in composition of the cast base-metal alloys have some effect on their hardness, as indicated by the values given in Table 10-13. In general, cast base-metal alloys have hardness values about one third greater than gold alloys used for the same purpose.

Hardness is an indication of the ease of finishing the structure and its resistance to scratching in service. The higher hardness of the cast base-metal alloys as compared with gold alloys requires the use of different polishing equipment and compounds, which may be considered a disadvantage, but the finishing operation can be completed without difficulty by experienced operators.

FATIGUE

The fatigue resistance of alloys used for removable dental prostheses is important when it is considered that these prostheses are placed and removed daily. At these times, the clasps are strained as they slide around the retaining tooth, and the alloy undergoes fatigue. Comparisons among cobalt-chromium, titanium, and gold alloys shows that cobalt-chromium alloys possess superior fatigue resistance, as indicated by a higher number of cycles required to fracture a clasp. Any procedures that result in increasing the porosity or carbide content of the alloy will reduce fatigue resistance. Also, soldered joints, which often contain inclusions or pores, represent weak links in the fatigue resistance of the prosthesis.

Corrosion

Recent research on dental casting alloys has been dominated by studies on corrosion and potential biological effects of metal ion release. In general, in vitro corrosion tests have evaluated a number of important variables, including effects of electrolytic media and artificial saliva, alloy composition, alloy microstructure, and surface state of the metal. These variables account for 2 to 4 orders of magnitude variation in the amount of species released. The surface state of the metal is an extremely important factor influencing corrosion, because the surface composition is almost always different from that of the bulk alloy.

Another important consideration is corrosion coupled with wear. Up to three times the mass of metal ions, such as nickel (Ni), is released during occlusal rubbing in combination with corrosion than during corrosion alone for nickel-chromium (Ni-Cr) alloys. No long-term studies have been performed to monitor the impact of the release of such large concentrations of metal ions on the overall health of patients.

Base-Metal Casting Alloys for Fixed Prosthodontics

Most of the nickel-chromium alloys contain 60% to 80% nickel, 10% to 27% chromium, and 2% to 14% molybdenum. As a comparison, cobalt-chromium alloys contain 53% to 67% cobalt, 25% to 32% chromium, and 2% to 6% molybdenum. They may also contain small amounts of aluminum, carbon, cobalt, copper, cerium, gallium, iron, manganese, niobium, silicon, tin, titanium, and zirconium. The range of compositions of base metal alloys for ceramic-metal restorations are given in Table 10-14, and typical properties of these alloys are listed in Table 10-15. Considerable variation in composition and properties are shown in these tables.

Base-metal casting alloys exhibit a higher hardness and elastic modulus than do noble alloys, but they require a slightly different approach in casting and soldering to accommodate their higher solidification shrinkage and generally lower densities than noble alloys.

NICKEL-CHROMIUM (Ni-Cr) ALLOYS

Chromium provides tarnish and corrosion resistance, whereas alloys containing aluminum (Al) are strengthened by the formation of coherent

TABLE 10.14 Composition Ranges of Base Metals for Ceramic-Metal Restorations (wt%)

Type	Ni	Cr	Co	Ti	Mo	Al	V	Fe	Be	Ga	Mn	Nb	W	B	Ru
Ni-Cr	69-77	13-16	—	—	4-14	0-4	—	0-1	0-2	0-2	0-1	—	—	—	—
Co-Cr	—	15-25	55-58	—	0-4	0-2	—	0-1	—	0-7	—	0-3	0-5	0-1	0-6
Ti	—	—	—	90-100	—	0-6	0-4	0-0.3	—	—	—	—	—	—	—

Al, *Aluminum*; B, *boron*; Be, *beryllium*; Co, *cobalt*; Cr, *chromium*; Fe, *iron*; Ga, *gallium*; Mo, *molybdenum*; Mn, *manganese*; Nb, *niobium*; Ni, *nickel*; Ru, *ruthenium*; Ti, *titanium*; V, *vanadium*; W, *tungsten*.

TABLE 10.15 Properties of Base-Metal Alloys for Ceramic-Metal Restorations

Type	Ultimate Tensile Strength (MPa)	Yield Strength at 0.2% Offset (MPa)	Elastic Modulus (GPa)	Elongation (%)	VHN (kg/mm^2)	Density (g/cm^3)	Casting Temperature (° C)
Ni-Cr	400-1000	255-730	150-210	8-20	210-380	7.5-7.7	1300-1450
Co-Cr	520-820	460-640	145-220	6-15	330-465	7.5-7.6	1350-1450
Ti	240-890	170-830	103-114	10-20	125-350	4.4-4.5	1760-1860

Co, *Cobalt*; Cr, *chromium*; Ni, *nickel*; Ti, *titanium*; VHN, *Vickers hardness number*.

precipitates of Ni_3Al. Molybdenum (Mo) is added to decrease the thermal coefficient of expansion. Note that because of the wide differences in atomic weight of nickel, and chromium, 2 wt% is roughly equal to 6 at%.

These alloys are harder than noble alloys but usually have lower yield strengths. They also have higher elastic moduli, and it was hoped thinner copings and frameworks could result. They have much lower densities (7 to 8 g/cm^3) and generally higher casting temperatures. Adequate casting compensation is at times a problem, as is the fit of the coping.

COBALT-CHROMIUM (Co-Cr) ALLOYS

Again, chromium provides tarnish and corrosion resistance. Unlike Co-Cr removable dental prosthesis alloys, the alloys for ceramic-metal restorations are strengthened by solution hardening rather than carbide formation. Molybdenum helps lower the coefficient of expansion, and ruthenium improves castability. Co-Cr alloys are stronger and harder than noble and Ni-Cr alloys and have roughly the same densities and casting temperature as Ni-Cr alloys. Casting and soldering of these alloys is more difficult than for noble alloys, as is obtaining a high degree of accuracy in the castings.

TITANIUM (Ti) AND TITANIUM ALLOYS

Pure titanium (Ti) and titanium alloyed with aluminum and vanadium (Ti-6Al-4V) may become important for cast restorations in the future, but they are currently important only in implant and orthodontic wire applications. They have superior biocompatibility compared with the other base metal alloys, but Ti and Ti-6Al-4V present processing difficulties, as indicated by their casting temperatures of $1760°$ to $1860°$ C, low densities, and ease of oxidation. Newer techniques, such as machine duplication and spark erosion to fabricate copings, may increase the use of these metals. Additional discussion of titanium and titanium alloys appear below.

Other Applications of Cast Base-Metal Alloys

Cast cobalt-chromium alloys serve a useful purpose in prostheses other than removable dental prostheses. In the surgical repair of bone fractures, alloys of this type have been used for bone plates, screws, various fracture appliances, and splints. Metallic obturators and implants for various purposes can be formed from cast base-metal alloys. The use of cobalt-chromium alloys for surgical purposes is well established, and these alloys have numerous oral surgical uses. They can be implanted directly into the bone structure for long periods without harmful reactions. This favorable response of the tissue is probably attributable to the low solubility and electrogalvanic action of the alloy; the metal is inert and produces no inflammatory response. The product known as surgical Vitallium is used extensively for this purpose. The primary metal used in dental implants today is titanium (see Chapter 16).

Advanced rapid manufacturing technology called *direct metal laser sintering (DMLS)* is being used to create pure cobalt-chrome crowns and fixed dental prosthesis frameworks. This method uses a high-power laser to fuse successive 0.02-mm-thick layers of powdered metal. After all layers are built, the solid copings and frameworks are removed from the machine, sand blasted, polished, and cleaned, ready for ceramic application. Cobalt-chrome can also be machined using computer aided design and manufacturing processes. High-speed milling machines under numerical control reproduce geometries created in software originating from scanners or other dental computer-aided design (CAD) systems. These devices process zirconium, cobalt-chromium, titanium, and plastics. Five-axis machining enables the creation of embrasures, undercuts, and other intricate geometries without the need for manual trimming and adjustment.

Titanium and Titanium Alloys

Titanium's resistance to electrochemical degradation; benign biological response elicited; relatively light weight; and low density, low modulus, and high strength make titanium-based materials attractive for use in dentistry. Titanium forms a very stable oxide layer with a thickness on the order of angstroms, and it repassivates in a time on the order of nanoseconds (10^{-9} second). This oxide formation is the basis for the corrosion resistance and biocompatibility of titanium. Titanium has therefore been called the material of choice in dentistry.

Commercially pure titanium (CP Ti) is used for dental implants, surface coatings, and more recently, for crowns, partial removable dental prostheses, and orthodontic wires. Several titanium alloys are also used. Of these alloys, Ti-6Al-4V is the most widely used. Wrought alloys of titanium and nickel and titanium and molybdenum are used for orthodontic wires. The term *titanium* is often used to include all types of pure and alloyed titanium. However, it should be noted that the processing, composition, structure, and properties of the various titanium alloys are quite different, and also that differences exist between the wrought and cast forms of a given type of titanium.

Commercially Pure Titanium

Commercially pure titanium (CP Ti) is available in four grades, which vary according to the oxygen (0.18 to 0.40 wt%) and iron (0.20 to 0.50 wt%) content (Table 10-16). These apparently slight concentration

TABLE 10.16   Composition of CP Titanium and Alloy (weight percent)

Titanium	N	C	H	Fe	O	Al	V	Ti
CP grade I	0.03	0.10	0.015	0.02	0.18			balance
CP grade II	0.03	0.10	0.015	0.03	0.25			balance
CP grade III	0.03	0.10	0.015	0.03	0.35			balance
CP grade IV	0.03	0.10	0.015	0.05	0.40			balance
Ti-6Al-4V alloy	0.05	0.08	0.012	0.25	0.13	5.50-6.50	3.50-4.50	balance

C, *Carbon*; CP, *commercially pure*; Fe, *iron*; H, *hydrogen*; N, *nitrogen*; O, *oxygen*; Ti, *titanium. Data from McCracken M. J Prosthodont 1999 8(1):40-43.*

TABLE 10.17   Mechanical Properties of Titanium and Other Selected Materials

Material	Elastic Modulus (GPa)	Ultimate Tensile Strength (MPa)	Yield Strength (MPa)
316L SS	200	965	690
Co-Cr-Mo	240	700	450
Type IV gold	90	770	>340
CP grade 1 Ti	102	240	170
CP grade 4 Ti	104	550	483
Ti-6Al-4V	113	930	860

Co, *cobalt*; CP, *commercially pure*; Cr, *chromium*; Mo, *molybdenum*; Ti, *titanium*.
Data from McCracken M: *J Prosthodont* 8(1):40-43, 1999 and Wataha J: *J Prosth Dent* 87:351-63, 2002.

differences have a substantial effect on the physical and mechanical properties.

At room temperature, CP Ti has a hexagonal close-packed (HCP) crystal lattice, which is denoted as the alpha (α) phase. On heating, an allotropic phase transformation occurs. At 883° C, a body-centered cubic (BCC) phase, which is denoted as the beta (β) phase, forms. A component with predominantly β phase is stronger but more brittle than a component with α-phase microstructure. As with other metals, the temperature and time of processing and heat treatment dictate the amount, ratio, and distribution of phases, overall composition and microstructure, and resultant properties. As a result, casting temperature and cooling procedure are critical factors in ensuring a successful casting.

The density of CP Ti (4.5 g/cm³) is about half the value of many of the other base metals. The modulus (100 GPa) is also about half the value of the other base metals. The yield and ultimate strengths vary, respectively, from 170 to 480 MPa and 240 to 550 MPa, depending on the grade of titanium. Table 10-17 lists the mechanical properties for CP grades 1 and 4 Ti for comparison with noble alloys and other base-metal alloys.

Titanium Alloys: General

Alloying elements are added to stabilize either the α or the β phase, by changing the β-transformation temperature. For example, in Ti-6Al-4V, aluminum is an α stabilizer, which expands the α-phase field by increasing the (α + β) to β-transformation temperature, whereas vanadium, as well as copper and palladium, are β stabilizers, which expand the β-phase field by decreasing the (α + β) to β-transformation temperature.

In general, alpha-titanium is weldable, but difficult to form or work with at room temperature. Beta-titanium, however, is malleable at room temperature and is thus used in orthodontics. The (α + β) alloys are strong and formable but difficult to weld. Thermal and thermochemical treatments can refine the postcast microstructures and improve properties.

Ti-6AL-4V

At room temperature, Ti-6Al-4V is a two-phase (α + β) alloy. At about 975° C, an allotropic phase transformation takes place, transforming the microstructure to a single-phase BCC β alloy. Thermal treatments dictate the relative amounts of the α and β phases and the phase morphologies and yield a variety of microstructures and a range of mechanical properties. Microstructural variations depend on whether working and heat treatments were performed above or below the β-transition temperature and on the cooling rate.

Following forging at temperatures in the range of 700° to 950° C, thermal treatments below the β-transition temperature (typically performed at approximately 700° C) produce recrystallized microstructures having fine equiaxed α grains (Figure 10-13). Equiaxed microstructures are characterized by small (3 to 10 µm), rounded grains that have aspect ratios near unity. This class of microstructure is recommended for Ti-6Al-4V surgical implants.

The mechanical properties of (α + β) titanium alloys are dictated by the amount, size, shape, and morphology of the α phase and the density of α/β interfaces. The tensile and fatigue properties of Ti-6Al-4V have been studied extensively.

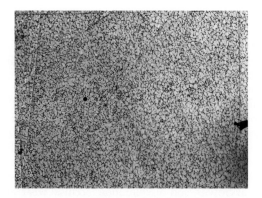

FIGURE 10.13 **Microstructure of equiaxed Ti-6Al-4V (×200).** Equiaxed microstructures are characterized by small, rounded α-grains, with aspect ratios near unity.

Microstructures with a small (less than 20 μm) α-grain size, a well-dispersed β phase, and a small α/β interface area, such as in equiaxed microstructures, resist fatigue crack initiation best and have the best high-cycle fatigue strength (approximately 500 to 700 MPa). Lamellar microstructures, which have a greater α/β surface area and more oriented colonies, have lower fatigue strengths (approximately 300 to 500 MPa) than do equiaxed microstructures.

Machined Titanium for Dental Implants

Endosseus dental implants are machined from billets of titanium. Typical materials are CP Ti or the Ti-6Al-4V alloy. Studies have been published on the potential for replacing vanadium with niobium, which might improve cell attachment. Recent research has focused on altering the surface texture of machined titanium to improve both the degree of osseointegration as well as improving the adaptation of soft tissue to the collar of the implant. To increase surface area for contact by bone cells, machined titanium can be grit blasted with metal oxide or hydroxyapatite particles. The surface can also be plasma sprayed with titanium or coated with hydroxyapatite. More discussion of implant surface modifications can be found in Chapter 16.

Cast Titanium

Based on the attributes, extensive knowledge, and clinical success of wrought titanium implants, interest has developed in cast titanium for dental applications. Although titanium has been cast for more than 50 years, only recently have nearly precision castings been attainable. For aerospace and medical components, hot isostatic pressing and specific finishing techniques are routinely practiced. However, these techniques are beyond the capabilities and affordability of most dental laboratories.

The two most important factors in casting titanium-based materials are its high melting point (1700° C for CP Ti) and chemical reactivity. Because of the high melting point, special melting procedures, cooling cycles, mold material, and casting equipment to prevent metal contamination are required. Titanium readily reacts with gaseous elements such as hydrogen, oxygen, and nitrogen, particularly at high temperatures (greater than 600° C). As a result, any manipulation of titanium at elevated temperatures must be performed in a well-controlled vacuum or inert atmosphere. Without such controls, titanium surfaces will be contaminated with α case, an oxygen-enriched and hardened surface layer, which can be as thick as 100 μm. Surface layers of this thickness reduce strength and ductility and promote cracking because of the embrittling effect of the oxygen. The technology required to overcome these factors is what makes casting titanium relatively more expensive.

Because of the high affinity titanium has for hydrogen, oxygen, and nitrogen, standard crucibles and investment materials cannot be used. Investment materials or face coats for the wax patterns must have oxides that are more stable than the very stable titanium oxide, and must also be able to withstand a temperature sufficient to melt titanium. If this is not the case, oxygen is likely to diffuse into the molten metal. Investment materials using a combination of ZrO_2 type face coat that is backed up by a phosphate-bonded silica investment or phosphate investment materials involving inert fillers (ZrO_2, Al_2O_3, MgO) achieve this goal.

Because of the low density of titanium, it is difficult to cast in conventional, centrifugal-force casting machines. In the last 10 to 15 years, advanced casting techniques, which combine centrifugal, vacuum, pressure, and gravity casting, new investment materials and advanced melting techniques (e.g., electric arc melting) have been developed. These advances have improved the feasibility of casting titanium-based materials in the dental laboratory.

Pure titanium and Ti-alloys such as Ti-6Al-4V have been cast into crowns, and removable dental prosthesis frameworks. Titanium alloys have a lower melting point than pure titanium. By alloying titanium, the melting temperature can be lowered to the same temperature as that of nickel-chromium and cobalt-chromium alloys. For example, the Ti-Pd and Ti-Cu alloys have melting points of 1350° C. Lower casting temperatures may also reduce the reactivity of titanium with oxygen and other gases. Other titanium alloys, such as Ti-6Al-4V, Ti-15V, Ti-20Cu, Ti-30Pd, Ti-Co, Ti-Cu, and Ti-Cu-Ni, are still in the experimental stages and have not yet been evaluated in any large clinical studies.

Microstructures of cast titanium materials are similar to those described previously, namely coarse lamellar grains, a result of slow cooling through the β to α or β to (α + β) transformation temperature (Figure 10-14).

The mechanical properties of cast CP Ti are similar to those of types III and IV gold alloy, whereas cast Ti-6Al-4V and Ti-15V exhibit properties, except for modulus, similar to those of nickel-chromium and cobalt-chromium alloys.

Recently, cast Ti-6Al-4V microstructures have been refined by temporary alloying with hydrogen. The resulting microstructures (Figure 10-15) can have α-grain sizes less than 1 μm, aspect ratios near unity, and discontinuous grain-boundary α, microstructural attributes that increase tensile and fatigue strength. These changes in microstructural form and structure result in significant increases in yield strength (974 to 1119 MPa), ultimate strength (1025 to 1152 MPa), and fatigue strength (643 to 669 MPa) as compared with respective values for lamellar (902, 994, and 497 MPa) and equiaxed microstructures (914, 1000, and 590 MPa).

Pure titanium has been cast with a pressure-vacuum casting machine. Other manufacturers have developed centrifugal casting machines that use

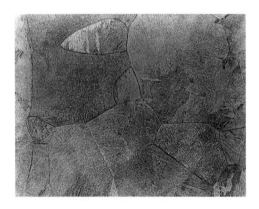

FIGURE 10.14 **Microstructure of as-cast Ti-6Al-4V.**

FIGURE 10.15 **Microstructure of hydrogen-alloy-treated Ti-6Al-4V (×200).**

an electric arc to melt the titanium in an argon or helium atmosphere. Melting is performed in a copper crucible, followed by centrifugal casting into a mold that uses investment. Such machines provide a relatively oxygen-free environment and, with the use of a tungsten arc, can reach temperatures of 2000° C. This latter casting regime has been used to cast CP Ti crowns. Crowns cast in this manner have been evaluated clinically, and results revealed that, although the fit was inferior to that of silver-palladium alloy, it was superior to that of nickel-chromium. Occlusal adjustment was no more difficult than with conventional crowns, and discoloration, occlusal wear, and plaque retention were similar to other metals.

Observations of randomly chosen cast crowns using old machines and silica-containing investments have revealed gross surface porosities, to a depth of 75 μm, on both the inside and outside of the surfaces. Mechanical polishing is insufficient to remove this porosity. Internal porosities, sometimes measuring up to 30% of the cross-sectional area, are also readily observed. Surfaces of castings can also be contaminated with α case. The cause of the α case is probably poor atmosphere control or contamination from crucible and mold materials. For optimum functionality of the final casting, the surface layer must be removed during finishing. However, even after the α case is removed, internal oxidation can remain and compromise the mechanical properties of the final prosthesis. Further examination of such castings has also revealed multiple microcracks at the edges of the margins. Some cracks are as long as 100 μm. Cracks of this length are catastrophic to a notch-sensitive material such as titanium.

As outlined, the difficulties with cast titanium for dental purposes include high melting point and high reactivity, low casting efficiency, inadequate expansion of investment, casting porosity, and difficulty in finishing this metal. From a technical standpoint, titanium is difficult to weld, solder, machine, finish, and adjust. Casting titanium requires expensive equipment.

Wrought Alloys

Alloys that are worked and adapted into prefabricated forms for use in dental restorations are described as *wrought alloys*. A wrought form is one that has been worked or shaped and fashioned into a serviceable form for a prosthesis (Figure 10-16). The work done to the alloy is usually at a temperature far below the solidus and is therefore referred to as *cold work*. Wrought forms may include precision attachments, backings for artificial teeth, and wire in various cross-sectional shapes. Wrought alloys are used in two ways in dental prostheses. First, they can be soldered to a previously cast restoration. An example is a wrought wire clasp on a removable dental prosthesis framework. Second, they can be embedded into a cast framework by casting to the alloy, as a precision attachment is cast to the retainer of a crown, bridge, or removable prosthesis. The physical properties required of the wrought alloy will depend on the technique used and the composition of the alloy in the existing prosthesis.

Microstructure

The microstructure of wrought alloys is fibrous. This fibrous structure results from the cold work applied during the operations that shape the alloy into its final form. Wires or other wrought forms normally have a measurable increase in tensile strength and hardness when compared with corresponding cast structures. The increase in these properties results from the entangled, fibrous internal structure created by the cold work.

Wrought forms will recrystallize during heating operations unless caution is exercised. During recrystallization, the fibrous microstructure is converted to a grained structure similar to the structure of a cast form. In general, the amount of recrystallization increases as both the heating time and temperature become excessive. For example, in most noble dental wires, a short heating cycle during the soldering operation is not sufficient to appreciably recrystallize the wire, even though the temperature approaches the fusion temperature. However, a prolonged heating period of 30 to 60 seconds or longer may cause recrystallization, depending on the time, temperature, alloy composition, and manner in which the

wire was fabricated. Recrystallization results in a reduction in mechanical properties in proportion to the amount of recrystallization. Severe recrystallization can cause wrought forms to become brittle in the area of recrystallization. Therefore, heating operations must be minimized when working with wrought forms.

Composition

By the current ADA definitions, all alloys used for wrought forms are high-noble alloys except one, which is a noble alloy (Table 10-18). As with the casting alloys, several strategies have been used to formulate alloys with appropriate properties. The compositions in Table 10-16 are not inclusive of all available wrought alloys, but are intended to demonstrate typical alloys. These compositions are designed to provide a range of melting ranges and mechanical properties that are appropriate for wrought alloy applications. The Pt-Au-Pd alloys contain primarily platinum with equal amounts (27 wt%) of palladium and gold. These PGP (platinum-gold-palladium) alloys have been commonly used as clasping wires on removable dental prostheses. The Au-Pt-Pd alloys are primarily gold with platinum and palladium. The Au-Pt-Cu-Ag, Au-Pt-Ag-Cu, and Au-Ag-Cu-Pd alloys contain approximately 60 wt% gold, but have adopted different strategies for the remaining 40% of the mass. The first two of these alloys contain about 15 wt% platinum with the balance in silver, copper, and palladium, whereas the third of these alloys contains no platinum and higher amounts of silver. The last alloy shown in Table 10-7 contains no appreciable gold or platinum, but consists of palladium and silver in approximately equal amounts with about 16 wt% copper. The Au-Ag-Cu-Pd wrought alloy (see Table 10-16) is similar to the Au-Cu-Ag-Pd-*II* casting alloy (see Table 10-5). These alloys differ only slightly in the

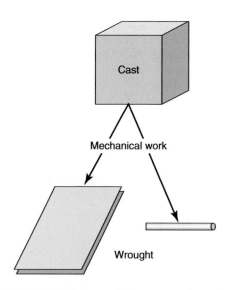

FIGURE 10.16 **Diagram of the process of mechanical work that transforms cast structures into wrought structures.** The microstructure and mechanical properties of cast and wrought forms are fundamentally different.

TABLE 10.18 Composition of Typical Wrought Dental Alloys (wt%)

Alloy	Ag	Au	Cu	Pd	Pt	Other
Pt-Au-Pd	—	27	—	27	45	
Au-Pt-Pd	—	60	—	15	24	Ir 1.0
Au-Pt-Cu-Ag	8.5	60	10	5.5	16	
Au-Pt-Ag-Cu	14	63	9	—	14	
Au-Ag-Cu-Pd	18.5	63	12	5	—	Zn 1.5
Pd-Ag-Cu	39	—	16	43	1	

Data from Lyman T: Metals handbook, vol 1. Properties and selection of metals, ed 8. American Society for Metals, Metals Park, Ohio, 1961.
Ag, Silver; Au, gold; Cu, copper; Ir, iridium; Pd, palladium; Pt, platinum; Zn, zinc.

gold/silver ratio. Other wrought alloys differ from the casting alloys primarily in their higher platinum contents and absence of iridium or ruthenium grain refiners. Platinum is added to increase the melting temperature of the alloys. The grain refinement is not necessary because these alloys are cold-worked into their final forms.

Properties

The properties of alloys used for wrought applications are shown in Table 10-19. The solidus of these alloys ranges from 875° C for Au-Ag-Cu-Pd to 1500° C for Pt-Au-Pd. If the wrought form is to be cast to or soldered to, the solidus must be sufficiently high so the form does not melt or lose its fibrous structure during burnout or casting operations. The solidus required will depend on the metals to be joined, the solder, and the burnout and casting temperatures to be used. In general, alloys with high solidus temperatures also have higher recrystallization temperatures. These alloys are mostly white because of the high platinum and palladium contents. Exceptions are the Au-Pt-Ag-Cu and Au-Ag-Cu-Pd alloys, which are light yellow and yellow, respectively. Yield strength, elongation, and hardness are properties relevant to wrought alloys (see Table 10-19). The wrought form must generally have yield strength low enough to allow for adjustment (of a clasp or attachment), but be high enough that permanent distortion does not occur in service. Furthermore, the elongation must be sufficient to allow for adjustment without fracture. Three of the wrought alloys shown in Table 10-19 can be hardened by formation of ordered phases. The Au-Pt-Ag-Cu and Au-Ag-Cu-Pd alloys are hardened by an Au-Cu ordered phase, whereas the Pd-Ag-Cu alloys are hardened by a Pd-Cu ordered phase. As with the casting alloys, the ordered phase imparts significantly more strength and hardness to the alloy and lower elongation.

Wrought Stainless Steel Alloys

Steel is an iron-carbon alloy. The term *stainless steel* is applied to alloys of iron and carbon that contain chromium, nickel, manganese, and perhaps other metals to improve properties and give the stainless quality to the steel. These alloys differ in composition from the cobalt-chromium, nickel-chromium, and titanium casting alloys. Usually, stainless steel alloys are not cast, but instead are used in the wrought form in dentistry, which represents the second way that stainless steel differs from the cast base-metal alloys. As a result, the types of prostheses formed from these two materials differ. The most common applications of stainless steel for dental purposes at present are in the preparation of orthodontic appliances and fabrication of endodontic instruments, such as files and reamers. Some specialized applications of stainless steel exist for temporary space maintainers, prefabricated crowns, or other prostheses placed in the mouth, and for various clinical and laboratory instruments.

Composition

Several broad classifications of stainless steel are generally recognized. The various groups are referred to as *ferritic, martensitic,* and *austenitic,* and they have different compositions, properties, and applications. The ferritic stainless steels are chromium steels employed in the manufacture of instruments or equipment parts in which some degree of tarnish resistance is desirable. A wide range of compositions is available in this group, in which amounts of chromium, the principal element contributing to stainless qualities, may vary from 15% to 25%. Elements such as carbon, silicon, and molybdenum are included but are all held within narrow limits.

The martensitic steels also are primarily chromium steels with a lower chromium content (about 12% to 18%). These steels can be hardened to some

TABLE 10.19   Properties of Typical Wrought Dental Alloys

Alloy	Solidus (° C)	Color	Property 0.2% Yield (Soft/Hard) (MPa)	Elongation (Soft/Hard) (%)	Vickers Hardness (Soft/Hard) (kg/mm^2)
Pt-Au-Pd	1500	White	750	14	270
Au-Pt-Pd	1400	White	450	20	180
Au-Pt-Cu-Ag	1045	White	400	35	190
Au-Pt-Ag-Cu	935	Light yellow	450/700	30/10	190/285
Au-Ag-Cu-Pd	875	Yellow	400/750	35/8	170/260
Pd-Ag-Cu	1060	White	515/810	20/12	210/300

Data from Lyman T: Metals handbook, vol. 1. Properties and Selection of Metals, ed 8. American Society for Metals, Metals Park, Ohio, 1961.
Ag, *Silver;* Au, *gold;* Cu, *copper;* Pd, *palladium;* Pt, *platinum.*

degree by heat treatment, and they have a moderate resistance to tarnish. They are used chiefly in the manufacture of instruments and, to a limited degree, for orthodontic appliances.

The austenitic steels represent the alloys used most extensively for dental prostheses. The most common austenitic steel used in dentistry is 18–8 stainless steel, so named because it contains approximately 18% chromium and 8% nickel. The carbon content is between 0.08% and 0.20%, and titanium, manganese, silicon, molybdenum, niobium, and tantalum are present in minor amounts to give important modifications to the properties. The balance (≈72%) is iron.

Function of Alloying Elements and Chemical Resistance

The corrosion resistance of stainless steel is attributed largely to the presence of chromium in the alloy, and no other element added to iron is as effective in producing resistance to corrosion. Iron cannot be used without chromium additions because iron oxide (Fe_2O_3), or rust, is not adherent to the bulk metal. About 11% chromium is needed to produce corrosion resistance in pure iron, and the necessary proportion is increased with the addition of carbon to form steel. Chromium resists corrosion well because of the formation of a strongly adherent coating of oxide on the surface, which prevents further reaction with the metal below the surface. The formation of such an oxide layer is called *passivation.* The surface coating is not visible, even at high magnification, but the film adds to the metallic luster of the metal. The degree of passivity is influenced by a number of factors, such as alloy composition, heat treatment, surface condition, stress in the prosthesis, and the environment in which the prosthesis is placed. In dental applications, the stainless characteristics of the alloys can therefore be altered or lost by excessive heating during assembly or adaptation; using abrasives or reactive cleaning agents, which can alter the surface conditions of the prosthesis; and even by poor oral hygiene practices over prolonged periods.

Of the stainless steel alloys in general use, the austenitic type of 18–8 stainless steel shows the greatest resistance to corrosion and tarnish. In these alloys, chromium and nickel form solid solutions with the iron, which gives corrosion protection. The chromium composition in these alloys must be between 13% and 28% for optimal corrosion resistance. If the chromium content is less than 13%, the adherent chromium oxide layer does not form. If there is more than 28% chromium, chromium carbides form at the grain boundaries, embrittling the steel. The amount of carbon must also be tightly controlled. If not, carbon will react

with chromium, forming these grain-boundary chromium-carbides, which lead to depletion of grain-boundary chromium and decrease corrosion resistance in a process known as *sensitization.* Molybdenum increases the resistance to pitting corrosion.

The elements present in small amounts tend to prevent the formation of carbides between the carbon present in the alloy and the iron or chromium and, as a result, often are described as *stabilizing elements.* Some steels, termed *stabilized stainless steels,* contain titanium, niobium, or tantalum, so the carbides that do form are titanium carbides rather than chromium carbides.

The chemical resistance of stainless steel alloys is improved if the surface is clean, smooth, and polished. Irregularities promote electrochemical action on the surface of the alloy. Soldering operations on stainless steel with gold and silver solder may contribute to a reduction in stainless qualities because of electrogalvanic action between dissimilar metals or because of localized, improper composition of the stainless steel wire.

Stress-Relieving Treatments

The 18–8 alloys are not subject to an increase in properties by heat treatment, but they do respond to strain hardening as a result of cold work during adjustment or adaptation of the alloy to form the prosthesis. Heat treatment above 650° C results in recrystallization of the microstructure, compositional changes, and formation of chromium-carbides, three factors that can reduce mechanical properties and corrosion resistance.

Prostheses formed from these alloys may, however, be subjected to a stress-relieving operation to remove the effects of cold working during fabrication, increase ductility, or produce some degree of hardening with some alloys. If heat treatment is to be performed, it should be held to temperatures between 400° and 500° C for 5 to 120 seconds, depending on the temperature, type of prosthesis, and alloy being heated. A time of 1 minute at 450° C would represent an average treatment to be used on an orthodontic appliance. Keep in mind that temperatures above 650° C will soften or anneal the alloy, and the properties cannot be restored by further treatment. The main advantage of a low-temperature heat-treating operation is that it establishes a uniformity of properties throughout the prosthesis after adaptation and fabrication, which may reduce the tendency toward breakage in service. Factors affecting an alloy's ability to be heat-treated and stress-relieved include alloy composition, working history (i.e., fabrication procedure), and the duration, temperature, and atmosphere of the heat treatment.

Wrought Nickel-Titanium Alloy

A wrought nickel-titanium alloy known as Nitinol is used as a wire for orthodontic appliances. Nitinol is characterized by its high resiliency, limited formability, and thermal memory.

Composition and Shape-Memory Effect

The industrial alloy is 55% nickel and 45% titanium and possesses a temperature transition range (TTR). At temperatures below the TTR, the alloy can be deformed plastically. When the alloy is then heated from below to above the TTR, a temperature-induced crystallographic transformation from a martensitic to an austenitic microstructure occurs and the alloy will return to its original shape. Hence, nickel-titanium is called a *shape-memory alloy.* The orthodontic alloy contains several percent cobalt to lower the TTR. A number of variations of the Ni-Ti alloy have been developed in dentistry. Compositional variations lead to changes in the martensitic and austenitic start and finish temperatures and mechanical properties. Only those wires with austenitic finish temperatures less than 37° C exhibit super-elasticity.

Properties and Manipulation

Mechanical properties of an orthodontic nickel-titanium alloy are compared with those of stainless steel and a beta-titanium alloy in tension, bending, and torsion in Table 10-20. The nickel-titanium alloy has the lowest elastic modulus and yield strength but the highest springback (maximum elastic deflection). As shown in Figures 10-17 and 10-18, nickel-titanium has the lowest spring rate but the highest resiliency in bending and torsion of the three alloys used for orthodontic wires. Clinically, the low elastic modulus and high resiliency mean that lower and more constant forces can be applied with activations and an increased working range. The high springback is important if large deflections are needed, such as with poorly aligned teeth. Nitinol wire requires special bending techniques and cannot be bent over a sharp edge or into a complete loop; thus the wire is more suited for use with pretorqued, preangulated brackets. The alloy is brittle and therefore cannot be soldered or welded, so wires must be joined mechanically.

Wrought Beta-Titanium Alloy

Composition and Microstructure

A titanium-molybdenum alloy known as *beta-titanium* is used as a wrought orthodontic wire. As discussed previously, CP Ti exists in a hexagonal, close-packed crystal lattice at temperatures below 883° C and in a body-centered cubic crystal lattice at higher temperatures. These structures are referred to

TABLE 10.20 Properties of Orthodontic Wires in Tension, Bending, and Torsion

Property	18-8 Stainless Steel	Nickel-Titanium	Beta-Titanium
TENSION			
Yield strength, 0.1% offset, MPa	1200	343	960
Elastic modulus, GPa	134	28.4	68.6
Springback (σ_s/E), 10^{-2}	0.89	1.40	1.22
BENDING			
Yield strength, 2.9 degree offset, MPa	1590	490	1080
Elastic modulus, GPa	122	32.3	59.8
Spring rate, mm-N/degree	0.80	0.17	0.37
TORSION			
Spring rate, mm-N/degree	0.078	0.020	0.035

Modified from Drake SR, Wayne DM, Powers JM, et al: Am. J. Orthod. 82, 206, 1982. Values are for a 0.43 × 0.64-mm rectangular wire.

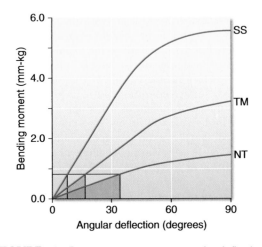

FIGURE 10.17 **Bending moment vs angular deflection.** Stored energy at a fixed bending moment below the proportional limit for 0.48-mm by 0.64-mm wires of alloys stainless steel (*SS*), beta- titanium (*TM*), and nickel-titanium (*NT*). The stored energy is equal to the shaded areas under the curve for each wire. The spring rate is equal to the slope of each curve. (*From Drake SR, Wayne DM, Powers JM, et al: Am. J. Orthod. 82, 206, 1982.*)

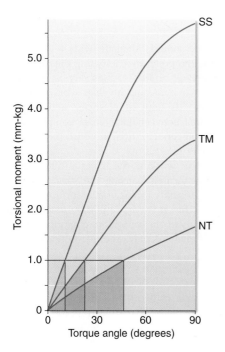

FIGURE 10.18 **Stored energy at a fixed torsional moment below the proportional limit for 0.48-mm by 0.64-mm wires of alloys stainless steel (SS), beta-titanium (TM), and nickel-titanium (NT).** The stored energy is equal to the shaded area under the curve for each wire. The spring rate is equal to the slope of each curve. *(From Drake SR, Wayne DM, Powers JM, et al: Am. J. Orthod. 82, 206, 1982.)*

as *alpha-titanium* and *beta-titanium,* respectively. The beta form of Ti can be stabilized at room temperature by alloying with certain elements. Beta-titanium alloy for dental use has the composition 78% titanium, 11.5% molybdenum, 6% zirconium, and 4.5% tin and is supplied as wrought wire.

Properties

Compared with stainless steel wires, beta-titanium wire has lower force magnitudes, a lower elastic modulus, higher springback (maximum elastic deflection), a lower yield strength, and good ductility, weldability, and corrosion resistance. The mechanical properties of beta-titanium alloy in tension, bending, and torsion are compared with stainless steel and nickel-titanium alloys in Table 10-20 and Figures 10-17 and 10-18. Beta-titanium alloy has values of yield strength, modulus of elasticity, and springback intermediate to those of stainless steel and Nitinol. Its formability and weldability are advantages over Nitinol, and it has a larger working range than do stainless steel wires.

SELECTED PROBLEMS

Amalgam

PROBLEM 1

An amalgam mix is difficult to remove from the capsule and appears excessively wet. What can be done to obtain a better mix?

Solution a

The most common cause is related to overtrituration. Trituration time should be decreased by 1 or 2 seconds, and the mix should then be tested for plasticity.

Solution b

The speed of trituration may have been too fast; a slower speed should be selected for the next mix. Remember that the energy of trituration is important in obtaining a normal mix and that the energy is a function of the speed and the duration of trituration; increasing either increases the energy of trituration.

PROBLEM 2

Mixes of amalgam are consistently on the dry side and lack plasticity during condensation. What can cause a dry mix to occur, and how can it be corrected?

Solution a

In contrast to Problem 1, a dry mix is often caused by undertrituration. Several mixes should be made at increased trituration times (an additional 1 to 2 seconds), and each one should be tested for plasticity. Listen for significant sound changes during trituration; the pestle can become wedged for the first few seconds, and the work-energy during that time is lost. Another choice would be to use a higher speed on the amalgamator.

Solution b

A dry mix can result from loss of mercury from the capsule during trituration. The two portions of most premeasured capsules are held together by a friction fit and occasionally some mercury can leak out during mixing. Check the inside of the housing covering the capsule area for small droplets of mercury, which also may appear like dust. Changing to a hermetically sealed capsule is suggested if the problem persists with the product being used.

PROBLEM 3

When larger restorative procedures are performed with amalgam, the amalgam is difficult to carve and seems to set before an adequate carving can be completed. What can cause this problem?

Solution a

The working time of an alloy can be influenced by the specific composition or particle size of an alloy and by the aging treatment during manufacturing. If the working characteristics of a particular alloy appear to change from those previously experienced, the cause may be an alteration made by the manufacturer. On the other hand, if the faster reaction rate occurs at initial trials with a new or unfamiliar alloy, this may simply indicate that the alloy has a short setting time and is unsuitable for use by certain operators or with specific techniques.

Solution b

The two most common manipulative variables that can accelerate the reaction and make carving difficult are overtrituration and decreased mercury/ alloy ratios. An overtriturated mix is recognizable by its shiny and very wet appearance and by its high initial plasticity. A low mercury/alloy ratio appears quite dry during condensation and presents difficulty in handling.

Solution c

The increased rate of the reaction may be compensated for by making several smaller mixes as material is used. Do not try to complete large restorations from a single mix or continue to use a mix after it has exceeded the usable range for plasticity. Also, the technique should be evaluated; most carving problems can be remedied by obtaining assistance and improving operator speed.

PROBLEM 4

When trying a new alloy, some amalgams may appear dry and brittle at the carving stage and tend to break away in large increments rather than to carve smoothly. What can cause this problem?

Solution a

A check should be made with a stopwatch to determine the point after initiating the mix at which this brittleness or loss of plasticity is first noticed. Prolonged condensation involves working the material beyond its limit of plasticity, and the loss of cohesiveness between increments complicates carving. Delayed condensation, in which there is a short, unavoidable interruption during the procedure, can also result in working the material after significant matrix has formed, causing the structure to break down. The result is a weak, friable surface that will not carve smoothly. It is very important to condense and carve an alloy in one continuous operation and within the time framework of the setting reaction for the alloy being used.

Solution b

The setting or working time of the alloy could be too short for the particular procedure being performed. Newer alloys appear to be faster setting and somewhat less consistent with respect to working time. The causes for a shortened setting time or an increased reaction rate are reviewed in Problem 3.

Solution c

In certain instances a lack of condensation force can result in a restoration with a large number of air voids or poor cohesion between increments. This often occurs when the cavity preparation is not confining and an unstable matrix technique is used. It can also occur when moisture contamination interferes with cohesion between increments.

PROBLEM 5

What factors are related to excessive tarnish and corrosion that appear several years after placement?

Solution a

A high residual mercury level in the final restoration can lead to increased corrosion as a result of an increase in the tin-mercury (γ_2) phase. This situation can result from a mercury/alloy ratio that is too high in the initial mix or from inadequate condensation to remove excessive mercury.

Solution b

Patients on a high-sulfur diet or dietary supplement show increased tarnish on amalgam restorations. A well-polished surface is the best preventive measure to minimize tarnishing.

Solution c

Surface texture is also important in preventing corrosion. Small scratches and exposed voids develop concentration cells, with saliva being the electrolyte. Thus corrosion weakens the amalgam in critical areas such as the margin interface and begins the breakdown process. One of the major advantages of polishing amalgam surfaces to a smooth texture is that polishing minimizes the effects of corrosion and thus enhances clinical performance.

Solution d

Galvanic action can also develop in the mouth when two dissimilar metals come into contact. The most common cause of galvanic action is gold and amalgam placed in adjacent teeth. The effects can be seen in the darkened corrosion products appearing on the surface of the amalgam. This does not occur in every mouth, and the severity may relate to salivary composition and its function as an electrolyte.

Solution e

Moisture contamination during condensation causes air voids to develop throughout the mass of the restoration and causes corrosion to progress at a faster rate.

PROBLEM 6

As amalgam restorations wear, the marginal integrity is usually the first area to show signs of failure. Small increments of amalgam or unsupported enamel fracture and crevices develop, thus leading to increased leakage and eventual secondary caries. What factors contribute to marginal deterioration of this type?

Solution a

Initially, every margin of a preparation should be examined for potential areas of enamel failure. Unsupported enamel rods and undercut walls are potential sites for fracture when subjected to occlusal forces. All cavosurface margins should be smooth-flowing curves and be free of unsupported enamel. Cavity walls should meet the external surface of the tooth at a 90-degree angle to provide optimum support for the tooth and sufficient bulk in the amalgam to resist fracture along the margin.

Solution b

Carving of the amalgam should be continuous with existing tooth form and should provide an accurate adaptation to the exposed cavity margin. Thin overextensions of amalgam beyond the margins and onto enamel can fracture readily into the bulk of amalgam and leave a crevice.

Solution c

Inadequate condensation of the amalgam in areas adjacent to the margins, especially in the areas of occlusal overpacking, causes a high residual mercury level to remain at the margin interface. The excessive γ_2 phase in that area leads to an increase in flow and corrosion and a decrease in strength that predisposes the restoration to fracture.

Solution d

Use of an alloy with a higher creep value, such as a microcut, results in evidence of early marginal fractures when subjected to occlusal function. The high-copper content alloys have less creep and demonstrate more durable marginal adaptation.

PROBLEM 7

Small interproximal restorations often fail by fracturing across the occlusal isthmus. How can this type of failure be avoided?

Solution a

The major cause of gross fracture of amalgam restorations is usually found in the design of the cavity preparation. Sufficient bulk of material must be provided to support occlusal forces. This can best be accomplished by keeping the isthmus narrow and providing adequate cavity depth; however, on occasion the reverse might be necessary to avoid pulpal involvement. The axiopulpal line angle should be rounded to reduce stress concentration in that area.

Solution b

Occlusal contacts should be adjusted to avoid excessive contact on the marginal ridge. A torquing action places the isthmus under tension and results in fracture sooner.

Solution c

A smaller condenser must be used in the isthmus area so that adequate condensation can be accomplished. Inadequately condensed amalgam results in a weakening of the area and a predisposition to fracture.

Solution d

If enough dentin is removed during cavity preparation to require the placement of a cement base, a sufficiently rigid material must be selected for use. Zinc phosphate cement is the best material having a high enough modulus to minimize deflection of the amalgam. Other dental cements, particularly zinc oxide–eugenol types, have low moduli; under occlusal function they allow too much deflection and brittle failure is likely to occur in the amalgam. The axiopulpal line angle is a critical area and should be reconstructed in a supporting base of zinc phosphate cement.

PROBLEM 8

A high-copper, fast-setting amalgam could not be finished by the early polishing procedure until 20 minutes after amalgamation and a satisfactory finish could not be obtained. What was the cause, and what would be the proper clinical procedure at this point?

Solution

For amalgams of this type to be polished at the first appointment, finishing should be started 8 to 10 minutes after trituration, depending on the alloy. If the finishing is delayed until 20 minutes after trituration, the setting of the amalgam has proceeded too far, and strength of the alloy is too great to complete the finishing with triple-x silex and water. If the finishing is delayed too long, attempts at early finishing should be stopped, and final finishing should be done in the standard manner at a second appointment.

PROBLEM 9

A spherical amalgam mix was condensed with a 2-mm diameter condenser to obtain a high condensation pressure and a well-condensed restoration. However, a low-strength amalgam restoration and failure resulted. Why?

Solution

Spherical alloys triturated with mercury do not resist small condenser tips well, but allow them to penetrate the mass and thus reduce the condensation pressure. Condensers with larger diameter tips that do not penetrate the mass as readily should be used, thus allowing higher pressures and better condensation. These amalgams appear to condense easily and there is a tendency to use less than the desired condensation force. For optimum strength, a condensation pressure of 7 MPa should be used.

PROBLEM 10

Why should scrap amalgam be stored in a sodium thiosulfate solution such as photographic fixer rather than just water?

Solution

Any mercury vapor released will react with the thiosulfate ions and lower the vapor pressure of mercury to levels below the instrument detection level of 0.01 mg/m^3. If scrap amalgam is stored under water only, the amount of mercury in the air above the water increases with the log of time.

PROBLEM 11

What assurances can you give a patient to dispel fears of mercury toxicity from dental amalgams?

Solution

Except for the rare allergic reaction, there is no scientific documentation of local or systemic effects of dental amalgams. Patients with nine occlusal surfaces of amalgam will inhale less than 1% of the mercury that a person would inhale in a workplace having a level allowed by Occupational Safety and Health Administration (OSHA). Ingested mercury is eliminated through feces and urine. The daily intake of mercury from air, water, and food exceeds that from dental amalgams.

Noble Alloys

PROBLEM 12

Table 10-7 shows that cast 24k gold has a hardness and strength that are not sufficient for dental restorations, yet gold foil, which is also 24k gold, has three times the hardness and more than twice the tensile strength. Why?

Solution

The manufacturing of gold foil starts with the cast form of the element, then imparts severe cold work until it is very thin. Thus gold foil has a wrought microstructure and exhibits superior mechanical properties because of its fibrous form. Condensation of the foil into the restoration imparts further work hardening to the metal. Note, however, that the elongation of the gold foil is less than half of the original cast 24k gold. Thus, by strengthening the gold through work hardening, it has also become more brittle. This trend is typical of wrought metals relative to their cast counterparts.

PROBLEM 13

A review of Table 10-5 indicates that most noble casting alloys are based on either gold, palladium, or silver, with smaller amounts of copper, platinum, and zinc added. Why do dental manufacturers pick these elements for noble dental casting alloys?

Solution

Gold and palladium are selected as major elements for noble casting alloys because they impart corrosion resistance to the alloys and are miscible (freely soluble) with the other elements (see Figure 10-7). In the past, palladium was often used because it was considerably cheaper than gold, and maintained corrosion resistance of the alloy. However, palladium prices have approached and even surpassed those of gold in recent times. Nevertheless, palladium is used to add strength and hardness without sacrificing corrosion resistance. Silver is used as a less expensive alternative to palladium, but cannot provide as much corrosion resistance because it is not a noble metal. Furthermore, silver is not miscible with copper. The other elements in Table 10-5 (copper, zinc, gallium, iridium, ruthenium, and indium) are inappropriate as major elements. Copper, zinc, gallium, and indium lack corrosion resistance, and iridium and ruthenium have extremely high melting points and are very expensive. These minor elements are used because they enhance the properties of the major elements. For example, copper provides solid-solution hardening, zinc is a deoxidizer during casting, and iridium is a grain refiner. Platinum, although a noble metal, is not generally used as a major element because of its cost and because it is not miscible with Au or Pd (see Figure 10-7).

PROBLEM 14

An alloy was listed by a manufacturer as an 11k alloy containing 4.2% Pd, 25% Cu, and 25% Ag (all wt%). What is the atomic percentage of Au in this alloy? Is the carat based on the atomic or weight percent?

Solution

The alloy contains 25.9 at% of gold. The answer is arrived at in the following manner: an 11-carat alloy contains $11/24 \times 100 = 45.8$ wt% gold. Thus the carat is based on weight percentage. The weight percentage of each element is divided by the respective atomic weight, giving the following results: Au $45.8/197 = 0.232$; Cu $25/63.5 = 0.394$; Ag $25/208 = 0.231$; Pd $4.2/106.5 = 0.039$. The atomic percentage of Au is $0.232 \times 100/(0.232 + 0.394 + 0.231 + 0.039) = 25.9$ at%.

PROBLEM 15

Upon inspection of the elements in Table 10-6, which elements do you think would be candidates as grain refiners and why? (Hint: Evaluate the melting range of most alloys in Table 10-9 before answering this question.)

Solution

Because Table 10-9 shows that the liquidus of most noble and high-noble casting alloys is below 1200° C, any grain refiner would have to have a melting point well above (greater than 500° to 600° C) this value. The elements that are best in this regard are ruthenium, rhodium, osmium, and iridium. All but osmium, which is much too expensive to justify its use over the others, are used in practice.

PROBLEM 16

A dentist tells a laboratory technician that he wants a type III alloy for a restoration. The laboratory then asks the dentist whether he wants a high-noble or noble alloy. The dentist believes that the laboratory's question is unnecessary, because type III specifies composition of the alloy. Who is right?

Solution

In this case, the laboratory is correct in asking about the composition of the alloy. Table 10-4 shows that a type III alloy is a hard alloy suitable for restorations subject to high stress, but type III gives no indication of composition. Therefore, a number of compositions, noble or high-noble, might meet the requirements for a type III alloy, and the laboratory is correct in asking. Confusion about this issue comes from the past definition of the term *type III*. In the past, alloy typing for gold-based alloys specified composition and physical properties. However, when the use of alloys other than gold-based varieties became common, the compositions and physical properties were separated. This change still causes confusion among dentists.

PROBLEM 17

In Table 10-5, the atomic percentages of elements in the alloys are sometimes different than their corresponding weight percentages and sometimes quite similar. Why?

Solution

If an alloy contains elements with vastly different atomic weights, then the atomic percentages and weight percentages will be significantly different. The heaviest elements will be lower in atomic percentage than weight percentage and the lightest elements will be higher in atomic percentages than weight percentages. If an alloy contains elements that are comparable in atomic weights, the atomic and weight percentages of the elements will not differ as much. Thus, in Table 10-5, the atomic and weight percentages of the Ag-Pd alloys are similar because the majority of the alloy is composed of silver, palladium, and indium, which are very close in atomic weight (Ag = 107.9, Pd = 106.4, and In = 114.8). The other element in this alloy, zinc, does not change much because it is a minor component. If zinc were more prevalent in this alloy, its atomic and weight percentages would be significantly different because its atomic weight (Zn = 65.4) is quite different than that of the other components.

PROBLEM 18

A gold crown made of Au-Cu-Ag-Pd-*I* alloy was inadvertently allowed to slowly cool to room temperature after casting. Because the crown was then in the hardened condition, it was placed into an oven at 400° C for 20 minutes and then quenched in water. However, the casting was still as difficult to finish. Why?

Solution

To convert the hardened alloy to the softened condition, it must be heated above 424° C to affect the conversion (see phase diagram in Figure 10-7, *A*). Alloys of this composition are often heated to 700° C, which is above the transition temperature of the ordered phase but well below the solidus, to affect the conversion. At this temperature, the alloy converts to the softened condition, then quenching maintains it in the softened condition by cooling it so fast that it does not have enough time to form the ordered phase.

Base-Metal Alloys

PROBLEM 19

The elastic modulus values of nickel-chromium and cobalt-chromium alloys are about twice those of gold alloys; thus the thickness of a restoration in the direction of a bending force can be about halved and still have the same deflection. Is this a justifiable conclusion? Defend your answer.

Solution

No. Although a stress-strain curve in tension might lead you to respond affirmatively, it should be remembered that although the deflection of a beam is directly proportional to the modulus, it is inversely proportional to the cube of the thickness. As a result, halving the thickness of the nickel-chromium beam will dramatically increase the deflection as compared with that of the gold beam, even though it has twice the elastic modulus. It can be shown that only small decreases in thickness of the nickel-chromium beam can be made and yet maintain the same stiffness as the gold alloy beam.

PROBLEM 20

During the soldering of a cobalt-chromium removable dental prosthesis, the temperature of the torch became very high. What might be the expected effect on the properties of the cast framework?

Solution

Excessive heating of the framework will result in a decrease in the yield strength and the percent elongation. This can result from migration of atoms and formation of carbides, resulting in chromium depletion in the grains, which can cause increased corrosion.

PROBLEM 21

Nickel-chromium alloys that can be cast into gypsum-bonded investments contain up to 2% beryllium to reduce the melting temperature. An alloy labeled as containing 77% nickel, 21% chromium, and 2% beryllium (Be) will contain 2 at% of Be. Is that statement correct? Defend your response.

Solution

No. The values listed are weight percentages. To obtain the atomic percentage, you must first divide the weight percent of each element by the respective atomic number. These quotients are then added, and the atomic percentage calculated by dividing each quotient by the sum times 100. For example, 77 wt% Ni 59 = 1.305, 21 wt% Cr ÷ 52 = 0.404, and 2 wt% Be ÷ 9 = 0.222. The sum of the quotients is 1.931, and 0.222 ÷ 1.931 × 100 = 11.5 at% Be.

Bibliography

Amalgam—Review Articles

Allen EP, Bayne SC, Becker IM, et al: Annual review of selected dental literature: report of the committee on scientific investigation of the American Academy of Restorative Dentistry, *J Prosthet Dent* 82:54, 1999.

Allen EP, Bayne SC, Donovan TE, et al: Annual review of selected dental literature, *J Prosthet Dent* 76:82, 1996.

Bryant RW: γ_2 Phase in conventional dental amalgams—discrete clumps or continuous network? A review, *Aust Dent J* 29:163, 1984.

De Rossi SS, Greenberg MS: Intraoral contact allergy: a literature review and case reports, *J Am Dent Assoc* 129:1435, 1998.

Halbach S: Amalgam tooth fillings and man's mercury burden [Review], *Human Exper Toxicol* 13:496, 1994.

Jendresen MD, Allen EP, Bayne SC, et al: Annual review of selected dental literature: report of the committee on scientific investigation of the American Academy of Restorative Dentistry, *J Prosthet Dent* 80:109, 1998.

Jendresen MD, Allen EP, Bayne SC, et al: Annual review of selected dental literature: report of the committee on scientific investigation of the American Academy of Restorative Dentistry, *J Prosthet Dent* 78:82, 1997.

Jendresen MD, Allen EP, Bayne SC, et al: Annual review of selected dental literature: report of the committee on scientific investigation of the American Academy of Restorative Dentistry, *J Prosthet Dent* 74:83, 1995.

Lloyd CH, Scrimgeour SN, editors: Dental materials: 1994 literature review, *J Dent* 24:159, 1996.

Lloyd CH, Scrimgeour SN, editors: Dental materials: 1995 literature review, *J Dent* 25:180, 1997.

Mitchell RJ, Okabe T: Setting reactions in dental amalgam: part 1. Phases and microstructures between one hour and one week [Review], *Crit Rev Oral Biol and Med* 7:12, 1996.

Okabe T, Mitchell RJ: Setting reactions in dental amalgam: part 2. The kinetics of amalgamation [Review], *Crit Rev Oral Biol Med* 7:23, 1996.

Strang R, Whitters CJ, Brown D, et al: Dental materials: 1996 literature review, *J Dent* 26:196, 1998.

Whitters CJ, Strang R, Brown D, et al: Dental materials: 1997 literature review, *J Dent* 27:407, 1999.

Amalgam—Reactions and Properties

Allan FC, Asgar K, Peyton FA: Micro-structure of dental amalgam, *J Dent Res* 44:1002, 1965.

Asgar K: Amalgam alloy with a single composition behavior similar to Dispersalloy, *J Dent Res* 53:60, 1974.

Asgar K, Sutfin L: Brittle fracture of dental amalgam, *J Dent Res* 44:977, 1965.

Baran G, O'Brien WJ: Wetting of amalgam alloys by mercury, *J Am Dent Assoc* 94:898, 1977.

Boyer DB, Edie JW: Composition of clinically aged amalgam restorations, *Dent Mater* 6:146, 1990.

Branstromm M, Astrom A: The hydrodynamics of the dentine: Its possible relationship to dentinal pain, *Int Dent J* 22:219, 1972.

Brockhurst PJ, Culnane JT: Organization of the mixing time of dental amalgam using coherence time, *Aust Dent J* 32:28, 1987.

Brown IH, Maiolo C, Miller DR: Variation in condensation pressure during clinical packing of amalgam restorations, *Am J Dent* 6:255, 1993.

Brown IH, Miller DR: Alloy particle shape and sensitivity of high-copper amalgams to manipulative variables, *Am J Dent* 6:248, 1993.

Corpron R, Straffon L, Dennison J, et al: Clinical evaluation of amalgams polished immediately after insertion: 5-year results, *J Dent Res* 63:178, 1984.

Dunne SM, Gainsford ID, Wilson NH: Current materials and techniques for direct restorations in posterior teeth. Part 1: silver amalgam, *Int Dent J* 47:123, 1997.

Farah JW, Hood JA, Craig RG: Effects of cement bases on the stresses in amalgam restorations, *J Dent Res* 54:10, 1975.

Farah JW, Powers JM, editors: High copper amalgams, *Dent Advis* 4(2):1, 1987.

Farah JW, Powers JM, editors: Dental amalgam and mercury, *Dent Advis* 8(2):1, 1991.

Gottlieb EW, Retief DH, Bradley EL: Microleakage of conventional and high copper amalgam restorations, *J Prosthet Dent* 53:355, 1985.

Hero H: On creep mechanisms in amalgam, *J Dent Res* 62:44, 1983.

Jensen SJ, Jÿrgensen KD: Dimensional and phase changes of dental amalgam, *Scand J Dent Res* 93:351, 1985.

Johnson GH, Bales DJ, Powell LV: Clinical evaluation of high-copper dental amalgams with and without admixed indium, *Am J Dent* 5:39, 1992.

Johnson GH, Powell LV: Effect of admixed indium on properties of a dispersed phase high-copper dental amalgam, *Dent Mater* 8:366, 1992.

Jÿrgensen KD: The mechanism of marginal fracture of amalgam fillings, *Acta Odont Scand* 23:347, 1965.

Jÿrgensen KD, Esbensen AL, Borring-Moller G: The effect of porosity and mercury content upon the strength of silver amalgam, *Acta Odont Scand* 24:535, 1966.

Jÿrgensen KD, Wakumoto S: Occlusal amalgam fillings; marginal defects and secondary caries, *Odont Tskr* 76:43, 1968.

Katz JL, Grenoble DE: A composite model of the elastic behavior of dental amalgam, *J Biomed Mater Res* 5:515, 1971.

Kawakami M, Staninec M, Imazato S, et al: Shear bond strength of amalgam adhesives to dentin, *Am J Dent* 7:53, 1994.

Leinfelder KF: Dental amalgam alloys, *Curr Opin Dent* 1:214, 1991.

Letzel H, Van't Hof MA, Marshall GW, et al: The influence of the amalgam alloy on the survival of amalgam restorations: a secondary analysis of multiple controlled clinical trials, *J Dent Res* 76:1787, 1997.

Lloyd CH, Adamson M: Fracture toughness (KlC) of amalgam, *J Oral Rehabil* 12:59, 1985.

Mahler DB: *Amalgam, International State-of-the-Art Conference on Restorative Dental Materials*, Bethesda, 1986, Md.

Mahler DB: Slow compressive strength of amalgam, *J Dent Res* 51:1394, 1972.

Mahler DB: The high-copper dental amalgam alloys, *J Dent Res* 76:537, 1997.

Mahler DB, Adey JD: Factors influencing the creep of dental amalgam, *J Dent Res* 70:1394, 1991.

Mahler DB, Adey JD, Marantz RL: Creep versus microstructure of gamma 2 containing amalgams, *J Dent Res* 56:1493, 1977.

Mahler DB, Adey JD, Marek M: Creep and corrosion of amalgam, *J Dent Res* 61:33, 1982.

Mahler DB, Adey JD, Marshall SJ: Effect of time at 37 degrees C on the creep and metallurgical characteristics of amalgam, *J Dent Res* 66:1146, 1987.

Mahler DB, Marantz RL, Engle JH: A predictive model for the clinical marginal fracture of amalgam, *J Dent Res* 59:1420, 1980.

Mahler DB, Nelson LW: Factors affecting the marginal leakage of amalgam, *J Am Dent Assoc* 108:50, 1984.

Mahler DB, Nelson LW: Sensitivity answers sought in amalgam alloy microleakage study, *J Am Dent Assoc* 125:282, 1984.

Mahler DB, Terkla LG, van Eysden J, et al: Marginal fracture vs mechanical properties of amalgam, *J Dent Res* 49:1452, 1970.

Mahler DB, van Eysden J, Terkla LG: Relationship of creep to marginal fracture of amalgam, *J Dent Res* 54:183, 1975.

Malhotra ML, Asgar K: Physical properties of dental silver-tin amalgams with high and low copper contents, *J Am Dent Assoc* 96:444, 1978.

Martin JA, Bader JD: Five-year treatment outcomes for teeth with large amalgams and crowns, *Oper Dent* 22:72, 1997.

McCabe JF, Carrick TE: Dynamic creep of dental amalgam as a function of stress and number of applied cycles, *J Dent Res* 66:1346, 1987.

Meletis EI, Gibbs CA, Lian K: New dynamic corrosion test for dental materials, *Dent Mater* 5:411, 1989.

O'Brien WJ, Greener EH, Mahler DB: Dental amalgam. In Reese JA, Valega TM, editors: *Restorative dental materials: an overview*, London, 1985, Quintessence.

Ogura H, Miyagawa Y, Nakamura K: Creep and rupture of dental amalgam under bending stress, *Dent Mater J* 8:65, 1989.

Osborne JW, Gale EN: Failure at the margin of amalgams as affected by cavity width, tooth position, and alloy selection, *J Dent Res* 60:681, 1981.

Papathanasiou AG, Curzon ME, Fairpo CG: The influence of restorative material on the survival rate of restorations in primary molars, *Paediatr Dent* 16:282, 1994.

Powers JM, Farah JW: Apparent modulus of elasticity of dental amalgams, *J Dent Res* 54:902, 1975.

Ryge G, Telford RF, Fairhurst CW: Strength and phase formation of dental amalgam, *J Dent Res* 36:986, 1957.

Sarkar NK, Eyer CS: The microstructural basis of creep of gamma 1 in dental amalgam, *J Oral Rehabil* 14:27, 1987.

Smales RJ, Hawthorne WS: Long-term survival of extensive amalgams and posterior crowns, *J Dent* 25:225, 1997.

Watkins JH, Nakajima H, Hanaoka K, et al: Effect of zinc on strength and fatigue resistance of amalgam, *Dent Mater* 11:24, 1995.

Wilson NH, Wastell DC, Norman RD: Five-year performance of high-copper content amalgam restorations in a multiclinical trial of a posterior composite, *J Dent* 24:203, 1996.

Wing G, Ryge G: Setting reactions of spherical-particle amalgam, *J Dent Res* 44:1325, 1965.

Young FA Jr, Johnson LB: Strength of mercury-tin phase in dental amalgam, *J Dent Res* 46:457, 1967.

Zardiackas LD, Anderson L Jr: Crack propagation in conventional and high copper dental amalgam as a function of strain rate, *Biomaterials* 7:259, 1986.

Amalgam—Retention and Bonding

Barkmeier WW, Gendusa NJ, Thurmond JW, et al: Laboratory evaluation of Amalgambond and Amalgambond Plus, *Am J Dent* 7:239, 1994.

Ben-Amar A, Liberman R, Rothkoff Z, et al: Long term sealing properties of Amalgambond under amalgam restorations, *Am J Dent* 7:141, 1994.

Boyer DB, Roth L: Fracture resistance of teeth with bonded amalgams, *Am J Dent* 7:91, 1994.

Eakle WS, Staninec M, Yip RL, et al: Mechanical retention versus bonding of amalgam and gallium alloy restorations, *J Prosthet Dent* 72:351, 1994.

Edgren BN, Denehy GE: Microleakage of amalgam restorations using Amalgambond and Copalite, *Am J Dent* 5:296, 1992.

Fischer GM, Stewart GP, Panelli J: Amalgam retention using pins, boxes, and Amalgambond, *Am J Dent* 6:173, 1993.

Hadavi R, Hey JH, Strasdin RB, et al: Bonding amalgam to dentin by different methods, *J Prosthet Dent* 72:250, 1994.

Ianzano JA, Mastrodomenico J, Gwinnett AJ: Strength of amalgam restorations bonded with Amalgambond, *Am J Dent* 6:10, 1993.

Nuckles DB, Draughn RA, Smith TI: Evaluation of an adhesive system for amalgam repair: bond strength and porosity, *Quint Int* 25:829, 1994.

Santos AC, Meiers JC: Fracture resistance of premolars with MOD amalgam restorations lined with Amalgambond, *Oper Dent* 19:2, 1994.

Staninec M, Holt M: Bonding of amalgam to tooth structure: tensile, adhesion and microleakage tests, *J Prosthet Dent* 59:397, 1988.

Staninec M: Retention of amalgam restorations: undercuts versus bonding, *Quint Int* 20:347, 1989.

Amalgam—Mercury and Biocompatibility Issues

Abraham JE, Svare EW: The effect of dental amalgam restorations on blood mercury levels, *J Dent Res* 63:71, 1984.

American Dental Association Council on Scientific Affairs: Dental amalgam—update on safety concerns, *J Am Dent Assoc* 129:494, 1998.

Arenholt-Bindslev D: Environmental aspects of dental filling materials, *Eur J Oral Sci* 106:713, 1998.

Berglund A: Estimation of the daily dose of intra-oral mercury vapor inhaled after release from dental amalgam, *J Dent Res* 69:1646, 1990.

Berglund A, Bergdahl J: Hansson Mild K: Influence of low frequency magnetic fields on the intra-oral release of mercury vapor from amalgam restorations, *Eur J Oral Sci* 106:671, 1998.

Berlin MH, Clarkston TW, Friberg LT, et al: Maximum allowable concentrations of mercury vapor in air, *Lakartidningen* 64:3628, 1967.

Berry TG, Nicholson J, Troendle K: Almost two centuries with amalgam: where are we today? *J Am Dent Assoc* 125:392, 1994.

Berry TG, Summitt JB, Chung AK, et al: Amalgam at the new millennium, *J Am Dent Assoc* 129:1547, 1998.

Bolewska J, Holmstrup P, Moller-Madsen B, et al: Amalgam-associated mercury accumulations in normal oral mucosa, oral mucosal lesions of lichen planus and contact lesions associated with amalgam, *J Oral Pathol Med* 19:19, 1990.

Burrows D: Hypersensitivity to mercury, nickel and chromium in relation to dental materials, *Int Dent J* 36:30, 1986.

Chang SB, Siew C, Gruninger SE: Factors affecting blood mercury concentrations in practicing dentists, *J Dent Res* 71:66, 1992.

Chew CL, Soh G, Lee AS, et al: Comparison of release of mercury from three dental amalgams, *Dent Mater* 5:244, 1989.

Clarkson TW: The toxicology of mercury, *Crit Rev Clinical Lab Sci* 34:369, 1997.

Council on Dental Materials and Devices: Recommendations in mercury hygiene, *J Am Dent Assoc* 92:1217, 1976.

Council on Dental Materials: Instruments, and Equipment: Safety of dental amalgam, *J Am Dent Assoc* 106:519, 1983.

Corbin SB, Kohn WG: The benefits and risks of dental amalgam: current findings reviewed, *J Am Dent Assoc* 125:381, 1994.

Cox SW, Eley BM: Further investigations of the soft tissue reaction to the gamma 1 phase (Ag_2Hg_3) of dental amalgam, including measurements of mercury release and redistribution, *Biomaterials* 8:296, 1987.

Cox SW, Eley BM: Further investigations of the soft tissue reaction to the gamma 2 phase ($Sn_{7-8}Hg$) of dental amalgam, including measurements of mercury release and redistribution, *Biomaterials* 8:301, 1987.

Cox SW, Eley BM: Mercury release, distribution and excretion from subcutaneously implanted conventional and high-copper amalgam powders in the guinea pig, *Arch Oral Biol* 32:257, 1987.

Cox SW, Eley BM: Microscopy and x-ray microanalysis of subcutaneously implanted conventional and high-copper dental amalgam powders in the guinea pig, *Arch Oral Biol* 32:265, 1987.

Cox SW, Eley BM: The release, tissue distribution and excretion of mercury from experimental amalgam tattoos, *Br J Exp Pathol* 67:925, 1986.

Craig RG: Biocompatibility of mercury derivatives, *Dent Mater* 2:91, 1986.

Ekstrand J, Bjorkman L, Edlund C, et al: Toxicological aspects on the release and systemic uptake of mercury from dental amalgam, *Eur J Oral Sci* 106:678, 1998.

Ferracane JL, Adey JD, Nakajima H, et al: Mercury vaporization from amalgams with varied alloy compositions, *J Dent Res* 74:1414, 1995.

Ferracane JL, Engle JH, Okabe T, et al: Reduction in operatory mercury levels after contamination or amalgam removal, *Am J Dent* 7:103, 1994.

FDI Commission: Environmental issues in dentistry—mercury, *Int Dent J* 47:105, 1997.

Forsell M, Larsson B, Ljungqvist A, et al: Mercury content in amalgam tattoos of human oral mucosa and its relations to local tissue reactions, *Eur J Oral Sci* 106:582, 1998.

Gronka PA, Bobkoskie RL, Tomchick GJ, et al: Mercury vapor exposures in dental offices, *J Am Dent Assoc* 81:923, 1970.

Guthrow CE, Johnson CB, Lawless KB: Corrosion of dental amalgam and its component phases, *J Dent Res* 46:1372, 1967.

Haikel Y, Gasser P, Salek P, et al: Exposure to mercury vapor during setting, removing, and polishing amalgam restorations, *J Biomed Mater Res* 24:1551, 1990.

Heintze U, Edwardsson S, Derand T, et al: Methylation of mercury from dental amalgam and mercuric chloride by oral streptococci in vitro, *Scand J Dent Res* 91:150, 1983.

Holland GA, Asgar K: Some effects of the phases of amalgam induced by corrosion, *J Dent Res* 53:1245, 1974.

Johansson C, Moberg LE: Area ratio effects on metal ion release from amalgam in contact with gold, *Scand J Dent Res* 99:246, 1991.

Kaaber S: Allergy to dental materials with special reference to the use of amalgam and polymethylmethacrylate, *Int Dent J* 40:359, 1990.

Kaga M, Seale NS, Hanawa T, et al: Cytotoxicity of amalgams, *J Dent Res* 67:1221, 1988.

Kaga M, Seale NS, Hanawa T, et al: Cytotoxicity of amalgams, alloys, and their elements and phases, *Dent Mater* 7:68, 1991.

Kingman A, Albertini T, Brown LJ: mercury concentrations in urine and whole blood associated with amalgam exposure in a US military population, *J Dent Res* 77:60, 1998.

Kuntz WD: Maternal and cord blood background mercury level, *Am J Obstet Gynecol* 143:440, 1982.

Kurland LT, Faro SN, Siedler H: Minamata disease, *World Neurol* 1:370, 1960.

Laine J, Kalimo K, Forssell H, et al: Resolution of oral lichenoid lesions after replacement of amalgam restorations in patients allergic to mercury compounds, *Br J Dermatol* 126:10, 1992.

Langolf GD, Chaffin DB, Henderson R, et al: Evaluation of workers exposed to elemental mercury using quantitative test of tremor and neuromuscular function, *Am Ind Hyg Assoc J* 39:976, 1978.

Langworth S, Elinder CG, Gothe CJ, et al: Biological monitoring of environmental and occupational exposure to mercury, *Int Arch Occup Environ Health* 63:161, 1991.

Lyttle HA, Bowden GH: The level of mercury in human dental plaque an interaction in vitro between biofilms of *Streptococcus mutans* and dental amalgam, *J Dent Res* 72:1320, 1993.

Lyttle HA, Bowden GH: The resistance and adaptation of selected oral bacteria to mercury and its impact on their growth, *J Dent Res* 72:1325, 1993.

Mackert JR Jr: Dental amalgam and mercury, *J Am Dent Assoc* 122:54, 1991.

Mackert JR Jr, Berglund A: Mercury exposure from dental amalgam fillings: absorbed dose and the potential for adverse health effects, *Crit Rev Oral Biol Med* 8:410, 1997.

Mackert JR Jr, Leffell MS, Wagner DA, et al: Lymphocyte levels in subjects with and without amalgam restorations, *J Am Dent Assoc* 122:49, 1991.

Mandel ID: Amalgam hazards: an assessment of research, *J Am Dent Assoc* 122:62, 1991.

Marek M: Acceleration of corrosion of dental amalgam by abrasion, *J Dent Res* 63:1010, 1984.

Marek M: Corrosion test for dental amalgam, *J Dent Res* 59:63, 1980.

Marek M: The effect of the electrode potential on the release of mercury from dental amalgam, *J Dent Res* 72:1315, 1993.

Marek M: The release of mercury from dental amalgam: the mechanism and in vitro testing, *J Dent Res* 69:1167, 1990.

Marek M, Hockman RF, Okabe T: In vitro corrosion of dental amalgam phases, *J Biomed Mater Res* 10:789, 1976.

Marshall SJ, Lin JHC, Marshall GW: Cu_2O and $CuCl_2 \cdot 3Cu(OH)_2$ corrosion products on copper rich dental amalgams, *J Biomed Mater Res* 16:81, 1982.

Martin MD, Naleway C, Chou H-N: Factors contributing to mercury exposure in dentists, *J Am Dent Assoc* 126:1502, 1995.

Miller JM, Chaffin DB, Smith RG: Subclinical psychomotor and neuromuscular changes exposed to inorganic mercury, *Am Ind Hyg Assoc J* 36(10):725, 1975.

Mueller HJ, Bapna MS: Copper-, indium-, tin-, and calcium-fluoride admixed amalgams: release rates and selected properties, *Dent Mater* 6:256, 1990.

Okabe T, Ferracane J, Cooper C, et al: Dissolution of mercury from amalgam into saline solution, *J Dent Res* 66:33, 1987.

Okabe T, Yomashita T, Nakajima H, et al: Reduced mercury vapor release from dental amalgams prepared with binary Hg-In liquid alloys, *J Dent Res* 73:1711, 1994.

Olsson S, Bergman M: Daily dose calculations from measurements of intra-oral mercury vapor, *J Dent Res* 71:414, 1992.

Olsson S, Berhlund A, Bergman M: Release of elements due to electrochemical corrosion of dental amalgam, *J Dent Res* 73:33, 1994.

Olstad ML, Holland RI, Pettersen AH: Effect of placement of amalgam restorations on urinary mercury concentration, *J Dent Res* 69:1607, 1990.

Pohl L, Bergman M: The dentist's exposure to elemental mercury vapour during clinical work with amalgam, *Act Odont Scand* 53:1023, 1995.

Powell LV, Johnson GH, Bales DJ: Effect of admixed indium on mercury vapor release from dental amalgam, *J Dent Res* 68:1231, 1989.

Powell LV, Johnson GH, Yashar N, et al: Mercury vapor release during insertion and removal of dental amalgam, *Oper Dent* 19:70, 1994.

Sandborough-Englund G, Elinder C-G, Landworth S, et al: Mercury in biological fluids after mercury removal, *J Dent Res* 77:615, 1998.

Sarkar NK, Park JR: Mechanism of improved corrosion resistance of Zn-containing dental amalgams, *J Dent Res* 67:1312, 1988.

Saxe SR, Snowdon DA, Wekstein MW, et al: Dental amalgam and cognitive function in older women: findings from the nun study, *J Am Dent Assoc* 126:1495, 1995.

Scarlett JM, Gutenmann WH, Lisk DJ: A study of mercury in the hair of dentists and dental-related professionals in 1985 and subcohort comparison of 1972 and 1985 mercury hair levels, *J Toxicol Environ Health* 25:373, 1988.

Schmalz G, Schmalz C: Toxicity tests on dental filling materials, *Int Dent J* 31:185, 1981.

Skare I, Engqvist A: Urinary mercury clearance of dental personnel after a long-term intermission in occupational exposure, *Swed Dent J* 14:255, 1990.

Snapp KR, Boyer DB, Peterson LC, et al: The contribution of dental amalgam to mercury in blood, *J Dent Res* 68:780, 1989.

Takaku S: Studies of mercury concentration in saliva with particular reference to mercury dissolution from dental amalgam into saliva, *Gakho Shikwa* 82:285, 1982.

Veron C, Hildebrand HF, Martin P: Dental amalgams and allergy, *J Biol Buccale* 14:83, 1986.

von Mayenburg J, Rakoski J, Szliska C: Patch testing with amalgam at various concentrations, *Contact Dermatitis* 24:266, 1991.

Casting Alloys

ADA Council on Scientific Affairs: Proper use of beryllium-containing alloys, *J Am Dent Assoc* 134:476, 2003.

Anusavice KJ: *Phillips' science of dental materials*, ed 11, St Louis, 2003, Saunders.

Böning K, Walter M: Palladium alloys in prosthodontics: selected aspects, *Int Dent J* 40:289, 1990.

Cartwright CB: Gold foil restorations, *J Mich Dent Assoc* 43:231, 1961.

Corso PP, German RM, Simmons HD: Corrosion evaluation of gold-based dental alloys, *J Dent Res* 64:854, 1985.

Council on Dental Materials, Instruments, and Equipment: Classification system for cast alloys, *J Am Dent Assoc* 109:766, 1984.

Council on Dental Materials, Instruments, and Equipment: Revised ANSI/ADA Specification No. 5 for dental casting alloys, *J Am Dent Assoc* 118:379, 1989.

Powers JM, Wataha JC: *Dental materials: properties and manipulations*, ed 9, St. Louis, 2008, Mosby.

Federation Dentaire Internationale: Alternative casting alloys for fixed prosthodontics, *Int Dent J* 40:54, 1990.

German RM, Wright DC, Gallant RF: In vitro tarnish measurement on fixed prosthodontic alloys, *J Prosthet Dent* 47:399, 1982.

Gettleman L: Noble alloys in dentistry, *Curr Opin Dent* 2:218, 1991.

Givan DA: Precious metals in dentistry, *Dent Clin N Am* 51:591, 2007.

Glantz PO: Intraoral behaviour and biocompatibility of gold versus non precious alloys, *J Biol Buccale* 12:3, 1984.

Hodson JT: Compaction properties of various gold restorative materials, *J Am Acad Gold Foil Op* 12:52, 1969.

Hollenback GM, Collard AW: An evaluation of the physical properties of cohesive gold, *J Calif Dent Assoc* 29:280, 1961.

Johansson BI, Lemons JE, Hao SQ: Corrosion of dental copper, nickel, and gold alloys in artificial saliva and saline solutions, *Dent Mater* 5:324, 1989.

Keller JC, Lautenschlager EP: Metals and alloys. In von Recum AF, editor: *Handbook of biomaterials evaluation*, New York, 1986, Macmillan.

Leinfelder KF: An evaluation of casting alloys used for restorative procedures, *J Am Dent Assoc* 128:37, 1997.

Leinfelder KF, Price WG, Gurley WH: Low-gold alloys: a laboratory and clinical evaluation, *Quint Dent Technol* 5:483, 1981.

Mahan J, Charbeneau GT: A study of certain mechanical properties and the density of condensed specimens made from various forms of pure gold, *J Am Acad Gold Foil Op* 8:6, 1965.

Malhotra ML: Dental gold casting alloys: a review, *Trends Tech Contemp Dent Lab* 8:73, 1991.

Malhotra ML: New generation of palladium-indium-silver dental cast alloys: a review, *Trends Tech Contemp Dent Lab* 9:65, 1992.

Mezger PR, Stols AL, Vrijhoel MM, et al: Metallurgical aspects and corrosion behavior of yellow low-gold alloys, *Dent Mater* 5:350, 1989.

Moffa JP: Alternative dental casting alloys, *Dent Clin North Am* 27:733, 1983.

Morris HF, Manz M, Stoffer W, et al: Casting alloys: the materials and "The Clinical Effects" per PubMed, *Adv Dent Res* 6:28, 1992.

Nielsen JP, Tuccillo JJ: Grain size in cast gold alloys, *J Dent Res* 45:964, 1966.

O'Brien WJ: *Dental materials and their selection*, ed 2, Carol Stream, IL, 1997, Quintessence.

Richter WA, Cantwell KR: A study of cohesive gold, *J Pros-thet Dent* 15:772, 1965.

Richter WA, Mahler DB: Physical properties vs clinical performance of pure gold restorations, *J Prosthet Dent* 29:434, 1973.

Roberts HW, Berzins DW, Moore BK, Charlton DG: Metal-ceramic alloys in dentistry, a review, *J Pros* 18:188, 2009.

Sarkar NK, Fuys RA Jr, Stanford JW: The chloride corrosion of low-gold casting alloys, *J Dent Res* 58:568, 1979.

Shell JS, Hollenback GM: Tensile strength and elongation of pure gold, *J Calif Dent Assoc* 34:219, 1966.

Stub JR, Eyer CS, Sarkar NK: Heat treatment, microstructure and corrosion of a low-gold casting alloy, *J Oral Rehabil* 13:521, 1986.

U.S. Department of Labor, Occupational Safety and Health Administration: Hazard Information Bulletin 02-04-19 (rev. 05-14-02), Preventing adverse health effects from exposure to beryllium in dental laboratories, 2002.

Vermilyea SG, Cai Z, Brantley WA, et al: Metallurgical structure and microhardness of four new palladium-based alloys, *J Prosthodont* 5:288, 1996.

Wataha JC: Biocompatibility of dental casting alloys, *J Pros-thet Dent* 83:223, 2000.

Wataha JC: Alloys for prosthodontic restorations, *J Prosthet Dent* 87:351–363, 2002.

Watanabe I, Watanabe E, Cai Z: Effect of heat treatment on mechanical properties of age-hardenable gold alloy at intraoral temperature, *Dent Mater* 17(5):388–393, 2001.

Wendt SL: Nonprecious cast-metal alloys in dentistry, *Cur Opin Dent* 1:222, 1991.

Cast Base-Metal Alloys

Asgar K, Allan FC: Microstructure and physical properties of alloy for partial denture castings, *J Dent Res* 47:189, 1968.

Asgar K, Peyton FA: Effect of casting conditions on some mechanical properties of cobalt-base alloys, *J Dent Res* 40:73, 1961.

Asgar K, Peyton FA: Effect of microstructure on the physical properties of cobalt-based alloys, *J Dent Res* 40:63, 1961.

Asgar K, Peyton FA: Flow and fracture of dental alloys determined by a microbend tester, *J Dent Res* 41:142, 1962.

Asgar K, Techow BO, Jacobson JM: A new alloy for partial dentures, *J Prosthet Dent* 23:36, 1970.

Baran GR: The metallurgy of Ni-Cr alloys for fixed prosthodontics, *J Prosthet Dent* 50:639, 1983.

Bates JF: Studies related to the fracture of partial dentures, *Br Dent J* 118:532, 1965.

Bumgardner JD, Lucas LC: Surface analysis of nickel-chromium dental alloys, *Dent Mater* 9:252, 1993.

Ben-Ur Z, Pataei H, Cardash HS, et al: The fracture of cobalt-chromium alloy removable partial dentures, *Quint Int* 17:797, 1986.

Bergman M, Bergman B, Soremark R: Tissue accumulation of nickel released due to electrochemical corrosion of non-precious dental casting alloys, *J Oral Rehabil* 7:325, 1980.

Brune D, Beltesbrekke H: Dust in dental laboratories: types and levels in specific operations, *J Prosthet Dent* 43:687, 1980.

Cecconi BT: Removable partial denture research and its clinical significance, *J Prosthet Dent* 39:203, 1978.

Cecconi BT, Asgar K, Dootz ER: Fit of the removable partial denture base and its effect on abutment tooth movement, *J Prosthet Dent* 25:515, 1971.

Cheng TP, Tsai WT, Chern Lin JH: The effect of beryllium on the corrosion resistance of nickel-chromium dental alloys, *J Mater Sci Mater Med* 1:211, 1990.

Council on Dental Materials, Instruments, and Equipment: Report on base metal alloys for crown and bridge applications: benefits and risks, *J Am Dent Assoc* 111:479, 1985.

Cunningham DM: Comparison of base metal alloys and Type IV gold alloys for removable partial denture frameworks, *Dent Clin North Am* 17:719, 1973.

Frank RP, Brudvik JS, Nicholls JI: A comparison of the flexibility of wrought wire and cast circumferential clasps, *J Prosthet Dent* 49:471, 1983.

Geis-Gerstorfer J, Passler K: Studies of the influence of Be content on corrosion behaviour and mechanical properties of Ni25Cr10Mo alloys, *Dent Mater* 9:177, 1993.

Hinman RW, Lynde TA, Pelleu GB Jr, et al: Factors affecting airborne beryllium concentrations in dental space, *J Prosthet Dent* 33:210, 1975.

Lucas LC, Lemons JE: Biodegradation of restorative metal systems, *Adv Dent Res* 65:32, 1992.

Mohammed H, Asgar K: A new dental super alloy system, I, II, III, *J Dent Res* 52:136, 145, 151, 1973.

Morris HF, Asgar K: Physical properties and microstructure of four new commercial partial denture alloys, *J Prosthet Dent* 33:36, 1975.

Morris HF, Asgar K, Rowe AP, et al: The influence of heat treatments on several types of base-metal removable partial denture alloys, *J Prosthet Dent* 41:388, 1979.

Roach M: Base metal alloys used for dental restorations and implants, *Dent Clin N Am* 51:603, 2007.

Rowe AP, Bigelow WC, Asgar K: Effect of tantalum addition to a cobalt-chromium-nickel base alloy, *J Dent Res* 53:325, 1974.

Smith DC: Tissue reaction to noble and base metal alloys. In Smith DC, William DF, editors: *Biocompatibility of dental materials*, vol, 4 Boca Raton, 1982, CRC Press.

Strandman E: Influence of different types of acetylene-oxygen flames on the carbon content of dental Co-Cr alloy, *Odontol Rev* 27:223, 1976.

Vallittu PK, Kokkonen M: Deflection fatigue of cobalt-chromium, titanium, and gold alloy cast denture clasps, *J Prosthet Dent* 74:412, 1995.

Wakasa K, Yamaki M: Dental application of the 30Ni-30Cu-40Mn ternary alloy system, *J Mater Sci Mater Med* 1:44, 1990.

Wakasa K, Yamaki M: Corrosive properties in experimental Ni-Cu-Mn based alloy systems for dental purposes, *J Mater Sci: Mater Med* 1:171, 1990.

Wakasa K, Yamaki M: Tensile behaviour in 30Ni-30Cu-30Mn based alloys for a dental application, *J Mater Sci Mater Med* 2:71, 1991.

Wataha JC, Craig RG, Hanks CT: The release of elements of dental casting alloys into cell-culture medium, *J Dent Res* 70:1014, 1991.

Wataha JC, Craig RG, Hanks CT: The effects of cleaning on the kinetics of in vitro metal release from dental casting alloys, *J Dent Res* 71:1417, 1992.

Waterstrat RM: New alloys, *J Am Dent Assoc* 123:33, 1992.

Yong T, De Long B, Goodkind RJ, et al: Leaching of Ni, Cr and Be ions from base metal alloys in an artificial oral environment, *J Prosthet Dent* 68:692, 1992.

Wrought Base-Metal Alloys

Alapati SB, Brantley WA, Svec TA, et al: Observations of nickel-titanium rotary endodontic instruments that fractured during clinical use, *J Endod* 31:40, 2005.

Alapati SB, Brantley WA, Svec TA, et al: Scanning electron microscope observations of new and used nickel-titanium rotary files, *J Endod* 29:667, 2003.

Andreasen GF, Barrett RD: An evaluation of cobalt-substituted Nitinol wire in orthodontics, *Am J Orthod* 63:462, 1973.

Andreasen GF, Brady PR: A use hypothesis for 55 Nitinol wire for orthodontics, *Angle Orthod* 42:172, 1972.

Andreasen GF, Morrow RE: Laboratory and clinical analyses of Nitinol wire, *Am J Orthod* 73:142, 1978.

Andreasen GF, Bigelow H, Andrews JG: 55 Nitinol wire: force developed as a function of œelastic memory, *Aust Dent J* 24:146, 1979.

Braff MH: A comparison between stainless steel crowns and multisurface amalgams in primary molars, *J Dent Child* 46:474, Nov-Dec 1975.

Brantley WA, Augat WS, Myers CL, et al: Bending deformation studies of orthodontic wires, *J Dent Res* 57:609, 1978.

Brantley WA, Svec TA, Iijima M, et al: Differential scanning calorimetric studies of nickel-titanium rotary endodontic instruments after simulated clinical use, *J Endod* 28:774, 2002.

Brantley WA, Svec TA, Iijima M, et al: Differential scanning calorimetric studies of nickel titanium rotary endodontic instruments, *J Endod* 28:567, 2002.

Burstone CJ, Goldberg AJ: Beta titanium: a new orthodontic alloy, *Am J Orthod* 77:121, 1980.

Chen R, Zhi YF, Arvystas MG: Advanced Chinese NiTi alloy wire and clinical observations, *Angle Orthod* 62:15, 1992.

Dolan DW, Craig RG: Bending and torsion of endodontic files with rhombus cross sections, *J Endod* 8:260, 1982.

Drake SR, Wayne DM, Powers JM, et al: Mechanical properties of orthodontic wires in tension, bending, and torsion, *Am J Orthod* 82:206, 1982.

Goldberg J, Burstone CJ: An evaluation of beta titanium alloys for use in orthodontic appliances, *J Dent Res* 58:593, 1979.

Goldberg AJ, Burstone CJ, Hadjinikolaoa I, et al: Screening of matrices and fibers for reinforced thermoplastics intended for dental applications, *J Biomed Mater Res* 28:167, 1994.

Ha'kel Y, Serfaty R, Bateman G, et al: Dynamic and cyclic fatigue of engine-driven rotary nickel-titanium endodontic instruments, *J Endod* 25:434, 1999.

Kapila S, Sachdeva R: Mechanical properties and clinical applications of orthodontic wires, *Am J Orthod Dentofac Orthop* 96:100, 1989.

Kusy RP: Comparison of nickel-titanium and beta titanium wire sizes to conventional orthodontic arch wire materials, *Am J Orthod* 79:625, 1981.

Neal RG, Craig RG, Powers JM: Cutting ability of K-type endodontic files, *J Endod* 9:52, 1983.

Neal RG, Craig RG, Powers JM: Effect of sterilization and irrigants on the cutting ability of stainless steel files, *J Endod* 9:93, 1983.

Newman JG, Brantley WA, Gorstein H: A study of the cutting efficiency of seven brands of endodontic files in linear motion, *J Endod* 9:316, 1983.

Parmiter OK: Wrought stainless steels. In *ASM metals handbook, Cleveland,* 1948, American Society for Metals.

Patel AP, Goldberg AJ, Burstone CJ: The effect of thermoforming on the properties of fiber-reinfroced composite wires, *J Appl Biomat* 3:177, 1992.

Peterson DS, Jubach TS, Katora M: Scanning electron microscope study of stainless steel crown margins, *ASDC J Dent Child* 45:376, Sept-Oct 1978.

Schwaninger B, Sarkar NK, Foster BE: Effect of long-term immersion corrosion on the flexural properties of Nitinol, *Am J Orthod* 82:45, 1982.

Shastry CV, Goldberg AJ: The influence of drawing parameters on the mechanical properties of two beta-titanium alloys, *J Dent Res* 62:1092, 1983.

Stokes OW, Fiore PM, Barss JT, et al: Corrosion in stainless-steel and nickel-titanium files, *J Endod* 25:17, 1999.

Svec TA, Powers JM: The deterioration of rotary nickel-titanium files under controlled conditions, *J Endod* 28:105, 2002.

Svec TA, Powers JM: A method to assess rotary nickel-titanium files, *J Endod* 26:517–518, 2000.

Thompson SA: An overview of nickel-titanium alloys used in dentistry, *Int Endod J* 33:297, 2000.

Waters NE: Superelastic nickel-titanium wires, *Br J Orthod* 19:319, 1992.

Wilkinson JV: Some metallurgical aspects of orthodontic stainless steel, *Am J Orthod* 48:192, 1962.

Wilson DF, Goldberg AJ: Alternative beta-titanium alloys for orthodontic wires, *Dent Mater* 3:337, 1987.

Yoneyama T, Doi H: Superelasticity and thermal behaviour of NiTi orthodontic archwires, *Dent Mater* 11:1, 1992.

Titanium

Ducheyne P, Kohn D, Smith TS: Fatigue properties of cast and heat treated Ti-6Al-4V alloy for anatomic hip prostheses, *Biomaterials* 8:223, 1987.

Ida K, Togaya T, Tsutsumi S, et al: Effect of magnesia investments on the dental casting of pure titanium or titanium alloys, *Dent Mater J* 1:8, 1982.

Ida K, Tani Y, Tsutsumi S, et al: Clinical applications of pure titanium crowns, *Dent Mater J* 4:191, 1985.

Kimura H, Izumi O, editors: *Titanium '80 science and technology,* Warrendale, PA, 1980, The Metallurgical Society of AIME.

Kohn DH, Ducheyne P: A parametric study of the factors affecting the fatigue strength of porous coated Ti-6Al-4V implant alloy, *J Biomed Mater Res* 24:1483, 1990.

Kohn DH, Ducheyne P: Microstructural refinement of beta-sintered and porous coated Ti-6Al-4V by temporary alloying with hydrogen, *J Mater Sci* 26:534, 1991.

Kohn DH, Ducheyne P: Tensile and fatigue strength of hydrogen treated Ti-6Al-4V alloy, *J Mater Sci* 26:328, 1991.

Lutjering G, Gysler A: Critical review-fatigue. In Lutjering G, Zwicker U, Bunk W, editors: *Titanium, science and technology,* Oferursel, West Germany, 1985, Deutsche Gesellschaft fur Metallkunde.

McCracken M: Dental implant materials: commercially pure titanium and titanium alloys, *J Prosthodont* 8(1):40–43, 1999.

Moser JB, Lin JH, Taira M, et al: Development of dental Pd-Ti alloys, *Dent Mater* 1:37, 1985.

Okabe T, Hero H: The use of titanium in dentistry, *Cells Mater* 5:211, 1995.

Peters M, Gysler A, Lutjering G: Influence of microstructure on the fatigue behavior of Ti-6Al-4V. In Kimura H, Izumi O, editors: *Titanium '80 science and technology,* Warrendale, PA, 1980, The Metallurgical Society of AIME.

Szurgot KC, Marker BC, Moser JB, et al: The casting of titanium for removable partial dentures, *Dent Mater Sci QDT Yearbook* 171, 1988.

Taira M, Moser JB, Greener EH: Studies of Ti alloys for dental castings, *Dent Mater* 5:45, 1989.

Voitik AJ: Titanium dental castings, cold worked titanium restorations—yes or no? *Trends and Techniques* 8(10):23, Dec 1991.

Waterstrat RM: *Comments on casting of Ti-13Cu-4.5Ni alloy,* Washington, DC, 1977, DHEW, Pub No (NIH) 77–1227, p 224.

Yamauchi M, Sakai M, Kawano J: Clinical application of pure titanium for cast plate dentures, *Dent Mater J* 7:39, 1988.

Restorative Materials—Ceramics

The term *ceramic* refers to any product made from a nonmetallic inorganic material usually processed by firing at a high temperature to achieve desirable properties. The more restrictive term *porcelain* refers to a specific compositional range of ceramic materials originally made by mixing kaolin (hydrated aluminosilicate), quartz (silica), and feldspars (potassium and sodium aluminosilicates), and firing at high temperature. Dental ceramics for *metal-ceramic* restorations belong to this compositional range and are commonly referred to as *dental porcelains.*

The laboratory portion of ceramic restorations is usually made in a commercial dental laboratory by skilled technicians working with specialized equipment to shape and tint the restoration to the specifications provided by the dentist. Skilled technicians and artisans are also employed by the manufacturers of artificial denture teeth to produce the many forms, types, and shades necessary in this application of porcelain. However, a variety of machinable ceramics are also available for chair-side fabrication of all-ceramic restorations by computer-aided design/computer-aided manufacturing (CAD/CAM). A discussion of CAD/CAM systems is presented in Chapter 14.

CLASSIFICATION OF DENTAL CERAMICS

Dental ceramics can be classified according to their applications, fabrication method, or crystalline phase (Table 11-1).

TABLE 11.1   Classification of Dental Ceramic Materials with Examples of Products and Their Manufacturers

Application	Fabrication	Crystalline phase	Products	Manufacturers
ALL-CERAMIC	Soft-machined	Zirconia (3Y-TZP)	Cercon®	Dentsply International
			Lava™	3M ESPE
			IPS e.max ZirCAD	Ivoclar Vivadent
			In-Ceram® YZ	Vident
		Alumina (Al_2O_3)	Procera	Nobel Biocare
			In-Ceram® AL	Vident
	Soft-machined & glass-infiltrated			
		Alumina (Al_2O_3)	In-Ceram® Alumina	Vident
		Spinel ($MgAl_2O_4$)	In-Ceram® Spinell	Vident
		Zirconia (12Ce-TZP/Al_2O_3)	In-Ceram® Zirconia	Vident
	Hard-machined	Lithium disilicate ($Li_2Si_2O_5$)	IPS e.max CAD	Ivoclar Vivadent
		Feldspar ((Na, K)$AlSi_3O_8$)	Vita Mark II	Vident
		Leucite ($KAlSi_2O_6$)	IPS Empress CAD	Ivoclar Vivadent
	Slip-cast	Alumina (Al_2O_3)	In-Ceram® Alumina	Vident
		Spinel ($MgAl_2O_4$)	In-Ceram® Spinell	Vident
		Zirconia (12Ce-TZP/Al_2O_3)	In-Ceram® Zirconia	Vident
	Heat-pressed	Leucite ($KAlSi_2O_6$)	IPS Empress	Ivoclar Vivadent
		Lithium disilicate ($Li_2Si_2O_5$)	IPS e.max Press	Ivoclar Vivadent
		Fluorapatite ($Ca_5(PO_4)_3F$)	IPS e.max ZirPress	Ivoclar Vivadent
	Sintered	Leucite ($KAlSi_2O_6$)	IPS Empress layering ceramic	Ivoclar Vivadent
		Alumina (Al_2O_3)	Procera Allceram	Nobel Biocare
		Fluorapatite ($Ca_5(PO_4)_3F$)	IPS e.max Ceram layering ceramic	Ivoclar Vivadent
METAL-CERAMIC	Sintered	Leucite ($KAlSi_2O_6$)	VMK-95	Vident
DENTURE TEETH	Manufactured	Feldspar	Trubyte®	Dentsply International
		Feldspar	Vita Lumin® Vacuum	Vident

Classification by Application

Ceramics have two major applications in dentistry: (1) ceramics for metal-ceramic crowns (Figure 11-1, *right*) and fixed partial prostheses, (2) all-ceramic crowns (Figure 11-1, *left*), inlays, onlays, veneers, and fixed partial prostheses. Additionally, ceramic orthodontic brackets, dental implant abutments, and ceramic denture teeth are available.

Classification by Fabrication Method

The classification by fabrication method is summarized in Table 11-1, which also includes examples of commercial ceramics and their manufacturers. The most common fabrication technique for metal-ceramic restorations is called *sintering*. Sintering is the process of firing the compacted ceramic powder at high temperature to ensure optimal densification. This occurs by pore elimination and viscous flow when the firing temperature is reached. All-ceramic restorations can also be produced by sintering, but they encompass a wider range of processing techniques, including slip-casting, heat-pressing, and CAD/CAM machining. Some of these techniques, such as machining and heat-pressing, can also be combined to produce the final restoration.

Classification by Crystalline Phase

Regardless of their applications or fabrication technique, after firing, dental ceramics are composed of a glassy (or vitreous) phase and one or more crystalline phases, together with various amounts of porosity. Depending on the nature and amount of crystalline phase and porosity present, the mechanical and optical properties of dental ceramics vary widely. Increasing the amount of crystalline phase may lead to crystalline reinforcement and increase the resistance to crack propagation but also can decrease translucency. Materials for all-ceramic restorations have increased amounts of crystalline

phase (between 35% for leucite-reinforced ceramics and up to 99% for polycrystalline zirconia ceramics such as 3Y-TZP) for better mechanical properties, but they are usually more opaque than dental porcelains for metal-ceramic restorations with low crystallinity. Table 11-1 lists the various combinations of fabrication techniques and crystalline phases found in dental ceramics.

GENERAL APPLICATIONS OF CERAMICS IN PROSTHETIC DENTISTRY

Ceramics remain the best material available for matching the esthetics of a complex human tooth. Their applications in dentistry are steadily expanding as new materials and manufacturing techniques are being introduced. They are used in single and multiunit metal-ceramic restorations. With all-ceramic systems, their applications include inlays, onlays, veneers, and crowns. The development of high-strength zirconia-based systems has made possible the fabrication of dental implant abutments and fixed partial prostheses. In addition, ceramics are still used to fabricate denture teeth. However, ceramics are generally brittle, weak in tension, and their performance is highly dependent on both their microstructure and the quality of the processing from the raw components to the final staining or glazing step.

Metal-Ceramic Crowns and Fixed Partial Prostheses

Ceramic is widely used as the veneering material in metal-ceramic crowns and fixed partial prostheses. This development was the result of successfully matching the coefficients of thermal expansion of porcelain with metal alloys and achieving a proper metal-ceramic bond. The finished glazed restoration is color-stable, tissue-friendly, biologically inert, and chemically durable. Metal-ceramic restorations are still widely used. However, while the survival rate of most all-ceramic crown systems compares favorably to that of metal-ceramic crowns for single restorations, the survival rate of multiunit all-ceramic fixed dental prostheses at 10 years is considerably lower. Meanwhile, survival rates at 5 years for zirconia-based all-ceramic systems appear promising.

All-Ceramic Crowns, Inlays, Onlays, and Veneers

Ceramics have been used to fabricate jacket crowns since the early 1900s. At that time feldspathic porcelain was used in the fabrication. Alumina-reinforced ceramics with improved mechanical

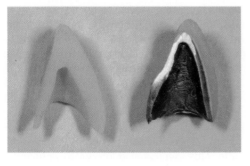

FIGURE 11.1 **Cutaways of all-ceramic crown (*left*) and porcelain fused to metal crown (*right*).** (*Courtesy of Dr. Charles Mark Malloy, Portland, Oregon.*)

properties were developed in the early 1960s. During the past 30 years, numerous novel materials and techniques for fabricating all-ceramic restorations have been introduced. As mentioned earlier in this chapter, they include heat-pressed, slip-cast, and machined all-ceramic materials. These new materials and techniques have widened the range of applications of ceramics, and in some cases made their processing easier.

Ceramic inlays and onlays are becoming increasingly popular as an alternative to posterior resin composites. They have better abrasion resistance than posterior composite resins and therefore are more durable. However, occlusal adjustments are more difficult and can lead to subsequent wear of the opposing tooth if not properly adjusted and polished. The marginal gap is clinically acceptable, yet greater than with gold inlays or onlays.

A ceramic esthetic veneer (laminate veneer) is a layer of ceramic bonded to the facial surface of a prepared tooth to cover an unsightly area. Ceramic veneers are custom made and are fabricated in a dental laboratory. Initially, ceramic veneers were made of feldspathic porcelain and sintered. Currently, most ceramic veneers are fabricated by heat-pressing or machining, using either a leucite-reinforced or lithium disilicate ceramic. To obtain sufficient adhesion, the tooth enamel is etched with phosphoric acid and the bonding surface of the ceramic is etched with 5% to 9% hydrofluoric acid gel and treated with a silane coupling agent. Resin composites specifically formulated for bonding to ceramic are used as the adhesive.

MECHANICAL AND THERMAL PROPERTIES OF DENTAL CERAMICS

Toughening Methods

Toughening methods for glasses and ceramics can be "built-in" or intrinsic to the material composition or crystalline phase. Crystalline reinforcement and transformation toughening are examples of built-in toughening mechanisms. Specific processing steps, such as tempering, chemical strengthening, or glaze application can also be involved to obtain strengthening.

The principle of toughening by crystalline reinforcement is to increase the resistance of the ceramic to crack propagation by introducing a dispersed crystalline phase with high toughness. Crystals can also act as crack deflectors when their coefficient of thermal expansion is greater than that of the surrounding glassy matrix, placing them under tangential compressive stresses after the ceramic has been cooled to room temperature.

Transformation toughening is obtained, for example, in ceramics containing partially stabilized tetragonal zirconia. Zirconia (ZrO_2) exists under several crystallographic forms. The monoclinic form is stable at all temperatures below 1170° C. The tetragonal form is stable between 1170° and up to 2370° C. The transformation from the tetragonal to the monoclinic form upon cooling is associated with a volume *increase* of the unit cell. This is the reason compacts of pure unalloyed zirconia cannot be obtained at room temperature; the compact would spontaneously crack upon cooling due to the transformation. The tetragonal form can be partially stabilized to room temperature by doping with various oxides, such as yttria oxide (Y_2O_3) or cerium oxide (CeO_2). Zirconia-based dental ceramics produced by machining followed by sintering at high temperature contain tetragonal zirconia polycrystals, partially stabilized with 3 mole percent yttrium (3Y-TZP). This partial stabilization or metastability of the tetragonal phase allows the transformation from tetragonal to monoclinic to occur under external applied stresses. The transformation is also called *stress-induced* and is accompanied by a volume increase with associated compressive stresses in the vicinity of the crack tip, eventually leading to a closing of the crack in the transformed zone (Figure 11-2). Transformation toughening is responsible for the excellent mechanical properties of 3Y-TZP. Figure 11-3 shows a Vickers indentation in a 3Y-TZP dental ceramic under a 98.1-N load. Only one short crack can be seen emanating from one corner of the indentation.

Tempering and chemical strengthening are extrinsic strengthening techniques based on the creation of a compressive stress layer at the surface of a glass or a ceramic. Tempering is obtained by using rapid but controlled cooling rates whereas chemical strengthening relies on the replacement of small ions with larger ions by diffusion from a molten salt bath in which the ceramic or glass is immersed. Although widely used in the glass industry, neither of these two techniques is used for dental ceramics.

Glazing is the final step in the fabrication of metal-ceramic restorations. This standard technique, also called *self-glazing*, does not significantly improve the flexural strength of feldspathic dental porcelains. However, a low-expansion glass called *glaze* can also be applied at the surface of the ceramic, then fired to high temperature. Upon cooling, this glaze layer is placed under compression from the greater contraction of the underlying ceramic. This layer is also known to reduce depth and width of the surface flaws, thereby improving the overall resistance of the ceramic to crack propagation.

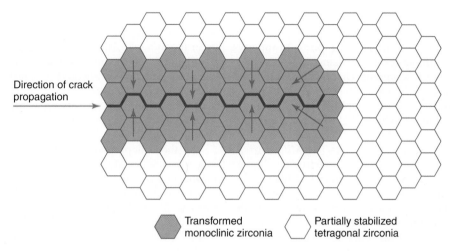

FIGURE 11.2 **Schematic of transformation toughening mechanism in partially stabilized zirconia.**

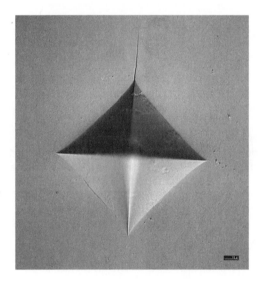

FIGURE 11.3 **Vickers indentation under a 98.1-N load on a zirconia-based dental ceramic.**

Test Methods

Numerous test methods are available to evaluate the mechanical properties of ceramics. Studies of the influence of test method on the failure stress of brittle dental materials have shown that important test parameters are the specimen thickness, contact zone at loading, homogeneity and porosity of the material, and loading rate. For this reason, discrepancies exist among the published values of mechanical properties for a given material. Manufacturers evaluate dental ceramics using a standard (ISO 6872) published and regularly revised by the International Organization for Standardization. Set protocols are proposed to evaluate radioactivity, flexural strength, linear coefficient of thermal expansion, glass transition temperature, and chemical solubility.

Sometimes, researchers use devices that try to simulate dental morphology. However, the experimental variables can become extremely complex and difficult to reproduce in this type of testing. Finite element analysis (FEA) constitutes another approach to the simulation of clinical conditions. Failure predictions of ceramic inlays by the FEA technique have successfully matched fractographic analyses of clinically failed restorations. Fractography is well established as a failure-analysis technique for glasses and ceramics. It has been recognized as a powerful analytical tool in dentistry. The *in vivo* failure stress of clinically failed all-ceramic crowns can be determined using fractography (see more discussion in Chapter 5.

Comparative Data

Flexural strength data for dental ceramics are summarized in Table 11-2. Feldspathic porcelains for metal-ceramic restorations have a mean flexural strength between 60 and 80 MPa. This value is lower than those listed for all-ceramic materials; however, because metal-ceramic restorations are supported by a metallic framework, their long-term probability of survival is usually higher.

Among the currently available all-ceramic materials, zirconia (3Y-TZP) ceramics exhibit the highest values (800-1300 MPa), followed by slip-cast ceramics (378 to 630 MPa), and lithium disilicate–reinforced ceramics (262 to 306 MPa). The flexural strength of leucite-reinforced ceramics is around 100 MPa. As mentioned previously, the nature and amount of the crystalline phase present in the ceramic material strongly influences the mechanical properties of the final product. The shear strength of feldspathic porcelain is 110 MPa, and the diametral tensile strength is lower at 34 MPa. The compressive strength is about 172 MPa, and the Knoop hardness is 460 kg/mm^2.

Fracture toughness is also an important property of ceramics; it measures the resistance to brittle fracture when a crack is present. The fracture toughness of conventional feldspathic porcelains is very similar to that of soda lime glass (0.78 MPa · m$^{0.5}$). Leucite-reinforced ceramics exhibit slightly higher fracture toughness values (1.2 MPa · m$^{0.5}$), followed by lithium disilicate–reinforced ceramics (3.0 MPa · m$^{0.5}$). 3Y-TZP ceramics have the highest fracture toughness of all-ceramic materials (greater than 5.0 MPa · m$^{0.5}$).

The elastic constants of dental ceramics are needed in the calculations of both flexural strength and fracture toughness. Poisson's ratio lies between 0.21 and 0.26 for dental ceramics. The modulus of elasticity is about 70 GPa for feldspathic porcelain, 110 GPa for lithium disilicate heat-pressed ceramics, and 210 GPa for 3Y-TZP ceramics and reaches 350 GPa for alumina-based ceramics.

Shrinkage remains an issue for all-ceramic materials with the exception of machined ceramics from fully sintered ceramic blocks and heat-pressed ceramics. Shrinkage of the veneering ceramics applied on all-ceramic cores has to be carefully compensated for during porcelain buildup. The large shrinkage of machined zirconia restorations during the subsequent sintering at very high temperature (about 25%) is compensated for at the design-stage by computerized enlargement of the restorations.

The density of fully sintered feldspathic porcelain is around 2.45 g/cm^3 and will vary with the porosity of the material. The density of ceramic materials also depends on the amount and nature of crystalline phase present. The theoretical density of 3Y-TZP dental ceramics is 6.08 g/cm^3, assuming that the material is pore free. A density greater than 98.7% of the theoretical density is required for medical grade 3Y-TZP ceramics.

The thermal properties of feldspathic porcelain include a conductivity of 0.0030 cal/sec/cm^2 (° C/cm), a diffusivity of 0.64 mm^2/sec, and a linear coefficient of thermal expansion (CTE) of about 12.0 × 10^{-6}/° C between 25° and 500° C. The CTE is about 10 × 10^{-6}/° C for aluminous ceramics and lithium disilicate ceramics, 10.5 × 10^{-6}/° C for zirconia-based ceramics (3Y-TZP), and 14 to 18 × 10^{-6}/° C for leucite-reinforced ceramics.

OPTICAL PROPERTIES OF DENTAL CERAMICS

Shade matching is a critical problem in replacing natural teeth. In addition, porcelain, being mostly amorphous in structure, cannot match the optical properties of crystalline enamel completely. As a result, ultraviolet (UV) and visible light rays are reflected and absorbed in different manners by the combination dentin/enamel, compared to porcelain,

TABLE 11.2   Flexural Strength of Selected Dental Ceramics

Processing Technique	Crystalline Phase	Flexural Strength (MPa)	Percent Crystallinity
Soft-machined	Zirconia (3Y-TZP)	1087 ± 173	Highly crystalline
	Alumina (Al$_2$O$_3$)	≈ 700*	Highly crystalline
Hard-machined	Feldspar ([Na, K]AlSi$_3$O$_8$)	122 ± 13	≈ 30
	Lithium disilicate (Li$_2$Si$_2$O$_5$)	262 ± 88	65
	Leucite (KAlSi$_2$O$_6$)	≈ 160*	≈ 35
Slip-cast	Alumina (Al$_2$O$_3$)	594 ± 52	65-68
	Spinel (MgAl$_2$O$_4$)	378 ± 65	67-68
	Zirconia (ZrO$_2$)	630 ± 58	67
Heat-pressed	Leucite (KAlSi$_2$O$_6$)	106 ± 17	35
	Lithium disilicate (Li$_2$Si$_2$O$_5$)	306 ± 29	65
Sintered	Leucite (KAlSi$_2$O$_6$)	104	35-40
	Fluorapatite (Ca$_5$[PO$_4$]$_3$F)	≈ 80*	10
Sintered metal-ceramic	Leucite (KAlSi$_2$O$_6$)	61 ± 5	15-25

Data from: Guazzato M, Albakry M, Ringer SP, et al: Dent. Mater. 20, 441-448, 2004; Guazzato M, Albakry M, Ringer SP, et al: Dent. Mater. 20, 449-456, 2004; Denry IL, Holloway JA, Tarr LA: J. Biomed. Mater. Res. (Appl. Biomater.), 48, 791-796, 1999; Della Bona A, Mecholsky Jr. JJ, Anusavice KJ: Dent. Mater. 20, 956-962, 2004; Höland W, Beall G: Glass-ceramic technology. The American Ceramic Society, Westerville, OH, 2002.
*Data from manufacturer.

and restorations viewed from one incidence angle may not appear the same as they do when viewed from a different incidence angle. The cementing medium is an important factor in the final appearance of an all-ceramic restoration. Because of its opacity, an aluminous all-ceramic restoration may be cemented with a wide range of luting agents. However, more translucent all-ceramic restorations such as leucite-reinforced heat-pressed or machined inlays, crowns, or veneers, or a machined inlay or veneer, usually require the use of translucent resin luting agents that are available in different shades.

The shades of commercial premixed dental porcelain powders are in the yellow to yellow-red range. Because the range of shades of natural teeth is much greater than the range available in a kit of premixed porcelains, modifier porcelains are also supplied for adjustments. These modifiers are strongly pigmented porcelains usually supplied in blue, yellow, pink, orange, brown, and gray. The dental technician may add the modifier porcelain to the opaque and body porcelains during the building of the crown. Extrinsic surface staining, another way of changing the appearance of a ceramic crown, involves the application of highly pigmented glazes. The main disadvantages of surface staining are a lowered durability (a result of solubility) and the reduction of translucency.

Translucency is another critical property of dental ceramics. The translucency of opaque, dentin (body), and enamel (incisal) porcelains differs considerably. Opaque porcelains have very low translucency, allowing them to mask metal substructure surfaces. Tin oxide (SnO_2) and titanium oxide (TiO_2) are important opacifying oxides for dental ceramics. Dentin porcelain translucency values range between 18% and 38%, as seen in Table 11-3. Enamel porcelains have the highest values of translucency, ranging between 45% and 50%. The translucency of materials for all-ceramic restorations varies with the nature of the reinforcing crystalline phase. Alumina- and some zirconia-based systems are opaque, whereas leucite-reinforced systems are more translucent. Recently, translucent zirconia systems have become available.

The translucency of spinel-based systems is comparable to that of lithium disilicate–based systems and intermediate between alumina-based and leucite-reinforced systems. In order to mimic the optical properties of human enamel, opalescence is often desirable. Opalescence is a form of scattering and occurs when the crystal size is equal or smaller than the wavelength of light. In reflected light, the shorter blue-violet wavelengths are transmitted, whereas in transmitted light, the longer red-orange wavelengths are transmitted through the porcelain.

Dental enamel also exhibits fluorescence. This characteristic is achieved in dental porcelains by adding rare earth oxides (such as cerium oxide). Because the outer layers of a ceramic crown are translucent, the apparent color is affected by reflectance from the inner opaque or core ceramic. For metal-ceramic restorations, shade mixing results from combining the light reflected from the inner, opaque porcelain surface and the light transmitted through the body porcelain. The thickness of the body porcelain layer determines the shade obtained with an opaque porcelain. This thickness effect may be minimized if the body porcelain and the opaque porcelain are the same color as that of some commercial systems.

ALL-CERAMIC RESTORATIONS

Materials for all-ceramic restorations use a wide variety of crystalline phases as reinforcing agents and contain up to 99% by volume of crystalline phase. The nature, amount, and particle size distribution of the crystalline phase directly influence the mechanical and optical properties of the material. The match between the refractive indexes of the crystalline phase and glassy matrix is an important factor for controlling the translucency of the porcelain.

As mentioned earlier, several processing techniques are available for fabricating all-ceramic restorations: sintering, heat-pressing, slip-casting, and CAD/CAM. Figure 11-1, *left*, illustrates the cross section of an all-ceramic crown.

TABLE 11.3 Percent Light Transmission of 1-mm Thick Dentin Porcelains

Shade	Ceramco	Vita	Neydium	Will-Ceram	Steeles
59	29.97	22.66	31.93	26.06	27.23
62	27.85	—	—	27.88	—
65	23.31	20.39	35.39	33.50	22.10
67	26.32	18.04	23.58	19.03	23.42
91	31.81	—	38.41	—	—

Adapted from Brodbelt RHW, O'Brien WJ, Fan PL: J. Dent. Res. 59, 70, 1980.

Sintered All-Ceramic Materials

Two main types of all-ceramic materials are available for the sintering technique: alumina-based ceramic and leucite-reinforced ceramic.

Alumina-Based Ceramic

The aluminous core ceramic used in the aluminous porcelain crown developed by McLean in 1965 is a typical example of strengthening by dispersion of a crystalline phase. Alumina has a high modulus of elasticity (350 GPa) and relatively high fracture toughness (3.5 to 4 MPa $\cdot$ m$^{0.5}$), compared to feldspathic porcelains. Its dispersion in a glassy matrix of similar thermal expansion coefficient leads to a significant strengthening effect. It has been proposed that the excellent bond between the alumina and the glass phase is responsible for this increase in strength compared with leucite-containing ceramics. The first aluminous core porcelains contained 40% to 50% alumina by weight, dispersed in a low-fusing glassy matrix. The core was baked on a platinum foil and later veneered with matched-expansion porcelain. Aluminous core ceramic is now baked directly on a refractory die. Aluminous core porcelains have flexural strengths approximately twice that of feldspathic porcelains (139 to 145 MPa).

Densely sintered alumina-based ceramics can also be produced by dry pressing, followed by sintering. In order to compensate for sintering shrinkage (12% to 20% linear), an enlarged die is generated by computer-aided design. A high purity alumina-based ceramic is then fabricated by dry pressing and sintering at high temperature (1550° C). The final product is a highly crystalline ceramic with a mean grain size of about 4 μm and a flexural strength of about 600 MPa. The entire process has to be carefully controlled by the manufacturer. The last steps consist of veneering with translucent porcelain, staining, and glazing. The clinical performance of this ceramic *in vivo* at 15 years is considered excellent. The same technology is also available for zirconia-based core ceramics.

Leucite-Reinforced Ceramic

Leucite-reinforced ceramics containing up to 45% by volume tetragonal leucite are available for fabricating all-ceramic sintered restorations. Leucite acts as a reinforcing phase; the greater leucite content (compared with conventional feldspathic porcelain for metal-ceramic restorations) leads to higher flexural strength (104 MPa) and compressive strength. The large amount of leucite in the material also contributes to a high thermal contraction coefficient. In addition, the large mismatch in thermal contraction between leucite (20 to 25 × 10^{-6}/° C) and the glassy matrix (8 × 10^{-6}/° C) results in the development of tangential compressive stresses in the glass around the leucite crystals

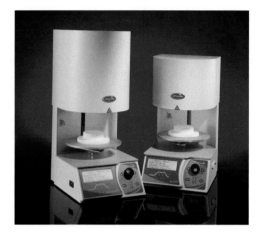

FIGURE 11.4 **Porcelain furnace.** *(Modified from Whip Mix Corporation, Louisville, KY)*

upon cooling, because the crystals contract more than the surrounding glassy matrix. These stresses can act as crack deflectors and contribute to increased resistance of the ceramic to crack propagation.

Sintered all-ceramic restorations are now being replaced by heat-pressed or machined all-ceramic restorations with better-controlled processing steps.

Heat-Pressed All-Ceramic Materials

Heat-pressing relies on the application of external pressure at high temperature to sinter and shape the ceramic. Heat-pressing is used in dentistry to produce all-ceramic crowns, inlays, onlays, veneers, and more recently, fixed partial prostheses. During heat-pressing, ceramic ingots are brought to high temperature in a phosphate-bonded investment mold produced by the lost wax technique. The heat-pressing temperature is chosen near the softening point of the ceramic. A pressure of 0.3 to 0.4 MPa is then applied through a refractory plunger. This allows filling of the mold with the softened ceramic. The high temperature is held for durations between 10 and 20 minutes. Heat-pressing requires a specially designed automated pressing furnace (Figure 11-4) and classically promotes a good dispersion of the crystalline phase within the glassy matrix. The mechanical properties of many ceramic systems are maximized with excellent crystal dispersion, higher crystallinity, and smaller crystal size, compared to sintered all-ceramics.

Leucite-Based Ceramic

First-generation heat-pressed ceramics contain leucite ($KAlSi_2O_6$ or $K_2O \cdot Al_2O_3 \cdot 4SiO_2$) as a reinforcing phase, in amounts varying from 35% to 55% by volume. Heat-pressing temperatures for this system are between 1150° and 1180° C with a dwell at temperature of about 20 minutes. The ceramic ingots

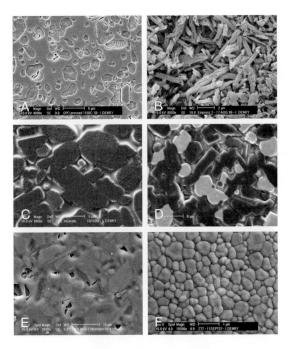

FIGURE 11.5 **Scanning electron micrographs showing the microstructure of selected all-ceramic materials (polished and etched surfaces). A,** Leucite-reinforced heat-pressed ceramic; **B,** lithium disilicate heat-pressed ceramic; **C** slip-cast alumina ceramic; **D,** slip-cast zirconia/alumina ceramic; **E,** feldspar-based machinable ceramic; **F,** soft-machined zirconia ceramic (3Y-TZP).

are available in a variety of shades. The final microstructure of these heat-pressed ceramics consists of leucite crystals, 1 to 5 μm, dispersed in a glassy matrix (Figure 11-5, *A*). The amount of porosity in the heat-pressed ceramic is 9 vol%. Two techniques are available: a staining technique and a layering technique involving the application of veneering ceramic. The two techniques lead to comparable mean flexural strength values for the resulting ceramic. To ensure compatibility with the thermal expansion coefficient of the veneering ceramic, the thermal expansion coefficient of the core material for the veneering technique ($14.9 \times 10^{-6}/^\circ$ C) is lower than that of the core material for the staining technique ($18 \times 10^{-6}/^\circ$ C). The flexural strength of these ceramics (120 MPa) is about double that of conventional feldspathic porcelains. This increase in strength can be explained by the fact that these ceramics possess a higher crystallinity and that the heat-pressing process generates an excellent dispersion of these fine leucite crystals. In addition, as mentioned earlier, thermal stresses around the leucite crystals promote crack deflection and contribute to improved mechanical performance. The main disadvantages are the initial cost of the equipment and relatively low strength compared with other all-ceramic systems.

Lithium Disilicate–Based Materials

The second generation of heat-pressed ceramics contain lithium disilicate ($Li_2Si_2O_5$) as a major crystalline phase. They are heat-pressed in the 890° to 920° C temperature range, using the same equipment as for the leucite-based ceramics. The heat-pressed restorations are later veneered with ceramics of matching thermal expansion. The final microstructure consists of about 65% by volume of highly interlocking prismatic lithium disilicate crystals (5.2 μm in length, 0.8 μm in diameter) dispersed in a glassy matrix (Figure 11-5, *B*). The amount of porosity after heat-pressing is about 1 vol%. Compared to first-generation leucite-based ceramics, the main advantage of the lithium disilicate–based ceramics is their enhanced flexural strength (300 MPa) and fracture toughness (2.9 MPa · m$^{0.5}$). This can be explained by the fact that, similar to leucite-based ceramics, there is a thermal expansion mismatch between the lithium disilicate crystals and the glassy matrix, potentially responsible for crack deflection. In addition, the microstructure consisting of elongated highly interlocked crystals is likely to lead to multiple crack deflections, thereby increasing the resistance to crack propagation. Finally, several studies have reported that heat-pressing promotes crystal alignment along the direction of pressing because of the high aspect ratio of the crystals. This leads to an even higher resistance to crack propagation in the direction perpendicular to crystal alignment. The enhanced mechanical properties of these second-generation heat-pressed ceramics have extended their range of applications making possible the fabrication of fixed partial prostheses.

Slip-Cast All-Ceramic Materials

Slip-casting was introduced in dentistry in the 1990s. The first step of the process involves the condensation of a porcelain slip on a refractory die. The term *slip* refers to an aqueous slurry containing fine ceramic particles. The porosity of the refractory die helps condensation by absorbing the water from the slip by capillary action. The restoration is incrementally built up, shaped, and finally sintered at high temperature on the refractory die. Usually the refractory die shrinks more than the condensed slip so that the restoration can be separated easily after sintering. The sintered porous core is later glass-infiltrated, a unique process in which molten glass is drawn into the pores by capillary action at high temperature. This leads to a microstructure consisting of two interpenetrating networks, one formed by the crystalline infrastructure and the other being the glassy phase. Three types of ceramics are available for slip-casting: alumina-based (Al_2O_3), spinel-based ($MgAlO_4$), and zirconia-toughened alumina ($12Ce-TZP-Al_2O_3$).

Alumina and Spinel-Based Slip-Cast Ceramics

The alumina content of the slip for alumina-based ceramics is more than 90%, with a particle size between 0.5 and 3.5 μm. After drying at 120° C for 6 hours and sintering for 2 hours at 1120° C and 2 hours at 1180° C, the porous alumina coping is infiltrated with a lanthanum-containing glass during a third firing at 1140° C for 2 hours. After removal of the excess glass, the restoration is veneered using matched-expansion veneering ceramic. This processing technique is unique in dentistry and leads to a high-strength material because of the presence of densely packed alumina particles. The microstructure of this material is shown in Figure 11-5, C. It consists of 68 vol% alumina, 27 vol% glass, and 5 vol% porosity. Blocky alumina grains of various sizes and shapes appear in dark contrast. The flexural strength of this slip-cast alumina material is around 600 MPa. Because of the high strength of the core, short-span anterior fixed partial prostheses can be made using this process. However, the presence of alumina crystals with a high refractive index, together with 5% porosity, account for some degree of opacity in this all-ceramic system. Spinel-based slip-cast ceramics are more translucent, because the spinel phase allows better sintering, but the flexural strength is slightly lower (378 MPa) than that of the alumina-based system.

Zirconia-Toughened Alumina Slip-Cast Ceramics

After processing, the zirconia-toughened alumina slip-cast ceramic comprises 34 vol% alumina, 33 vol% zirconia stabilized with 12 mol% ceria (12Ce-TZP), 23 vol% glassy phase, and 8 vol% residual porosity. The microstructure is shown in Figure 11-5, D. The alumina grains appear in darker contrast whereas zirconia grains are brighter. The combination of alumina and zirconia allows two types of strengthening mechanisms. The stress-induced transformation of 12Ce-TZP and the associated increase in volume produces compressive stresses within the zirconia grains. Additionally, the large alumina grains promote crack deflection. The flexural strength of this system has been reported at 630 MPa.

The main advantage of slip-cast ceramics is their high strength; disadvantages include high opacity (with the exception of the spinel-based materials) and long processing times.

Machinable All-Ceramic Materials

Hard machining of machinable all-ceramic materials is performed in the fully sintered state. In this case, the restoration is machined directly to final size. Some all-ceramic materials can also be machined in a partially sintered state and later fully sintered, this

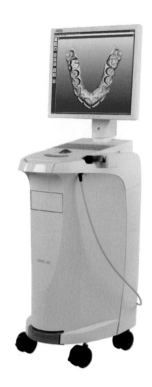

FIGURE 11.6 **Chair-side CAD/CAM system for all-ceramic restorations fabrication.** *(Courtesy of Sirona Dental Systems, LLC, Charlotte, NC)*

is called *soft machining*. This latter technique requires milling of an enlarged restoration to compensate for sintering shrinkage and is well adapted to ceramics that are difficult to machine in the fully sintered state, such as alumina and zirconia.

Hard Machining

Machinable ceramics can be milled to form inlays, onlays, veneers, and crowns using CAD/CAM technology to produce restorations in one office visit. After the tooth is prepared, the preparation is optically scanned and the image is computerized. The restoration is designed with the aid of a computer, as shown in Figure 11-6. The restoration is then machined from ceramic blocks by a computer-controlled milling machine. The milling process takes only a few minutes. Restorations are bonded to the tooth preparation with resin cements. The most recent versions of digital impression software (3M ESPE Lava Chairside Oral Scanner C.O.S., 3M ESPE; CEREC AC, Sirona Dental Systems, LLC; E4D Dentist, D4D Technologies; iTero, Cadent, Inc.) allow complete tridimensional visualization of the projected restoration with *virtual seating* capabilities. The various surfaces of the virtual restoration can be modified in all three dimensions prior to machining.

Further information on digital impression systems can be found in Chapter 14.

Another system for machining ceramics is to form inlays, onlays, veneers, and crowns using copy milling (Celay®, Mikrona Technologie AG). In this system, a hard resin pattern is made on a traditional stone die. This handmade pattern is then copied and machined from a ceramic block using a pantographic device similar in principle to those used for duplicating house keys.

Several machinable ceramics are presently available for use with these systems: feldspar, leucite, and lithium disilicate–based. The feldspar-based ceramic contains approximately 30 vol% feldspar ($Na,K\ AlSi_3O_8$) as a major crystalline phase, dispersed in a glassy matrix (see Figure 11-5, E). Its flexural strength is ranked as moderate (120 MPa). Leucite-reinforced and lithium disilicate ceramic blocks are also available for hard machining by CAD/CAM. The leucite-reinforced ceramic blocks are similar in microstructure and mechanical properties to the first-generation heat-pressed, leucite-reinforced ceramics. The lithium disilicate ceramic blocks are machined in the fully sintered but partially crystallized state, which is more easily machined than the fully crystallized state. In the partially crystallized state, the ceramic contains crystal nuclei of both lithium metasilicate (Li_2SiO_3) and lithium disilicate ($Li_2Si_2O_5$). The translucency of the ceramic can be adjusted by varying the crystallization heat treatment, which dictates crystal size and crystallinity. Low, medium, and high translucency blocks are proposed. After full crystallization heat treatment at 850° C for 10 minutes, the high translucency ceramic exhibits lithium disilicate crystals ($1.5 \times 0.8\ \mu m$) in a glassy matrix, whereas the low translucency ceramic exhibits a high number density of small ($0.8 \times 0.2\ \mu m$) interlocked lithium disilicate crystals. The flexural strength after full crystallization heat treatment is 360 MPa, according to manufacturer's data. One study reported a flexural strength (three-point bending) of 262 ± 88 MPa after full crystallization.

Soft Machining Followed by Sintering

The CAD/CAM and copy-milling systems can also be used to machine presintered alumina, spinel, or zirconia-toughened-alumina blocks to fabricate copings for crowns and fixed partial prostheses. The copings are further glass-infiltrated, resulting in a microstructure similar to that of slip-cast ceramics. The mechanical properties of these materials are comparable to those of the slip-cast version, with a final marginal accuracy within 50 μm.

In 2002, the first zirconia-based ceramic for soft machining was introduced on the dental market. The material consists of tetragonal zirconia polycrystals partially stabilized by addition of 3 mole percent yttrium (3Y-TZP). Single or multiunit restorations are produced by direct ceramic machining (DCM) of presintered 3Y-TZP blocks. The blocks are easy to mill, which leads to substantial savings in time and tool wear. The process involves the fabrication of a full contour wax-up of the restoration, which is later digitized with a laser scanner. Restorations are oversized at the design and machining stages, to compensate for the large shrinkage (20% to 25%) that occurs during the sintering process at high temperature (1350° C for 2 hours).

Since the introduction of the DCM technique, a wide variety of partially sintered 3Y-TZP blocks have become available for soft machining by CAD/CAM. In this case, the wax-up step is eliminated, a digital impression of the preparation is made and the restoration design is accomplished by computer. Similarly to the DCM technique, machined restorations are fully sintered at high temperature.

The microstructure of these polycrystalline 3Y-TZP ceramics consists of densely packed tetragonal zirconia grains with a mean grain size of 0.2 to 0.7 μm, depending on sintering temperature and duration (Figure 11-5, F). Depending on the manufacturer, recommended sintering temperatures vary from 1350° to 1550° C and durations from 2 to 6 hours. They exhibit the highest flexural strength (900-1500 MPa) and highest fracture toughness (greater than $5\ MPa \cdot m^{0.5}$) of all currently available dental ceramics. In all systems, the last step consists of veneering the core 3Y-TZP ceramic with porcelain of matched thermal expansion. Importantly, most of the clinical problems encountered so far with these systems consist of crazing or cracking at the interface between veneering porcelain and core ceramic. These findings have been explained by a destabilization of the tetragonal phase at the core/veneer interface, with transformation to the monoclinic phase leading to local stresses due to the difference in coefficient of thermal expansion between the two crystallographic phases.

The metastability of 3Y-TZP ceramics should be kept in mind when surface-altering treatments such as grinding or sandblasting are performed. Depending on the grain size, such treatments have the potential to trigger the tetragonal to monoclinic transformation with the immediate beneficial consequence of producing surface compressive stresses. However, long-term effects may be detrimental because of the presence of underlying tensile stresses. This is why extreme care should be taken to follow manufacturer's instructions with partially stabilized zirconia-based systems.

Hard machining techniques make it possible to fabricate the restoration chair side in one office visit. However, all-ceramic materials available with these techniques exhibit only low to moderate strength, restricting the applications to single-unit restorations.

The benefit of fabricating the restoration in one office visit is lost with soft machining techniques, because restorations require sintering at high temperature after they are machined. This disadvantage is counterbalanced by the unique mechanical properties of 3Y-TZP, making possible the realization of both single and multiunit anterior and posterior restorations. Initially a concern, marginal accuracy is currently acceptable with these techniques. The negative impact of the high opacity of zirconia is attenuated by the ability to decrease coping thickness to 0.4 to 0.5 mm.

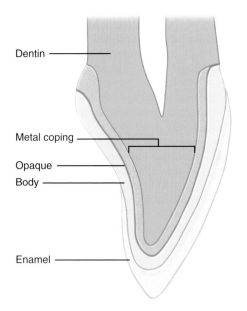

Dentin ——————

Metal coping ——————

Opaque ——————

Body ——————

Enamel ——————

FIGURE 11.7 Cross section of a metal-ceramic crown showing metal coping, opaque porcelain layer, body (*dentin*), and enamel porcelain layers.

METAL-CERAMIC RESTORATIONS

Metal-ceramic restorations consist of a cast metallic framework (or core) on which at least two layers of ceramic are baked (Figure 11-7). The first layer applied is the opaque layer, consisting of porcelain modified with opacifying oxides. Its role is to mask the darkness of the oxidized metal framework to achieve adequate esthetics. This thin opaque layer also contributes to the metal-ceramic bond. The next step is the buildup of dentin and enamel (most translucent) porcelains to obtain an esthetic appearance similar to that of a natural tooth. The dentin or enamel porcelain powder is mixed with modeling liquid (mainly distilled water) to a creamy consistency and is applied on the opaque layer. The porcelain is then condensed by vibration and removal of the excess water with absorbent tissue, and slowly dried to allow for water diffusion and evaporation. The porcelain buildup has to be oversized to compensate for the large shrinkage (25%-30%) associated with the sintering process. After building up of the porcelain powders, metal-ceramic restorations are sintered under vacuum in a porcelain furnace. Sintering under vacuum helps eliminate pores. As the furnace door closes, the pressure is lowered to 0.01 MPa (0.1 atmosphere). The temperature is raised until the sintering temperature is reached, the vacuum is then released, and the furnace pressure returns to 0.1 MPa (1 atmosphere). In combination with viscous flow at high temperature, the increase in pressure helps close residual pores. The result is a dense, relatively pore-free porcelain, as illustrated in Figure 11-8. Studies have shown that sintering under vacuum reduces the amount of porosity from 5.6% in air-fired porcelains to 0.56%. Opaque, dentin, and enamel porcelains are available in various shades.

Figure 11-9 shows two three-unit metal-ceramic fixed partial prostheses. When fabricated by skilled

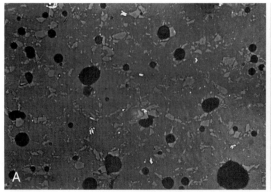
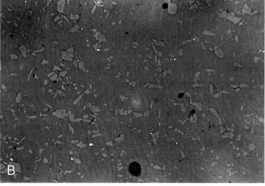

FIGURE 11.8 **Air-fired and vacuum-fired porcelain. A,** Optical micrograph of air-fired porcelain, showing porosity. **B,** Optical micrograph of vacuum-fired porcelain showing minimal porosity. *(Courtesy of J.O. Semmelman, York, PA, 1959, Dentsply International.)*

technicians, these restorations provide excellent esthetics, along with adequate strength because of the metal framework support. The alloys used for casting the substructure are usually gold-based containing tin and indium.

It is essential that the coefficient of thermal expansion of the veneering porcelain be slightly lower than that of the alloy to ensure that the ceramic is in slight compression after cooling. This will establish a better resistance to crack propagation of the ceramic part of the restoration.

REQUIREMENTS FOR A METAL-CERAMIC SYSTEM

1. The alloy must have a high melting temperature. The melting range must be substantially higher (greater than 100° C) than the firing temperature of the veneering porcelain and solders used to join segments of a fixed partial prosthesis.
2. The veneering porcelain must have a low fusing temperature so that no creep, sag, or distortion of the framework takes place during sintering.
3. The porcelain must wet the alloy readily when applied as a slurry to prevent voids forming at the metal-ceramic interface. In general, the contact angle should be 60 degrees or less.
4. A good bond between the ceramic and metal is essential and is achieved by chemical reaction of the porcelain with metal oxides on the surface of metal (see Figure 10-10) and by mechanical interlocking made possible by roughening of the metal coping.
5. Coefficients of thermal expansion (CTE) of the porcelain and metal must be compatible so that the veneering porcelain never undergoes tensile stresses, which would lead to cracking. Metal-ceramic systems are therefore designed so that the CTE of the metal is slightly higher

than that of the porcelain, thus placing the veneering porcelain in compression (where it is stronger) following cooling (see Figure 10-11). This is assuming that linear coefficients of thermal expansion of both porcelain and metal are identical to linear coefficients of thermal contraction.

6. Adequate stiffness and strength of the metal framework are especially important for fixed partial dental prostheses and posterior crowns. High stiffness of the metal reduces tensile stresses in the porcelain by limiting deflection amplitude and deformation (strain). High strength is essential in the interproximal connector areas of fixed partial prostheses.
7. High resistance to deformation at high temperature is essential. Metal copings are relatively thin (0.4 to 0.5 mm); no distortion should occur during firing of the porcelain, or the fit of the restorations would be compromised.
8. Adequate design of the restoration is critical. The preparation should provide for adequate thickness of the metal coping (see #7 below), as well as enough space for an adequate thickness of the porcelain to yield an esthetic restoration. During preparation of the metal framework, prior to porcelain application, it is important that all sharp angles be eliminated and rounded to later avoid stress concentration in the porcelain. If full porcelain coverage is not used (e.g., a metal occlusal surface), the position of the metal-ceramic junction should be located at least 1.5 mm from all centric occlusal contacts.

METAL-CERAMIC BONDING

The bond strength between porcelain and metal is an important requirement for good long-term performance of metal-ceramic restorations. In general, the bond is a result of chemisorption by diffusion between the surface oxide layer on the alloy and the porcelain. For metal alloys that do not oxidize easily, this oxide layer is formed during a special firing cycle prior to opaque porcelain application. For metal alloys that do oxidize easily, the oxide layer is formed during wetting of the alloy by the porcelain and subsequent firing cycle. The most common mechanical failure for metal-ceramic restorations is debonding of the porcelain from the metal. Many factors control metal-ceramic adhesion: the formation of strong chemical bond, mechanical interlocking between the two materials, and thermal residual stresses. In addition, as noted earlier, the porcelain must wet and fuse to the surface to form a uniform interface with no voids. These factors are also important for ceramic coatings on metallic implants.

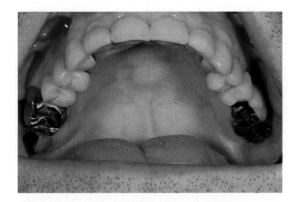

FIGURE 11.9 **View of metal-ceramic fixed partial dental prostheses.** *(Courtesy of Dr. Charles Mark Malloy, Portland, OR.)*

From a practical standpoint, the surface roughness at the metal-ceramic interface has a large effect on the quality of the metal-ceramic bond. Airborne particle abrasion is routinely used on metal frameworks for metal-ceramic restorations to produce a clean surface with controlled roughness. During the firing cycle, the porcelain softens, its viscosity decreases, and the porcelain first wets the metal surface before interlocking between porcelain and metal is created. The increased area of the rough metal surface also permits the formation of a greater density of chemical bonds. The contact angle between the porcelain and metal is a measure of the wetting and, to some extent, the quality of the bond that forms. Low contact angles indicate good wetting. The contact angle of porcelain on a gold (Au) alloy is about 60 degrees. A scanning electron micrograph of the oxidized surface of a gold (Au)-platinum (Pt)-palladium (Pd) 98% noble alloy is shown in Figure 10-10. However, rough surfaces can reduce adhesion if the porcelain does not wet the surface and voids are present at the interface.

The formation of an oxide layer at the surface of the metal has been shown to be the key to an adequate metal-ceramic bond. Noble metal alloys, which are resistant to oxidizing, usually have other more easily oxidized elements added, such as indium (In) and tin (Sn), to form an oxide layer and improve the bond. The oxide layer is formed during a special firing cycle prior to porcelain application. Some noble alloys containing silver have been shown to lead to porcelain discoloration or greening, explained by ionic diffusion of silver in the porcelain. Base-metal alloys contain elements, such as nickel (Ni) and chromium (Cr), that oxidize easily, and care must be taken to avoid the formation of too thick an oxide layer. Manufacturers specify firing conditions for the formation of an optimal oxide layer and often indicate the color of the oxide. Oxides rich in nickel (NiO) tend to be dark gray, whereas those rich in chromium (Cr_2O_3) are greenish. If firing recommendations are not followed, these oxides may dissolve in the porcelain during firing, leading to discoloration visible in areas where the porcelain is thinnest, for example near the gingival margin of the restoration. Some alloys form oxide layers rich in Cr_2O_3, which do not bond or adhere well to the alloy. These alloys typically require the application of a bonding agent to the alloy surface to modify the type of oxide formed. In some cases, manufacturers recommend an oxidation firing under reduced pressure to limit the thickness of the oxide layer. An oxidation firing in air may lead to a thicker oxide layer.

High thermal residual stresses between the metal and porcelain can lead to failure. If the metal and ceramic have largely different thermal expansion coefficients, the two materials will contract at different rates during cooling and large thermal residual stresses will form along the metal-ceramic interface. If these stresses are very high (whether tensile or compressive), the porcelain will crack and/or delaminate from the metal. Even if these stresses do not cause immediate failure, they can still weaken the bond, and lead to delayed failure. To avoid these problems, porcelains and alloys are formulated to have adequately matched thermal expansion coefficients. Most porcelains have coefficients of thermal expansion between 13.0 and 14.0 × $10^{-6}/°$ C, and metals between 13.5 and 14.5 × $10^{-6}/°$ C. The difference of 0.5 × $10^{-6}/°$ C in thermal contraction between metal and porcelain causes the metal to contract slightly more than does the ceramic during cooling. This condition places the porcelain under slight residual compression, which makes it less sensitive to the tensile stresses induced by mechanical loading.

A metal-ceramic bond may fail in any of three possible locations (Figure 11-10). Knowing the location of failure provides considerable information on the quality of the bond. The highest bond strength leads to failure within the porcelain when tested (see Figure 11-10, C); this is observed with some alloys that were properly prepared with excellent wetting by the porcelain and is also called a *cohesive failure*. Testing these high-strength specimens using the push-through shear test shows that the bond strength is approximately the same as the shear strength of the porcelain. Another possible cohesive failure is within the oxide layer (see Figure 11-10, B). Failures occurring at the interface between metal and oxide layer (see Figure 11-10, A) are called *adhesive failures* and are commonly observed with metal alloys that are resistant to forming surface oxides, such as

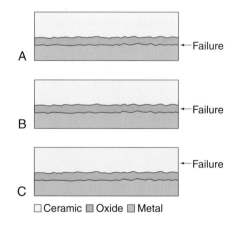

FIGURE 11.10 **Diagram showing three observed types of bond failure in metal-ceramic systems. A,** Metal-metal oxide (adhesive); **B,** metal oxide–metal oxide (cohesive); and **C,** ceramic-ceramic (cohesive). NOTE: The dimensions of the layers are not to scale.

pure gold or platinum, and exhibit poor bonding. Base-metal alloys commonly exhibit failures within the oxide layer if an excessively thick oxide layer is present.

CERAMICS FOR METAL-CERAMIC RESTORATIONS

Ceramics for metal-ceramic restorations must fulfill five requirements: (1) they must simulate the appearance of natural teeth, (2) they must fuse at relatively low temperatures, (3) they must have thermal expansion coefficients compatible with alloys used for metal frameworks, (4) they must age well in the oral environment, and (5) they must have low abrasiveness. Porcelains are carefully formulated to achieve these requirements. These ceramics are composed of a crystalline phase (leucite) dispersed in a glassy (amorphous) matrix. Their chemical composition includes silica (SiO_2), alumina (Al_2O_3), sodium oxide (Na_2O), and potassium oxide (K_2O) (Table 11-4). Opacifiers (TiO_2, ZrO_2, SnO_2), various heat-stable coloring oxides and small amounts of fluorescing oxides (CeO_2) are added to match the appearance of the dentin/enamel complex structure. The presence of a large amount of glassy phase in dental porcelains (80-90 vol%) permits a translucency similar to that of enamel. Coloring oxides and opacifiers allow fine tuning of the final appearance and shade control. Porcelain is supplied as a fine powder.

DENTAL PORCELAIN COMPOSITION AND MANUFACTURE

Composition

The quality of any ceramic depends on the choice of components, correct proportioning of each component, and control of the firing procedure. Only the purest components are used in the manufacture of dental porcelains because of the stringent requirements of optical properties and chemical inertness, combined with adequate strength, toughness, and thermal expansion.

In its mineral state, feldspar, the main raw component of dental porcelains for metal-ceramic restorations, is crystalline and opaque. Chemically it is designated as potassium aluminosilicate, with a composition of $KAlSi_3O_8$ or $K_2O \cdot Al_2O_3 \cdot 6SiO_2$. Feldspar melts incongruently at about 1150° C, forming leucite ($KAlSi_2O_6$ or $K_2O \cdot Al_2O_3 \cdot 4SiO_2$) and molten glass.

Manufacture

Many dental porcelain manufacturers buy feldspar as powder already screened and cleaned from impurities to their specifications. Other raw materials used in the manufacture of dental porcelains are various types of silica (SiO_2) in the form of fine powder, alumina (Al_2O_3), as well as alkali and alkaline earth carbonates as fluxes. During the manufacturing process, the ground components are carefully mixed

TABLE 11.4 Composition of Dental Ceramics for Fusing to High-Temperature Alloys

Compound	Biodent Opaque BG 2 (%)	Ceramco Opaque 60 (%)	V.M.K. Opaque 131 (%)	Biodent Dentin BD 27 (%)	Ceramco Dentin T 69 (%)
SiO_2	52.0	55.0	52.4	56.9	62.2
Al_2O_3	13.55	11.65	15.15	11.80	13.40
CaO	—	—	—	0.61	0.98
K_2O	11.05	9.6	9.9	10.0	11.3
Na_2O	5.28	4.75	6.58	5.42	5.37
TiO_2	3.01	—	2.59	0.61	—
ZrO_2	3.22	0.16	5.16	1.46	0.34
SnO_2	6.4	15.0	4.9	—	0.5
Rb_2O	0.09	0.04	0.08	0.10	0.06
BaO	1.09	—	—	3.52	—
ZnO	—	0.26	—	—	—
UO_3	—	—	—	—	—
B_2O_3, CO_2, and H_2O	4.31	3.54	3.24	9.58	5.85

From Nally JN, Meyer JM: Schweiz. Monatsschr. Zahnheilked. 80, 25, 1970.

together and heated to about 1200° C in large crucibles. As mentioned earlier, feldspar melts incongruently at about 1150° C to form a glassy phase with an amorphous structure, as illustrated in Figure 11-11, and a crystalline phase consisting of leucite, a potassium aluminosilicate ($KAlSi_2O_6$).

The mix of leucite and glassy phase is then cooled very rapidly (quenched) in water that causes the mass to shatter in small fragments. The product obtained, called a *frit*, is ball-milled to achieve proper particle size distribution. Coloring pigments in small quantities are added at this stage to obtain the delicate shades necessary to mimic natural teeth. The metallic pigments include titanium oxide for yellow-brown shades, manganese oxide for lavender, iron oxide for brown, cobalt oxide for blue, copper or chromium oxides for green, and nickel oxide for brown. In the past, uranium oxide was used to provide fluorescence; however, because of the small amount of radioactivity, lanthanide oxides (such as cerium oxide) have been substituted for this purpose. Tin, titanium, and zirconium oxides are used as opacifiers.

After the manufacturing process is completed, feldspathic dental porcelain consists of a glassy (or amorphous) phase and leucite ($KAlSi_2O_6$) as a crystalline phase. The glassy phase formed during the manufacturing process has properties typical of glass, such low toughness and strength, and high translucency. The crystalline structure of leucite is tetragonal at room temperature (Figure 11-12). Leucite undergoes a reversible crystallographic phase transformation at 625° C, temperature above which its structure becomes cubic. This transformation is accompanied by a thermal expansion resulting in a 1.2 vol% increase of the unit cell. This explains the high thermal expansion coefficient associated with tetragonal leucite (greater than $20 \times 10^{-6}/°$ C). As a result, the amount of leucite present (10 to 20 vol%) controls the thermal expansion coefficient of the porcelain so that it is adequately matched to that of dental alloys.

The microstructure of conventional feldspathic porcelain is shown in Figure 11-13; the glassy phase has been lightly acid-etched to reveal the leucite crystals. Typical compositions for opaque and dentin porcelain powders are given in Table 11-4.

For a discussion on Porcelain application please go to the website http://evolve.elsevier.com/sakaguchi/restorative ⊖

Feldspathic porcelains have other qualities that make them well suited for metal-ceramic restorations.

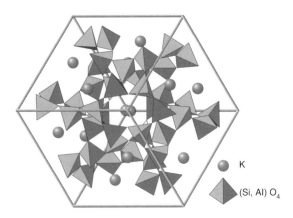

FIGURE 11.12 **Three-dimensional structure of leucite ($KAlSi_2O_6$).** *K, potassium; Si, silicon; Al, aluminum; O, oxygen.*

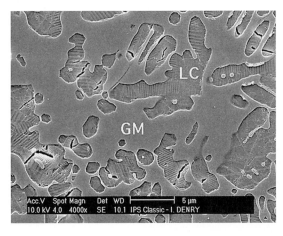

FIGURE 11-13 **Scanning electron micrograph showing the microstructure of feldspathic porcelain for metal-ceramic restorations.** *GM, Glassy matrix; LC, leucite crystal.*

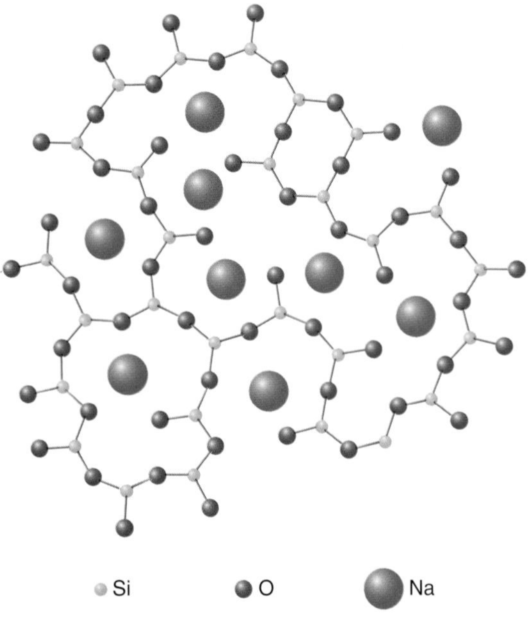

FIGURE 11.11 **Two-dimensional structure of sodium silicate glass.** *Si, silicon; O, oxygen; Na, sodium. (Modified from Warren BE, Biscoe J: J. Am. Ceram. Soc. 21,259, 1938.)*

They fuse at lower temperatures than do many other ceramic materials, lessening the potential for distortion of the metal coping. This is made possible by the presence of alkali oxides (Na_2O and K_2O) in the glassy matrix, these oxides are responsible for the creation of nonbridging oxygens in the glass network, thereby lowering the fusing temperatures to the range 930° to 980° C. Porcelains having an even lower fusing temperature (760° to 780° C) and high coefficient of thermal expansion ($15.8 \times 10^{-6}/°$ C) are also available. These porcelains are designed to be compatible for bonding to yellow high-Au alloys, which have coefficients of thermal expansion between 16.1 and $16.8 \times 10^{-6}/°$ C). They can, however, be abrasive to opposing teeth because of their hardness; this becomes a significant problem if the porcelain surface is roughened by occlusal adjustments or sensitivity to aging in the oral environment.

EFFECT OF DESIGN ON METAL-CERAMIC RESTORATIONS

Because ceramics are weak in tension and can withstand very little strain before fracturing, the metal framework must be rigid to minimize deformation of the porcelain. However, copings should be as thin as possible to allow space for the porcelain to mask the metal framework without over-contouring the porcelain. This consideration is especially true for alloys that appear gray. This might lead to the conclusion that nickel-chromium (Ni-Cr) or cobalt-chromium (Co-Cr) alloys would be superior to the noble alloys because their moduli of elasticity (stiffness) are 1.5 to 2 times greater and the thickness of the coping could be halved. However, loading the restoration places it in bending, and the bending deflection is a function of only the first power of the modulus, whereas it is a function of the cube of the thickness. It can be shown that for a typical dental metal-ceramic restoration, the thickness of a base-metal coping can be reduced only about 7% because of the higher modulus of elasticity. Thus the advantage of the higher modulus for the base-metal alloys is minimal.

The labial margin of metal-ceramic prostheses is a critical area regarding design because there is little porcelain thickness at the margin to mask the appearance of the metal coping and to resist fracture. Recommended margin designs include a 90-degree shoulder, a 120-degree shoulder, or a shoulder bevel. Provided that the shoulder depth is at least 1.2 mm, these designs should all provide for sufficient porcelain thickness to minimize the risk of porcelain fracture.

When using partial porcelain coverage, such as when a metal occlusal surface is desired, the position of the metal-ceramic joint is critical. Because of the large difference in modulus of elasticity between porcelain and metal, stresses occur at the interface when the restoration is loaded. These stresses should be minimized by placing the metal-ceramic junction at least 1.5 mm from centric occlusal contacts.

The geometry of the interproximal connector area between abutment crown and pontic is critical in the design of a metal-ceramic fixed partial prosthesis. The incisocervical thickness of the connector should be large enough to prevent deformation or fracture because deflection is decreased as the cube of the thickness; greater thickness will minimize deflection of the framework, which may lead to debonding or fracture of the porcelain. It should be remembered that a fixed partial prosthesis is not a uniform beam; maximum deflection on loading will occur at the thinnest cross section, which is the interproximal connector area. However, connector thickness cannot impinge on gingival tissues or restrict access for oral hygiene procedures.

FAILURE AND REPAIR OF METAL-CERAMIC RESTORATIONS

Metal-ceramic restorations remain the most popular materials combination selected for crown and bridge applications and have a 10-year success rate of about 95%. The majority of retreatments are due to biological failures, such as tooth fracture, periodontal disease, and secondary caries. Prosthesis fracture and esthetic failures account for only 20% of retreatment cases for single-unit restorations. For metal-ceramic fixed partial prostheses (FPP), prosthesis fracture is the most common reason for retreatment, with long-span FPPs (five or more units) having approximately twice the incidence of failure compared to short-span FPPs.

When metal-ceramic prosthesis fails, it is often due to adhesive failure between porcelain and metal or cohesive failure within the ceramic near the metal-ceramic interface. Ideally, the prosthesis should be retrieved, metal surfaces should be cleaned, and a new oxide layer should be formed on the exposed area of metal prior to porcelain application and firing. However, this cannot be achieved intra-orally, and removal of the prosthesis is both unpleasant for the patient and time consuming. Thus a variety of techniques have been developed for porcelain repair using dental composite. All of these techniques present the challenge of bonding chemically dissimilar materials. When porcelain fragments are available and no functional loading is exerted on the fracture site, silane coupling agents can be used to achieve good adhesion between the composite and porcelain; however, metal alloys have no such bonding agent and this type of repair is considered only temporary. Systems are available for coating the metal surface with silica particles through airborne particle abrasion. The particles are embedded in the metal surface upon impact, then a silane coupling agent can be applied. Alternatively, base metal alloys can be coated with tin followed by the application of an acidic primer. Both methods achieve adequate bond strength and may delay the eventual need for remaking the prosthesis.

SELECTED PROBLEMS

All-Ceramic Crowns

PROBLEM 1

A heat-pressed leucite-reinforced crown fractured after firing of the veneering ceramic. Explain the probable cause.

Solution a

Improper core material was used. Heat-pressed ceramic ingots are available either for the staining technique or for the veneering technique. These ingots have different coefficients of thermal expansion. If the veneering ceramic was fired on a core material for the staining technique, the thermal expansion mismatch between the two ceramics can lead to fracture or cracking upon cooling.

Solution b

Improper veneering ceramic was used; for example, an aluminous veneering ceramic with unmatched coefficient of thermal expansion.

PROBLEM 2

A heat-pressed, all-ceramic crown pressed incompletely. Explain the possible causes of incomplete pressing.

Solution a

The pressing temperature was not reached because of an erroneous temperature calibration. Heat-pressing furnaces should be calibrated regularly. If the pressing temperature was not reached, the viscosity of the ceramic ingot was too high to allow complete pressing of the crown.

Solution b

The air pressure in the heat-pressing furnace was too low. Ideal pressure should be at least 0.45 MPa (65 psi) for proper heat-pressing.

Solution c

Only one ceramic ingot was used when two were needed. Wax-patterns should be weighed before pressing to ensure that enough material is available for pressing.

PROBLEM 3

A sintered all-ceramic crown fractured as a result of excessive porosity. What can be done to avoid porosity?

Solution a

Care should be taken to mix the porcelain with modeling liquid to a creamy consistency without entrapping air bubbles.

Solution b

Porcelain should be heated gradually when first fired to evaporate the water holding the particles together without creating steam. If the rate of water evaporation is greater than the rate of water diffusion, the steam produced can create porosity.

Solution c

The vacuum level in the porcelain furnace was improperly set. Vacuum-firing reduces the furnace pressure to about 0.1 atm, when the firing temperature is reached, the vacuum is released and furnace pressure becomes atmospheric pressure (1 atm). This favors sintering and pore elimination. Air-firing does not allow proper elimination of pores during sintering.

PROBLEM 4

A veneering ceramic that normally glazes at 982° C was found to require 1010° C for glazing. Explain why.

Solution a

A porcelain furnace requires periodic temperature calibration. This is usually done with silver disks or threads that melt at a fixed temperature of 962° C and are supplied by the furnace manufacturer.

Solution b

If the particle size of the porcelain powder is altered, the sintering and glazing temperatures are also altered. It is important to shake the porcelain powder bottle before using it, to counteract any settling of large particles at the bottom of the bottle and ensure a uniform particle size distribution.

PROBLEM 5

Which all-ceramic systems can be chemically etched?

Solution

Any ceramic system with a silica-rich glass phase can be chemically etched with hydrofluoric acid-based etching solutions. These include both leucite-reinforced and lithium disilicate–reinforced all-ceramic systems. Alumina-based or zirconia-based all-ceramic systems do not offer a silica-rich glass phase and therefore cannot be etched with hydrofluoric acid-based etching solutions, independently of their concentration.

Metal-Ceramic Systems—Porcelain

PROBLEM 6

A patient presented with considerable enamel wear on natural teeth opposing metal-ceramic restorations. Explain the possible causes.

Solution

Dental porcelain is harder than human enamel and can cause excessive wear. This is particularly true if occlusal adjustments have been performed on porcelain surfaces without careful polishing to smooth the surface. Metal-ceramic restorations with occlusal metallic surfaces result in less wear. Occlusal porcelain surfaces are to be avoided in case of bruxism.

PROBLEM 7

The surface of a finished metal-ceramic crown exhibits several dark inclusions. What are the possible causes of these defects?

Solution a

The inclusions are metallic inclusions created during framework preparation and grinding. They were not eliminated because of inadequate cleaning after grinding. They were then incorporated in the porcelain during porcelain buildup and became embedded in the porcelain during subsequent firing.

Solution b

Spatulas or brushes contaminated with metal shavings were used to mix or apply the porcelain mix on the metal framework.

Solution c

Metallic instruments were used at any time during porcelain preparation or application.

PROBLEM 8

The ceramic of a metal-ceramic crown placed in the mouth fractured from the metallic substructure. What factors might have produced such a failure, and how can it be avoided?

Solution a

Surface contamination of the alloy before applying the porcelain may be a factor. Impurities on the metal surface, such as organic powder from the grinding stones or grease and oils from fingers, may prevent a good wetting of the metal, and air bubbles will be present at the metal-ceramic interface. This problem can be avoided by using vitrified grinding stones and carefully cleaning the metal surface from all debris and contaminants.

Solution b

An improperly sintered opaque layer may be a factor. When the opaque porcelain has not reached its fusing temperature, a complete wetting of the metal surface cannot be achieved, leading to a poor bond between metal and porcelain. Respecting manufacturer's recommended firing schedule and regularly calibrating porcelain furnaces will prevent this problem.

Solution c

Another cause for the fracture may be improper metal thickness. A uniform metal thickness is very important to prevent failures in the metal-ceramic bond. A minimum thickness of 0.4 mm is allowable. Thinner metal substructures could cause porcelain failure.

Solution d

The reuse of metal alloys may be detrimental to the quality of the oxide layer. When sprue buttons are recycled and used to cast a new substructure, the amounts of tin or indium may be significantly decreased, and a very weak bonding with the porcelain is the result. The use of fresh alloys for casting the substructure is ideal, but a combination of a 50% (75% is better) fresh alloy and 25% to 50% recycled alloy may be used without detrimental effects on the metal-ceramic bond.

PROBLEM 9

When a metal-ceramic restoration was removed from the oven, cracks in the porcelain were observed. What factors may have caused this failure, and how could it be avoided?

Solution a

Improper selection of porcelain and alloy will cause such cracks. Manufacturers design porcelains with specific characteristics to match the thermal expansion properties of a particular alloy. When another alloy is used with the same porcelain, the mismatch in thermal expansion coefficients may be sufficient to cause cracking. Only the alloy and matching porcelain suggested by the manufacturer should be used.

Solution b

Another factor may be overglazed or overfired porcelain that no longer matches the alloy properly. This could be due, for example, to a furnace malfunction.

Solution c

When the metal-ceramic restoration is allowed to cool in the furnace after the porcelain has been baked, cracks in the porcelain material will be produced. A metal-ceramic restoration should not be cooled in the furnace because slow cooling may change some physical properties of the ceramic, creating a mismatch with the alloy.

Solution d

When the porcelain is touched with a cold instrument while still hot, the thermal shock can produce cracks.

PROBLEM 10

A metal-ceramic restoration was completed, but the shade appears too gray. What could be the cause of the shade mismatch, and how could it be avoided?

Solution a

When the opaque porcelain layer is too thin, the translucency of the body porcelain will allow the oxidized dark metal framework to show through. The opaque layer should be examined for dark areas that may show through and a second opaque bake should be performed if any are present.

Solution b

If the opaque layer is baked too many times, the opaque porcelain may have become too glazed and lost some of its opacifying qualities, thereby allowing the metal to show through the opaque layer, creating a gray shade. The manufacturer's suggested technique for baking the opaque should be carefully followed.

Solution c

The darker shade could also be due to the metal itself. When a crucible contaminated by a different alloy containing base metals is used, a dark shade may be obtained. To avoid this problem, do not use a crucible that has been used to cast any other alloy. Only clean crucibles without ceramic liners or fluxes should be employed to cast the alloys for metal-ceramic restorations.

Solution d

Non-noble alloys may contaminate the oven. Another source of oven contamination is the formation of volatilized impurities when the porcelain furnace has been used often for degassing and soldering operations. When the contamination accumulates in the oven, the porcelain may be discolored or appear gray. To avoid this problem, the porcelain furnace should be purged regularly.

Bibliography

Albakry M, Guazzato M, Swain MV: Influence of hot pressing on the microstructure and fracture toughness of two pressable dental glass–ceramics, *J Biomed Mater Res* 71B:99–107, 2004.

Andersson M, Oden A: A new all-ceramic crown. A dense-sintered, high-purity alumina coping with porcelain, *Acta Odontol Scand* 51:59–64, 1993.

Anusavice KJ, Dehoff PH, Hojjatie B, et al: Influence of tempering and contraction mismatch on crack development in ceramic surfaces, *Journal of Dental Research* 68:1182–1187, 1989.

Anusavice KJ, Gray A, Shen C: Influence of initial flaw size on crack growth in air-tempered porcelain, *Journal of Dental Research* 70:131–136, 1991.

Ban S: Reliability and properties of core materials for all-ceramic dental restorations, *Jpn Dent Sci Rev* 44:3–21, 2008.

Baran GR, Obrien WJ, Tien TY: Colored emission of rare-earth ions in a potassium feldspar glass, *Journal of Dental Research* 56:1323–1329, 1977.

Barreiro MM, Riesgo O, Vicente EE: Phase identification in dental porcelains for ceramo-metallic restorations, *Dent Mater* 5:51–57, 1989.

Brodbelt RH, Obrien WJ, Fan PL: Translucency of dental porcelains, *Journal of Dental Research* 59:70–75, 1980.

Chevalier J: What future for zirconia as a biomaterial? *Biomaterials* 27:535–543, 2006.

Chevalier J, Grémillard L, Virkar AV, et al: The Tetragonal-Monoclinic Transformation in Zirconia: Lessons Learned and Future Trends, *J Am Ceram Soc* 92:1901–1920, 2009.

Denry I, Holloway J: Ceramics for Dental Applications: A Review, *Materials* 3:351–368, 2010.

Denry I, Kelly JR: State of the art of zirconia for dental applications, *Dent Mater* 24:299–307, 2008.

Denry IL: Recent advances in ceramics for dentistry, *Critical Reviews in Oral Biology & Medicine* 7:134–143, 1996.

Denry IL, Holloway JA, Colijn HO: Phase Transformations in a Leucite-Reinforced Pressable Dental Ceramic, *J Biomed Mater Res* 54:351–359, 2001.

Dong JK, Luthy H, Wohlwend A: Heat-pressed ceramics: technology and strength, *Int J Prosthodont* 5:9–16, 1992.

Duret F, Blouin JL, Duret B: CAD-CAM in dentistry, *Journal of the American Dental Association* 117:715–720, 1988.

Filser F, Kocher P, Gauckler LJ: Net-shaping of ceramic components by direct ceramic machining, *Assembly Autom* 23:382–390, 2003.

Garvie RC, Hannink RH, Pascoe RT: Ceramic steel? *Nature* 258:703–704, 1975.

Gray H: The porcelain jacket crown, *New Zealand Dental Journal* 283, 1963.

Haag P, Andersson M, Vult Von Steyern P, et al: 15 Years of Clinical Experience with Procera® Alumina, *Appl Osseoint Res* 4:7–12, 2004.

Hannink RHJ, Kelly PM, Muddle BC: Transformation toughening in zirconia-containing ceramics, *J Am Ceram Soc* 83:461–487, 2000.

Hodson JT: Some physical properties of three dental porcelains, *J Prosth Dent* 9:325–335, 1959.

Höland W, Apel E, Van't hoen C, et al: Studies of crystal phase formations in high-strength lithium disilicate glass-ceramics, *J Non-Cryst Solids* 352:4041–4050, 2006.

Höland W, Beall G: *Glass-ceramic technology*, Westerville, OH, 2002, The American Ceramic Society.

Holand W, Schweiger M, Rheinberger VM, et al: Bioceramics and their application for dental restoration, *Advances in Applied Ceramics* 108:373–380, 2009.

ISO 2008. International Standard - Dental Ceramics. *6872- (E), Geneva, Switzerland*, 1, 6-15.

Kelly JR, Campbell SD, Bowen HK: Fracture surface analysis of dental ceramics, *Journal of Prosthetic Dentistry* 62:536–541, 1989.

Kelly JR, Denry I: Stabilized zirconia as a structural material, *Dent Mater* 24:289–298, 2008.

Kelly JR, Nishimura I, Campbell SD: Ceramics in dentistry: historical roots and current perspectives, *J Prosthet Dent* 75:18–32, 1996.

Kelly JR, Tesk JA, Sorensen JA: Failure of all-ceramic fixed partial dentures in vitro and in vivo: analysis and modeling, *Journal of Dental Research* 74:1253–1258, 1995.

Kingery WD, Bowen HK, Uhlmann DR: *Introduction to ceramics*, New York, 1976, John Wiley & Sons.

Kosmac T, Oblak C, Jevnikar P, et al: Strength and reliability of surface treated Y-TZP dental ceramics, *J Biomed Mater Res* 53:304–313, 2000.

Lawn BR, Pajares A, Zhang Y, et al: Materials design in the performance of all-ceramic crowns, *Biomaterials* 25:2885–2892, 2004.

Leone EF, Fairhurst CW: Bond strength and mechanical properties of dental porcelain enamels, *Journal of Prosthetic Dentistry* 18:155, 1967.

Mackert JR Jr, Rueggeberg FA, Lockwood PE, et al: Isothermal anneal effect on microcrack density around leucite particles in dental porcelains, *J Dent Res* 73:1221–1227, 1994.

Mackert JR Jr, Twiggs SW, Evans-Williams AL: Isothermal anneal effect on leucite content in dental porcelains, *J Dent Res* 74:1259–1265, 1995.

May K, Russell M, Razzoog M, et al: Precision of fit: the Procera AllCeram crown, *J Prosthet Dent* 80:394–404, 1998.

Mclaren EA, Sorensen JA: High-strength alumina crowns and fixed partial dentures generated by copy-milling technology, *Quint Dent Technol* 18:310, 1995.

Mclean J, Hughes T: The reinforcement of dental porcelain with ceramic oxides, *Br Dent J* 119:251–267, 1965.

Mclean JW: Alumina reinforced porcelain jacket crown, *Journal of the American Dental Association* 75:621, 1967.

Meyer JM, O'Brien WJ, Cu Y: Sintering of dental porcelain enamels, *J Dent Res* 55:696–699, 1976.

Milleding P, Ortengren U, Karlsson S: Ceramic inlay systems: some clinical aspects, *Journal of Oral Rehabilitation* 22:571–580, 1995.

Mora GP, OBrien WJ: Thermal-shock resistance of core reinforced all-ceramic crown systems, *Journal of Biomedical Materials Research* 28:189–194, 1994.

Morena R, Lockwood PE, Fairhurst CW: Fracture toughness of commercial dental porcelains, *Dent Mater* 2:58–62, 1986.

O'Brien W: Ceramics, *Dent Clin North Am* 29:851, 1985.

Paravina R, Powers J: *Esthetic color training in dentistry*, St Louis, 2004, Mosby.

Piche PW, O'Brien WJ, Groh CL, et al: Leucite content of selected dental porcelains, *Journal of Biomedical Materials Research* 28:603–609, 1994.

Probster L: Survival rate of In-Ceram restorations, *Int J Prosthodont* 6:259–263, 1993.

Rekow ED: A review of the developments in dental CAD/CAM systems, *Current Opinion in Dentistry* 2:25–33, 1992.

Sailer I, Feher A, Filser F, et al: Five-year clinical results of zirconia frameworks for posterior fixed partial dentures, *Int J Prosthodont* 20:383–388, 2007.

Sherrill CA, Brien WJ: Transverse strength of aluminous and feldspathic porcelain, *J Dent Res* 53:683–690, 1974.

Spear F, Holloway J: Which all-ceramic system is optimal for anterior esthetics? *Journal of the American Dental Association* 139:19S–24S, 2008.

Tholey MJ, Swain MV, Thiel N: SEM observations of porcelain Y-TZP interface, *Dent Mater* 25:857–862, 2009.

Thompson JY, Anusavice KJ, Naman A, et al: Fracture surface characterization of clinically failed all-ceramic crowns, *Journal of Dental Research* 73:1824–1832, 1994.

Tinschert J, Zwez D, Marx R, et al: Structural reliability of alumina-, feldspar-, leucite-, mica- and zirconia-based ceramics, *J Dent* 28:529–535, 2000.

Vines R, Semmelman J: Densification of dental porcelain, *J Dent Res* 36:950–956, 1957.

Von Steyern PV, Carlson P, Nilner K: All-ceramic fixed partial dentures designed according to the DC-Zircon® technique. A 2-year clinical study, *J Oral Rehabil* 32: 180–187, 2005.

Weinstein M, Weinstein LK, Katz S, et al: Fused porcelain-to-metal teeth, *United States patent application*, 1962.

Zhang Y, Lawn BR: Long-term strength of ceramics for biomedical applications, *J Biomed Mater Res* 69B:166–172, 2004.

Metal Ceramic Systems

Anthony DH, Burnett AP, Smith DL, et al: Shear test for measuring bonding in cast gold alloy-porcelain composites, *J Dent Res* 49:27, 1970.

Anusavice KJ: Reducing the failure potential of ceramic-based restorations. Part 1: Metal-ceramic crowns and bridges, *Gen Dent* 44:492, 1996.

Anusavice KJ, Dehoff PH, Fairhurst CW: Comparative evaluation of metal-ceramic bond tests using finite element stress analysis, *J Dent Res* 59:608, 1980.

Anusavice KJ, Hojjatie B: Stress distribution in metal-ceramic crowns with a facial porcelain margin, *J Dent Res* 66:1493, 1987.

Anusavice KJ, Ringle RD, Fairhurst CW: Bonding mechanism evidence in a ceramic non-precious alloy system, *J Biomed Mater Res* 11:701, 1977.

Anusavice KJ, Ringle RD, Fairhurst CW: Identification of fracture zones in porcelain-veneered-to-metal bond test specimens by ESCA analysis, *J Prosthet Dent* 42:417, 1979.

Anusavice KJ, Ringle RD, Morse PK, et al: A thermal shock test for porcelain metal systems, *J Dent Res* 60:1686, 1981.

Baran GR: Phase changes in base metal alloys along metal-porcelain interfaces, *J Dent Res* 58:2095, 1979.

Baran GR: Oxide compounds on Ni-Cr alloys, *J Dent Res* 63:1332, 1984.

Baran GR, Meraner M, Farrell P: Transient oxidation of multiphase Ni-Cr base alloys, *Oxides of Metals* 29:409, 1988.

Baran GR, Woodland EC: Forming of cast precious metal alloys, *J Dent Res* 60:1767, 1981.

Bartolotti RL, Moffa JP: Creep rate of porcelain-bonding alloys as a function of temperature, *J Dent Res* 59:2062, 1980.

Butel EM, DiFiore PM: Crown margin design: a dental school survey, *J Prosthet Dent* 65:303, 1991.

Council on Dental Materials and Devices: How to avoid problems with porcelain-fused-to-metal restorations, *J Am Dent Assoc* 95:818, 1977.

Dent RJ, Preston JD, Moffa JP, et al: Effect of oxidation on ceramometal bond strength, *J Prosthet Dent* 47:59, 1982.

Donachie MJ Jr, editor: *Titanium, a technical guide*, Metals Park, OH, 1988, ASM International.

Donovan T, Prince J: An analysis of margin configurations for metal-ceramic crowns, *J Prosthet Dent* 53:153, 1985.

Dorsch P, Ingersoll C: *A review of proposed standards for metal-ceramic restorations*, Liechtenstein, Feb 4, 1988, Ivoclar-Vivadent Report, Ivoclar AG, Schoen.

Duncan JD: Casting accuracy of nickel-chromium alloys: marginal discrepancies, *J Dent Res* 59:1164, 1980.

Duncan JD: The casting accuracy of nickel-chromium alloys for fixed prostheses, *J Prosthet Dent* 47:63, 1982.

Duncanson MG Jr: Nonprecious metal alloys for fixed restorative dentistry, *Dent Clin North Am* 20:422, 1976.

Eden GT, Franklin OM, Powell JM, et al: Fit of porcelain fused-to-metal crown and bridge casting, *J Dent Res* 58:2360, 1979.

Fairhurst CW, Anusavice KJ, Hashinger DT, et al: Thermal expansion of dental alloys and porcelains, *J Biomed Mater Res* 14:435, 1980.

Farah JW, Craig RG: Distribution of stresses in porcelain-fused-to-metal and porcelain jacket crowns, *J Dent Res* 54:255, 1975.

Faucher RR, Nicholls JI: Distortion related to margin design in porcelain-fused-to-metal restorations, *J Prosthet Dent* 43:149, 1980.

German RM: Hardening reactions in a high-gold content ceramo-metal alloy, *J Dent Res* 59:1980, 1960.

Haselton DR, Diaz-Arnold AM, Dunne JT: Shear bond strengths of 2 intraoral porcelain repair systems to porcelain or metal substrates, *J Prosthet Dent* 86:526, 2001.

Heintze SD, Rousson V: Survival of zirconia- and metal-supported fixed dental prostheses: a systematic review, *Int J Prosthodont* 23:493, 2010.

Huget EF, Dvivedi N, Cosner HE Jr: Characterization of gold-palladium-silver and palladium-silver for metal-ceramic restoration, *J Prosthet Dent* 36:58, 1976.

Huget EF, Dvivedi N, Cosner HE Jr: Properties of two nickel-chromium crown and bridge alloys for porcelain veneering, *J Am Dent Assoc* 94:87, 1977.

Johnson T, van Noort R, Stokes CW: Surface analysis of porcelain fused to metal systems, *Dent Mater* 22:330, 2006.

Jones DW: Coatings of ceramics on metals. In Ducheyne P, Lemons JE, editors: *Bioceramics: materials characteristics versus in vivo behavior*, vol 523, New York, 1988, New York Academy of Science.

Kànànen M, Kivilahti J: Bonding of low-fusing dental porcelain to commercially pure titanium, *J Biomed Mater Res* 28:1027, 1994.

Lautenschlager EP, Greener EH, Elkington WE: Microprobe analysis of gold-porcelain bonding, *J Dent Res* 48:1206, 1969.

Leibrock A, Degenhart M, Behr M, et al: in vitro study of the effect of thermo- and load-cycling on the bond strength or porcelain repair systems, *J Oral Rehabil* 26:130, 1999.

Lenz J, Schwarz S, Schwickerath H, et al: Bond strength of metal-ceramics systems in three-point flexure bond test, *J Appl Biomater* 6:55, 1955.

Lubovich RP, Goodkind RJ: Bond strength studies of precious, semiprecious, and non-precious metal-ceramic alloys with two porcelains, *J Prosthet Dent* 37:288, 1977.

Mackert JR Jr, Twiggs SW, Evans-Williams AL: Isothermal anneal effect on leucite content in dental porcelains, *J Dent Res* 74:1259, 1995.

Malhotra ML, Maickel LB: Shear bond strength of porcelain-fused-to-alloys of varying noble metal contents, *J Prosthet Dent* 44:405, 1980.

Meyer JM, Payan J, Nally JM: Evaluation of alternative alloys to precious ceramic alloys, *J Oral Rehabil* 6:291, 1979.

Nâpânkangas R, Salonen-Kemppi MA, Raustia AM: Longevity of fixed metal ceramic bridge prostheses: a clinical follow-up study, *J Oral Rehabil* 29:140, 2002.

O'Brien WJ: Ceramics, *Dent Clin North Am* 29:851, 1985.

Ohno H, Kanzawa I, Kawashima I, et al: Structure of high-temperature oxidation zones of gold alloys for metal-porcelain bonding containing small amounts of In and Sn, *J Dent Res* 62:774, 1983.

Özcan M, Niedermeier W: Clinical study on the reasons for and location of failures of metal-ceramic restorations and survival of repairs, *Int J Prosthodont* 15:299, 2002.

Ringle RD, Fairhurst CW, Anusavice KJ: Microstructures in non-precious alloys near the porcelain-metal interaction zone, *J Dent Res* 58:1979, 1987.

Robin C, Scherrer SS, Wiskott HWA, et al: Weibull parameters of composite resin bond strengths to porcelain and noble alloy using the Rocatec system, *Dent Mater* 18:389, 2002.

Saxton PL: Post soldering of non-precious alloys, *J Prosthet Dent* 43:592, 1980.

Shell JS, Nielsen JP: Study of the bond between gold alloys and porcelain, *J Dent Res* 41:1424, 1962.

Shimoe S, Tanoue N, Yanagida H, et al: Comparative strength of metal-ceramic and metal-composite bonds after extended thermocycling, *J Oral Rehabil* 31:689, 2004.

Smith DL, Burnett AP, Brooks MS, et al: Iron-platinum hardening in casting golds for use with porcelain, *J Dent Res* 49:283, 1970.

Valega TM, editor: *Alternatives to gold alloys in dentistry*, proceedings of a conference held at NIH, Bethesda, MD, January 1977, DHEW Publication No (NIH) 77–1227.

Vermilyea SG, Huget EF, Vilca JM: Observations on gold-palladium-silver and gold-palladium alloys, *J Prosthet Dent* 44:294, 1980.

Walton TR: A 10-year longitudinal study of fixed prosthodontics: clinical characteristics and outcome of single-unit metal-ceramic crowns, *Int J Prosthodont* 12:519, 1999.

Zarone F, Russo S, Sorrentino R: From porcelain-fused-to-metal to zirconia: clinical and experimental considerations, *Dent Mater* 27:83, 2011.

Replicating Materials— Impression and Casting

Impression materials are used to register or reproduce the form and relationship of the teeth and oral tissues. Hydrocolloids and synthetic elastomeric polymers are among the materials most commonly used to make impressions of various areas of the dental arch. Each of these classes of materials has certain advantages and disadvantages. An understanding of the physical characteristics and the limitations of each material is necessary for their successful use in clinical dentistry. Digital impressions are described in Chapter 14. Waxes and dental pattern materials are discussed on the website. http://evolve.elsevier.com/sakaguchi/restorative ☉

PURPOSE OF IMPRESSION MATERIALS

Impression materials are used to make an accurate replica or mold of the hard and soft oral tissues. The area involved may vary from a single tooth to the whole dentition, or an impression may be made of an edentulous mouth. The impression is a negative reproduction of the tissues, and by filling the impression with dental stone or other model material, a positive cast is made that can be removed after the model material has set. An impression and a stone cast made from the impression are shown in Figure 12-1. Casts of the mouth are used to evaluate the dentition when orthodontic, occlusal, or other problems are involved, and in the laboratory fabrication of restorations and prostheses.

Usually the impression material is carried to the mouth in an unset (plastic) condition in a tray and applied to the area under treatment. When the impression material has set, it is removed from the mouth with the tray. The cast is made by filling the impression with dental stone or other model material. The accuracy, detail, and quality of this final replica are of greatest importance. When the positive reproduction takes the form of the tissues of the upper or lower jaw and serves for the construction of dentures, crowns, fixed dental prostheses, and other restorations, it is described as a *cast*. The positive reproduction of the form of a prepared tooth constitutes a die for the preparation of inlays or fixed dental prostheses. When a positive likeness of the arch or certain teeth is reproduced for orthodontic treatment, it is sometimes described as a *model*, although the term *cast* is the more proper term. On other occasions and in other branches of dentistry, these terms are used interchangeably. Sometimes impression materials are used to duplicate a cast or model that has been formed when more than one positive reproduction is

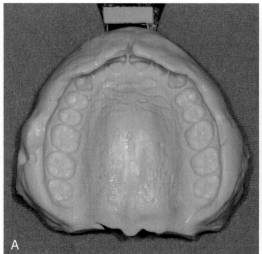
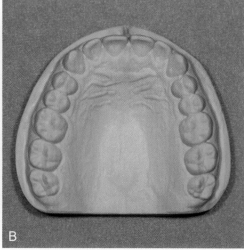

FIGURE 12.1 Alginate impression (**A**) and gypsum stone cast (**B**). *(Courtesy of Dr. Charles Mark Malloy and Dr. Kyle Malloy, Portland, OR.)*

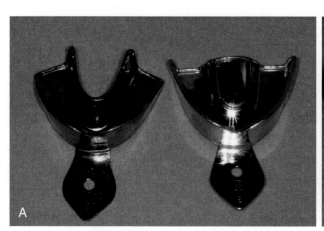
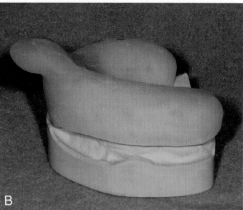

FIGURE 12.2 **A,** Mandibular and maxillary rim-lock impression trays. **B,** Custom impression tray. *(Courtesy of Dr. Charles Mark Malloy, Portland, OR.)*

required. Such impression materials are referred to as *duplicating* materials (refer to website for addition information).

A variety of impression trays are used to make impressions. Examples of typical impression trays are shown in Figure 12-2. The tray is placed so the material is supported and brought into contact with the oral tissues, then held without movement until the impression material has set. The tray with the impression material is then removed from the mouth, and the impression is ready for disinfection and pouring with a cast material to make a positive replica. The clinical impression technique and the production of the cast vary with each impression material. The properties of custom trays are discussed later in this chapter.

DESIRABLE QUALITIES

Affording safe contact with tissues in the mouth and having the ability to fulfill the needs of clinical procedures are critical requirements that dictate the physical properties of dental impression materials. No impression material fulfills every requirement, and selection of the material best suited for a particular clinical situation and technique rests with the dentist. The desirable properties of an impression can be summarized briefly as follows:

1. A pleasant odor, taste, and acceptable color
2. Absence of toxic or irritant constituents
3. Adequate shelf life for requirements of storage and distribution

4. Economically commensurate with the results obtained
5. Easy to use with the minimum of equipment
6. Setting characteristics that meet clinical requirements
7. Satisfactory consistency and texture
8. Readily wets oral tissues
9. Elastic properties that allow easy removal of the set material from the mouth and good elastic recovery
10. Adequate strength to avoid breaking or tearing upon removal from the mouth
11. Dimensional stability over temperature and humidity ranges normally found in clinical and laboratory procedures for a period long enough to permit the production of a cast or die
12. Compatibility with cast and die materials
13. Accuracy in clinical use
14. Readily disinfected without loss of accuracy
15. No release of gas or other byproducts during the setting of the impression or cast and die materials

TYPES OF IMPRESSION MATERIALS

Alginate hydrocolloid and elastomeric impression materials are the most widely used today, and the properties of these are examined first. Elastomeric impression materials have replaced rigid setting materials such as plaster, impression compound, and zinc oxide–eugenol for recording soft-tissue and occlusal relationships. Information on plaster, impression compound, and zinc oxide–eugenol

impression materials can be found on the website http://evolve.elsevier.com/sakaguchi/restorative ⊜

ALGINATE HYDROCOLLOIDS

Dental alginate impression materials change from the sol phase to the gel phase because of a chemical reaction. Once gelation is completed, the material cannot be re-liquefied to a sol. These hydrocolloids are called *irreversible* to distinguish them from the agar reversible hydrocolloids. Agar impression materials are described on the website. Alginate impressions are widely used to form study casts used to plan treatment, monitor changes, and fabricate provisional restorations and removable dental prostheses. http://evolve.elsevier.com/sakaguchi/restorative ⊜

Alginate impression products have acceptable elastic properties. Preparation for use requires only the mixing of measured quantities of powder and water. The resulting paste flows well and registers acceptable anatomical detail. Gypsum casts and models are made by pouring dental plaster or stone into the impression; no separating medium is necessary. The powder is supplied in bulk containers along with suitable measures for dispensing the correct quantities of powder and water. The powder is also available in small sealed packets containing a quantity suitable for a single impression and ready for mixing with a measured quantity of water. These methods of packaging, together with the measuring devices supplied by the manufacturer, are shown in Figure 12-3.

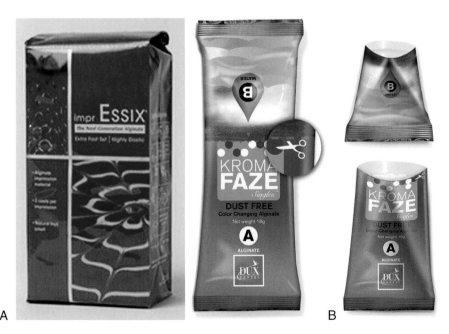

FIGURE 12.3 Alginate impression products. (*A, Courtesy of Dentsply Raintree Essix, Bradenton, FL; and B, Courtesy of DUX Dental, Oxnard, CA*)

Composition and Chemistry

Potassium and sodium salts of alginic acid have properties that make them suitable for compounding a dental impression material. Alginic acid, which is prepared from a marine plant, is a high-molecular-weight block copolymer of anhydro-β-d-mannuronic acid and anhydro-β-d-guluronic acid, as shown in the top part of the formula for alginate below. The properties of alginate raw material depend largely on the degree of polymerization and the ratio of guluronan and mannuronan blocks in the polymeric molecules. The mannuronan regions are stretched and flat, whereas the guluronan regions contribute less flexibility. Also, mainly guluronan blocks bind with Ca^{2+}. Therefore, alginates rich in guluronan form strong, brittle gels, whereas those rich in mannuronan form weaker and more elastic gels.

Alginic Acid   Sol (Chains)

Na-/Ca-Alginate   Gel (Cross-Linked Chains)

$$CaSO_4 - 2H_2O(s) \longrightarrow Ca^{2+}(aq) + SO_4^{2-}(aq)$$
$$Na - Alginate(s) \longrightarrow Na^+(aq) + Alginate^-(aq)$$
$$Na_4P_2O_7(s) \text{ (retarder)} \longrightarrow 4Na^+(aq) + P_2O_7^{4-}(aq)$$
$$2Ca^{2+}(aq) + P_2O_7^{4-}(aq) \longrightarrow Ca_2P_2O_7(s)$$

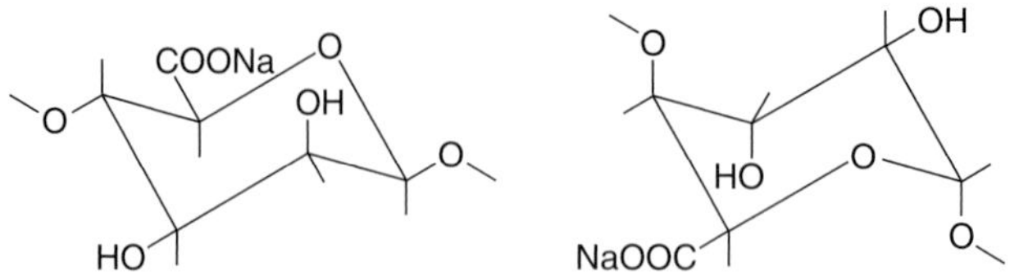

Mannuronate   Guluronate

sol

$$Ca^{2+}(aq) + Alginate^-(aq) \longrightarrow Ca - Alginate^+$$

gel

network

Solutions of these soluble salts, when reacted with a calcium salt, produce an insoluble elastic gel commonly called *calcium alginate*; the structures are shown above. Upon mixing with water, the alginate impression material first forms a sol. Following the chemical reaction described above, a gel is formed to create the set impression material. The gel-forming ability of alginates is mainly related to the proportion of L-guluronan blocks. The concept of sols and gels is presented in the discussion of colloids in Chapter 4.

The nature of this chemical reaction is shown above for the sodium salt. The equally common potassium salt reacts similarly. In an alginate impression compound, the calcium sulfate dihydrate, soluble alginate, and sodium phosphate are included in the powder. When water is added to the powder, compounds disassociate as shown. Calcium ions from the calcium sulfate dihydrate react preferentially with phosphate ions from the sodium phosphate and pyrophosphate to form insoluble calcium phosphate. Calcium phosphate is formed rather than calcium alginate because it has a lower solubility; thus the sodium phosphate is called a *retarder* and provides working time for the mixed alginate.

After the phosphate ions are depleted, the calcium ions react with the soluble alginate to form the insoluble calcium alginate, which together with water forms the irreversible calcium alginate gel. The calcium alginate is insoluble in water, and its formation causes the mixed material to gel. This reaction is irreversible; it is not possible to convert the calcium alginate to a sol after it has set.

To meet the critical requirements of a dental impression material, this reaction must be controlled to attain the desirable properties of consistency, working time, setting time, strength, elastic quality, and smooth, hard surfaces on gypsum casts. These requirements are achieved by adding agents to control the rate of the reaction, develop strength and elasticity in the gel, and counteract the delaying effect of alginate on the setting of gypsum products. The use of suitable fillers in correct quantities produces a consistency that is suitable for various clinical uses.

The composition of a typical alginate impression material and the function of its ingredients are shown in Table 12-1. Manufacturers adjust the concentration of sodium phosphate to produce regular- and fast-set alginates. They also adjust the concentration of filler to control the flexibility of the set impression material from soft-set to hard-set. Although alginate impressions are usually made in a tray, injection types are much more fluid after mixing and more flexible after setting. Manufacturers add organic glycols to the alginate powder to reduce dust. Diatomaceous earth or fine siliceous particles are used as fillers. Because these particles can be a respiratory irritant, inhalation of the dust should be minimized. Impressions should be disinfected with a spray solution after removal from the mouth and before pouring with a casting material. Other ingredients in some products include antimicrobials agents and pH indicators that change color when setting has occurred.

Proportioning and Mixing

The proportioning of the powder and water before mixing is critical to obtaining consistent results. Changes in the water/powder ratio will alter

TABLE 12.1 Ingredients in an Alginate Impression Powder and Their Functions

Ingredient	Weight (%)	Function
Potassium alginate	18	To dissolve in water and react with calcium ions
Calcium sulfate dihydrate	14	To react with potassium alginate to form an insoluble calcium alginate gel
Potassium sulfate, potassium zinc	10	To counteract the inhibiting effect of the hydrocolloid on the fluoride, silicates, or borates setting of gypsum, giving a high-quality surface to the die
Sodium phosphate	2	To react preferentially with calcium ions to provide working time before gelation
Diatomaceous earth or silicate	56	To control the consistency of the mixed alginate and the powder flexibility of the set impression
Organic glycols	Small	To make the powder dustless
Wintergreen, peppermint, anise	Trace	To produce a pleasant taste
Pigments	Trace	To provide color
Disinfectants (e.g., quaternary ammonium salts and chlorhexidine)	1-2	To help in the disinfection of viable organisms

TABLE 12.2 Typical Properties of Alginate and Heavy-Bodied Agar Hydrocolloid Impression Materials

	Working Time (min)	Setting Time (min)	Gelation (°C)	Recovery* (%)	Flexibility† (%)	Compressive Strength‡ (MPa)	Tear Strength§ (kN/m)
Alginate	1.25-4.5	1.5-5.0	—	98.2	8-15	0.49-0.88	0.4-0.7
Agar	—	—	37-45	99.0	4-15	0.78	0.8-0.9

*At 10% compression for 30 seconds; †At a stress of 1000 g/cm²; ‡at a loading rate of 10 kg/min; §ASTM Tear Die C at 25 cm/min.

the consistency and setting times of the mixed material and also the strength and quality of the impression. Usually the manufacturers provide suitable containers for proportioning the powder and water by volume, and these are sufficiently accurate for clinical use.

The mixing time for regular alginate is 1 minute; the time should be carefully measured, because both undermixing and overmixing are detrimental to the strength of the set impression. Fast-set alginates should be mixed with water for 45 seconds. The powder and water are best mixed vigorously in a flexible rubber bowl with an alginate spatula or a spatula of the type used for mixing plaster and stone. Mechanical mixing devices are also available.

Properties

Some typical properties of a tray-type alginate impression material are listed in Table 12-2.

Working Time

The fast-set materials have working times of 1.25 to 2 minutes, whereas time of the regular-set materials is usually 3 minutes, but may be as long as 4.5 minutes. With a mixing time of 45 seconds for the fast-set types, 30 to 75 seconds of working time remain before the impression needs to be completely seated. For the regular-set materials, a mixing time of 60 seconds leaves 2 to 3.5 minutes of working time for materials that set at 3.5 to 5 minutes. In both cases, the mixed alginate must be loaded into the tray and the impression made promptly.

Setting Time

Setting times range from 1 to 5 minutes. The ANSI/ADA (American National Standards Institute/American Dental Association) specification No. 18 (ISO [International Organization for Standardization] 1563) requires that it be at least that value listed by the manufacturer and at least 15 seconds longer than the stated working time. Lengthening the setting time is better accomplished by reducing the temperature of the water used with the mix than by reducing the proportion of powder. Reducing the ratio of powder to water reduces the strength and accuracy of the alginate. Selecting an alginate with a different setting time is a better alternative than changing the water/powder ratio.

The setting reaction is a typical chemical reaction, and the rate can be approximately doubled by a temperature increase of 10° C. However, using water that is cooler than 18° C or warmer than 24° C is not advisable. The clinical setting time is detected by a loss of surface tackiness. If possible, the impression should be left in place 2 to 3 minutes after the loss of tackiness, because the tear strength and elastic recovery (recovery from deformation) increase significantly during this period.

Color-changing alginates provide a visual indication of working time and setting time. The mechanism of the color change is a pH-related change of a dye. One such alginate changes its color from light pink to white.

Elastic Recovery

A typical alginate impression is compressed about 10% in areas of undercuts during removal. The actual magnitude depends on the extent of the undercuts and the space between the tray and the teeth. The ANSI/ADA specification requires that the elastic recovery be more than 95% when the material is compressed 20% for 5 seconds at the time it would normally be removed from the mouth. As indicated in Table 12-2, a typical value for elastic recovery is 98.2%. The corresponding permanent deformation is 1.8%.

The permanent deformation, indicated as percent compression set, is a function of percent compression, time under compression, and time after removal of the compressive load, as illustrated in Figure 12-4. Note that permanent deformation is a time-dependent property. Lower permanent deformation (higher elastic recovery) occurs (1) when the percent compression is lower, (2) when the impression is under compression a shorter time, and (3) when the recovery time is longer, up to about 8 minutes after the release of the load. Clinically these factors translate into requirements for a reasonable bulk of alginate between the tray and the teeth, appropriate retention of the alginate in the tray, and a rapid removal of the impression from the mouth. The usual procedures followed to disinfect the impression and produce a gypsum model provide adequate time for any recovery that might occur.

Flexibility

The ANSI/ADA specification permits a range of 5% to 20% at a stress of 0.1 MPa, and most alginates have a typical value of 14%. However, some of the

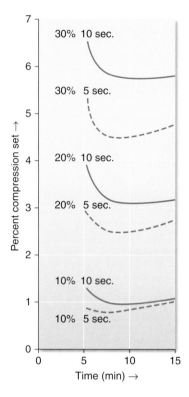

FIGURE 12.4 Variation of compression set with time of an alginate impression material at strains of 10%, 20%, and 30% applied for 5 and 10 seconds. *(Modified from Wilson HJ: Br. Dent. J. 121, 466, 1966.)*

hard-set materials have values from 5% to 8%. A reasonable amount of flexibility is required for ease of removal of the impression.

Strength

The compressive and tear strengths of alginates are listed in Table 12-2. Both properties are time dependent, with higher values obtained at higher rates of loading. Compressive strengths range from approximately 0.5 to 0.9 MPa. The ANSI/ADA specification requires that certified products have a compressive strength of at least 0.35 MPa. Tear strengths vary from 0.4 to 0.7 kN/m, and this property is probably more important than the compressive strength. The tear strength is a measure of the force/thickness ratio needed to initiate and continue tearing and is often determined on a specimen of the shape shown in Figure 12-5. Tearing occurs in the thin sections of the impression, and the probability of tearing decreases with increasing rates of removal. The effect of loading rate on the tear strength of several alginates is shown in Figure 12-6. Values for tray materials range from 0.38 to 0.48 N/mm at 20 mm/min to 0.6 to 0.7 N/mm at 500 mm/min. The lower tear strength at corresponding rates for the

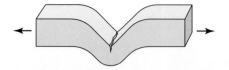

FIGURE 12.5 Sketch of tear strength specimen with load applied in the directions of the arrows; the specimen tears at the V-notch.

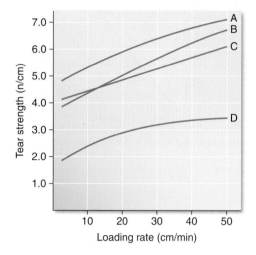

FIGURE 12.6 **Tear strength (N/cm) of alginate impression materials as a function of rate of loading (cm/min).** Materials *A, B,* and *C* are designed to be used in a tray; *D* is a syringe material. *(Modified from MacPherson GW, Craig RG, Peyton FA: J. Dent. Res. 46, 717, 1967.)*

syringe materials reflects the decreased alginate in the syringe material.

Compatibility with Gypsum

The selection of an alginate-gypsum combination that produces good surface quality and detail is highly important. The surface quality and ability of alginate-gypsum combinations to reproduce fine V-shaped grooves are shown in Figure 12-7, *A* and *B*. A type III model plaster was poured against an alginate in Figure 12-7, *A*, and type IV dental stone was poured against the same alginate in Figure 12-7, *B*. The finest groove was 0.025 mm wide in each instance. The combination in Figure 12-7, *B*, was not as compatible as the one in Figure 12-7, *A*, with respect to either surface quality or detail. For purposes of comparison, in Figure 12-7, *C*, the same type IV dental stone used in Figure 12-7, *B*, was poured against a polysulfide impression.

The impression must be rinsed well in cold water to remove saliva and any blood, and then disinfected. Next, all free surface water should be removed before preparing a gypsum model. Saliva and blood

interfere with the setting of gypsum, and if free water accumulates, it tends to collect in the deeper parts of the impression and dilute the gypsum model material, yielding a soft, chalky surface. The excess surface water has been removed when the reflective surface becomes dull. If the alginate impression is stored for 30 minutes or more before preparing the model, it should be rinsed with cool water to remove any exudate on the surface caused by syneresis of the alginate gel; exudate will retard the setting of the gypsum. Thereafter, it should be wrapped loosely in a moist paper towel and sealed in a plastic bag to avoid moisture loss.

The set gypsum model should not remain in contact with the alginate impression for periods of several hours because contact of the slightly soluble calcium sulfate dihydrate with the alginate gel containing a great deal of water is detrimental to the surface quality of the model.

Dimensional Stability

Alginate impressions lose water by evaporation and shrink when standing in air. Impressions left on the bench for as short a time as 30 minutes may become inaccurate enough to require remaking the impression. Even if the impression stored for more than 30 minutes in air were immersed in water, it would not be feasible to determine when the correct amount of water had been absorbed, and in any case the previous dimensions would not be reproduced. For maximum accuracy, the model material should be poured into the alginate impression as soon as possible. If for some reason the models cannot be prepared directly, the impressions should be stored in 100% relative humidity in a plastic bag or wrapped in a damp (but not wringing-wet) paper towel. There is a greater chance for distortion the longer the impression is stored (Figure 12-8). New alginates have improved long-term storage ranging from 48 to 120 hours when stored in a plastic bag. Now, orthodontists routinely send alginate impressions to companies that offer digital fabrication of appliances.

Disinfection

Disinfection of impressions is a concern with respect to viral diseases such as hepatitis B, acquired immunodeficiency syndrome, and herpes simplex, because the viruses may be transferred to gypsum models and present a risk to dental laboratory and operating personnel.

All alginate impressions should be disinfected before pouring with gypsum to form a cast. The most common form of disinfection is spraying, but studies have shown that such impressions can be immersed in disinfectant also. The effect of disinfection in 1% sodium hypochlorite or 2%

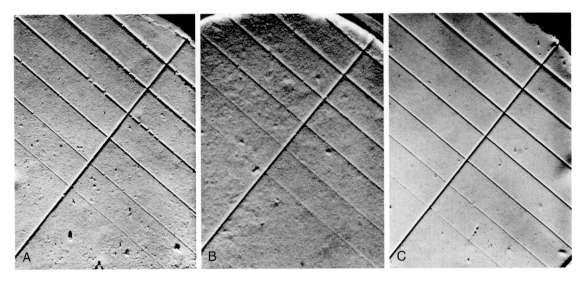

FIGURE 12.7 **Surface quality and reproduction using model plaster and dental stone. A,** Model plaster poured against alginate; **B,** dental stone poured against the same alginate; and **C,** the same dental stone poured against polysulfide. It should be emphasized that another alginate with the same plaster and stone could yield opposite results. *(From Craig RG, MacPherson GW: University of Michigan School of Dentistry, Ann Arbor, 1965.)*

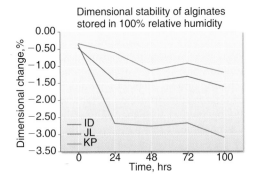

FIGURE 12.8 Dimensional change of alginate impression materials stored in 100% relative humidity. *(Modified from Lu H, Frey GN, Powers JM. Unpublished data.)*

potentiated glutaraldehyde solutions on accuracy and surface quality has been measured after 10- to 30-minute immersion. Statistically significant dimensional changes were observed; however, the changes were on the order of 0.1% and the quality of the surface was not impaired. Such changes would be insignificant for clinical applications such as the preparation of study models and working casts. In another study, immersion disinfection of alginates demonstrated little effect on accuracy and surface quality, but it was shown that one alginate product was best immersed in iodophor and another brand in glyoxal glutaraldehyde. The effect of disinfection on agar impression materials has not been reported, but considering the similarity of the two hydrocolloids, similar recommendations are reasonable.

ELASTOMERIC IMPRESSION MATERIALS

Four types of synthetic elastomeric impression materials are available to record dental impressions: polysulfides, condensation silicones, addition silicones (polyvinylsiloxanes), and polyethers. Polysulfides were the first synthetic elastomeric impression material introduced (1950). Condensation silicones were made available to dentists in 1955, polyether in 1965, and addition silicones in 1975. Polysulfide and condensation silicone impression materials are described on the website. Polyvinylsiloxanes and polyethers form the vast majority of elastomeric impressions used worldwide today. Changes in recent years have provided greater choice of consistency and new mixing techniques. http://evolve.elsevier.com/sakaguchi/restorative ⊜

Consistencies

Elastomeric impression materials are typically supplied in several consistencies (viscosities) to accommodate a range of impression techniques. Addition silicones are available: extra-low, low (syringe or wash), medium (regular), monophase, high (tray), and putty (extra-high) consistencies. Polyether impression materials are now available in low, medium, and high consistencies.

Mixing Systems

Two types of systems are available to mix the catalyst and base thoroughly before taking the impression: static *automixing* and dynamic *mechanical mixing*

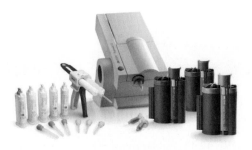

FIGURE 12.9 Addition silicone impression materials packaged with automixed cartridges, mixing gun, and static mixing tips, and dynamic mechanical mixer. *(Courtesy of 3M ESPE Dental Products, St. Paul, MN)*

A very popular means of mixing the catalyst and base is with a so-called *automixing system*. The base and catalyst are in separate cylinders of the plastic cartridge. The cartridge is placed in a mixing gun containing two plungers that are advanced by a ratchet mechanism to extrude equal quantities of base and catalyst. The base and catalyst are forced through the static-mixing tip containing a stationary plastic internal spiral; the two components are folded over each other many times as they are pushed through the spiral, resulting in a uniform mix at the tip end. Because one cylinder may be filled slightly more that the other, the first part of the mix from a new cartridge should be discarded.

The mixed material can be extruded directly into an injection syringe or into the impression tray. Intraoral delivery tips can be placed on the end of the static mixing tip, and the mixed material can be injected into and around the cavity preparation. The tip can be removed, and additional mixed material can be extruded into the impression tray. The automixing systems have been shown to result in mixes with many fewer voids than hand mixes. Although for each mix the material left in the mixing tip is wasted, the average loss is only 1 to 2 mL, depending on the manufacturer's tip, whereas three to four times this much is wasted in a hand mix as a result of overestimating the amount needed. Initially, automixing was used for low consistencies, but new designs of guns and mixing tips allow all consistencies except putty to be used with this system. Addition silicones and polyethers are available with this means of mixing.

The second and newest system is a dynamic, mechanical mixer, illustrated in Figure 12-9. The catalyst and base are supplied in large plastic bags housed in a cartridge, which is inserted into the top of the mixing machine. A new, plastic mixing tip is placed on the front of the machine, and when the button is depressed, parallel plungers push against the collapsible plastic bags, thereby opening the bags and forcing material into the dynamic mixing tip. This mixing tip differs from automixing in that the internal spiral is motor driven so it

rotates. Thus mixing is accomplished by this rotation plus forward motion of the material through the spiral. In this manner, thorough mixing can be ensured and higher viscosity material can be mixed with ease. The advantage of this system is ease of use, speed, and thoroughness of mixing, but more must be invested in the purchase of the system compared with hand and automixing. In addition, there is slightly more material retained in the mixing tip than with automixing, but less than that wasted when mixed by hand. Polyether and addition silicone impression materials are available for mixing with this system.

One variation in mixing is with the addition silicone two-putty systems mixed by hand. Scoops are supplied by the manufacturer for dispensing, and the putties are most often kneaded with fingers until free from streaks. The putty materials that have a liquid catalyst are initially mixed with a spatula until the catalyst is reasonably incorporated, and mixing is completed by hand. It should be noted that latex gloves may interfere with setting of addition silicone impression materials, as discussed later.

Impression Techniques

Three common methods for making impressions for fixed restorations are a simultaneous, dual-viscosity technique, a single-viscosity or monophase technique, and a putty-wash technique. In nearly all cases, impression material is injected directly on and into the prepared teeth and a tray containing the bulk of the impression material is placed thereafter. After the impression is set, the tray is removed.

The simultaneous, dual-viscosity technique is one in which low-consistency material is injected with a syringe into critical areas and the high-consistency material is mixed and placed in an impression tray. After injecting the low-viscosity material, the tray containing the higher-viscosity material is placed in the mouth. In this manner, the more viscous tray impression material forces the lower-viscosity material to flow into fine aspects of the areas of interest. Because they are both mixed at nearly the same time, the materials join, bond, and set together. After the materials have set, the tray and the impression are removed. An example of an impression using this procedure is shown in Figure 12-10.

In the single-viscosity or monophase technique, impressions are often taken with a medium-viscosity impression material. Addition silicone and polyether impression materials are well suited for this technique because both have a capacity for shear thinning. As described in Chapter 4, pseudoplastic materials demonstrate a decreased viscosity when subjected to high shear rates such as occurs during mixing and syringing. When the medium viscosity material is forced through an impression syringe, the viscosity is reduced, whereas

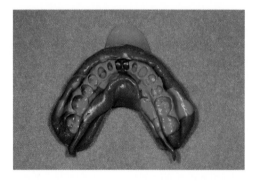

FIGURE 12.10 An elastomeric addition silicone impression. Turquoise material is of a low or injection consistency, and maroon material of a high or tray consistency. *(Courtesy of Dr. Charles Mark Malloy, Portland, OR.)*

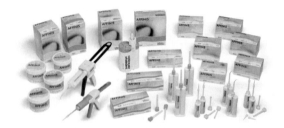

FIGURE 12.11 Various consistencies and types of packaging of an addition silicone impression material. *(Courtesy of Coltene/Whaledent Inc, Cuyahoga Falls, OH.)*

Composition and Reactions

The next two sections describe the general composition and setting reactions of addition silicone and polyether impression materials. The following section describes their physical properties, permitting a more direct comparison of the various types and their properties.

Addition Silicone

Addition silicone is available in extra low, low, medium, heavy, and very heavy (putty) consistencies. A representative product line of addition silicones is shown in Figure 12-11. The base paste of this class of impression materials contains a moderately low-molecular-weight polymer (polymethylhydrosiloxane) with more than 3 and up to 10 pendant or terminal hydrosilane groups per molecule (see formulas below and addition silicone formula 1 [AS1]). The base also contains filler.

the viscosity of the same material residing in the tray is unaffected. In this manner, such materials can be used for syringing and for trays, as previously described for the simultaneous, dual-viscosity technique. The mechanism for shear thinning is discussed in the later section on the viscosity of impression materials.

The putty-wash technique is a two-step impression procedure whereby a preliminary impression is taken in high- or putty-consistency material before the cavity preparation is made. Space is provided for a low-consistency material by a variety of techniques, and after cavity preparation, a low-consistency material is syringed into the area and the preliminary impression reinserted. The low- and high-consistency materials bond, and after the low-consistency material sets, the impression is removed. This procedure is sometimes called a *wash technique*. The putty-consistency material and this technique were developed for condensation silicones to minimize the effects of dimensional change during polymerization. Most of the shrinkage during polymerization takes place in the putty material when the preliminary impression is made, confining final shrinkage to the thin wash portion of the impression. Care must be taken so the wash material can freely escape via vents in the putty material when the wash impression is made. If not, the wash material can compress the putty in the second-stage impression, inducing permanent distortion and inaccuracies to the impression. The putty-wash technique was extended to addition silicones after their introduction, even though their polymerization shrinkage is significantly lower.

Manufacturers add coloring agents to the accelerator or base as an aid in determining the thoroughness of the mix. Normally a different color is used for each consistency of a particular product line so one can distinguish the wash (low) consistency from the tray consistency in the set impression. Retarders may be added as well to control working and setting time of the products.

Pendant hydrosilane groups   Terminal hydrosilane groups

$$-O-\underset{\underset{H}{|}}{\overset{\overset{CH_3}{|}}{Si}}-O- \qquad\qquad -O-\underset{\underset{CH_3}{|}}{\overset{\overset{CH_3}{|}}{Si}}-H-$$

Polymethylhydrosiloxane

$$CH_3-\underset{\underset{CH_3}{|}}{\overset{\overset{CH_3}{|}}{Si}}-\left[O-\underset{\underset{CH_3}{|}}{\overset{\overset{CH_3}{|}}{Si}}\right]_x\left[\underset{\underset{H}{|}}{\overset{\overset{CH_3}{|}}{Si}}-O\right]_y\underset{\underset{CH_3}{|}}{\overset{\overset{CH_3}{|}}{Si}}-CH_3$$

AS1   Vinylpolysiloxane

$$CH_2=CH-\underset{\underset{CH_3}{|}}{\overset{\overset{CH_3}{|}}{Si}}-\left[O-\underset{\underset{CH_3}{|}}{\overset{\overset{CH_3}{|}}{Si}}\right]_n CH=CH_2$$

The accelerator (catalyst) and the base paste contain a dimethylsiloxane polymer with vinyl terminal groups, plus filler. The accelerator also contains a platinum catalyst of the so-called *Karstedt type*, which is a complex compound consisting of platinum and

1,3-divinyltetramethyldisiloxane. Unlike the condensation type, the addition reaction does not normally produce a low-molecular-weight byproduct, as indicated in the reaction shown below (AS2).

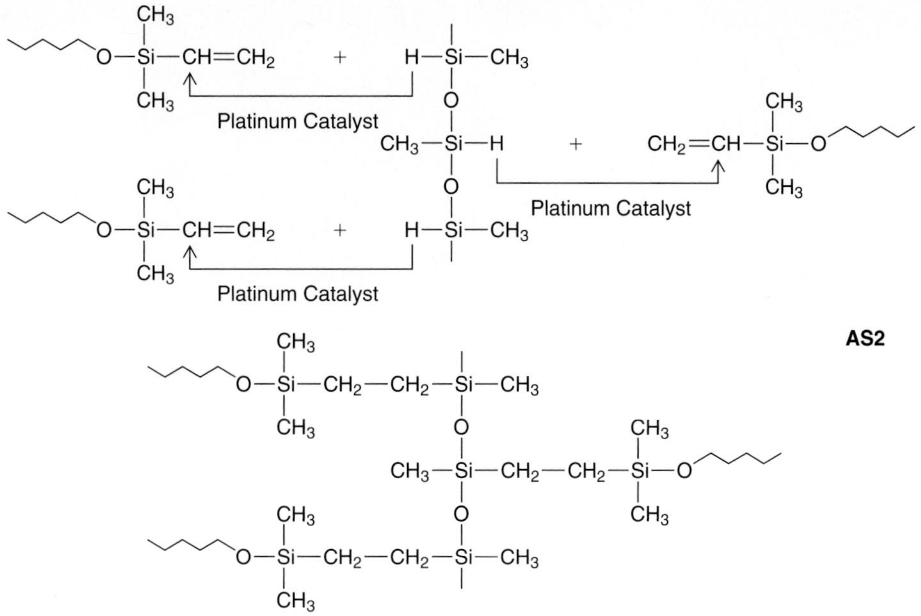

$$
\begin{array}{c}
\text{CH}_3 \\
\text{O—Si—CH=CH}_2 \quad + \quad \text{H—Si—CH}_3 \\
\text{CH}_3 \\
\text{Platinum Catalyst}
\end{array}
$$

$$
\begin{array}{c}
\text{CH}_3\text{—Si—H} \quad + \quad \text{CH}_2\text{=CH—Si—O} \\
\text{O} \qquad\qquad \text{CH}_3 \\
\text{Platinum Catalyst}
\end{array}
$$

$$
\begin{array}{c}
\text{CH}_3 \\
\text{O—Si—CH=CH}_2 \quad + \quad \text{H—Si—CH}_3 \\
\text{CH}_3 \\
\text{Platinum Catalyst}
\end{array}
$$

AS2

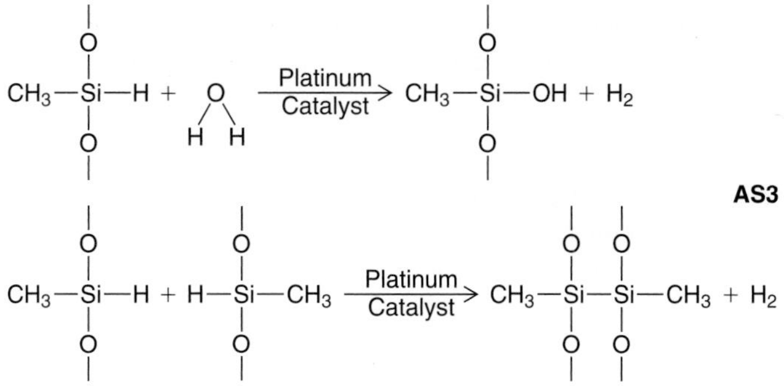

$$
\begin{array}{c}
\text{CH}_3 \\
\text{O—Si—CH}_2\text{—CH}_2\text{—Si—CH}_3 \\
\text{CH}_3 \qquad\qquad \text{O} \\
\text{CH}_3\text{—Si—CH}_2\text{—CH}_2\text{—Si—O} \\
\text{CH}_3 \qquad\qquad \text{O} \qquad\qquad \text{CH}_3 \\
\text{O—Si—CH}_2\text{—CH}_2\text{—Si—CH}_3 \\
\text{CH}_3
\end{array}
$$

$$
\text{CH}_3\text{—Si—H} + \text{O}\langle^{H}_{H} \xrightarrow[\text{Catalyst}]{\text{Platinum}} \text{CH}_3\text{—Si—OH} + \text{H}_2
$$

AS3

$$
\text{CH}_3\text{—Si—H} + \text{H—Si—CH}_3 \xrightarrow[\text{Catalyst}]{\text{Platinum}} \text{CH}_3\text{—Si—Si—CH}_3 + \text{H}_2
$$

A secondary reaction can occur, however, with the production of hydrogen gas if —OH groups are present. The most important source of —OH groups is water (H—OH), the reaction of which under consumption of Si—H-units is illustrated above (AS3). Another possible source of hydrogen gas is a side reaction of the Si—H units of the polymethylhydrosiloxane with each other, under the influence of the platinum catalyst, also shown above (AS3).

Not all addition silicone impression materials release hydrogen gas, and because it is not known which do, it is recommended that one wait at least 30 minutes for the setting reaction to be completed before the gypsum models and dies are poured. Epoxy dies should not be poured until the impression has stood overnight. The difference in the delay with gypsum and epoxy is that gypsum products have

much shorter setting times than epoxy die materials. Some products contain a hydrogen absorber such as palladium, and gypsum and epoxy die materials can be poured against them as soon as practical. Examples of high-strength stone poured after 15 minutes against addition silicone, with and without a hydrogen absorber, are shown in Figure 12-12.

Latex gloves have been shown to adversely affect the setting of addition silicone impressions. Sulfur compounds that are used in the vulcanization of latex rubber gloves can migrate to the surface of stored gloves. These compounds can be transferred onto the prepared teeth and adjacent soft tissues during tooth preparation and when placing tissue retraction cord. They can also be incorporated directly into the impression material when mixing two putties by hand. These compounds can poison

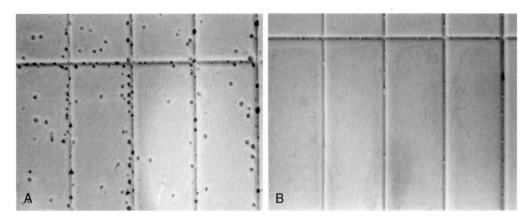

FIGURE 12.12 **Addition-silicone impressions poured in high-strength stone at 15 minutes. A,** Bubbles are caused by the release of hydrogen. **B,** No bubbles are apparent because palladium hydrogen absorber is included in the impression material.

the platinum-containing catalyst, which results in retarded or no polymerization in the contaminated area of the impression. Thorough washing of the gloves with detergent and water just before mixing sometimes minimizes this effect, and some brands of gloves interfere with the setting more than others. Vinyl and nitrile gloves do not have such an effect. Residual monomer in acrylic provisional restorations and resin composite cores has a similar inhibiting effect on the set of addition silicone materials. The preparation and adjacent soft tissues can also be cleaned with 2% chlorhexidine to remove contaminants.

Polyether

Polyethers are supplied in low-, medium-, and heavy-body consistency. The base paste consists of a long-chain polyether copolymer with alternating oxygen atoms and methylene groups ($O-[CH_2]_n$) and reactive terminal groups (see polyether 1 [PE1]). Also incorporated are a silica filler, compatible plasticizers of a nonphthalate type, and triglycerides. In the catalyst paste, the former 2,5-dichlorobenzene sulfonate was replaced by an aliphatic cationic starter as a cross-linking agent. The catalyst also includes silica filler and plasticizers. Coloring agents are added to base and catalyst to aid in the recognition of different material types. Examples of polyether impression materials are shown in Figure 12-9.

The reaction mechanism is shown (PE2) in a simplified form. The elastomer is formed by cationic polymerization by opening of the reactive terminal rings. The backbone of the polymer is believed to be a copolymer of ethylene oxide and tetramethylene oxide units. The reactive terminal rings open under the influence of the cationic initiator of the catalyst paste and can then, as a cation itself, attack and open additional rings. Whenever a ring is opened, the

TABLE 12.3 Setting Properties of Elastomeric Impression Materials

Material	Consistency	Temperature Rise (° C)	Viscosity 45 sec after Mixing (cp)	Working Time (min)	Setting Time (min)	Dimensional Change at 24 hr (%)
POLYSULFIDES						
	Low	3.4	60,000	4-7	7-10	−0.40
	Medium		110,000	3-6	6-8	−0.45
	High		450,000	3-6	6-8	−0.44
SILICONES						
Condensation	Low	1.1	70,000	2.5-4	6-8	−0.60
	Very high			2-2.5	3-6	−0.38
Addition	Low			2-4	4-6.5	−0.15
	Medium		150,000	2-4	4-6.5	−0.17
	High			2.5-4	4-6.5	−0.15
	Very high			1-4	3-5	−0.14
POLYETHERS						
	Low	4.2		3	6	−0.23
	Medium		130,000	2.5-3	6	−0.24
	High			2.5	5.5	−0.19

cation function remains attached, thus lengthening the chain (see PE3). Because of the identical chemical base, all polyether consistencies can be freely combined with each other. A chemical bond between all materials develops during curing.

Setting Properties

Typical values of the setting properties of elastomeric impression materials are presented in Table 12-3. The temperature rise in typical mixes of impression materials was pointed out in the previous section, but Table 12-3 illustrates that the temperature rise is small and of no clinical concern.

Viscosity

The viscosity of materials 45 seconds after mixing is listed in Table 12-3. As expected, the viscosity increases for the same type of material from low to high consistencies. Viscosity is a function of time after the start of mixing.

A shearing force can affect the viscosity of polyether and addition silicone impression materials, as was mentioned in the section on impression techniques. This effect is called *shear thinning* or *pseudoplasticity*. For impression materials possessing this characteristic, the viscosity of the unset material diminishes with an increasing outside force or shearing speed. When the influence is discontinued, the

viscosity immediately increases. This property is very important for the use of monophase impression materials, and is illustrated for polyether in Figure 12-13. In the case of polyether, shear-thinning properties are influenced by a weak network of triglyceride crystals. The crystals align when the impression material is sheared, as occurs when mixed or flowing through a syringe tip. The microcrystalline triglyceride network ensures that the polyether remains viscous in the tray or on the tooth but flows under pressure. This allows a single or monophase material to be used as a low- and medium-consistency material. Cooling of the pastes results in substantial viscosity increase. Before using, pastes have to be brought to room temperature.

The effect of shear rate (rotational speed of the viscometer) on the viscosity of single-consistency (monophase) addition silicones is shown in Figure 12-14. Although all products showed a decrease in viscosity with increasing shear rate, the effect was much more pronounced for two products, Ba and Hy, with about an eightfold to eleven-fold decrease from the lowest to the highest shear rate. The substantial decrease in viscosity at high shear stress, which is comparable with the decrease during syringing, permits the use of a single mix of material, with a portion to be used as syringe material and another portion to be used as tray material in the syringe-tray technique.

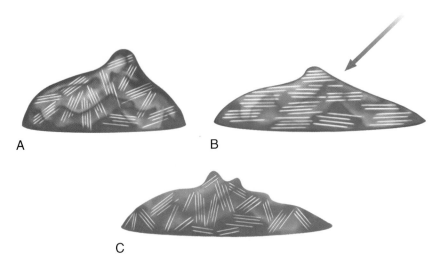

FIGURE 12.13 **Demonstration of the mechanism for the property of shear thinning or pseudoplasticity in poly-ethers.** The trigliceride network, **A,** within the impression material aligns when sheared as with syringing, and **B,** to achieve a lower viscosity. Once the shear force is removed, the viscosity increases with randomization of the triglyceride network, **C.**

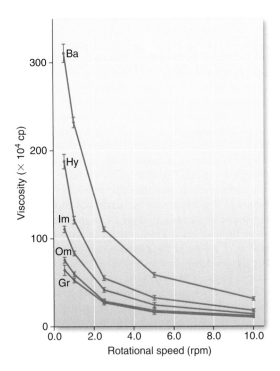

FIGURE 12.14 Viscosity in centipoise as a function of shear rate (rotational speed of the viscometer) for five single-consistency addition-silicone impression materials. A rotational speed of 0.5 rpm would represent a shear rate comparable with that observed when placing the material in a tray, and a speed of 10 rpm would represent a shear rate comparable with that experienced when syringing the material. *(Data from Kim KN, Craig RG, Koran A III: J. Prosthet. Dent. 67,794, 1992.)*

Working and Setting Times

The working and setting times of addition silicone and polyether impression materials are listed in Table 12-3. In general, for a given class of elastomeric impression materials by a specific manufacturer, the working and setting times decrease as the viscosity increases from low to high. Polyethers show a clearly defined working time with a sharp transition into the setting phase. This behavior is often called *snap-set.* This transition from plastic condition into elastic properties is rather short compared with older addition silicones, which was shown in investigations of rheological properties of setting materials (Figure 12-15).

Note that the working and setting times of the elastomeric impression materials are shortened by increases in temperature and humidity; on hot, humid days this effect should be considered in the clinical application of these materials.

The initial (or working) and final setting times can be determined fairly accurately by using a penetrometer with a needle and weight selected to suit these materials. The Vicat penetrometer, as shown in Figure 12-16, with a 3-mm diameter needle and a total weight of 300 g, has been used by a number of investigators. A metal ring, 8 mm high and 16 mm in diameter, is filled with freshly mixed material and placed on the penetrometer base. The needle is applied to the surface of the impression material for 10 seconds, and a reading is taken. This is repeated every 30 seconds. The initial set is that time at which the needle no longer completely penetrates the specimen to the bottom of the ring. The final set is the time of the first of three identical nonmaximum

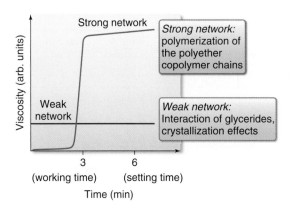

FIGURE 12.15 Illustration of the snap-set of polyether. The initial viscosity of the unset material is influenced by the structural triglycerides, whereas the polymerization of copolymer chains thereafter provides the quick increase in viscosity as the material sets.

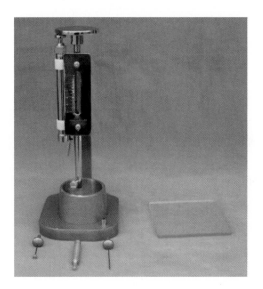

FIGURE 12.16 Vicat penetrometer used to determine setting time of impression materials and other restorative materials.

penetration readings. When the material has set, the elasticity still allows penetration of the needle, but it is the same at each application.

Dimensional Change on Setting

The impression material undergoes a dimensional change on setting. The major factor for contraction during setting is cross-linking and rearrangement of bonds within and between polymer chains. Impressions can expand if water sorption takes place and an impression can be distorted if seated after the material has set to any degree. Finally, distortion or creep will occur if the material does not recover elastically when the set impression is removed from undercuts.

Imbibition is discussed in the section on disinfecting impressions, and creep-induced distortion is discussed under elastic recovery.

Addition silicone and polyether impression materials undergo shrinkage due to polymerization. The linear dimensional change between a die and the impression after 24 hours is listed in Table 12-3. The addition silicones have the smallest change, about −0.15%, followed by the polyethers at about −0.2%. The contraction is low for these two products because there is no loss of byproducts.

The rate of shrinkage of elastomeric impression materials is not uniform during the 24 hours after removal from the mouth. In general, about half the shrinkage observed at 24 hours occurs during the first hour after removal; for greatest accuracy, therefore, the models and dies should be prepared promptly, although in air the elastomeric impression materials are much more stable than hydrocolloid products.

Mechanical Properties

Typical mechanical properties of elastomeric impression materials are listed in Table 12-4. The permanent deformation (in the current specification, elastic recovery, which is 100% minus the permanent deformation), strain in compression, and dimensional change are properties used in ANSI/ADA specification No. 19 (ISO 4823) to classify elastomeric impression materials as low, medium, high, or very high viscosity types. The requirements for these properties are given in Table 12-5. Further requirements of the specification for elastomeric impression materials are indicated in Table 12-6. The consistency diameter is used to classify viscosity by measuring the diameter of the disk formed when 0.5 mL of mixed material is subjected to a 5.6-N weight at 1.5 minutes after mixing for 12 minutes. Because the setting times of elastomeric impression materials vary, the consistency diameter is affected not only by the viscosity but also by the setting time. The classification of a material by the consistency diameter may be different from that by a true viscosity measurement.

Elastic Recovery

The order in which the permanent deformation of the elastomeric impression materials is listed in Table 12-4 demonstrates that addition silicones have the best elastic recovery during removal from the mouth, followed by polyethers. A material with a permanent deformation of 1% has an elastic recovery of 99%.

Strain in Compression

The strain in compression under a stress of 0.1 MPa is a measure of the flexibility of the material. Table 12-4 illustrates that, in general, the low-consistency

TABLE 12.4   Mechanical Properties of Elastomeric Impression Materials

Material	Consistency	Permanent Deformation[*] (%)	Strain in Compression (%)	Flow (%)	Shore A Hardness	Tear Strength (kN/m)
POLYSULFIDES						
	Low	3-4	14-17	0.5-2	20	2.5-7.0
	Medium	3-5	11-15	0.5-1	30	3.0-7.0
	High	3-6	9-12	0.5-1	35	—
SILICONES						
Condensation	Low	1-2	4-9	0.05-0.1	15-30	2.3-2.6
	Very high	2-3	2-5	0.02-0.05	50-65	—
Addition	Low	0.05-0.4	3-6	0.01-0.03	35-55	1.5-3.0
	Medium	0.05-0.3	2-5	0.01-0.03	50-60	2.2-3.5
	High	0.1-0.3	2-3	0.01-0.03	60-70	2.5-4.3
	Very high	0.2-0.5	1-2	0.01-0.1	50-75	—
POLYETHERS						
	Low	1.5	3	0.03	35-40	1.8
	Medium	1-2	2-3	0.02	40-60	2.8-4.8
	High	2	3	0.02	40-50	3.0

*Elastic recovery from deformation is 100% minus the percent permanent deformation.

TABLE 12.5   Elastic Recovery, Strain in Compression, and Dimensional Change Requirements for Elastomeric Impression Materials

Viscosity Type	Minimum Elastic Recovery (%)	Strain in Compression (%)		Maximum Dimensional Change in 24 Hours (%)
		Minimum	Maximum	
Low	96.5	2.0	20	1.5
Medium	96.5	2.0	20	1.5
High	96.5	0.8	20	1.5
Very high	96.5	0.8	20	1.5

Modified from ISO Specification No. 4823.

TABLE 12.6   Requirements by ANSI/ADA Specification No. 19 (ISO 4823) for the Various Viscosities of Elastomeric Impression Materials

Viscosity	Maximum Mixing Time (min)	Minimum Working Time (min)	Diameter of Consistency Disk (mm)		Reproduction of Detail	
			Minimum	Maximum	Line Width in Impression (mm)	Line Width in Gypsum (mm)
Low	1	2	36	—	0.020	0.020
Medium	1	2	31	41	0.020	0.020
High	1	2	—	35	0.050	0.050
Very High	1	2	—	35	0.075	0.075

Modified from ISO Specification No. 4823.

materials of each type are more flexible than the high-consistency elastomeric impressions. For a given consistency, polyethers are generally the stiffest, followed by addition silicones.

Flow

Flow is measured on a cylindrical specimen 1 hour old, and the percent flow is determined 15 minutes after a load of 1 N is applied. As seen in Table 12-4, silicones and polyethers have low values of flow.

Typical elastomeric impression materials apparently have no difficulty meeting the mechanical property requirements of ANSI/ADA specification No. 19 (see Table 12-6). Although the flow, hardness, and the tear strengths of elastomeric impression materials are not mentioned in the specification, these are important properties; they are also listed in Table 12-4.

Hardness

The Shore A hardness increases from low to high consistency. When two numbers are given, the first represents the hardness 1.5 minutes after removal from the mouth, and the second number is the hardness after 2 hours. The low-, medium-, and high-viscosity addition silicones do not change hardness significantly with time, whereas the hardness of polyethers does increase with time. In addition, the hardness and strain in compression affect the force necessary to remove the impression from the mouth. Low flexibility and high hardness can be compensated for clinically by producing more space for the impression material between the tray and the teeth. This can be accomplished with additional block-out for custom trays or by selecting a larger tray when using disposable trays.

A new variation in polyether provides less resistance to deformation during removal of the impression from the mouth and the gypsum cast from the impression. To achieve this, the filler content was reduced from 14 to 6 parts per unit, thereby reducing the Shore A hardness from 46 to 40 after 15 minutes, and from 61 to 50 after 24 hours. The ratio of high-viscous softener to low-viscous softener was changed to achieve a consistency similar to that of the conventional monophase polyether.

Tear Strength

Tear strength is important because it indicates the ability of a material to withstand tearing in thin interproximal areas and margins of periodontally involved teeth. The tear strengths listed in Table 12-4 are a measure of the force needed to initiate and continue tearing a specimen of unit thickness. As the consistency of the impression type increases, tear strength undergoes a small increase, but most of the values are between 2.0 and

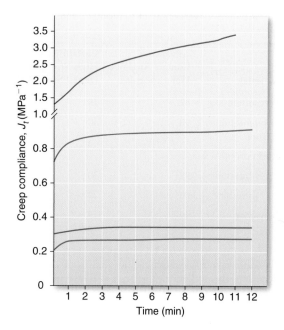

FIGURE 12.17 Creep compliance of elastomeric impression materials at the time recommended for removal from the mouth. Curves from top to bottom: polysulfide, condensation silicone, addition silicone, and polyether. *(Data from Craig RG: J. Mich. Dent. Assoc. 59, 259, 1977.)*

3.9 kN/m. Values for very high consistency types are not listed because this property is not important for these materials. Higher tear strengths for elastomeric impression materials are desirable, but compared with the values for hydrocolloid impression materials of 0.3 to 0.7 kN/m, they are a major improvement.

Creep Compliance

Elastomeric impression materials are viscoelastic, and their mechanical properties are time dependent. For example, the higher the rate of deformation, the higher the tear strength; and the longer the impressions are deformed, the higher the permanent deformation. As a result, plots of creep compliance versus time describe the properties of these materials better than stress-strain curves. Creep-compliance time curves for low-consistency polysulfide, condensation silicone, addition silicone, and medium-consistency polyether are shown in Figure 12-17. The initial creep compliance illustrates polysulfide is the most flexible and polyether is the least flexible. The flatness or parallelism of the curves with respect to the time axis indicates low permanent deformation and excellent recovery from deformation during the removal of an impression material; addition silicones and polyethers have the best elastic recovery.

TABLE 12.7   Wettability of Elastomeric Impression Materials

Material	Advancing Contact Angle of Water (degrees)	Castability of High-Strength Dental Stone (%)
Polysulfide	82	44
Condensation silicone	98	30
Addition silicone		
Hydrophobic	98	30
Hydrophilic	53	72
Polyether	49	70

The recoverable viscoelastic quality of the materials is indicated by differences between the initial creep compliance and the creep compliance value obtained by extrapolation of the linear portion of the curve to zero time. As a result, addition silicones have the lowest viscoelastic quality and require less time to recover viscoelastic deformation, followed by the polyethers.

Detail Reproduction

The requirements of elastomeric impression materials are listed in Table 12-6. Except for the very high-viscosity products, all should reproduce a V-shaped groove and a 0.02-mm wide line in the elastomeric. The impression should be compatible with gypsum products so the 0.02-mm line is transferred to gypsum die materials. Low-, medium-, and high-viscosity elastomeric impression materials have little difficulty meeting this requirement.

Wettability and Hydrophilization of Elastomeric Impression Materials

Wettability may be assessed by measuring the advancing contact angle of water on the surface of the set impression material or by using a tensiometer to measure forces as the material is immersed and removed (Wilhelmy technique). The advancing contact angles for elastomeric impression materials are listed in Table 12-7. Of all the impression materials discussed in this chapter, only alginates can be considered truly hydrophilic. All of the elastomeric impression materials possess advancing and receding contact angles greater than 45 degrees. There are, however, differences in wetting among and within types of elastomeric impression materials. Traditional addition silicone is not as wettable as polyether. When mixes of gypsum products are poured into hydrophobic addition silicone, high contact angles are formed, making the preparation of bubble-free models difficult.

Surfactants have been added to addition silicones by manufacturers to reduce the contact angle, improve wettability, and simplify the pouring of gypsum models. This class with improved wetting characteristics is most accurately called *hydrophilized addition silicone*. Most commonly, nonionic surfactants have gained importance in this area. These molecules consist of an oligoether or polyether substructure as the hydrophilic part and a silicone-compatible hydrophobic part (Figure 12-18, *A*). The mode of action of these wetting agents is believed to be a diffusion-controlled transfer of surfactant molecules from the polyvinylsiloxane into the aqueous phase, as shown, thereby altering the surface tension of the surrounding liquid. As a result, a reduction in surface tension and therefore greater wettability of the polyvinylsiloxane is observed (Figure 12-18, *B*). This mechanism differs from polyethers, which possess a high degree of wettability because their molecular structure contains polar oxygen atoms, which have an affinity for water. Because of this affinity, polyether materials flow onto hydrated intraoral surfaces and are therefore cast with gypsum more easily than are addition silicones. This affinity also allows polyether impressions to adhere quite strongly to soft and hard tissues.

By observing water droplets on impression surfaces, it has been shown that hydrophilized addition silicones and polyethers are wetted the best, and condensation silicones and conventional addition silicones the least. Wettability was directly correlated to the ease of pouring high-strength stone models of an extremely critical die, as shown in Table 12-7. Using a tensiometer to record forces of immersed impression specimens (Wilhelmy method), polyether was shown to wet significantly better than hydrophilized addition silicones for both advancing (74° versus 108° C) and receding contact angles (50° versus 81° C).

To evaluate the ability of impression materials to reproduce detail under wet and dry surface conditions, impressions were made of a standard wave pattern used to calibrate surface analyzers. The surfaces of impressions were scanned for average roughness (Ra) after setting to determine their ability to reproduce the detail of the standard, the value of which is shown with a double line in Figure 12-19. From a clinical standpoint, most impression materials produced acceptable detail under wet and dry conditions. Polyethers produced slightly better detail than did addition silicones, and were generally unaffected by the presence of moisture, whereas detail decreased some for addition silicones under wet conditions, even if hydrophilized.

Disinfection of Elastomeric Impressions

All impressions should be disinfected upon removal from the mouth to prevent transmission of organisms to gypsum casts and to laboratory

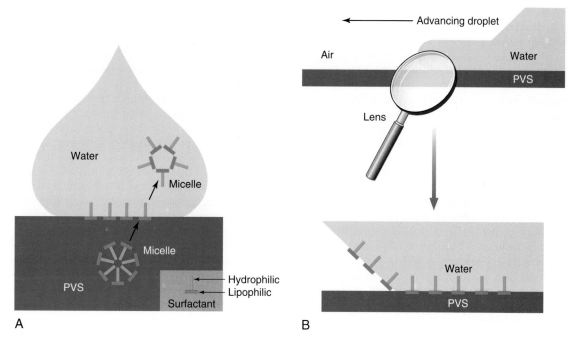

FIGURE 12.18 **Hydrophilization of addition silicones. A,** The hydrophilization of addition silicones is gained with the incorporation of nonionic surfactants shown as micelles. These molecules consist of a hydrophilic part and a silicone-compatible hydrophobic part. The mode of action of these surfactants is thought to be a diffusion-controlled transfer of surfactant molecules from the polyvinylsiloxane into the aqueous phase, as shown. In this manner, the surface tension of the surrounding liquid is altered. **B,** This increased wettability allows the addition silicone to spread more freely along the surface. *PVS,* Polyvinylsiloxane.

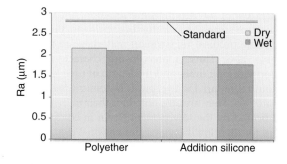

FIGURE 12.19 **Ability of polyether and hydrophilized addition silicone materials to reproduce detail under dry and wet conditions.** The average roughness, Ra, of the standard from which impressions were made is shown *(double line).* Polyethers produced the best detail and were unaffected by moisture. The detail captured by addition silicones decreased slightly in the presence of moisture. *(Data from Johnson GH, Lepe X, Berg JC: J. Dent. Res. 77 [Spec Issue B], 798, 1998.)*

personnel. Several studies confirm that addition silicone and polyether impressions can be disinfected by immersion in several different disinfectants for up to 18 hours without a loss of surface quality and accuracy.

Relationship of Properties and Clinical Application

Accuracy, the ability to record detail, ease of handling, and setting characteristics are of prime importance in dental impressions.

Silicones generally have shorter working times than polysulfides but somewhat longer times than polyethers. Single-mix materials have some advantage in that, as a result of shear thinning, they have low viscosities when mixed or syringed but higher viscosities when inserted in a tray. The time of placement of an elastomeric impression material is critical, because viscosity increases rapidly with time as a result of the polymerization reaction. If the material is placed in the mouth after the consistency or viscosity has increased via polymerization, internal stresses induced in the impression are released after the impression is removed from the mouth, resulting in an inaccurate impression.

Thorough mixing is essential; otherwise portions of the mix could contain insufficient accelerator to polymerize thoroughly or may not set at the same rate as other portions of the impression. In this event, removal of the impression would cause less elastic recovery and result in an inaccurate impression. Automixing and mechanical mixing systems produce mixes with fewer bubbles than hand mixing, save time in mixing, and result in a more bubble-free impression.

Polymerization of elastomeric impression materials continues after the material has set, and the mechanical properties improve with time. Removal too early may result in high permanent deformation; however, excessively long times in the mouth are unacceptable to the patient. The manufacturer usually recommends a minimum time for leaving the impression in the mouth, and this minimum is used for testing the materials according to ANSI/ADA specification No. 19.

Dimensional changes on setting can be compensated for by use of a double-impression or putty-wash technique. When using a double-impression technique, a preliminary impression is taken in the high- or puttylike-consistency material, providing some space for the final impression in low-consistency material. The preliminary impression is removed, the cavity prepared, and the final impression taken with the low-consistency material, using the preliminary impression as a tray. In this way, the dimensional change in the high consistency or puttylike consistency is negligible, and although the percent dimensional change of the low-consistency material is still large, the thickness is so small that the actual dimensional change is small. The double-impression technique is suitable for use with a stock impression tray, because the preliminary impression serves as a custom tray. With the monophase and simultaneous dual-viscosity technique, a slight improvement in accuracy results when a custom-made tray is used because it provides a uniform thickness of impression material. Several studies have shown, however, that relatively stiff stock plastic or metal trays yield nearly the same accuracy.

Clinical studies have shown that the viscosity of the impression material is the most important factor in producing impressions and dies with minimal bubbles and maximum detail. As a result, the syringe-tray technique produced superior clinical results in the reproduction of fine internal detail of proximal boxes or grooves.

The accuracy of the impression may be affected when the percentage of deformation and the time involved in removing the impression are increased. In both instances, permanent deformation increases, the amount depending on the type of elastomeric impression material.

Because elastomeric impressions recover from deformation for a period after their removal, some increase in accuracy can be expected during this time. However, polymerization shrinkage is also occurring, and the overall accuracy is determined by a combination of these two effects. Insignificant elastic recovery occurs after 20 to 30 minutes; therefore, dies should be prepared promptly after that time for greatest accuracy. Addition silicones that release hydrogen are an exception to this guideline.

Second pours of gypsum products into elastomeric impressions produce dies that are not quite as accurate as the first, because the impression can be deformed during the removal of the first die; however, they are usually sufficiently accurate to be used as a working die.

OCCLUSAL REGISTRATION MATERIALS

Elastomeric Registration Materials

Addition silicones and polyethers have been formulated for use as occlusal registration materials. Most of the products are addition silicones and most are supplied in automix cartridges. Properties of these occlusal registration materials are listed in Table 12-8. These materials are characterized by short working times and the length of time left in the mouth compared with typical elastomeric impression materials. They are also noted for their high stiffness, indicated by the low percent strain in compression, and for their low flow and dimensional change even after 7 days. The property that distinguishes addition silicones from polyethers is their lower dimensional change after removal; however, either is superior to the stability of waxes for making occlusal records.

TABLE 12.8   Properties of Elastomeric Impression Materials Used for Occlusal Registrations

Material	Mixing Type	Working Time (min)	Time in Mouth (min)	Strain in Compression (%)	Dimensional Change		
					Flow (%)	1 Day (%)	7 Days (%)
Addition silicone	Automix	0.5-3.0	1.0-3.0	1.0-2.9	0.0-0.01	0.0 to −0.15	−0.04 to −0.20
Addition silicone	Handmix	1.4	2.5	0.92	0.0	−0.06	−0.08
Polyether	Handmix	2.1	3.0	1.97	0.0	−0.29	−0.32

IMPRESSION TRAYS

Custom impression trays provide a nearly constant distance between the tray and the tissues, allowing a more even distribution of the impression material during the impression procedure, and improved accuracy. Light-activated and vacuum-formed polymers are now used more frequently than chemically accelerated acrylic to produce custom impression trays because of the volatility of the acrylic monomer and sensitivity to the monomer reported by dental staff. Vacuum-formed polystyrene is popular with commercial laboratories because the trays can be made rapidly. These trays must be handled carefully because they are more flexible than acrylic trays and can be deformed easily by the application of heat. Prefabricated impression trays are very popular. These stock trays vary considerably between manufacturers. When a stock tray is chosen, care must be taken to ensure that the tray is well adapted to the tissues and is adequately reinforced to prevent flexing during impression fabrication and removal.

Light-activated tray materials have many advantages over chemically accelerated acrylic. They are similar to light-activated denture base materials but are of a different color. The trays are strong, easy to make, contain no methylmethacrylate, and have negligible polymerization shrinkage in the light chamber. They can be used soon after processing because there is no clinically significant dimensional change after polymerization.

DIE, CAST, AND MODEL MATERIALS

Dental stones, plaster, epoxy resin, and refractory materials are some of the materials used to make casts or dies from dental impressions. The selection of one of these is determined by the particular impression material in use and by the purpose for which the die or cast is to be used.

Impressions in alginate hydrocolloid can be used only with a gypsum material, such as plaster, stone, or casting investment. Various elastomeric impression materials can be used to prepare gypsum or epoxy dies.

Desirable Qualities of a Cast or Die Material

Cast and die materials must reproduce an impression accurately and remain dimensionally stable under normal conditions of use and storage. Setting expansion, contraction, and dimensional variations in response to changes in temperature must be held to a minimum. Not only should the cast be accurate, but it should also satisfactorily reproduce fine detail and have a smooth, hard surface. Such an accurate cast or die must also be strong and durable and withstand the subsequent manipulative procedures without fracture or abrasion of the surface. Qualities of strength, resistance to shearing forces or edge strength, and abrasion resistance are therefore important and are required in varying degrees, according to the purpose for which the cast or die is to be used. For example, because it will not be subjected to much stress in use, a satisfactory study cast might be formed from dental model plaster in which the aforementioned qualities are at a minimum. However, an elastomeric impression used to produce an indirect inlay could be poured in high-strength stone or epoxy, thereby producing a die in which these qualities are sufficient to withstand the carving and finishing procedures that are a part of this technique.

The color of a cast or die can facilitate manipulative procedures, such as waxing inlay patterns, by presenting a contrast in color to the inlay wax. The ease with which the material can be adapted to the impression and the time required before the cast or die is ready for use are of considerable practical significance.

Dental Plaster and Stone

The chemistry and physical properties of dental plaster, stone, and high-strength stone are discussed later in this chapter. Gypsum materials are used extensively to make casts and dies from dental impressions and can be used with any impression material. Stone casts, which are stronger and resist abrasion better than plaster casts, are used whenever a restoration or appliance is to be made on the cast. Plaster may be used for study casts, which are for record purposes only.

Hardening solutions, usually about 30% silica sols in water, are mixed with stone. The increase in hardness of stone dies poured against impressions varies from 2% for silicones to 110% for polyether. The dimensional change on setting of stones mixed with hardener is slightly greater than when mixes are made with water, 0.07% versus 0.05%. In most instances the abrasion or scraping resistance of mixes of stone made with hardening solutions is higher than comparable mixes made with water. A range of effects in the abrasion resistance of surface treatments of stone has been reported. Model and die sprays generally increase the resistance to scraping, whereas lubricants can decrease surface hardness and resistance to scraping.

High-strength dental stones make excellent casts or dies, readily reproduce the fine detail of a dental impression, and are ready for use after approximately

1 hour. The resulting cast is dimensionally stable over long periods and withstands most of the manipulative procedures involved in the production of appliances and restorations.

When wax patterns constructed on high-strength stone dies are to be removed, some separating agent or die lubricant is necessary to prevent the wax from adhering. The lubricant is applied liberally to the high-strength stone die and allowed to soak in; usually several applications can be made before any excess accumulates on the surface. The excess is blown off with an air blast before proceeding to make the wax pattern.

Epoxy Die Materials

Until recently, epoxy materials were supplied in the form of a paste to which a liquid activator (amine) was added to initiate hardening. Because the activators are toxic, they should not come into contact with the skin during mixing and manipulation of the unset material. Shrinkage of 0.1% has occurred during hardening, which may take up to 24 hours. The hardened resin is more resistant to abrasion and stronger than a high-strength stone die. The viscous paste is not as readily introduced into the details of a large impression as high-strength dental stone is; a centrifugal casting machine has been developed to assist in the pouring of epoxy resins. Fast-setting epoxy materials have been supplied in automixing systems similar to those described for automixing addition silicones. The epoxy resin is in one cartridge, and the catalyst in the other. Forcing the two pastes through the static mixing tip thoroughly mixes the epoxy material, which can be directly injected into a rubber impression. A small intraoral delivery tip may be attached to the static-mixing tip if desired for injecting into detailed areas of the impression. The fast-setting epoxy hardens rapidly, so dies can be waxed 30 minutes after injecting into the impression. Because water retards the polymerization of resin, epoxy resins cannot be used with water-containing agar and alginate impression materials, and thus are limited to use with elastomeric impression materials.

Comparison of Impression and Die Materials

High-strength stone dies may be from 0.35% larger to 0.25% smaller than the master, depending on the location of the measurement and the impression material used. In general, occlusogingival (vertical) changes are greater than buccolingual or mesiodistal (horizontal) changes. The shrinkage of the impression material toward the surfaces of the tray in the horizontal direction usually results in dimensions larger than the master. In the vertical direction, shrinkage is away from the free surface of the impression and toward the tray, and dimensions smaller than the master are obtained.

The accuracy of elastomeric impression materials is in the following order from best to worst, regardless of whether stone or metal dies are used: addition silicone and polyether.

Epoxy dies all exhibit some polymerization shrinkage, with values ranging from 0.1% to 0.3%, and as a result the dies are undersized.

Ranking materials by the ability of an impression-die combination to reproduce surface detail produces different results than does ranking by values for dimensional change. If a release agent is not needed on the surface of the impression, epoxy dies are best for reproducing detail (10 μm), followed by high-strength stone dies (170 μm). The silicone-epoxy combination produces the sharpest detail, although not all epoxy die materials are compatible with all silicone impression materials.

Resistance to abrasion and scraping should also be considered. Epoxy dies have good resistance and high-strength stone dies have the least resistance.

GYPSUM PRODUCTS

Gypsum products probably serve the dental profession more adequately than any other materials. Dental plaster, stone, high-strength/high-expansion stone, and casting investment constitute this group of closely related products. With slight modification, gypsum products are used for several different purposes. For example, impression plaster is used to make impressions of edentulous mouths or to mount casts, whereas dental stone is used to form a die that duplicates the oral anatomy when poured into any type of impression. Gypsum products are also used as a binder for silica in gold alloy casting investment, soldering investment, and investment for low-melting-point nickel-chromium alloys. These products are also used as a mold material for processing complete dentures. The main reason for such diversified use is that the properties of gypsum materials can be easily modified by physical and chemical means.

The dihydrate form of calcium sulfate, called *gypsum*, usually appears white to milky yellowish and is found in a compact mass in nature. The mineral gypsum has commercial importance as a source of plaster of Paris. The term *plaster of Paris* was given this product because it was obtained by burning the gypsum from deposits near Paris, France. Deposits of gypsum, however, are found in most countries.

CHEMICAL AND PHYSICAL NATURE OF GYPSUM PRODUCTS

Most gypsum products are obtained from natural gypsum rock. Because gypsum is the dihydrate form of calcium sulfate ($CaSO_4 \cdot 2H_2O$), on heating, it loses 1.5 g mol of its 2 g mol of H_2O and is converted to calcium sulfate hemihydrate ($CaSO_4 \cdot \frac{1}{2}H_2O$), sometimes written ($CaSO_4)_2 \cdot H_2O$. When calcium sulfate hemihydrate is mixed with water, the reverse reaction takes place, and the calcium sulfate hemihydrate is converted back to calcium sulfate dihydrate. Therefore, partial dehydration of gypsum rock and rehydration of calcium sulfate hemihydrate constitute a reversible reaction. Chemically, the reaction is expressed as shown below.

$$CaSO_4 \cdot \frac{1}{2}H_2O + 1\frac{1}{2}H_2O \rightarrow$$
Plaster of Paris   Water

$$CaSO_4 \cdot 2H_2O + 3900 \text{ cal/g mol}$$
Gypsum

The reaction is exothermic, and whenever 1 g mol of calcium sulfate hemihydrate is reacted with 1.5 g mol of water, 1 g mol of calcium sulfate dihydrate is formed, and 3900 calories of heat are developed. This chemical reaction takes place regardless of whether the gypsum material is used as an impression material, a die material, or a binder in casting investment.

Manufacture of Dental Plaster, Stone, and High-Strength Stone

Three types of base raw materials are derived from partial dehydration of gypsum rock, depending on the nature of the dehydration process. *Plasters* are fluffy, porous, and least dense, whereas the *hydrocal* variety has a higher density and is more crystalline. *Densite* is the densest of the raw materials. These three types of raw materials are used to formulate the four types of relatively pure gypsum products used in dentistry. They are classified as plasters (model and laboratory), low- to moderate-strength dental stones, high-strength/low-expansion dental stones, and high-strength/high-expansion dental stones, or alternatively as types 2, 3, 4, and 5 in ANSI/ADA specification No. 25 (ISO 6873).

Although these types have identical chemical formulas of calcium sulfate hemihydrate, $CaSO_4 \cdot \frac{1}{2}H_2O$, they possess different physical properties, which makes each of them suitable for a different dental purpose. All four forms are derived from natural gypsum deposits, with the main difference being the manner of driving off part of the water of the calcium sulfate dihydrate. Synthetic gypsum can also be used to formulate some products, but is less popular because of higher manufacturing costs.

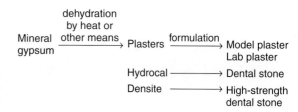

Plasters are produced when the gypsum mineral is heated in an open kettle at a temperature of about 110° to 120° C. The hemihydrate produced is called β-*calcium sulfate hemihydrate.* Such a powder is known to have a somewhat irregular shape and is porous in nature. These plasters are used in formulating model and lab plasters. Crystals of model plaster are shown in Figure 12-20.

If gypsum is dehydrated under pressure and in the presence of water vapor at about 125° C, the product is called *hydrocal.* The powder particles of this product are more uniform in shape and denser than the particles of plaster. Crystals of a dental stone are shown in Figure 12-21. The calcium sulfate hemihydrate produced in this manner is designated as α-*calcium sulfate hemihydrate.* Hydrocal is used in making low- to moderate-strength dental stones.

Types 4 and 5 high-strength dental stones are manufactured with a high-density raw material called *densite.* This variety is made by boiling gypsum rock in a 30% calcium chloride solution, after which the chloride is washed away with hot water (100° C) and the material is ground to the desired fineness. The powder obtained by this process is the densest of the types. These materials are generally formulated as high-strength/low-expansion

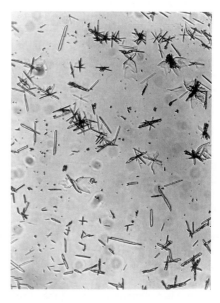

FIGURE 12.20 **Crystals of model plaster.**

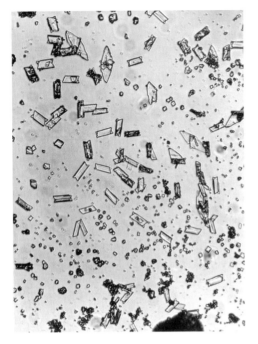

FIGURE 12.21 **Crystal structure typical of dental stone.**

dental stone or high-strength/high-expansion dental stone.

Gypsum products may be formulated with chemicals that modify their handling characteristics and properties. Potassium sulfate, K_2SO_4, and terra alba (set calcium sulfate dihydrate) are effective accelerators. Sodium chloride in small amounts shortens the setting reaction but increases the setting expansion of the gypsum mass. Sodium citrate is a dependable retarder. Borax, $Na_2B_4O_7$, is both a retarder and accelerator. A mixture of calcium oxide (0.1%) and gum arabic (1%) reduces the amount of water necessary to mix gypsum products, resulting in improved properties. Type 4 gypsum differs from type 5 in that type 4 contains extra salts to reduce its setting expansion.

Chemical Reaction

The chemical reaction that takes place during the setting of gypsum products determines the quantity of H_2O needed for the reaction. The reaction of 1 g mol of plaster with 1.5 g mol of water produces 1 g mol of gypsum material. In other words, 145 g of plaster requires 27 g of water to react and form 172 g of gypsum or 100 g of plaster requires 18.6 g of water to form 118 g of calcium sulfate dihydrate. As seen in practice, however, model plaster cannot be mixed with such a small amount of water and still develop a mass suitable for manipulation. Table 12-9 shows the recommended mixing water, required water, and

excess water for model plaster, dental stone, and high-strength dental stone.

For example, to mix 100 g of model plaster to a usable flowable consistency, use 45 g of water. Note that only 18.6 g of 45 g of water reacts with the 100 g of model plaster; the excess (45 g − 18.6 g = 26.4 g) is distributed as free water in the set mass without taking part in the chemical reaction. When the set material is dried, the excess water evaporates and leaves porosity in the structure, weakening it. Therefore, set model plaster is weaker than dental stone, which in turn is weaker than high-strength dental stone. If 100 g of model plaster is mixed with 50 g of water, the resultant mass is thinner and mixes and pours easily into a mold, but the quality of the set gypsum is inferior and weaker than when 45 g of water is used. When model plaster is mixed with a lesser amount of water, the mixed mass is thicker, is more difficult to handle, and traps air bubbles easily when it is poured into a mold, but the set gypsum is usually stronger. Thus careful control of the proper amount of water in the mix is necessary for proper manipulation and quality of the set mass.

Water/Powder Ratio of Dental Stone and High-Strength Dental Stone

The reason for the differences among the recommended amounts of mixing water for model plaster, dental stone, and high-strength dental stone is in the shape and form of the calcium sulfate hemihydrate crystals. Some calcium sulfate hemihydrate crystals are comparatively irregular in shape and porous in nature, as are the crystals in model plaster, whereas the crystals of dental stone and the two high-strength dental stones are dense and more regular in shape, as shown in Figures 12-20 and 12-21. This difference in the physical shape and nature of the crystals makes it possible to obtain the same consistency with less excess water with dental stone and high-strength dental stones than with model plaster.

When mixed with water, model plaster, dental stone, or high-strength dental stones set to a hard mass of gypsum. The gypsum products known as high-strength dental stones (types 4 and 5) are the strongest, the mass produced as model plaster is the weakest, and dental stone produces an intermediate strength material. Note, however, that all gypsum products have the same chemical formula, and that the chemical nature of the masses produced by mixing them with water is also identical; the differences among them are primarily in their physical properties.

Mechanism of Setting

The most important and well-recognized theory for the mechanism of the setting is the crystalline theory. It was originated in 1887 by Henry Louis

TABLE 12.9   Required and Excess Water for Gypsum Materials[*]

Gypsum	Mixing Water (mL/100 g of powder)	Required Water (mL/100 g of powder)	Excess Water (mL/100 g of powder)
Model plaster	37-50	18.6	18-31
Dental stone	28-32	18.6	9-13
High-strength dental stone	19-24	18.6	0-5

Water-powder ratio varies with each product.

Le Chatelier, a French chemist. The theory received the full support of Jacobus Hendricus van't Hoff, a famous Dutch chemist in Berlin at the turn of the century. According to the explanation of van't Hoff, the setting reaction of water with calcium sulfate hemihydrate to from calcium sulfate dihydrate is caused by the difference in solubility between these two components. Calcium sulfate dihydrate is less soluble than the hemihydrate form. When the hemihydrate dissolves in water, the dihydrate, being of lower solubility, is then supersaturated and precipitates out of solution from points of nucleation in the form of needle-like crystals. Bonding between contacting crystals results in the final cohesive structure.

Volumetric Contraction

Theoretically, calcium sulfate hemihydrate should contract volumetrically during the setting process. However, experiments have determined that all gypsum products expand linearly during setting. As indicated earlier, when 145.15 g of calcium sulfate hemihydrate reacts with 27.02 g of water, the result is the production of 172.17 g of calcium sulfate dihydrate. However, if the volume rather than the weight of calcium sulfate hemihydrate is added to the volume of water, the sum of the volumes will be about 7% less than the volume of calcium sulfate dihydrate. In practice about 0.2% to 0.4% linear expansion is obtained. According to the crystalline theory of Le Chatelier and van't Hoff, the expansion results from the thrusting action of gypsum crystals, $CaSO_4 \cdot 2H_2O$, during their growth from a supersaturated solution. The fact that the contraction of gypsum is not visible does not invalidate its existence, and when the volumetric contraction is measured by a dilatometer, it is determined to be about 7%. Because of the linear expansion of the outer dimensions, which is caused by the growth of calcium sulfate dihydrate, with a simultaneous true volumetric contraction of calcium sulfate dihydrate, these materials are porous when set.

Effect of Spatulation

The mixing process, called *spatulation*, has a definite effect on the setting time and setting expansion of the material. Within practical limits an increase in the amount of spatulation (either speed of spatulation or time or both) shortens the setting time. Obviously when the powder is placed in water, the chemical reaction starts, and some calcium sulfate dihydrate is formed. During spatulation the newly formed calcium sulfate dihydrate breaks down to smaller crystals and starts new centers of nucleation, from which the calcium sulfate dihydrate can be precipitated. Because an increased amount of spatulation causes more nuclei centers to be formed, the conversion of calcium sulfate hemihydrate to dihydrate is accelerated.

Effect of Temperature

The temperature of the water used for mixing, as well as the temperature of the environment, has an effect on the setting reaction of gypsum products. The setting time probably is affected more by a change in temperature than by any other physical property. Evidently the temperature has two main effects on the setting reaction of gypsum products.

The first effect of increasing temperature is a change in the relative solubilities of calcium sulfate hemihydrate and calcium sulfate dihydrate, which alters the rate of the reaction. The ratio of the solubilities of calcium sulfate dihydrate and calcium sulfate hemihydrate at 20° C is about 4.5. As the temperature increases, the solubility ratios decrease, until 100° C is reached and the ratio becomes 1. As the ratio of the solubilities becomes lower, the reaction is slowed, and the setting time is increased. The solubilities of calcium sulfate hemihydrate and calcium sulfate dihydrate are shown in Table 12-10.

The second effect is the change in ion mobility with temperature. In general, as the temperature increases, the mobility of the calcium and sulfate ions increases, which tends to increase the rate of the reaction and shorten the setting time.

Practically, the effects of these two phenomena are superimposed, and the total effect is observed. Thus, by increasing the temperature from 20° to 30° C, the solubility ratio decreases from 0.90/0.200 = 4.5 to 0.72/0.209 = 3.4, which ordinarily should retard the reaction. At the same time, however, the mobility of the ions increases, which should accelerate the setting reaction. Thus, according to the solubility

TABLE 12.10   Solubility of Calcium Sulfate Hemihydrate and Calcium Sulfate Dihydrate at Different Temperatures

Temperature (° C)	$CaSO_4 \cdot {}^{1}/_{2}H_2O$ (g/100 g water)	$CaSO_4 \cdot 2H_2O$ (g/100 g water)
20	0.90	0.200
25	0.80	0.205
30	0.72	0.209
40	0.61	0.210
50	0.50	0.205
100	0.17	0.170

Modified from Partridge EP, White AH: J. Am. Chem. Soc. 51, 360, 1929.

values, the reaction should be retarded, whereas according to the mobility of the ions, the reaction should be accelerated. Experimentation has shown that increasing the temperature from room temperature of 20° C to body temperature of 37° C increases the rate of the reaction slightly and shortens the setting time. However, as the temperature is raised over 37° C, the rate of the reaction decreases, and the setting time is lengthened. At 100° C the solubilities of dihydrate and hemihydrate are equal, in which case no reaction occurs, and plaster does not set.

Effect of Humidity

When the relative humidity increases to 70% and above, moisture in the air can cause some conversion of hemihydrate to dihydrate. Because dihydrate crystals can accelerate the reaction by providing more nuclei for crystallization, the initial result is acceleration of setting. However, further contamination by moisture can reduce the amount of hemihydrate remaining to form gypsum and retardation of setting will occur. Therefore, all gypsum products should be kept in a closed container and well protected from moisture in the air.

Effect of Colloidal Systems and pH

Colloidal systems such as agar and alginate retard the setting of gypsum products. If these materials are in contact with $CaSO_4 \cdot {}^{1}\!\!/_2H_2O$ during setting, a soft, easily abraded surface is obtained. Accelerators such as potassium sulfate are added to improve the surface quality of the set $CaSO_4 \cdot 2H_2O$ against agar or alginate.

These colloids do not retard the setting by altering the solubility ratio of the hemihydrate and dihydrate forms, but rather by being adsorbed on the hemihydrate and dihydrate nucleation sites, thus interfering in the hydration reaction. The adsorption of these materials on the nucleating sites retards the setting reaction more effectively than adsorption on the calcium sulfate hemihydrate.

Liquids with low pH, such as saliva, retard the setting reaction. Liquids with high pH accelerate setting.

PROPERTIES

The important properties of gypsum products include quality, fluidity at pouring time, setting time, linear setting expansion, compressive strength, hardness and abrasion resistance, and reproduction of detail. Some of these property requirements, described by ANSI/ADA specification No. 25 (ISO 6873), are summarized in Table 12-11.

Setting Time
Definition and Importance

The time required for the reaction to be completed is called the *final setting time*. If the rate of the reaction is too fast or the material has a short setting time, the mixed mass may harden before the operator can manipulate it properly. On the other hand, if the rate of reaction is too slow, an excessively long time is required to complete the operation. Therefore, a proper setting time is one of the most important characteristics of gypsum materials.

The chemical reaction is initiated at the moment the powder is mixed with water, but at the early stage only a small portion of the hemihydrate is converted to gypsum. The freshly mixed mass has a semifluid consistency and can be poured into a mold of any shape. As the reaction proceeds, however, more and more calcium sulfate dihydrate crystals are produced. The viscosity of the mixed mass increases, and the mass can no longer flow easily into the fine details of the mold. This time is called the *working time*.

The final setting time is defined as the time at which the material can be separated from the impression without distortion or fracture. The initial setting time is the time required for gypsum products to reach a certain arbitrary stage of firmness in their setting process. In the normal case, this arbitrary stage is represented by a semihard mass that has passed the working stage but is not yet completely set. At final setting, the conversion of calcium sulfate hemihydrate to calcium sulfate dihydrate is virtually completed.

Measurement

The initial setting time is usually measured arbitrarily by some form of penetration test, although occasionally other types of test methods have been designed. For example, the loss of gloss from the

TABLE 12.11   Property Requirements for Gypsum Materials

Type	Setting Time (min)	Setting Expansion Range (%)	Compressive Strength (MPa)		Reproduction of Detail (μm)
			Minimum	Maximum	
1. Impression plaster	2.5-5.0	0-0.15	4.0	8.0	75 ± 8
2. Model plaster	±20%*	0-0.30	9.0	—	75 ± 8
3. Dental stone	±20%	0-0.20	20.0	—	50 ± 8
4. High-strength/low-expansion dental stone	±20%	0-0.15	35.0	—	50 ± 8
5. High-strength/high-expansion dental stone	±20%	0.16-0.30	35.0	—	50 ± 8

*Setting time shall be within 20% of value claimed by manufacturer.

surface of the mixed mass of model plaster or dental stone is an indication of this stage in the chemical reaction and is sometimes used to indicate the initial set of the mass. Similarly, the setting time may be measured by the temperature rise of the mass, because the chemical reaction is exothermic.

The Vicat apparatus shown in Figure 12-16 is commonly used to measure the initial setting time of gypsum products. It consists of a rod weighing 300 g with a needle of 1-mm diameter. A ring container is filled with the mix, the setting time of which is to be measured. The rod is lowered until it contacts the surface of the material, then the needle is released and allowed to penetrate the mix. When the needle fails to penetrate to the bottom of the container, the material has reached the Vicat or the initial setting time. Other types of instruments, such as Gillmore needles, can be used to obtain the initial and final setting times of gypsum materials.

Control of Setting Time

Methods for controlling setting time have been discussed previously. Initially the manufacturer can add various components that act as either accelerators or retarders. The operator can alter setting time by changing the temperature of the mix water and by changing the degree of spatulation. Water-powder (W/P) ratio can also affect setting time; using more water in the mix can prolong the setting time as shown in Table 12-12.

The easiest and most reliable way to change the setting time is to add different chemicals. Potassium sulfate, K_2SO_4, is known as an effective accelerator, and the use of a 2% aqueous solution of this salt rather than water reduces the setting time of model plaster from approximately 10 minutes to about 4 minutes. On the other hand, sodium citrate is a dependable retarder. The use of a 2% aqueous solution of borax to mix with the powder may prolong the setting time of some gypsum products to a few hours.

TABLE 12.12   Effect of Water/Powder Ratio on Setting Time

Material	W/P Ratio (mL/g)	Spatulation Turns	Initial (Vicat) Setting Time (min)
Model plaster	0.45		8
	0.50	100	11
	0.55		14
Dental stone	0.27		4
	0.30	100	7
	0.33		8
High-strength dental stone	0.22		5
	0.24	100	7
	0.26		9

If a small amount of set calcium sulfate dihydrate is ground and mixed with model plaster, it provides nuclei of crystallization and acts as an accelerator. The set gypsum used as an accelerator is called *terra alba,* and it has a pronounced effect at lower concentrations. The setting time changes significantly if the amount of terra alba present in the mix is changed from 0.5% to 1%. However, terra alba concentrations above 1% have less effect on the setting time. Manufacturers usually take advantage of this fact and add about 1% terra alba to plaster. Thus the setting time of model plaster is altered less in normal use because of opening and closing the container.

The W/P ratio has a pronounced effect on the setting time. The more water in the mix of model plaster, dental stone, or high-strength dental stone, the longer the setting time, as shown in Table 12-12. The effect of spatulation on setting time of model plaster and dental stone is shown in Table 12-13. Increased

TABLE 12.13   Effect of Spatulation on Setting Time

Material	W/P Ratio (mL/g)	Spatulation Turns	Setting Time (min)
Model plaster	0.50	20	14
	0.50	100	11
	0.50	200	8
Dental stone	0.30	20	10
	0.30	100	8

TABLE 12.14   Properties of a High-Strength Dental Stone Mixed by Hand and by a Power-Driven Mixer with Vacuum

	Hand Mix	Power-Driven Mix with Vacuum
Setting time	8.0	7.3
Compressive strength at 24 hr (MPa)	43.1	45.5
Setting expansion at 2 hr (%)	0.045	0.037
Viscosity, centipoise (cp)	54,000	43,000

Modified from Garber DK, Powers JM, Brandau HE: J. Mich. Dent. Assoc. 67, 133, 1985.

TABLE 12.15   Viscosity of Several High-Strength Dental Stones and Impression Plaster

Material	Viscosity (cp)[†]
High-strength dental stone[*]	
A	21,000
B	29,000
C	50,000
D	54,000
E	101,000
Impression plaster	23,000

Modified from Garber DK, Powers JM, Brandau HE: J. Mich. Dent. Assoc. 67, 133, 1985.
*Stones were mixed with 1% sodium citrate solution to retard setting.
†Viscosity was measured 4 minutes from the start of mixing.

spatulation shortens the setting time. Properties of a high-strength dental stone mixed by hand and by a power-driven mixer with vacuum are shown in Table 12-14. The setting time is usually shortened for power mixing compared with hand mixing.

Viscosity

The viscosities of several high-strength dental stones and impression plaster are listed in Table 12-15. A range of viscosities from 21,000 to 101,000 centipoises (cp) was observed for five different high-strength stones. More voids were observed in casts made from the stones with the higher viscosities. Impression plaster is used infrequently, but it has a low viscosity, which makes it possible to take impressions with a minimum of force on the soft tissues (mucostatic technique).

Compressive Strength

When set, gypsum products show relatively high values of compressive strength. The compressive strength is inversely related to the W/P ratio of the mix. The more water used to make the mix, the lower the compressive strength.

Model plaster has the greatest quantity of excess water, whereas high-strength dental stone contains the least excess water. The excess water is uniformly distributed in the mix and contributes to the volume but not the strength of the material. Set model plaster is more porous than set dental stone, causing the apparent density of model plaster to be lower. Because high-strength dental stone is the densest, it shows the highest compressive strength, with model plaster being the most porous and thus the weakest.

The 1-hour compressive strength values are about 12.5 MPa for model plaster, 31 MPa for dental stone, and 45 MPa for high-strength dental stones. These values are representative for the normal mixes, but they vary as the W/P ratio is increased or decreased. The effect of the W/P ratio on the compressive strength of these materials is given in Table 12-16. As shown in Table 12-14, the compressive strength of a high-strength dental stone is improved slightly by vacuum mixing. Evidently, when stone is mixed with the same W/P ratio as model plaster, the compressive strength of dental stone is almost the same as that of model plaster. Similarly, the compressive strength of high-strength dental stone with W/P ratios of 0.3 and 0.5 is similar to the normal compressive strength of dental stone and model plaster.

At 1 or 2 hours after the final setting time, the hardened gypsum material appears dry and seems to have reached its maximum strength. Actually, this is not the case. The wet strength is the strength of gypsum materials with some or all of the excess water present in the specimen. The dry strength is the strength of the gypsum material with all of its excess water driven out. The dry compressive strength is usually about twice that of the wet strength. Notice that as the hardened mass slowly loses its excess water, the compressive strength of the material does not increase uniformly. The effect of drying on the compressive strength of dental stone is shown in Figure 12-22. Theoretically, about 8.8% of excess water is in the hardened mass of the stone. As

TABLE 12.16 Effect of Water/Powder Ratio on the Compressive Strength of Model Plaster, Dental Stone, and High-Strength Dental Stone[*]

Material	W/P Ratio (mL/g)	Compressive Strength (MPa)
Model plaster	0.45	12.5
	0.50	11.0
	0.55	9.0
Dental stone	0.27	31.0
	0.30	20.5
	0.50	10.5
High-strength dental stone	0.24	38.0
	0.30	21.5
	0.50	10.5

All mixes spatulated 100 turns and tested 1 hour after the start of mixing.

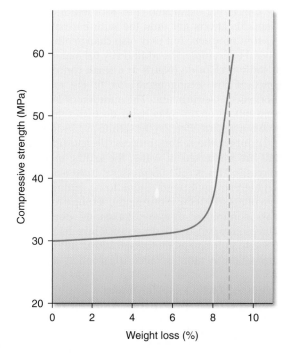

FIGURE 12.22 **Effect of loss of excess water on compressive strength of dental stone.**

the mass loses up to 7% of the water, no appreciable change develops in the compressive strength of the material. When the mass loses 7.5% of the excess water, however, the strength increases sharply, and when all of the excess (8.8%) is lost, the strength of the material is over 55 MPa.

The drying time for gypsum materials varies according to the size of the gypsum mass and the temperature and humidity of the storage atmosphere. At room temperature and average humidity, about 7 days are necessary for an average denture flask filled with gypsum materials to lose the excess water.

Surface Hardness and Abrasion Resistance

The surface hardness of unmodified gypsum materials is related in a general way to their compressive strength. High compressive strengths of the hardened mass correspond to high surface hardnesses. After the final setting occurs, the surface hardness remains practically constant until most excess water is evaporated from the surface, after which its increase is similar to the increase in compressive strength. The surface hardness increases at a faster rate than the compressive strength, because the surface of the hardened mass reaches a dry state earlier than the inner portion of the mass.

Attempts have been made to increase the hardness of gypsum products by impregnating the set gypsum with epoxy or methylmethacrylate monomer that is allowed to polymerize. Increases in hardness were obtained for model plaster but not for dental stone or high-strength dental stone. Increases in scratch resistance of 15% to 41% were observed for a high-strength dental stone impregnated with epoxy resins or a light-cured dimethacrylate resin. Generally, impregnating set gypsum with resin increases abrasion resistance, but decreases compressive strength and surface hardness.

The idea of drying molds, casts, or dies in an oven to obtain a quick, dry compressive strength and dry surface hardness of a material is not practical, because the gypsum would be dehydrated, which would reduce the strength instead of increasing it. Soaking the gypsum dies or casts in glycerin or different oils does not improve the surface hardness but rather makes the surface smoother, so that a wax carver or other instrument will not cut the stone as it slides over the surface. Mixing high-strength dental stone with a commercial hardening solution containing colloidal silica (about 30%) improves the surface hardness of the set gypsum. The Knoop hardnesses of two commercial high-strength dental stones were 54 and 77 kg/mm^2 when mixed with water. When the hardening solution was used, these values increased to 62 and 79 kg/mm^2, respectively. Increased surface hardness does not necessarily mean improved abrasion resistance because hardness is only one of many factors that can affect wear resistance. Two-body abrasion studies suggest that the commercial hardening solutions do not improve the abrasion resistance of high-strength dental stones. However, the clinical relevancy of the two-body abrasion test on gypsum has not been established. Further studies of abrasion resistance and methods of measurement are needed. As discussed in the chapter on impression materials, gypsum dies abrade more readily than epoxy dies, even though the gypsum dies are harder.

Although the use of disinfectant chemicals on gypsum dies effectively destroys potentially dangerous organisms, some can damage the surface of a die. Surfaces can be eroded, and the surface hardness can be adversely affected by treatment with some commonly used disinfectants. Other disinfectants, including sodium hypochlorite solutions, have very little effect on the surfaces of gypsum dies.

Reproduction of Detail

ANSI/ADA specification No. 25 requires that types 1 and 2 reproduce a groove 75 mm in width, whereas types 3, 4, and 5 reproduce a groove 50 mm in width (see Table 12-11). Gypsum dies do not reproduce surface detail as well as electroformed or epoxy dies because the surface of the set gypsum is porous on a microscopic level (Figure 12-23). Air bubbles are often formed at the interface of the impression and gypsum cast because freshly mixed gypsum does not wet some elastomeric impression materials (condensation silicones) well. The incorporation of nonionic surfactants in silicone impression materials improves the wetting of the impression by slurry water. The use of vibration during the pouring of a cast reduces the presence of air bubbles. Contamination of the impression in which the gypsum die is poured by saliva or blood can also affect the detail reproduction. Rinsing the impression and blowing away excess water can improve the detail recorded by the gypsum die material.

Setting Expansion

When set, all gypsum products show a measurable linear expansion. The percentage of setting expansion, however, varies from one type of gypsum material to another. Under ordinary conditions, plasters have 0.2% to 0.3% setting expansion, low- to moderate-strength dental stone about 0.15% to 0.25%, and high-strength dental stone only 0.08% to 0.10%. The setting expansion of high-strength/high-expansion dental stone ranges from 0.10% to 0.20%. Typically, over 75% of the expansion observed at 24 hours occurs during the first hour of setting.

The setting expansion may be controlled by different manipulative conditions and by the addition of some chemicals. Mechanical mixing decreases setting expansion. As shown in Table 12-14, a vacuum-mixed high-strength stone expands less at 2 hours than when mixed by hand. Power mixing appears to cause a greater initial volumetric contraction than is

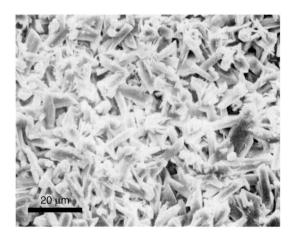

FIGURE 12.23 **Scanning electron photomicrograph of the surface of a set high-strength stone die.** *(From Craig RG, Powers JM, Wataha JC: Dental materials: properties and manipulation, ed 8. Mosby, St. Louis, 2004.)*

observed for hand mixing. The W/P ratio of the mix also has an effect, with an increase in the ratio reducing the setting expansion. The addition of different chemicals affects not only the setting expansion of gypsum products, but may also change other properties. For example, the addition by the manufacturer of sodium chloride (NaCl) in a small concentration increases the setting expansion of the mass and shortens the setting time. The addition of 1% potassium sulfate, on the other hand, decreases the setting time but has no effect on the setting expansion.

If during the setting process, the gypsum materials are immersed in water, the setting expansion increases. This is called *hygroscopic expansion.* A typical, high-strength dental stone has a setting expansion of about 0.08%. If during the setting process the mass is immersed in water, it expands about 0.10%. Increased expansion is observed when dental stone hardens as it comes in contact with a hydrocolloid impression. A more detailed explanation of hygroscopic expansion is presented later under casting investments with a gypsum binder.

MANIPULATION

When any of the gypsum products is mixed with water, it should be spatulated properly to obtain a smooth mix. Water is dispensed into a mixing bowl of an appropriate size and design (Figure 12-24). The powder is added and allowed to settle into the water for about 30 seconds. This technique minimizes the amount of air incorporated into the mix during initial spatulation by hand. Spatulation can be continued by hand using a spatula with a stiff blade (Figure 12-25) with the bowl on a vibrator (see Figure 12-25)

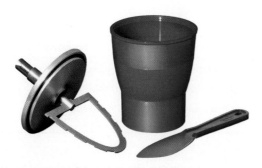

FIGURE 12.24 **Flexible rubber mixing bowl and metal spatula with a stiff blade.** *(Courtesy of Whip Mix Corporation, Louisville, KY.)*

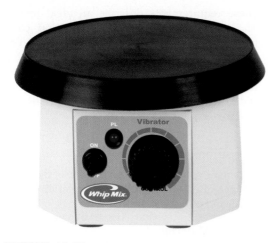

FIGURE 12.25 A Vibrator is designed to promote the release of bubbles in the gypsum mix and to facilitate pouring of the impression. *(Courtesy of Whip Mix Corporation, Louisville, KY.)*

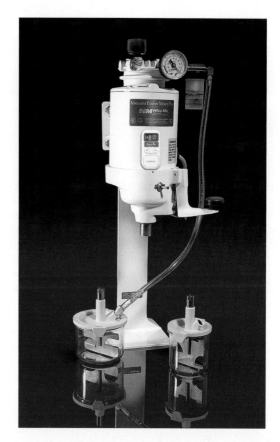

FIGURE 12.26 **Power-driven mechanical spatulator with a vacuum attachment.** *(Courtesy of Whip Mix Corporation, Louisville, KY.)*

or a power-driven mechanical spatulator (Figure 12-26). A summary of the effect of various manipulative variables on the properties of gypsum products is presented in Table 12-17.

Spatulation by hand involves stirring the mixture vigorously while wiping the inside surfaces of the bowl with the spatula. Spatulation to wet and mix the powder uniformly with the water requires about 1 minute at 2 revolutions per second.

Spatulation with a power-driven mechanical spatulator requires that the powder initially be wet by the water as with hand mixing. The mix is then spatulated for 20 seconds on the low-speed drive of the mixer. Vacuuming during mixing reduces the air entrapped in the mix. Vibration immediately after mixing and during pouring of the gypsum minimizes air bubbles in the set mass.

Pouring an impression with gypsum requires care to avoid trapping air in critical areas. The mixed gypsum should be poured slowly or added to the impression with a small instrument such as a wax spatula. The mass should run into the rinsed impression under vibration in such a manner that it pushes air ahead of itself as it fills the impressions of the teeth. Commonly, the teeth of a cast are poured in dental stone or high-strength dental stone, whereas the base is poured in model plaster for easier trimming.

Once poured, the gypsum material should be allowed to harden for 45 to 60 minutes before the impression and cast are separated and disinfected. Models can be disinfected by immersion in 1:10 dilution of sodium hypochlorite for 30 minutes or with a spray of iodophor following manufacturer's instructions.

CASTING INVESTMENTS

The adoption of the casting practice in dentistry for making gold alloy inlays, crowns, bridges, and other restorations represents one of the major advances in restorative dentistry. In recent years,

TABLE 12.17 · Summary of Effect of Manipulative Variables on Properties of Gypsum Products

Manipulative Variable	Setting Time	Consistency	Setting Expansion	Compressive Strength
Increase water/powder ratio	Increase	Increase	Decrease	Decrease
Increase rate of spatulation	Decrease	Decrease	Increase	No effect
Increase temperature of mixing water from 23° to 30° C	Decrease	Decrease	Increase	No effect

alloys with higher melting points, the palladium and base metal alloys, have been cast into crowns, and fixed and removable dental prostheses by using basically the same lost-wax technique used for dental gold alloys. All such casting operations involve (1) a wax pattern of the object to be reproduced; (2) a suitable mold material, known as investment, which is placed around the pattern and permitted to harden; (3) suitable furnaces for burning out the wax patterns and heating the investment mold; and (4) proper facilities to melt and cast the alloy. An *investment* can be described as a ceramic material that is suitable for forming a mold into which a metal or alloy is cast. The operation of forming the mold is described as *investing*. Details of the casting technique are described on the website http://evolve.elsevier.com/sakaguchi/restorative ⊜

Properties Required of an Investment

1. Easily manipulated: Not only should it be possible to mix and manipulate the mass readily and to paint the wax pattern easily, but the investment should also harden within a relatively short time.
2. Sufficient strength at room temperature: The investment should permit ease in handling and provide enough strength at higher temperatures to withstand the impact force of the molten metal. The inner surface of the mold should not break down at a high temperature.
3. Stability at higher temperatures: Investment must not decompose to give off gases that could damage the surface of the alloy.
4. Sufficient expansion: It must expand enough to compensate for shrinkage of the wax pattern and metal that takes place during the casting procedure.
5. Beneficial casting temperatures: Preferably the thermal expansion versus temperature curve should have a plateau of the thermal expansion over a range of casting temperatures.
6. Porosity: It should be porous enough to permit the air or other gases in the mold cavity to escape easily during the casting procedure.
7. Smooth surface: Fine detail and margins on the casting should be preserved.
8. Ease of divestment: The investment should break away readily from the surface of the metal and should not have reacted chemically with it.
9. Inexpensive.

These requirements describe an ideal investment. No single material is known that completely fulfills all these requirements. However, by blending different ingredients, one can develop an investment that possesses most of the required qualities. These ideal qualities are the basis for considering the behavior and characteristics of casting investments.

Composition

In general, an investment is a mixture of three distinct types of materials: refractory material, binder material, and other chemicals.

Refractory Material

Refractory material is usually a form of silicon dioxide, such as quartz, tridymite, or cristobalite, or a mixture of these. Refractory materials are contained in all dental investments, whether for casting gold or high-melting-point alloys.

Binder Material

Because the refractory materials alone do not form a coherent solid mass, some kind of binder is needed. The common binder used for dental casting gold alloy is α-calcium sulfate hemihydrate. Phosphate, ethyl silicate, and other similar materials also serve as binders for high-temperature casting investments. These latter investments are described later in conjunction with investment for casting high-melting-point alloys.

Other Chemicals

Usually a mixture of refractory materials and a binder alone is not enough to produce all the desirable properties required of an investment. Other chemicals, such as sodium chloride, boric acid, potassium sulfate, graphite, copper powder, or magnesium oxide, are often added in small quantities to modify various physical properties. For example, small amounts of chlorides or boric acid enhance the thermal expansion of investments bonded by calcium sulfate.

CALCIUM SULFATE–BONDED INVESTMENTS

The dental literature and patent references describe the quantity and purpose of each of a variety of ingredients in dental casting investments. In general, the investments suitable for casting gold alloys contain 65% to 75% quartz or cristobalite, or a blend of the two, in varying proportions; 25% to 35% of α-calcium sulfate hemihydrate; and about 2% to 3% chemical modifiers. With the proper blending of these basic ingredients, the manufacturer is able to develop an investment with an established group of physical properties that are adequate for dental gold casting practices. A list of specific compositions is of little value, however, because the final product's properties are influenced by both the ingredients present in the investment and the manner in which the mass is manipulated and used in making the mold.

Investments with calcium sulfate hemihydrate as a binder are relatively easy to manipulate, and more information about the effect of different additives, as well as various manipulative conditions, is available for this type than for other types, such as those that use silicates or phosphates as binders. The calcium sulfate–bonded investment is usually limited to gold castings and is not heated above 700° C. The calcium sulfate portion of the investment decomposes into sulfur dioxide and sulfur trioxide at temperatures over 700° C, tending to embrittle the casting metal. Therefore, the calcium sulfate type of binder is usually not used in investments for making castings of high-melting-point metals such as palladium or base metal alloys.

Properties of Calcium Sulfate–Bonded Investments

ANSI/ADA specification No. 126 (ISO 7490) for gypsum-bonded casting investments applies to two different types of investments suitable for casting dental restorations of gold alloys:

Type 1: For casting inlays and crowns
Type 2: For casting complete denture and partial removable dental prosthesis bases

Both types have calcium sulfate as a binder material. The physical properties included in this specification are appearance of powder, fluidity at working time, setting time, compressive strength, linear setting expansion, and linear thermal expansion. The values allowed for these properties are summarized in the specification. The manipulation of investments in the inlay casting procedure is discussed in detail on the website http://evolve.elsevier.com/sakaguchi/restorative ⊝

Effect of Temperature on Investment

In casting with the lost-wax process, the wax pattern is invested and placed in an oven at a temperature that melts and removes the pattern from the investment, thereby leaving a mold cavity into which the molten metal is cast. This oven temperature varies from one technique to another, but in no case is it lower than 550° C or higher than 700° C for calcium sulfate–bonded investments. During the heating process, the refractory material is affected differently by the thermal changes than is the gypsum binder.

Effect of Temperature on Silicon Dioxide Refractories

Each of the polymorphic forms of silica—quartz, tridymite, and cristobalite—expands when heated, but the percentage of expansion varies from one type to another. Pure cristobalite expands to 1.6% at 250° C, whereas quartz expands about 1.4% at 600° C, and the thermal expansion of tridymite at 600° C is less than 1%. The percentage of expansion of the three types of silica versus temperature is shown in Figure 4-41. As seen in Figure 4-41, none of the three forms of silica expands uniformly; instead they all show a break (nonlinearity) in their thermal expansion curves. In the case of cristobalite, the expansion is somewhat uniform up to about 200° C. At this temperature its expansion increases sharply from 0.5% to 1.2%, and then above 250° C it again becomes more uniform. At 573° C quartz also shows a break in the expansion curve, and tridymite shows a similar break at a much lower temperature.

The breaks on the expansion versus temperature curves indicate that cristobalite and quartz each exist in two polymorphic forms, one of which is more stable at a higher temperature and the other at a lower temperature. The form that is more stable at room temperature is called the α-*form*, and the more stable form at higher temperatures is designated as the β-*form*. Tridymite has three stable polymorphic forms. Thus the temperatures of 220° C for cristobalite, 573° C for quartz, and 105° and 160° C for tridymite are displacive transition temperatures. A displacive change involves expansion or contraction in the volume of the mass without breaking any bonds. In changing from the α-form (which is the more stable form at room temperature) to the β-form (which is stable at higher temperatures), all three forms of silica expand. The amount of expansion is highest for cristobalite and lowest for tridymite.

The quartz form of silica is found abundantly in nature, and it can be converted to cristobalite and tridymite by being heated through a reconstructive transition during which bonds are broken and a new crystal structure is formed. The α-quartz is converted to β-quartz at a temperature of 573° C. If the β-quartz is heated to 870° C and maintained at that temperature, it is converted to β-tridymite. From β-tridymite, it is possible to obtain either α-tridymite or β-cristobalite. If β-tridymite is cooled rapidly to

120° C and held at that temperature, it is changed to α-tridymite, which is stable at room temperature. On the other hand, if β-tridymite is heated to 1475° C and held at that temperature, it is converted to β-cristobalite. Further heating of β-cristobalite produces fused silica, but if it is cooled to 220° C and held at that temperature, α-cristobalite is formed. These transitions are shown in the following equation.

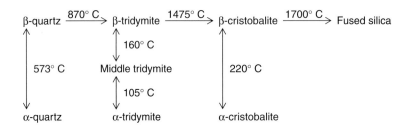

All forms of silica are in their α-forms in the investment, and during the heating process they are converted completely or in part to their corresponding β-forms. This transition involves an expansion of the mass, which helps to compensate for the casting shrinkages.

Effect of Temperature on Calcium Sulfate Binders

The binder used for gold alloy casting investments in dentistry is α-calcium sulfate hemihydrate. During the investing process, some of the water mixed with the investment reacts with the hemihydrate and is converted to calcium sulfate dihydrate, whereas the remainder of the water is uniformly distributed in the mix as excess water. During the early stages of heating, the excess water evaporates. As the temperature rises to about 105° C, calcium sulfate dihydrate starts losing water. The investment mass is then heated still further to the proper temperature for casting the metal. In this way, anhydrous calcium sulfate, silica, and certain chemical additives remain to form the mold into which the gold alloy is cast.

It has been observed experimentally that investment expands when it is first heated from room temperature to about 105° C, then contracts slightly or remains unchanged up to about 200° C, and registers varying degrees of expansion, depending on the silica composition of the investment, between 200° and 700° C. These properties are explained as follows. Up to about 105° C, ordinary thermal expansion occurs. Above 105° C, the calcium sulfate dihydrate is converted to anhydrous calcium sulfate. Dehydration of the dihydrate and a phase change of the calcium sulfate anhydrite cause a contraction. However, the α-form of tridymite (which might be present as an impurity) is expanding and compensates for the

contraction of the calcium sulfate sufficiently to prevent the investment from registering a serious degree of contraction. At elevated temperatures, the α-forms of silica present in the investment are converted to the β-forms, which cause some additional expansion.

The thermal expansion curves for a currently available hygroscopic type of investment containing quartz *(A)* and a thermal expansion type of investment containing cristobalite *(B)* are shown in Figure 12-27, which illustrates the expected degree of expansion at different temperatures. The expansion of the silica content of the investment must not only be sufficiently high to overcome all the contraction, but should also take place at temperatures close to the temperature at which contraction of the hemihydrate occurs.

Cooling of the Investment

When the investment is allowed to cool, the refractory and binder contract according to a thermal contraction curve that is different from the thermal expansion curve of the investment (Figure 12-28). On cooling to room temperature, the investment exhibits an overall contraction compared with its dimensions before heating. On reheating to the temperature previously attained, the investment does not expand thermally to the previous level; moreover, the process of cooling and reheating causes internal cracks in the investment that can affect the quality of the casting.

Setting Expansion of Calcium Sulfate–Bonded Investment

All the calcium sulfate–bonded investments currently available for casting gold alloys have both setting and thermal expansion. The sum of these two expansions results in a total dimensional change that

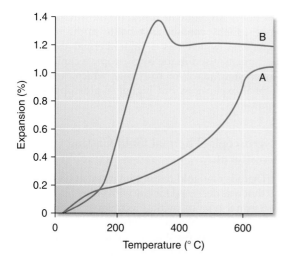

FIGURE 12.27 **Thermal expansion curves for calcium sulfate–bonded investments.** *A,* Hygroscopic type; *B,* thermal expansion type. *(Modified from Asgar, K., 1976. Casting restorations. In: Clark, J.W. (Ed.), 1976. Clinical dentistry, vol 4. Harper & Row, New York.)*

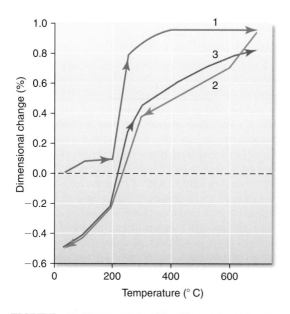

FIGURE 12.28 **Thermal expansion and contraction curves for calcium sulfate–bonded investment (thermal expansion type).** Curve 1 is first heating, curve 2 is cooling, and curve 3 is reheating.

is an essential property of dental casting investments because it provides compensation for the casting shrinkage of the casting alloys. The setting expansion of an investment, like that of other gypsum products discussed earlier in this chapter, is the linear expansion that takes place during the setting of the investment. If the investment is setting surrounded by air,

the expansion is referred to as *normal setting expansion.* On the other hand, if the mixed investment is setting in contact with water, the expansion is substantially greater and is called *hygroscopic setting expansion.* Such contact with water can be achieved in the commonly used casting techniques of (1) placing a wet liner inside the casting ring in which the investment is poured, or (2) if after investing, the casting ring is placed in a water bath. The presently accepted mechanism for hygroscopic setting expansion also relates to the normal setting expansion that occurs when the investment mix sets in contact with air. The basis for this mechanism lies in the role played by the surface tension of the mix water and can be described as follows. After the investment is mixed, water surrounds the components of the setting investment. As the reaction of the calcium sulfate binder progresses, the surrounding water is reduced and growing gypsum crystals impinge on the surface of the remaining water whose surface tension inhibits outward crystal growth. When the water needed for the reaction is used up and the reaction is virtually completed, the growth of gypsum crystals stops in its inhibited form.

If the investment is poured into a casting ring having a water-filled liner, the gypsum crystals can grow further, but only until the new water surface provided by the additional water in the liner is reached; surface tension then inhibits further growth. If water is supplied to the mixed investment mass by immersing the invested ring in a water bath, no new surface is close enough to provide inhibition of crystal growth. The resulting hygroscopic setting expansion for complete immersion as measured in an unconfined trough (ANSI/ADA specification No. 126) is more than twice that of normal expansion. However, when the investment is setting in a confined ring, hygroscopic expansion is limited by the confinement of the ring. For hygroscopic expansion, the additional water provided must be presented to the investment during setting. This is significantly different than adding more water to the premixture components (i.e., increasing the W/P ratio). Another requirement for hygroscopic expansion is that the additional water be presented before the observed loss of gloss, which is when the setting reaction is not complete and the mix water can still be observed on the surface of the setting investment. This allows the additional water to join the remaining mix water and extend the water surface so that the action of surface tension is either delayed or inactive.

Particle Size of Silica

The particle size of calcium sulfate hemihydrate has little effect on hygroscopic expansion, whereas the particle size of silica has a significant effect. Finer silica produces higher setting and hygroscopic expansions.

Silica/Binder Ratio

Investments usually contain 65% to 75% silica, 25% to 35% calcium sulfate hemihydrate, and about 2% to 3% of some additive chemicals to control the different physical properties and to color the investments. If the silica/stone ratio is increased, the hygroscopic expansion of the investment also increases, but the strength of the investment decreases.

Water/Powder Ratio

As with the setting expansion of gypsum products, the more water in the mix (the thinner the mix or the higher the W/P ratio), the less the normal and hygroscopic setting expansions. Less thermal expansion is also obtained with a thinner mix.

Spatulation

The effect of spatulation on the setting and hygroscopic expansion of the investment is similar to that on the setting expansion of all gypsum products.

Age of Investment

Investments that are 2 or 3 years old do not expand as much as freshly prepared investments. For this reason, the containers of investment must be kept closed as much as possible, especially if the investment is stored in a humid atmosphere.

Water-Bath Temperature

For the water-bath immersion technique, the temperature of the water bath has a measurable effect on the wax pattern. At higher water-bath temperatures, the wax pattern expands, requiring less expansion of the investment to compensate for the total casting shrinkage. In addition, higher water-bath temperatures soften the wax. The softened wax then provides less resistance to the expansion of the investment, thus making the setting expansion more effective. The net effect is higher expansion of the mold with higher water-bath temperatures.

THERMAL AND HYGROSCOPIC CASTING INVESTMENT

Casting techniques involving gypsum-bonded investments are often classified as thermal or hygroscopic techniques. The thermal technique directs placing the invested ring after setting into the burnout oven set for a relatively high temperature (649° C), whereas the hygroscopic technique directs immersing the invested ring before setting in a water bath and then, after setting, placing the ring into the burnout oven set for relatively low temperature (482° C). Although all gypsum-bonded investments exhibit both thermal and hygroscopic setting expansion, the relative proportion of these two expansions

can vary. Investments used in the thermal technique usually contain cristobalite as the refractory ingredient, which has a high thermal expansion. Investments used in the hygroscopic technique usually contain quartz or tridymite, which have lower thermal expansions but higher hygroscopic setting expansions.

Hygroscopic-Thermal Gold Casting Investment

There is one gold casting investment on the market that was designed for use with either hygroscopic or thermal type of casting techniques. Figure 12-29 shows the high thermal expansion of this investment in the range between 482° C and 649° C. This expansion is high enough to use the investment with the thermal casting technique, without water immersion. However, when immersed in a water bath, the investment expands hygroscopically (Figure 12-30). With the hygroscopic technique, the investment needs to be heated to only 482° C to provide the appropriate expansion.

Investment for Casting High-Melting-Point Alloys

Most palladium and base metal alloys used for removable dental prostheses and ceramic-metal restorations have high melting temperatures. They should be cast at a mold temperature greater than 700° C. For this reason, calcium sulfate–bonded investments are usually not used for casting these alloys. Only one base metal alloy for dental applications possesses a low enough melting point to be cast into a mold at 700° C with a calcium sulfate binder. This alloy is an exception, because base metal alloys are usually cast into molds at 850° to 110° C. To withstand these high temperatures, the molds require different types of binders, such as silicate and phosphate compounds. This type of investment usually has less than 20% binder, and the remainder of the investment is quartz or another form of silica.

Phosphate-Bonded Investment

The most common type of investment for casting high-melting point alloys is the phosphate-bonded investment. This type of investment consists of three different components. One component contains a water-soluble phosphate ion. The second component reacts with phosphate ions at room temperature. The third component is a refractory, such as silica. Different materials can be used in each component to develop different physical properties.

The binding system of a typical phosphate-bonded investment undergoes an acid-base reaction between acid monoammonium phosphate ($NH_4H_2PO_4$) and

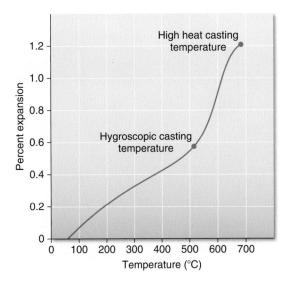

FIGURE 12.29 **Thermal expansion of mixed hygroscopic-thermal gold casting investment.** *(Courtesy of Whip Mix Corporation, Louisville, KY.)*

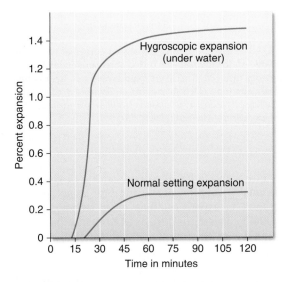

FIGURE 12.30 **Setting and hygroscopic expansion of mixed hygroscopic-thermal gold casting investment.** *(Courtesy of Whip Mix Corporation, Louisville, KY.)*

basic magnesia (MgO). The soluble phosphate in water reacts with the sparingly soluble magnesia at its surface, forming a binding medium with filler particles embedded in the matrix. The chemical reaction at room temperature can be expressed simply as follows:

$$NH_4H_2PO_4 + MgO + H_2O \rightarrow$$
$$NH_4MgPO_4 \cdot 6H_2O + H_2O$$

The water produced by this reaction at room temperature lowers the viscosity of the mix as spatulation continues.

As the reaction takes place, colloidal particles are formed with a strong interaction among the particles. During setting and burnout, the sequence of chemical and thermal reactions causes various phase changes, providing room-temperature strength (green strength) and high-temperature strength that enable the investment to withstand the impact of high-melting-point alloys. Phases formed at high temperatures include $Mg_2P_2O_7$ and subsequently $Mg_3(PO_4)_2$. To produce higher expansion, a combination of different particle sizes of silica is used.

These investments can be mixed with water or with a special liquid supplied by the manufacturer. The special liquid is a form of silica sol in water. As shown in Figure 12-31, phosphate-bonded investments possess higher setting expansion when they are mixed with the silica sol than when mixed with water. With a mix containing silica sol, the investment mass is capable of expanding hygroscopically, whereas if the mix is only water, the hygroscopic expansion of such an investment is negligible. Not all phosphate-bonded investments, however, can expand hygroscopically. Using silica sol instead of water with phosphate-bonded investment also increases its strength considerably. Figure 12-32 shows thermal expansion curves of two commercial phosphate-bonded investments mixed according to the manufacturers' recommended liquid/powder ratio. Both the setting and thermal expansions must be considered in selecting these investments.

ANSI/ADA specification No. 126 (ISO 9694) for dental phosphate-bonded casting investments specifies two types of investments for alloys having a solidus temperature above 1080° C:

Type 1: For inlays, crowns, and other fixed restorations
Type 2: For removable dental prostheses

The following properties and their specified values are described by the specification: fluidity, initial setting time, compressive strength, and linear thermal expansion. The setting time must not differ by more than 30% from the time stated by the manufacturer. The compressive strength at room temperature shall be not less than 2.5 MPa for type 1 investments and 3.0 MPa for type 2 investments. The linear thermal expansion must not differ by more than 15% from the time stated by the manufacturer.

Silica-Bonded Investment

Another type of binding material for investments used with casting high-melting-point alloys is a silica-bonding ingredient. This type of investment may derive its silica bond from ethyl silicate, an aqueous dispersion of colloidal silica, or from sodium silicate.

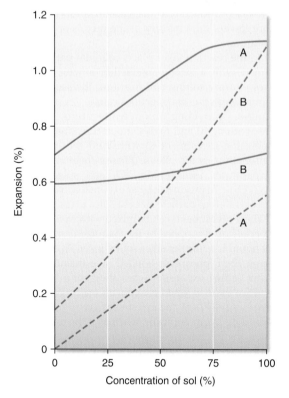

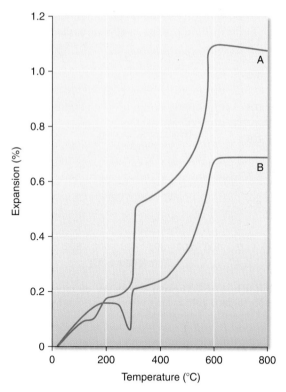

FIGURE 12.31 Effect of silica sol concentration on thermal expansion *(solid lines)* at 800° C and setting expansion *(dotted lines)* of two phosphate-bonded investments. *A,* Thermal expansion type; *B,* hygroscopic expansion type. *(Data from Zarb GA, Bergman G, Clayton JA, MacKay HF (Eds.): Prosthodontic treatment for partially edentulous patients. Mosby, St. Louis, 1978.)*

FIGURE 12.32 Thermal expansion curves of two phosphate-bonded investments mixed at recommended liquid/powder ratios. *A,* Thermal expansion type; *B,* hygroscopic expansion type. *(Data from Zarb GA, Bergman B, Clayton JA, MacKay HF (Eds.): Prosthodontic treatment for partially edentulous patients. Mosby, St. Louis, 1978.)*

One such investment consists of silica refractory, which is bonded by the hydrolysis of ethyl silicate in the presence of hydrochloric acid. The product of the hydrolysis is a colloidal solution of silicic acid and ethyl alcohol, which can be written as follows:

$$Si(OC_2H_5)_4 + 4H_2O \xrightarrow{HCl} Si(OH)_4 + 4C_2H_5OH$$

In practice, however, the reaction is more complicated, and instead of tetrasilicic acid, which is converted into $SiO_2 - 2H_2O$, a polymerized compound of silicon is formed with the following structure:

$$
\begin{array}{cc}
| & | \\
-Si-O-Si- \\
| & | \\
O & O \\
| & | \\
-Si-O-Si- \\
| & | \\
O & O \\
| & | \\
-Si-O-Si- \\
| & |
\end{array}
$$

This material has an even higher silica content and better refractory properties than the $SiO_2 \cdot 2H_2O$.

Ethyl silicate has the disadvantage of giving off flammable components during processing, and the method is expensive; thus other techniques and methods have been developed to reduce the use of this material. Sodium silicate and colloidal silica are more common binders of the silica type.

Today this investment is usually supplied with two bottles of special liquid, instead of water, with which the investment powder should be mixed. In one of the bottles the manufacturer usually supplies a properly diluted water-soluble silicate solution. The other bottle usually contains a properly diluted acid solution, such as a solution of hydrochloric acid. The contents of each bottle can be stored almost indefinitely. Before use, mix an equal volume from each bottle and allow the mixed liquids to stand for a prescribed time, according to the manufacturer's instructions, so hydrolysis can take place and freshly prepared silicic acid forms.

ANSI/ADA specification No. 126 (ISO 11246) for ethyl silicate casting investments specifies setting time, compressive strength, and linear thermal expansion. The setting time must not differ by more than 30% from the time stated by the manufacturer. The compressive strength at room temperature shall not be less than 1.5 MPa. The linear thermal expansion must not differ by more than 15% from the time stated by the manufacturer.

Brazing Investment

When brazing (soldering) the parts of a restoration, such as clasps on a removable dental prosthesis, the parts must be surrounded with a suitable ceramic or investment material before the heating operation. The assembled parts are temporarily held together with sticky wax until they are surrounded with the appropriate investment material, after which the wax is softened and removed. The portion to be soldered is left exposed and free from investment to permit wax removal and effective heating before it is joined with solder.

ANSI/ADA specification No. 126 (ISO 11244) for dental brazing investments defines two types of investment:

Type 1: Gypsum-bonded dental brazing investments
Type 2: Phosphate-bonded dental brazing investments

The specification specifies quality, fluidity, setting time, compressive strength, linear thermal expansion, and linear setting expansion. The setting time must not differ by more than 30% from the time stated by the manufacturer. The compressive strength shall be in the range of 2.0 to 10 MPa. The linear setting and thermal expansions must not differ by more than 15% from the time stated by the manufacturer.

The investment for soldering of low-melting-point alloys is similar to casting investments containing quartz and a calcium sulfate hemihydrate binder. For high-melting-point alloys, a phosphate-bonded investment is used.

Soldering investments are designed to have lower setting and thermal expansions than casting investments, a feature that is desirable so the assembled parts do not shift in position during the setting and heating of the investment. Soldering investments are often made of ingredients that do not have as fine a particle size as the casting investment, because the smoothness of the mass is less important. Relatively little information is available in the dental literature on the properties of soldering investments.

INVESTMENT FOR ALL-CERAMIC RESTORATIONS

Two types of investment materials have been developed recently for producing all-ceramic restorations. The first type is used for the cast glass technique. This investment is provided by the manufacturer of the glass casting equipment and is composed of phosphate-bonded refractories. The second type of investment for making all-ceramic restorations is the refractory die type of material, which is used for all-ceramic veneers, inlays, and crowns. Refractory dies are made by pouring the investment into impressions. When the investment is set, the die is removed, and is heated to remove gases that may be detrimental to the ceramic (degassing). A refractory die spacer may be added to the surface. Next, porcelain or other ceramic powders are added to the die surface and fired. These materials must accurately reproduce the impression, remain undamaged during the porcelain firing, and have a thermal expansion compatible with that of the ceramic (otherwise the ceramic could crack during cooling). These materials are also phosphate-bonded, and they generally contain fine-grained refractory fillers to allow accurate reproduction of detail. ANSI/ADA specification No. 126 (ISO 11245) for phosphate-bonded refractory die materials describes the required properties.

SELECTED PROBLEMS

PROBLEM 1

A mix of alginate was made, and the setting time was shorter than previously experienced with this brand. The material was too stiff at the time of insertion to obtain adequate seating and surface detail. What factors should be considered in the correction of this difficulty?

Solution a

The most common cause for the shorter setting time is too high a temperature of the mix water. The setting reaction is a typical chemical reaction that is accelerated by increases in temperature; a 10° C increase in temperature almost doubles the rate of the reaction. In many operations, a single water faucet is present with a mixing valve to control the temperature of the water. Gradual failure of the mixing valve can inadvertently result in the use of water substantially hotter than the 21° C usually recommended.

Solution b

The setting time can also be shortened by incorrect dispensing, resulting in too high a powder/liquid ratio. If the alginate powder is not aerated before each dispensing, the weight of each scoop will be too high, because the apparent density of the powder is higher after standing. The increased amount of powder causes the setting or gelation time to be less than normally experienced.

Solution c

Aging of the alginate powder in a warm, humid atmosphere can affect the setting by reducing the effectiveness of the retarder, resulting in a shorter than normal setting time.

PROBLEM 2

A mix of alginate was made, and it appeared thicker than normal. After the impression was taken, its surface seemed grainy and lacking in surface detail. What precautions should be taken to avoid this condition when the impression is retaken?

Solution

A thick consistency can result from lack of aeration of the powder before dispensing, or from an incorrect number of measures of powder or water. However, a thick, grainy mix can occur from inadequate mixing of the correct proportions of powder and water. Inadequate mixing may be caused by casual rather than vigorous spatulation or by not mixing for the full time recommended. Hot water used in combination with the two factors just mentioned accentuates the problem of thick, grainy mixes. If the next mix is carefully dispensed, the temperature of the water checked, and the length of mixing timed, a smooth, creamy consistency should result.

PROBLEM 3

An alginate impression was taken of a patient with a fixed appliance, and tearing of the impression occurred in critical areas as a result of severely undercut areas. What can be done to improve the next impression, because alginate impressions are supposed to be elastic?

Solution

It is true that alginate impressions are flexible, although they are not entirely elastic (they exhibit incomplete recovery) and have rather low resistance to tearing compared with elastomeric impression materials. Several precautions can be taken to improve the chances of an acceptable impression. The severely undercut areas can be blocked out, thus placing less stress on the alginate during removal. Recall that the strength of the alginate improves quite rapidly for 5 to 10 minutes after setting, and the impression can be left in the mouth a few extra minutes before removal. Also,

remember that the tear strength is a function of the rate of removal of the impression, and rapid rates enhance the chances of an acceptable impression. Finally, mixes with high powder/liquid ratios have higher tear strengths; however, to obtain a smooth consistency that will record the desired level of surface detail, the ratio must not be increased beyond the limit.

PROBLEM 4

An alginate impression is to be taken of a patient known to have a problem with gagging. What steps can be taken in materials management to reduce the problem and yet obtain a satisfactory impression?

Solution a

The viscosity of mixed alginates remains fairly constant until just before the setting time because the retardation reaction prevents the formation of the calcium alginate gel. When the working and setting times are known accurately, insertion of the impression material into the mouth can be delayed until just before the end of the working time, but allowing enough time to seat the impression. The impression should then be removed at the earliest possible time after it sets but while it still has adequate properties. Thus the impression is in the mouth the shortest possible time.

Solution b

A fast-setting alginate can be selected that not only sets in a shorter time but also has better mechanical properties in a shorter time than regular-setting material.

Solution c

Care should be taken during the loading of the maxillary impression tray to avoid excessive amounts of alginate in the posterior portion of the tray. The posterior part of the tray should be seated before the anterior portion, with the patient's head in a position to avoid excess alginate flowing in a posterior direction on the palate.

PROBLEM 5

The set alginate impression separated from the tray during removal from the mouth, resulting in distortion and tearing of the impression. What can be done to avoid this?

Solution

Two choices can be made. A change in the brand of alginate to one that adheres to the metal tray is one option. However, if a nonadhesive alginate is desired, select a tray with perforations that provides mechanical retention. Second, use commercial tray adhesives specifically formulated for retention of alginate impressions.

PROBLEM 6

An inaccurate model is obtained despite the use of the correct mixing technique for the alginate and the proper pouring procedure for the gypsum model. What possible factors might have resulted in the inaccurate impression?

Solution a

The tray selected may have been too small, thus providing too little alginate between the tray and the tissues. During the removal of the set alginate, the percent compression may have been too high when the bulge of the tooth compressed the alginate in the undercut areas. This excessive compression results in higher than normal permanent deformation. Correct the problem by selecting a tray that provides about 5 mm of space between the tray and tissues. With the same amount of undercut, the alginate is subjected to lower percent compression, and lower permanent deformation results.

Solution b

A second possible cause of the problem could be the premature removal of the impression. The permanent deformation of the impression on removal decreases with the time after setting. Therefore, premature removal of the impression, even though the material is no longer tacky, can be the cause of excessive permanent deformation of the impression in undercut areas.

Solution c

A third possible cause of the inaccurate impression might be a too slow rate of removal of the set impression material. With everything else being equal, a slow rate of removal rather than a snap removal results in higher than normal amounts of permanent deformation.

Solution d

A fourth reason for the difficulty might be overextension of the alginate to areas not supported by the tray. The weight of these overextended areas can deform the impression; if they are not cut away, deformation and permanent distortion of the impression in these areas can occur.

Solution e

Finally, the alginate impression can be permanently distorted if after removal it is stored in such a manner that the impression is deformed. Two possible conditions could cause this effect: placing the impression down with the weight of the tray on it, and wrapping the impression too tightly in a damp towel.

PROBLEM 7

When an addition silicone impression was withdrawn from the mouth, the impression material was separated from the tray in some areas. What caused this separation, and how accurate are the dies obtained from such an impression?

Solution

The adhesion of an impression material to the custom-made tray is obtained by coating the tray with an adhesive. To get good adhesion to the tray, use enough coats of the adhesive. It is also necessary to wait until the volatile organic solvent evaporates and the adhesive is dry. When the tray is filled with the high-consistency material too soon after applying the adhesive, the retention fails and the impression material separates from the tray. In this instance, a distortion of the impression is always present and results in a distorted model and dies. It is better to remake the impression than to continue with the procedure. When the failure is caused by the adhesive itself, better mechanical retention for the impression material can be obtained by making perforations with a bur in the same type of custom tray. These mechanical interlocks retain the impression material in position, and the uniform thickness of impression material in the custom tray helps control the polymerization shrinkage of the material.

PROBLEM 8

An impression of a dentulous quadrant was taken with a medium-consistency polyether impression material in a custom-made acrylic tray. The normal relief of 2 mm was provided between the tray and the oral structures. After removal of the impression, tearing was noted at several locations. What adjustments can be made so that the possibility of tearing will be minimized on retaking the impression?

Solution a

Polyethers adhere quite well to hard and soft tissues and the medium consistency is quite stiff when set (low strain in compression). The adhesion and stiffness, combined with moderate tear strength, increases the probability of tearing of the impression. Before removal, first break the seal of the impression to tissues by pulling the impression slightly in the vestibular area. Syringing water into the area can also help break the seal. Finally, increase the relief space between the tray and the tissues to at least 4 mm to allow greater flexibility of impression material, thereby improving the ease of removal.

Solution b

Use the new, softened, medium-consistency polyether impression material in the tray; it is less rigid and possesses reduced Shore A hardness in the set condition. Also, provide additional relief space between the tray and the tissues (at least 4 mm) to increase the effective flexibility of the elastomer.

PROBLEM 9

The manufacturer of an addition silicone impression specified that high-strength stone dies should not be poured until after 1 hour. An epoxy die was desired, and therefore pouring was delayed for 1 hour. On separation, the die was covered with negative bubbles. What caused the problem, and how can it be avoided?

Solution

Some brands of addition silicones release hydrogen after setting. Waiting 1 hour before pouring the fast-setting, high-strength stone allows the rate of hydrogen release to decrease sufficiently so bubble-free dies can be produced. However, many epoxy die materials set slowly compared with high-strength stone, and sufficient hydrogen is still being released at 1 hour to produce bubbles on the surface of the epoxy die. Even waiting 4 hours may not result in a bubble-free epoxy die. Allowing the impression to stand overnight before pouring the epoxy die solves the problem. Also, note that the accuracy of addition silicone impressions is excellent at 24 hours, even with the evolution of hydrogen.

PROBLEM 10

An impression, taken in a nonhydrophilized addition silicone, had been mixed by hand spatulation. The resulting high-strength stone die had enough positive and negative bubbles, especially along the internal line angles and finish lines of the preparation, so a retake of the impression was necessary. What could be done to reduce the number of bubbles?

Solution

Changing to an addition silicone supplied in auto-mixing cartridges substantially reduces the number of bubbles in the mix, compared with one prepared by hand spatulation, and minimizes the number of positive bubbles. In addition, changing to hydrophilized, automixing addition silicone decreases the number of negative bubbles in the die because of the better wetting of the impression by the mix of high-strength stone.

PROBLEM 11

A patient has fractured a lingual cusp and comes to the office for emergency care. You would like to prepare the tooth for a gold crown and have your dental assistant make a custom tray for the final impression while you are preparing the tooth. In terms of the dimensional accuracy of the tray, what must be considered?

Solution

Autopolymerizing tray materials continue to change dimensionally during the first few hours after they are made. Use of a tray before this polymerization is complete can affect the accuracy of the impression. Two things can be done to eliminate this problem: (1) have the dental assistant boil the tray for a short time to force the polymerization reaction to completion, or (2) use a light-activated tray material that experiences no significant dimensional change after processing.

PROBLEM 12

High-strength dental stone dies sometimes fracture during separation from elastomeric impressions. How can this difficulty be minimized?

Solution a

The recommended water/powder ratio should be used. The water/powder ratio can vary from 0.19 to 0.24 for various type 4 gypsum products. The water and powder should be dispensed accurately. Optimum strength is achieved only at the correct water/powder ratio.

Solution b

Vacuum mixing of high-strength dental stone ensures maximum strength by minimizing porosity.

Solution c

The poured die should be allowed to set for at least 20 minutes or until final set before it is removed from the impression.

Solution d

Increasing the thickness of stiffer impression materials (polyether) increases the ease of removal of the die.

PROBLEM 13

The occlusal surfaces of teeth of a type 3 gypsum model poured from an alginate impression were chalky and friable. What may have happened, and how can this problem be solved?

Solution

Excess water in the depressions of an alginate impression (or any impression) from rinsing will increase the water/powder ratio of the dental stone. Blood and saliva remaining on the impression retard the setting of the dental stone. Both conditions can cause the dental stone to be chalky and friable. Carefully rinse and remove excess water from an impression before pouring it in dental stone.

PROBLEM 14

The surface of a high-strength dental stone die was abraded during preparation of the wax pattern. Can type 4 gypsum be treated to create a more abrasion-resistant surface that is less susceptible to damage during construction of the pattern and finishing of the casting?

Solution

Apparently not, because the available hardening solutions and various impregnation techniques have little effect on the abrasion resistance of type 4 gypsum. Hardening solutions do result in a slightly higher setting expansion of high-strength dental stone dies.

PROBLEM 15

A dental stone master cast for a complete denture was placed in a bowl of water before it was mounted on an articulator. Inadvertently, the cast was left in the water overnight. After the cast was mounted and dried, an unusually rough surface appeared. What happened?

Solution

Dental stone is slightly soluble in water. Leaving the cast in water for an extended time can dissolve some of the surface, roughening the cast. This roughness is transferred to the surface of the denture. If the cast must be stored in water, use a saturated calcium sulfate dihydrate solution (slurry water).

PROBLEM 16

The boxing edge of a dental stone master cast was trimmed on a model trimmer several days after it had been poured. Trimming was much more difficult than when done soon after the dental stone had set. Why was the cast more difficult to trim, and how can this difficulty be corrected?

Solution

As dental stone dries over a period of several days, its compressive strength increases to about twice that when wet. The wet strength may be regained by soaking the cast in slurry water, which is used to minimize dissolution of the surface during soaking.

PROBLEM 17

A gypsum investment was mixed with water in the proportions recommended by the manufacturer, but the working time was too short to invest the wax pattern. What may have happened, and how can this problem be solved?

Solution a

The powder may have been contaminated by water, from high humidity or a wet dispensing spoon. Investment should be stored in an airtight and waterproof container.

Solution b

The temperature of the mixing water may have been higher than 23° C. Water at 20° to 23° C is recommended. Higher temperatures shorten the working time.

Solution c

The spatulation may have been done incorrectly with a mechanical mixer. Overmixing, too long or too rapid, shortens the working time.

Solution d

The mixing bowl or spatula may have been contaminated with particles of set investment containing calcium sulfate dihydrate, accelerating the reaction. Mixing implements should be cleaned before use.

PROBLEM 18

A full crown casting prepared by an immersion hygroscopic technique was too loose. What conditions might have caused this problem, and how can a tighter crown be obtained?

Solution a

The water bath may have been warmer than usual. When warmer water is used, the wax pattern offers less resistance to the expansion of the investment, producing a larger mold. The temperature of the water bath should be monitored regularly.

Solution b

A thicker-than-average mix of investment may have been used, causing an increased setting and hygroscopic expansion. The water/powder ratio recommended by the manufacturer should be used, and the water and powder accurately dispensed.

Bibliography

Review Articles—Impression Materials

Allen EP, Bayne SC, Becker IM, et al: Annual review of selected dental literature: report of the committee on scientific investigation of the American Academy of Restorative Dentistry, *J Prosthet Dent* 82:50, 1999.

Allen EP, Bayne SC, Donovan TE, et al: Annual review of selected dental literature, *J Prosthet Dent* 76:75, 1996.

Craig RG: Review of dental impression materials, *Adv Dent Res* 2:51, 1988.

Donovan TE, Chee WW: A review of contemporary impression materials and techniques, *Dent Clin North Am* 48:vi–vii, 445, 2004.

Jendresen MD, Allen EP, Bayne SC, et al: Annual review of selected dental literature: report of the committee on scientific investigation of the American Academy of Restorative Dentistry, *J Prosthet Dent* 80:105, 1998.

Whitters CJ, Strang R, Brown D, et al: Dental materials: 1997 literature review, *J Dent* 27:421, 1999.

Agar and Alginate Hydrocolloids

Bergman B, Bergman M, Olsson S: Alginate impression materials, dimensional stability and surface detail sharpness following treatment with disinfectant solutions, *Swed Dent J* 9:255, 1985.

Buchan S, Peggie RW: Role of ingredients in alginate impression compounds, *J Dent Res* 45:1120, 1966.

Craig RG: Mechanical properties of some recent alginates and tensile bond strengths of agar/alginate combinations, *Phillip's J Rest Zahnmed* 6:242, 1989.

Cserna A, Crist R, Adams A, et al: Irreversible hydrocolloids: a comparison of antimicrobial efficacy, *J Prosthet Dent* 71:387, 1994.

Ellis B, Lamb DJ: The setting characteristics of alginate impression materials, *Br Dent J* 151:343, 1981.

Farah JW, Powers JM: Alginate impression materials, *Dent Advis* 18(4):1, 2001.

Fish SF, Braden M: Characterization of the setting process in alginate impression materials, *J Dent Res* 43:107, 1964.

Ghani F, Hobkirk JA, Wilson M: Evaluation of a new antiseptic-containing alginate impression material, *Br Dent J* 169:83, 1990.

Hall BD, Munoz-Viveros CA, Naylor WP, et al: Effects of a chemical disinfectant on the physical properties of dental stones, *Int J Prosthodont* 17:65, 2004.

Hilton T, Schwartz R, Bradley D: Immersion disinfection of irreversible hydrocolloid impressions. Part II: effects on gypsum casts, *Int J Prosthodont* 7:424, 1994.

Hutchings MI, Vanderwalle K, Schwartz R, et al: Immersion disinfection of irreversible hydrocolloid impressions in pH-adjusted sodium hypochlorite. Part 2: effect on gypsum casts, *Int J Prosthodont* 9:223, 1996.

Johnson GH, Chellis KD, Gordon GE, et al: Dimensional stability and detail reproduction of alginate and elastomeric impressions disinfected by immersion, *J Prosthet Dent* 79:446, 1998.

MacPherson GW, Craig RG, Peyton FA: Mechanical properties of hydrocolloid and elastomeric impression materials, *J Dent Res* 46:714, 1967.

Miller MW: Syneresis in alginate impression materials, *Br Dent J* 139:425, 1975.

Murata H, Kawamura M, Hamada T, et al: Physical properties and compatibility with dental stones of current alginate impression materials, *J Oral Rehabil* 31:1115, 2004.

Peutzfeldt A, Asmussen E: Effect of disinfecting solutions on accuracy of alginate and elastomeric impressions, *Scand J Dent Res* 97:470, 1989.

Peutzfeldt A, Asmussen E: Effect of disinfecting solutions on surface texture of alginate and elastomeric impressions, *Scand J Dent Res* 98:74, 1990.

Schwartz R, Bradley D, Hilton T, et al: Immersion disinfection of irreversible hydrocolloid impressions. Part I: microbiology, *Int J Prosthodont* 7:418, 1994.

Vanderwalle K, Charlton D, Schwartz R, et al: Immersion disinfection of irreversible hydrocolloid impressions with sodium hypochlorite. Part II: effect on gypsum, *Int J Prosthodont* 7:315, 1994.

Wanis TM, Combe EC, Grant AA: Measurement of the viscosity of irreversible hydrocolloids, *J Oral Rehabil* 20:379, 1993.

Woodward JD, Morris JC, Khan Z: Accuracy of stone casts produced by perforated trays and nonperforated trays, *J Prosthet Dent* 53:347, 1985.

Properties and Use of Elastomeric Impression Materials

Baumann MA: The influence of dental gloves on the setting of impression materials, *Br Dent J* 179:130, 1995.

Boening KW, Walter MH, Schuette U: Clinical significance of surface activation of silicone impression materials, *J Dent* 26:447, 1998.

Braden M, Causton B, Clarke RL: A polyether impression rubber, *J Dent Res* 51:889, 1972.

Braden M, Inglis AT: Visco-elastic properties of dental elastomeric impression materials, *Biomaterials* 7:45, 1986.

Chai J, Pand IC: A study of the thixotropic property of elastomeric impression materials, *Int J Prosthodont* 7:155, 1994.

Chen SY, Liang WM, Chen FN: Factors affecting the accuracy of elastometric impression materials, *J Dent* 32:603, 2004.

Cho GC, Chee WW: Distortion of disposable plastic stock trays when used with putty vinyl polysiloxane impression materials, *J Prosthet Dent* 92:354, 2004.

Chong YH, Soh G: Effectiveness of intraoral delivery tips in reducing voids in elastomeric impressions, *Quint Int* 22:897, 1991.

Cook WD: Permanent set and stress relaxation in elastomeric impression materials, *J Biomed Mater Res* 15:44, 1981.

Cook WD: Rheological studies of the polymerization of elastomeric impression materials. I. Network structure of the set state, *J Biomed Mater Res* 16:315, 1982.

Cook WD: Rheological studies of the polymerization of elastomeric impression materials. II. Viscosity measurements, *J Biomed Mater Res* 16:331, 1982.

Cook WD: Rheological studies of the polymerization of elastomeric impression materials. III. Dynamic stress relaxation modulus, *J Biomed Mater Res* 16:345, 1982.

Cook WD, Liem F, Russo P, et al: Tear and rupture of elastomeric dental impression materials, *Biomaterials* 5:275, 1984.

Cook WD, Thomasz F: Rubber gloves and addition silicone materials, *Aust Dent J* 31:140, 1986.

Craig RG: Composition, characteristics and clinical and tissue reactions of impression materials. In Smith DC, Williams DF, editors: *Biocompatibility of dental materials*, vol 3, Boca Raton, 1982, CRC Press.

Craig RG: Evaluation of an automatic mixing system for an addition silicone impression material, *J Am Dent Assoc* 110:213, 1985.

Craig RG: Properties of 12 addition silicones compared with other rubber impression materials , *Phillip J Restaur Zahnmed* 3:244, 1986.

Craig RG, Sun Z: Trends in elastomeric impression materials, *Oper Dent* 19:138, 1994.

Craig RG, Urquiola NJ, Liu CC: Comparison of commercial elastomeric impression materials, *Oper Dent* 15:94, 1990.

Farah JW, Powers JM: Impression and bite registration materials, *Dent Advis* 28(2):5, 2011.

Goldberg AJ: Viscoelastic properties of silicone, polysulfide, and polyether impression materials, *J Dent Res* 53:1033, 1974.

Gordon GE, Johnson GH, Drennon DG: The effect of tray selection on the accuracy of elastomeric impression materials, *J Prosthet Dent* 63:12, 1990.

Herfort TW, Gerberich WW, Macosko CW, et al: Viscosity of elastomeric impression materials, *J Prosthet Dent* 38:396, 1977.

Herfort TW, Gerberich WW, Macosko CW, et al: Tear strength of elastomeric impression materials, *J Prosthet Dent* 39:59, 1978.

Hondrum S: Tear and energy properties of three impression materials, *Int J Prosthodont* 7:155, 1994.

Idris B, Houston F, Claffey N: Comparison of the dimensional accuracy of one-step techniques with the use of putty/wash addition silicone impression materials, *J Prosthet Dent* 74:535, 1995.

Inoue K, Wilson HJ: Viscoelastic properties of elastomeric impression materials. II. Variation of rheological properties with time, temperature and mixing proportions, *J Oral Rehabil* 5:261, 1978.

Johansson EG, Erhardson S, Wictorin L: Influence of stone mixing agents, impression materials and lubricants on surface hardness and dimensions of a dental stone die material, *Acta Odontol Scand* 33:17, 1975.

Johnson GH, Craig RG: Accuracy of four types of rubber impression materials compared with time of pour and a repeat pour of models, *J Prosthet Dent* 53:484, 1985.

Johnson GH, Craig RG: Accuracy of addition silicones as a function of technique, *J Prosthet Dent* 55:197, 1986.

Johnson GH, Lepe X, Aw TC: Detail reproduction for single versus dual viscosity impression techniques, *J Dent Res* 78(Spec Issue B):140, 1999:(Abstract 273).

Kim KN, Craig RG, Koran A III: Viscosity of monophase addition silicones as a function of shear rate, *J Prosthet Dent* 67:794, 1992.

Koran A, Powers JM, Craig RG: Apparent viscosity of materials used for making edentulous impressions, *J Am Dent Assoc* 95:75, 1977.

Lampe I, Marton S, Hegedus C: Effect of mixing technique on shrinkage rate of one polyether and two polyvinyl siloxane impression materials, *Int J Prosthodont* 17:590, 2004.

Laufer BZ, Baharav H, Ganor Y, et al: The effect of marginal thickness on the distortion of different impression materials, *J Prosthet Dent* 76:466, 1996.

Lee IK, Delong R, Pintado MR, et al: Evaluation of factors affecting the accuracy of impressions using quantitative surface analysis, *Oper Dent* 20:246, 1995.

Lepe X, Johnson GH, Berg JC, et al: Effect of mixing technique on surface characteristics of impression materials, *J Prosthet Dent* 79:495, 1998.

Lorren RA, Salter DJ, Fairhurst CW: The contact angles of die stone on impression materials, *J Prosthet Dent* 36:176, 1976.

Lu H, Nguyen B, Powers JM: Mechanical properties of 3 hydrophilic addition silicone and polyether elastomeric impression materials, *J Prosthet Dent* 92:151, 2004.

Mansfield MA, Wilson HJ: Elastomeric impression materials: a comparison of methods for determining working and setting times, *Br Dent J* 132:106, 1972.

McCabe JF, Arikawa H: Rheological properties of elastomeric impression materials before and during setting, *J Dent Res* 77:1998, 1874.

McCabe JF, Bowman AJ: The rheological properties of dental impression materials, *Br Dent J* 151:179, 1981.

McCabe JF, Storer R: Elastomeric impression materials. The measurement of some properties relevant to clinical practice, *Br Dent J* 149:73, 1980.

Michalakis KX, Pissiotis A, Anastasiadou V, et al: An experimental study on particular physical properties of several interocclusal recording media. Part III: Resistance to compression after setting, *J Prosthodont* 13:233, 2004.

Neissen LC, Strassler H, Levinson PD, et al: Effect of latex gloves on setting time of polyvinylsiloxane putty impression material, *J Prosthet Dent* 55:128, 1986.

Norling BK, Reisbick MH: The effect of nonionic surfactants on bubble entrapment in elastomeric impression materials, *J Prosthet Dent* 42:342, 1979.

Ohsawa M, Jorgensen KD: Curing contraction of addition-type silicone impression materials, *Scand J Dent Res* 91:51, 1983.

Pang IC, Chai J: The effect of a shear load on the viscosities of ten vinyl polysiloxane impression materials, *J Prosthet Dent* 71:177, 1994.

Pratten DH, Craig RG: Wettability of a hydrophilic addition silicone impression material, *J Prosthet Dent* 61:197, 1989.

Reusch B, Weber B: In *precision impressions—a guide for theory and practice, theoretical section*, Seefeld, Germany, 1999, ESPE Dental AG.

Rueda LJ, Sy-Munoz JT, Naylor WP, et al: The effect of using custom or stock trays on the accuracy of gypsum casts, *Int J Prosthodont* 9:367, 1996.

Salem NS, Combe EC, Watts DC: Mechanical properties of elastomeric impression materials, *J Oral Rehabil* 15:125, 1988.

Sandrik JL, Vacco JL: Tensile and bond strength of putty-wash elastomeric impression materials, *J Prosthet Dent* 50:358, 1983.

Schelb E, Cavazos E Jr, Troendle KB, et al: Surface detail reproduction of Type IV dental stones with selected polyvinyl siloxane impression materials, *Quint Int* 22:51, 1991.

Sneed WD, Miller R, Olean J: Tear strength of ten elastomeric impression materials, *J Prosthet Dent* 49:511, 1983.

Stackhouse JA Jr: The accuracy of stone dies made from rubber impression materials, *J Prosthet Dent* 24:377, 1970.

Stackhouse JA Jr: Relationship of syringe-tip diameter to voids in elastomeric impressions, *J Prosthet Dent* 53:812, 1985.

Tolley LG, Craig RG: Viscoelastic properties of elastomeric impression materials, *J Oral Rehabil* 5:121, 1978.

Vermilyea SG, Huget EF, de Simon LB: Apparent viscosities of setting elastomers, *J Dent Res* 59:1149, 1980.

Williams JR, Craig RG: Physical properties of addition silicones as a function of composition, *J Oral Rehabil* 15:639, 1988.

Disinfection of Elastomeric Impression Materials

Bergman M, Olsson S, Bergman B: Elastomeric impression materials: dimensional stability and surface sharpness following treatment with disinfection solutions, *Swed Dent J* 4:161, 1980.

Drennon DG, Johnson GH: The effect of immersion disinfection of elastomeric impressions on the sur-face detail reproduction of improved gypsum casts, *J Prosthet Dent* 63:233, 1990.

Drennon DG, Johnson GH, Powell GL: The accuracy and efficacy of disinfection by spray atomization on elastomeric impressions, *J Prosthet Dent* 62:468, 1989.

Johnson GH, Drennon DG, Powell GL: Accuracy of elastomeric impressions disinfected by immersion, *J Am Dent Assoc* 116:525, 1988.

Lepe X, Johnson GH: Accuracy of polyether and addition silicone after long-term immersion disinfection, *J Prosthet Dent* 78:245, 1997.

Lepe X, Johnson GH, Berg JC: Surface characteristics of polyether and addition silicone impression materials after long term disinfection, *J Prosthet Dent* 74:181, 1995.

Rios MP, Morgano SM, Stein RS, et al: Effects of chemical disinfectant solutions on the stability and accuracy of the dental impression complex, *J Prosthet Dent* 76:356, 1996.

Storer R, McCabe JF: An investigation of methods available for sterilising impressions, *Br Dent J* 151:217, 1981.

Thouati A, Deveraux E, Lost A, et al: Dimensional stability of seven elastomeric impression materials immersed in disinfectants, *J Prosthet Dent* 76:8, 1996.

Tray Materials

Carrotte PV, Johnson A, Winstanley RB: The influence of the impression tray on the accuracy of impressions for crown and bridge work—an investigation and review, *Br Dent J* 185:580, 1998.

Goldfogel M, Harvey WL, Winter D: Dimensional change of acrylic resin tray materials, *J Prosthet Dent* 54:284, 1985.

Martinez LJ, von Fraunhofer JA: The effects of custom try material on the accuracy of master casts, *J Prosthodont* 7:106, 1998.

Millstein P, Maya A, Segura C: Determining the accuracy of stock and custom tray impression/casts, *J Oral Rehabil* 25:645, 1998.

Pagniano RP, Scheid RC, Clowson RL, et al: Linear dimensional change of acrylic resins used in the fabrication of custom trays, *J Prosthet Dent* 47:279, 1982.

Dental Plaster and Stone

Buchanan AS, Worner HK: Changes in the composition and setting characteristics of plaster of paris on exposure to high humidity atmospheres, *J Dent Res* 24:65, 1945.

Chong JA, Chong MP, Docking AR: The surface of gypsum cast in alginate impression, *Dent Pract* 16:107, 1965.

Combe EC, Smith DC: Some properties of gypsum plasters, *Br Dent J* 117:237, 1964.

Docking AR: Gypsum research in Australia: the setting process, *Int Dent J* 15:372, 1965.

Docking AR: Some gypsum precipitates, *Aust Dent J* 10:428, 1965.

Earnshaw R: The consistency of gypsum products, *Aust Dent J* 18:33, 1973.

Earnshaw R, Smith DC: The tensile and compressive strength of plaster and stone, *Aust Dent J* 11:415, 1966.

Fairhurst CW: Compressive properties of dental gypsum, *J Dent Res* 39:812, 1960.

Fan PL, Powers JM, Reid BC: Surface mechanical properties of stone, resin, and metal dies, *J Am Dent Assoc* 103:408, 1981.

Garber DK, Powers JM, Brandau HE: Effect of spatulation on the properties of high-strength dental stones, *J Mich Dent Assoc* 67:133, 1985.

Hollenback GM, Smith DD: A further investigation of the physical properties of hard gypsum, *J Calif Dent Assoc* 43:221, 1967.

Jorgensen KD: Studies on the setting of plaster of paris, *Odont Tskr* 61:305, 1953.

Lindquist JT, Brennan RE, Phillips RW: Influence of mixing techniques on some physical properties of plaster, *J Prosthet Dent* 3:274, 1953.

Mahler DB: Hardness and flow properties of gypsum materials, *J Prosthet Dent* 1:188, 1951.

Mahler DB: Plasters of paris and stone materials, *Int Dent J* 5:241, 1955.

Mahler DB, Asgarzadeh K: The volumetric contraction of dental gypsum material on setting, *J Dent Res* 32:354, 1953.

Neville HA: Adsorption and reaction. I. The setting of plaster of paris, *J Phys Chem* 30:1037, 1926.

Peyton FA, Leibold JP, Ridgley GV: Surface hardness, compressive strength, and abrasion resistance of indirect die stones, *J Prosthet Dent* 2:381, 1952.

Phillips RW, Ito BY: Factors affecting the surface of stone dies poured in hydrocolloid impressions, *J Prosthet Dent* 2:390, 1952.

Sanad ME, Combe EC, Grant AA: The use of additives to improve the mechanical properties of gypsum products, *J Dent Res* 61:808, 1982.

Sarma AC, Neiman R: A study on the effect of disinfectant chemicals on physical properties of die stone, *Quint Int* 21:53, 1990.

Stern MA, Johnson GH, Toolson LB: An evaluation of dental stones after repeated exposure to spray disinfectants. Part I: Abrasion and compressive strength, *J Prosthet Dent* 65:713, 1991.

Sweeney WT, Taylor DF: Dimensional changes in dental stone and plaster, *J Dent Res* 29:749, 1950.

Torrance A, Darvell BW: Effect of humidity on calcium sulphate hemihydrate, *Aust Dent J* 35:230, 1990.

von Fraunhofer JA, Spiers RR: Strength testing of dental stone: a comparison of compressive, tensile, transverse, and shear strength tests, *J Biomed Mater Res* 17:293, 1983.

Wiegman-Ho L, Ketelaar JA: The kinetics of the hydration of calcium sulfate hemihydrate investigated by an electric conductance method, *J Dent Res* 61:36, 1982.

Williams GJ, Bates JF, Wild S: The effect of surface treatment of dental stone with resins, *Quint Dent Technol* 7:41, 1983.

Worner HK: Dental plasters. I. General, manufacture, and characteristics before mixing with water, *Aust J Dent* 46:1, 1942.

Worner HK: Dental plasters. II. The setting phenomenon, properties after mixing with water, methods of testing, *Aust J Dent* 46:35, 1942.

Worner HK: The effect of temperature on the rate of setting of plaster of paris, *J Dent Res* 23:305, 1944.

Casting Investments

Anderson JN: *Applied dental materials*, ed 5, Oxford, 1976, Blackwell Scientific.

Asgar K, Lawrence WN, Peyton FA: Further investigations into the nature of hygroscopic expansion of dental casting investments, *J Prosthet Dent* 8:673, 1958.

Asgarzadeh K, Mahler DB, Peyton FA: The behavior and measurement of hygroscopic expansion of dental casting investment, *J Dent Res* 33:519, 1954.

Chew CL, Land MF, Thomas CC, et al: Investment strength as a function of time and temperature, *J Dent* 27:297, 1999.

Delgado VP, Peyton FA: The hygroscopic setting expansion of a dental casting investment, *J Prosthet Dent* 3:423, 1953.

Docking AR: The hygroscopic setting expansion of dental casting investments. I, *Aust J Dent* 52:6, 1948.

Docking AR, Chong MP, Donnison JA: The hygroscopic setting expansion of dental casting investments. II, *Aust J Dent* 52:160, 1948.

Docking AR, Chong MP: The hygroscopic setting expansion of dental casting investments. IV, *Aust J Dent* 53:261, 1949.

Docking AR, Donnison JA, Chong MP: The hygroscopic setting expansion of dental casting investments. III, *Aust J Dent* 52:320, 1948.

Eames WB, Edwards CR Jr, Buck WH Jr: Scraping resistance of dental die materials: a comparison of brands, *Oper Dent* 3:66, 1978.

Earnshaw R: The effect of restrictive stress on the thermal expansion of gypsum-bonded investments. I. Inlay casting investments, "thermal expansion" type, *Aust Dent J* 11:345, 1966.

Earnshaw R: The effects of additives on the thermal behaviour of gypsum-bonded casting investments. I, *Aust Dent J* 20:27, 1975.

Earnshaw R, Morey EF, Edelman DC: The effect of potential investment expansion and hot strength on the fit of full crown castings made with phosphate-bonded investment, *J Oral Rehabil* 24:532, 1997.

Higuchi T: Study of thermal decomposition of gypsum bonded investment. I. Gas analysis, differential thermal analysis, thermobalance analysis, x-ray diffraction, *Kokubyo Gakkai Zasshi* 34:217, 1967.

Jones DW: Thermal analysis and stability of refractory investments, *J Prosthet Dent* 18:234, 1967.

Jones DW, Wilson HJ: Setting and hygroscopic expansion of investments, *Br Dent J* 129:22, 1970.

Lyon HW, Dickson G, Schoonover IC: Effectiveness of vacuum investing in the elimination of surface defects in gold castings, *J Am Dent Assoc* 46:197, 1953.

Lyon HW, Dickson G, Schoonover IC: The mechanism of hygroscopic expansion in dental casting investments, *J Dent Res* 34:44, 1955.

Luk HW-K, Darvell BW: Strength of phosphate-bonded investments at high temperature, *Dent Mater* 7:99, 1991.

Luk HW-K, Darvell BW: Effect of burnout temperature on strength of phosphate-bonded investments, *J Dent* 25:153, 1997.

Luk HW-K, Darvell BW: Effect of burnout temperature on strength of phosphate-bonded investments—part II, *J Dent* 25:423, 1997.

Mahler DB, Ady AB: An explanation for the hygroscopic expansion of dental gypsum products, *J Dent Res* 39:578, 1960.

Mahler DB, Ady AB: The influence of various factors on the effective setting expansion of casting investments, *J Prosthet Dent* 13:365, 1963.

Matsuya S, Yamane M: Thermal analysis of the reaction between II-CaSO4 and quartz in nitrogen flow, *Gypsum Lime* 164:3, 1980.

Miyaji T, Utsumi K, Suzuki E, et al: Deterioration of phosphate-bonded investment on exposure to 100% relative humidity atmosphere, *Bull Tokyo Med Dent Univ* 29:53, 1982.

Moore TE: Method of making dental castings and composition employed in said method, *U.S. Patent* 1,924,874, 1933.

Mori T: Thermal behavior of the gypsum binder in dental casting investments, *J Dent Res* 65:877, 1986.

Neiman R, Sarma AC: Setting and thermal reactions of phosphate investments, *J Dent Res* 59:1478, 1980.

Norling BK, Reisbick MH: Wetting of elastomeric impression materials modified by nonionic surfactant additions, *J Dent Res* 56B(abstr):148, 1977.

O'Brien WJ, Nielsen JP: Decomposition of gypsum investment in the presence of carbon, *J Dent Res* 38:541, 1959.

Phillips RW: Relative merits of vacuum investing of small castings as compared to conventional methods, *J Dent Res* 26:343, 1947.

Ryge G, Fairhurst CW: Hygroscopic expansion, *J Dent Res* 35:499, 1956.

Schilling ER, Miller BH, Woody RD, et al: Marginal gap of crowns made with a phosphate-bonded investment and accelerated casting method, *J Prosthet Dent* 81:129, 1999.

Schnell RJ, Mumford G, Phillips RW: An evaluation of phosphate bonded investments used with a high fusing gold alloy, *J Prosthet Dent* 13:324, 1963.

Shell JS, Dootz ER: Permeability of investments at the casting temperature, *J Dent Res* 40:999, 1961.

Shell JS, Hollenback GM: Setting and thermal investment expansion in longitudinal and transverse directions, *J Calif Dent Assoc* 41:511, 1965.

Tiara M, Okazaki M, Takahashi J, et al: Effects of four mixing methods on setting expansion and compressive strength of six commercial phosphate-bonded silica investments, *J Oral Rehabil* 27:306, 2000.

Weinstein LJ: Composition for dental molds, *U.S. Patent* 1,708,436, 1929.

Materials for Adhesion and Luting

Cementation is one of the final steps in the sequence of clinical procedures for indirect restorations. There are two objectives for the cementation, or luting, procedure: to help retain the restoration in place and to maintain the integrity of the remaining tooth structure. Retention is achieved by friction (or micromechanical interlocking), by an adhesive joint consisting of the prepared tooth, the cement, and the restoration, or a combination of both mechanisms. An effective interfacial seal depends on the ability of the cement to fill the irregularities between the tooth and the restoration and to resist the action of the oral environment, short and long term. Adhesion is also important in this context, because a strong bond between the luting agent and the dental substrates may help prevent bacteria from colonizing the interface and minimizing the transit of fluids that may cause dentin hypersensitivity.

This chapter presents the basic aspects of the application of adhesion science to dentistry and describes the composition, properties, manipulation, and indications for use of acid-base and resin-based cements. Acid-base cements are easy to use and, when correctly indicated, provide good long-term clinical service. Some release fluoride and bond to tooth structures. Resin cements have a chemistry based on resin composites. They show high bond strengths to tooth structures. Some products also contain monomers or are compatible with primers that enable bonding to metal alloys and ceramics. In general, resin cements have better mechanical properties than acid-base cements, but the cementation process is more technique sensitive.

The fundamental technologies and chemistries used to formulate the various types of adhesives and luting cements are derived from their corresponding restorative materials. However, in most cases modifications have been made to create formulations suitable for a particular clinical application in terms of viscosity and handling characteristics.

Different clinical situations require different luting agents and no one material is indicated for every case. Therefore, it is important to differentiate luting cements based on their mechanical properties and overall characteristics to identify the best options available for each clinical situation.

PRINCIPLES OF ADHESION

The creation of a strong, durable, and bonded interface with enamel or dentin provides important benefits. It significantly protects the restoration's interface against penetration of bacteria that may cause secondary caries. It reduces the need for retentive areas in the preparation that would require removal of sound tooth structure. In some cases, bonding may help strengthen the remaining tooth structure. The development of adhesive luting techniques also broadened the application of materials such as low-strength ceramics and indirect composites for crowns, inlays, and onlays.

The term *adhesion* refers to the establishment of molecular interactions between a substrate (*adherend*) and an adhesive brought into close contact, creating an adhesive joint (Figure 13-1). *Cohesion* is used to describe the interaction of similar atoms and molecules within a material, involving primary (i.e., covalent or ionic) or strong secondary forces (i.e., hydrogen bonding).

In dentistry, true chemical bonding between the tooth structure and restorative or luting materials is very difficult to achieve, because of the complex composition of some substrates such as dentin, the presence of contaminants, and the presence of water. Zinc polycarboxylate, glass ionomer, resin-modified glass ionomer, and self-adhesive resin cements are examples of dental materials capable of establishing chemical interaction with hydroxyapatite. However, in daily practice, adhesion is accomplished by micromechanical interlocking between the adhesive and the substrate. It is important to point out that when two materials are in close contact, physical bonding is always present (e.g., van der Waals dipoles); however, it is weak and does not really contribute significantly to the integrity of the adhesive joint.

A dental sealant attached to enamel is an example of a simple adhesive joint with one interface. Often times, however, adhesive joints involve more than

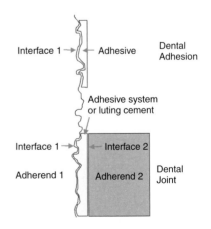

FIGURE 13.1 **Definitions of the terminology associated with adhesive systems (adhesives, adherends or substrates, and interfaces).** Most dental joints involve at least one adhesive, two substrates, and two interfaces.

one interface (e.g., tooth/adhesive and adhesive/ restorative or luting material), which presents an extra challenge because an adhesive does not necessarily bond equally well to different substrates (see Figure 2-1.

The most basic aspect to be observed in creating any adhesive joint is the cleanliness of the substrate. Saliva, biofilm, and other organic debris are always present on the tooth surface. The walls of a cavity preparation are covered with a smear layer. All of these contaminants reduce the surface energy of the bonding substrate and, consequently, its wettability. Therefore, it is very important for the surface that will contact the adhesive to be thoroughly clean and, in some cases, for the smear layer to be removed by acid etching. Indirect restorations also need to have their internal surface cleaned and free from films that may impede the penetration of the adhesive.

Wettability is the result of molecular interactions between the adhesive and the substrate, as well as the cohesion forces of the adhesive, particularly its surface tension. Liquids tend to form spheres when placed on a surface because that is the shape with the lowest surface area and, therefore, the minimum surface energy (Figure 13-2). Wetting is usually evaluated by the contact angle (θ), that is, the internal angle between the liquid and the substrate. Generally, small contact angles are achieved when a low surface tension liquid is placed on a high-energy surface substrate. Contact angles less than 90 degrees indicate a favorable wetting of the surface. Ideal wetting occurs when the liquid spreads over the surface with $\theta \approx 0$ degrees. Surface roughness increases the wettability of the surface by liquids.

Viscosity influences the contact of the adhesive with the substrate. It should be low enough to allow the adhesive to flow readily and penetrate into the details of the substrate surface, without leaving porosities at the interface. Finally, the adhesive must set sufficiently to create strong interlocks with the substrate microstructure to achieve micromechanical retention.

Adhesive Systems
Classification and Basic Components

Adhesive systems can rely on different approaches to obtain a strong and durable bond to dentin and enamel. They are classified according to the etching strategy as *etch-and-rinse* or *self-etch*. Etch-and-rinse (also referred to as *total-etch*) systems can be presented as three-step systems, that is, etching, priming, and bonding in separate application steps. Alternatively, two-step systems present primer and bonding resin mixed in a single component. Etching uses 30% to 40% phosphoric acid gels to demineralize the tooth structure. Acid etchants are also called *conditioners* to disguise the fact that most are relatively strong acids (pH less than 1.0). Originally, etching solutions were free-flowing liquids and were difficult to control during placement. Gel etchants were developed by adding small amounts of microfiller or cellulose thickening agents. These gels flow under slight pressure but do not flow under their own weight.

Primers are hydrophilic monomers, oligomers, or polymers, usually carried in a solvent. The solvents used in primers are acetone, ethanol-water, or primarily water. In some primers, the solvent levels can be as high as 90%. Therefore, primers have different evaporation rates, drying patterns, and penetration characteristics, all of which can influence the resulting bond strength. Dimethacrylate oligomers and lower-molecular-weight monomers can be added to the primer in two-step etch-and-rinse systems, or presented as a separate step in three-step systems or in self-etch two-step systems.

Self-etch systems contain ester monomers with grafted carboxylic or phosphate acid groups dissolved in water. According to their aggressiveness, these systems can be divided into *strong* (pH of 1 or less), *moderate* (pH between 1 and 2), or *mild* (pH of 2 or greater). They can be presented as two-step systems, with a hydrophobic bonding resin in a separate bottle (also known as *self-etching primers*) or single component systems (*all-in-one* systems).

Most bonding agents are light-cured and contain an activator such as camphorquinone and an organic amine. Dual-cured bonding agents include a catalyst to promote self-curing. Although most bonding

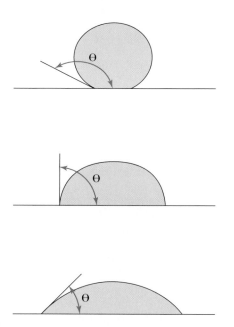

FIGURE 13.2 **Relation of contact angle to the spreading or wetting of a liquid on a solid.**

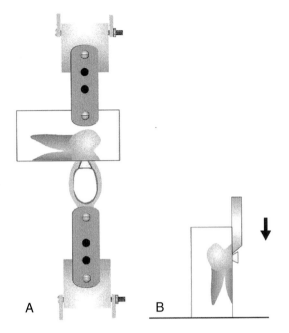

FIGURE 13.3 **Bond strength tests. A**, Diagram of the tensile test apparatus; **B**, diagram of the shear test apparatus. *(From Cardoso PEC, Braga RR, Carrilho MRO: Dent. Mater. 14, 394-398, 1998.)*

agents are unfilled, some products contain nanofillers and submicron glasses ranging from 0.5% to 40% by weight. Fillers are described in more detail in Chapter 9. Filled bonding agents may be easier to place on the tooth and may produce higher in vitro bond strengths. Bonding agents may contain fluoride, antimicrobial ingredients, or desensitizers, such as glutaraldehyde. The effectiveness of fluoride and antimicrobial release from a bonding agent has not been demonstrated.

In Vitro Evaluation of Bond Performance

Laboratory tests have been extensively used to compare the bond performance of adhesive systems. Though clinical relevance of in vitro evaluations is questionable, they certainly represent a valuable "screening" tool. Also, different than clinical studies, laboratory evaluations allow isolation of specific variables that may interfere with bond performance, for example, substrate conditions, contaminants, application procedures, and thermal and mechanical cycling.

Bond strength tests are, by far, the most popular among in vitro methods. ISO/TS11405 (2003) describes test protocols for both shear and tensile bond strength tests (Figure 13-3). Both tests use relatively large bonding areas (3-6 mm in diameter, 7-28 mm^2). Nominal (average) bond strength is calculated by dividing the failure load by the specimen cross-sectional area. The high incidence of cohesive

failures of the substrate observed with these tests prompted the development of *micro bond strength tests* (Figure 13-4), using specimens with much smaller bonding areas (1 mm^2). The main limitation of bond strength tests, despite their great popularity, is that results from different studies cannot be directly compared because of the lack of standardization among research groups. Also, because of the heterogeneous stress distribution along the bonded interface, the nominal bond strength value is far from representative of the true stress that initiated debonding.

The quality of the marginal seal obtained with adhesive systems can be estimated by different methods. Microleakage tests use the immersion of a restored tooth in a tracer solution (e.g., methylene blue or silver nitrate). The tooth is sectioned and the extent of dye penetration is evaluated, either qualitatively (using scores) or quantitatively. Interfacial gaps can be measured under a scanning electron microscope (SEM). Because processing of the real specimen for SEM viewing is critical and more gaps can be unintentionally created, replicas of the bonded interface in epoxy resin are preferred. The term *nanoleakage* applies to a method in which specimens previously immersed in silver nitrate are observed under a transmission electron microscope (TEM). The presence of silver deposits demonstrates the presence of gaps and voids at the bonded interface (Figure 13-5).

Other *in vitro* methods for evaluating the performance of bonding systems are fracture toughness tests that quantify the critical stress level responsible for initiating debonding, and fatigue testing in which the cyclic fatigue resistance after a predetermined number of loading cycles (usually 10^5 cycles) is calculated.

Biocompatibility

Solvents and monomers in bonding agents are typically skin irritants. For example, 2-hydroxyethylmethacrylate (HEMA) may produce local and systemic reactions in dentists and dental assistants sufficient to preclude their further use in the dental office. It is critical that dental personnel protect themselves from recurring exposure. Protective techniques include wearing gloves, immediately replacing contaminated gloves, using high-speed suction, keeping all bottles tightly closed or using unit-dose systems, and disposing of materials in such a way that the monomers cannot evaporate into the office air. Even with double gloves, contact with aggressive solvents and monomers will produce actual skin contact in a few minutes. All reasonable precautions should be followed, and if unwanted contact occurs, affected areas should be flushed immediately with copious amounts of water and soap. Once the materials are polymerized, there is very little risk of

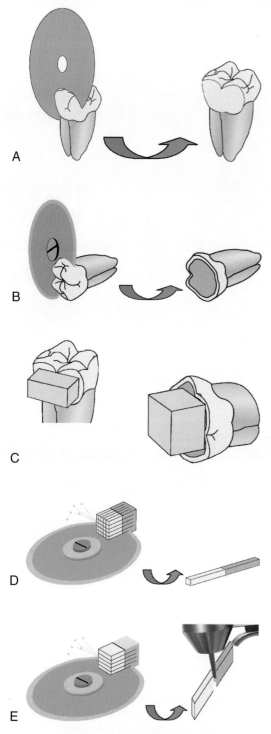

FIGURE 13.4 **Micro bond strength tests. A,** Enamel specimens preparation involved the removal of a portion of superficial tissue without exposing the underlying dentin. **B,** Tooth prepared for dentin test: the occlusal third was removed with a diamond disc, creating a flat surface. **C,** Resin build-up over the enamel and the dentin surface. **D,** Cutting of the tooth along the X- and Y-axis and the resulting sticks. **E,** Procedure for the preparation of hourglass-shaped specimens: the bonded tooth is sectioned in multiple slabs. On each slab the narrowest cross section is created at the interface by trimming with a bur. *(From Goracci C, Sadek FT, Monticelli F, et al: Dent. Mater. 20, 643-654, 2004.)*

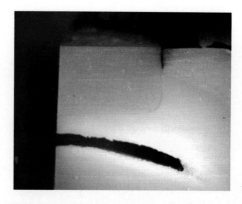

FIGURE 13.5 Section of restored tooth showing microleakage at the composite/enamel interface. *(Courtesy of Dr. Fernanda C. Calheiros, São Paulo, Brazil.)*

side effects. Although patients should be protected during bonding operations, properly polymerized materials have not been shown to be hazardous to the patient.

Clinical Performance

American Dental Association (ADA) guidelines require adhesives to be tested in restorations for non-retentive class 5 lesions. The lesions, which may be saucer- or notch-shaped, have enamel along the coronal margin and dentin along the apical margin. The success of a bonding agent is evaluated indirectly by examining the performance of the restorations for (1) postoperative sensitivity, (2) interfacial staining, (3) secondary caries, and (4) retention or fracture followed for 18 months. These clinical trials test short-term retention and initial sealing.

Most commercial adhesive systems are successful in clinical trials. However, these clinical trials generally combine enamel and dentin bonding. There is no acceptable clinical regimen for critically testing only dentin bonding in nonretentive preparations. Because clinical trials are usually highly controlled, they are often not predictive of routine clinical use in general practice. Longevity of the bond in general practice may be only 40% of that achieved in clinical trials. Long-term clinical performance of bonding systems for a wide range of materials has not yet been reported.

Sites of failure for most bonded restorations occur along cervical margins where the bonding is primarily to dentin (Figure 13-6). Studies of bonded composites in class 2 restorations have shown that 95% of all secondary caries associated with the composite restoration is in the interproximal area. These margins are the most difficult to seal during placement of the restoration because they are typically bonded to dentin and cementum rather than enamel, and are hard to access with a light guide for adequate polymerization.

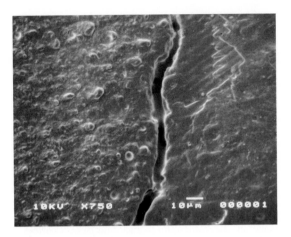

FIGURE 13.6 Scanning electron micrograph (SEM) micrograph of the epoxy replica showing a contraction gap between enamel (*right*) and resin cement (*left*) *(From Braga RR, Ferracane JL, Condon JR: J. Dent. 30, 333-340, 2002.)*

The three-step etch-and-rinse systems remain the "gold standard" for adhesive systems, both in laboratory and clinical evaluations.

Enamel Bonding

Bonding to enamel occurs by micromechanical retention after acid etching is used to preferentially dissolve hydroxyapatite crystals in the enamel outer surface (Figure 13-7). Fluid adhesive constituents penetrate into the newly produced surface irregularities and become locked into place after polymerization of the adhesive.

Gel etchants (typically phosphoric acid) are dispensed from a syringe onto tooth surfaces to be etched. Etching times for enamel vary depending on the type and quality of enamel. Generally, a 15-second etch with 30% to 40% phosphoric acid is sufficient to reach the characteristic clinical endpoint of a frosty enamel appearance. Deciduous unground enamel generally contains some prismless enamel that has not yet worn away and requires longer etching times (20-30 seconds) to create a retentive pattern. Enamel may have been rendered more insoluble as a result of fluorosis. In those cases, extended etching times (15-30 seconds) are required to ensure that sufficient micromechanical bonding can occur. The only caution is that dentin should be protected from exposure to acid because fluorotic dentin is more susceptible to acid than regular dentin.

After the intended etching time, the acid gel is rinsed away and the tooth structure is dried to receive the bonding resin. If a hydrophilic primer or a two-step etch-and-rinse system is used, the surface can be left moist for the next stage of bonding. Then, primer can be flowed onto the surface to penetrate into the available surface irregularities. After curing,

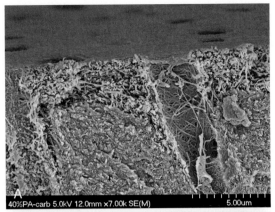

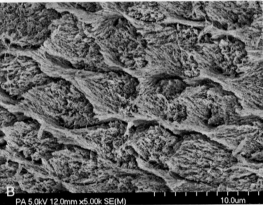

FIGURE 13.7 Scanning electron micrograph (SEM) of etched enamel and dentin. A, Field emission SEM of dentin etched with 40% phosphoric acid for 15 seconds. Note the collagen fibers deprived from hydroxyapatite crystals as a result of acid demineralization. The more intense decalcification around the peritubular area may be a result of both the high mineral content of the peritubular region and the easier penetration of the acid through the tubular lumen. B, Enamel etched with 38% phosphoric acid (Pulpdent) for 15 seconds. *(From Perdigão J: Dent. Clin. N. Am. 51, 333-357, 2007.)*

primer and adhesive produce resin *macrotags* by penetrating the space surrounding the enamel prisms. Microtags form where adhesive flows into the etched prisms involving individual hydroxyapatite crystals. Microtags are much more numerous and contribute to most of the micromechanical retention.

Strong self-etch adhesives produce a similar pattern on enamel as that obtained with phosphoric acid. Mild self-etch systems present lower bond strength to enamel compared to etch-and-rinse systems, probably because of a shallower etching pattern.

Dentin Bonding

The high water content in dentin represents an extra challenge for the establishment of an interdiffusion zone. To manage this problem, primers have hydrophilic components, such as HEMA, that wet dentin and penetrate its structure. In etch-and-rinse systems, etching with phosphoric acid removes the mineral content, creating microporosities within the collagen network. Once the hydroxyapatite component of the outer layer of dentin is removed, dentin contains about 50% unfilled space and about 20% remaining water. After acid is rinsed, drying of dentin must be done cautiously. Even a short air blast from an air-water spray can inadvertently dehydrate the outer surface and cause the remaining collagen scaffold to collapse onto itself. Once this happens, the collagen mesh readily excludes the penetration of primer and bonding will fail. However, excess moisture tends to dilute the primer and interfere with resin interpenetration. The ideal dentin moisture level varies according to the solvent present in the adhesive. With that respect, self-etch systems have the enormous advantage of eliminating this rather subjective step of the bonding procedure.

The infiltration of resin within the collagen scaffold is termed *hybridization* (Figure 13-8). The result of this diffusion process is called *resin-interpenetration zone* or *resin-interdiffusion zone* or simply *hybrid layer*. Concurrent with hybrid layer formation is the penetration of primer into the fluid-filled dentinal tubules. This generates quite large resin tags. However, these appear to be of little value to overall bonding. This material is generally undercured and behaves as soft flexible tags. If dentin is dehydrated before priming and bonding, these resin tags are more likely to be quite extensive.

Primers contain solvents to displace the water and carry the monomers into the microporosities in the collagen network. During application of the primer, most of the solvent evaporates quickly. Thus several layers usually must be applied to ensure a complete impregnation. The rule of thumb is that one should apply as many layers as are necessary to produce a persisting glistening appearance on dentin.

The thickness of a hybrid layer is not a critical requirement for success. Dentin bond strength is probably proportional to the interlocking between resin and collagen, as well as to the "quality" of the hybrid layer, not to its thickness. Effective etching of dentin does not require long times to produce acceptable dentin bond strengths. Usually, 15 seconds is employed. If etching time is too long and the etched zone is too deep, the decalcified dentin may not be fully impregnated. The etched but not impregnated space may reside as a mechanically weak zone and promote nanoleakage. Although this zone has been detected in laboratory experiments, the clinical results of this process have never been demonstrated to be a problem.

After priming the surface, an adhesive is applied and light cured. Surfaces of the cured bonding agents are initially air inhibited and do not immediately react. However, as composite is placed against the surface, the air is displaced and copolymerization occurs.

Self-etch systems have the great advantages of eliminating the risk of incomplete primer/adhesive penetration into the collagen scaffold and also eliminating the subjectivity when determining the amount of moisture on the dentin surface ideal for primer diffusion. With these systems, the smear layer is dissolved and incorporated into the hybrid layer. The bonding mechanism for strong self-etch adhesives is very similar to that of etch-and-rinse systems. Their bond strength, particularly for all-in-one systems, is relatively low, probably because of their high initial acidity and high water content. Mild self-etch systems demineralize dentin only superficially (a few microns) and leave residual hydroxyapatite attached to collagen fibers. Although the main bonding mechanism is the interlocking between collagen fibers and the polymerized resin, monomers such as 4-META (4-methacryloxyethyl-trimellitic anhydride) and 10-MDP (10-methacryloyloxydecyl dihydrogen phosphate) may bond to this residual hydroxyapatite. Also, the presence of hydroxyapatite may help protect the collagen against degradation, which weakens the bonded interface. Mild self-etch systems may present relatively low bond strength values when applied to sclerotic dentin. Another drawback associated with all-in-one systems is that, due to their high water content, they behave as semipermeable membranes, which increases degradation by hydrolysis.

Bonding to Other Substrates
Cast Alloys

Sandblasting with aluminum oxide is the most commonly used method to prepare metal substrates for receiving bonding resins or resin cements. It creates a micro-retentive, high energy surface. Electrolytic etching can be used with base metal alloys, but is not as effective with noble alloys because of its more homogeneous microstructure. Tin-plating can be used to improve the retention of noble alloys to resin cements. Commercial systems using silica-coating at high temperatures or tribochemical application of a silica layer using aluminum oxide modified by silicic acid have also been available for many years. In both cases, a silane solution is applied to the treated metal to create a surface capable of bonding to dimethacrylate-based resins.

Monomers such as 10-MDP and 4-META are used in formulations of resin cements to improve retention

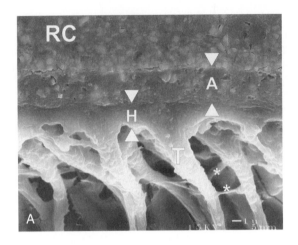

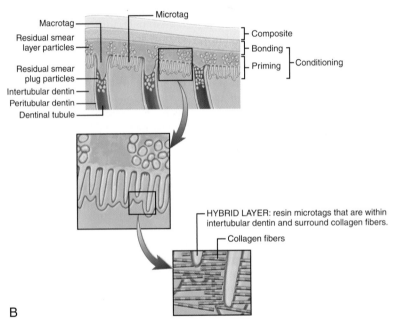

B

FIGURE 13.8 **Adhesion to dentin. A,** Scanning electron micrograph of interface bonded with a dental adhesive (final magnification: ×4000). Note the visible thickness of the adhesive layer (**A,** *arrowheads*) beneath the resin composite (*RC*). The hybrid layer (*H, arrowheads*) is 2 μm thick. The tubular resin tags (*T*) show lateral branches (*asterisks*). **B,** Schematic showing that etching removes hydroxyapatite crystals within intertubular dentin and along peritubular dentin. Primer penetrates intertubular spaces and fluid-filled tubular spaces. Cured primer forms microtags within intertubular dentin and macrotags within tubules. *(A, from Frankenberger R, Perdigão J, Rosa BT, et al: Dent. Mater. 17, 373-380, 2001.)*

of cast alloy restorations. They seem to be more effective with base metal alloys, compared to noble alloys. Metal primers developed for improving the bond strength between alloy and resin cements are also available. However, research results are inconsistent.

Ceramics

Low-strength, silica-based ceramics have been successfully bonded to resin cements by etching the restoration's inner surface with a hydrofluoric acid solution, followed by the application of a silane primer (Figure 13-9). Different acid concentrations are commercially available, from 2.5% to 10%, in liquid or gel forms, and recommended etching times vary from 1 to 4 minutes. Hydrofluoric acid attacks the glass phase of ceramics, to the point where crystals are removed, leaving a microretentive honeycomb-like, high-energy surface. Silane application improves the wettability of the resin cement on the ceramic surface and establishes covalent bonds with both the ceramic surface (via siloxane bonds, -Si-O-Si-) and the resin cement (by carbon double bond

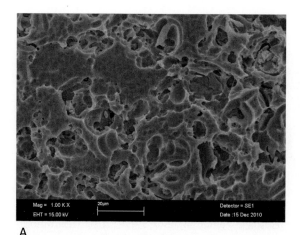

A

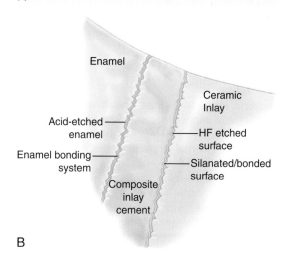

B

FIGURE 13.9 **Etched porcelain. A,** Scanning electron micrograph (SEM) of etched porcelain. **B,** Schematic of materials and interfaces involved in bonding all-ceramic restorations to tooth structure. *(Part A From Cesar PF, Yoshimura HN, Miranda Junior WG, et al: Correlations between fracture toughness and leucite content in dental porcelains. J. Dent. 33(9):721-729, 2005.)*

polymerization). Hydrolysis of the silane molecule is necessary to convert the methoxy groups ($-OCH_3$) to silanol ($-Si-OH$). Silanes are presented in a nonhydrolyzed form (two bottles) or prehydrolyzed (one bottle). In general, prehydrolyzed silanes are less stable, with shorter shelf-life than nonhydrolyzed solutions.

Bonding of high-strength ceramics remain a subject of debate among clinicians and researchers. The higher the crystalline content, the less efficient is acid etching. Airborne particle abrasion with 110 μm alumina and tribochemical silica coating are recommended with glass-infiltrated or densely-sintered alumina, as well as zirconia ceramics. Self-adhesive resin cements have also shown good results with zirconia restorations.

Indirect (Laboratory) Composites

A microretentive bonding surface is obtained with alumina sandblasting. Etching with 37% phosphoric acid is used to clean the surface from debris, prior to the application of the resin cement. Etching with hydrofluoric acid is not recommended, because it causes degradation of the composite surface.

Amalgam

Adhesive systems, filled adhesives, and resin cements can be used in association with amalgam in the so-called *bonded amalgam* restoration. The purpose of this technique is to reduce the need for macromechanical retention, which would save tooth structure, and reinforce the remaining structure by creating a bonded interface between the restorative material and the cavity walls. The bonding between the adhesive and the amalgam is achieved by the establishment of an interpenetration zone. Although laboratorial studies show better results for bonded amalgams compared to conventional, nonbonded amalgam in terms of bond strength, microleakage, and retention, these findings are not supported by clinical data, which show no difference between bonded restorations and those retained by mechanical undercuts.

Fiber Posts

Bonding fiber-reinforced resin posts to radicular dentin is one of the most challenging situations faced by the clinician. Adhesive application is critical, because it is virtually impossible to control moisture inside the root canal. The use of self-etching adhesives systems is not indicated, because their acidity would impede the chemical activation of the resin cement. The use of self-adhesive resin cements (see page 13-26) has shown promising results in laboratory evaluations. The surface treatment of the post has also been debated. Silanization, sandblasting, or the association of both treatments are often quoted as being effective procedures to improve the bonding between the resin cement and the fiber post.

Repair of Composite, Ceramic, and Ceramic-Metal Restorations

Repair of fractured restorations is indicated when the extent of the fracture does not recommend the replacement of the restoration or when there are other factors taken into consideration, such as conservation of the tooth structure, cost, time, or in case of fixed prostheses, the replacement of multiple units.

Aging of composite restorations in the oral environment severely decreases the composite-to-composite bond strength. Therefore, the use of adhesive systems to mediate the bond between the aged and the fresh composite is recommended. The surface can be roughened with the use of intra-oral sandblasters or a diamond bur, followed by phosphoric acid application for cleaning, prior to adhesive application.

The repair of chipped ceramic restorations includes conditioning with hydrofluoric acid, silanization, application of a bonding resin, and restoration with a resin composite. Intra-oral use of hydrofluoric acid must be performed with rubber dam isolation, because of its caustic effect on soft tissues.

Repair of metal-ceramic restorations includes bonding to different substrates. When there is a large area of the metal infrastructure exposed, sandblasting with alumina or alumina modified with silicic acid is recommended, followed by the application of silane and adhesive resin, prior to composite application. Porcelain fractured surface can be sandblasted and etched with hydrofluoric acid prior to silanization, adhesive application, and restoration with composite.

CLASSIFICATION AND CHARACTERISTICS OF LUTING AGENTS

Classification

Luting agents can be classified according to the length of time they are expected to stay in function as provisional or definitive. Provisional (temporary) cements are indicated for fixation of temporary restorations used between the clinical appointments necessary to finish the definitive restoration. Because temporary restorations often need to be removed during treatment, provisional cements must have a relatively low strength and be easily handled. Also, they must not irritate the pulp. Examples of temporary luting agents are zinc oxide–eugenol and noneugenol cements and calcium hydroxide pastes. Definitive cements are supposed to remain in function for the longest time possible and, for such, must have sufficient properties.

According to setting mechanism, luting agents are divided in those presenting an acid-base reaction (which include glass-ionomer, resin-modified glass ionomer, zinc oxide–eugenol, zinc polycarboxylate, and zinc phosphate) and those setting by polymerization (resin cements, compomers, and self-adhesive resin cements). In some cases, this classification refers to the predominant setting mechanism because resin-modified glass ionomers contain polymerizable groups, whereas compomers and self-adhesive resin cements may have an acid-base reaction.

The physical requirements of luting cements are described in the following standards from the International Association for Standardization: ISO 3107:2004 (zinc oxide–eugenol and noneugenol cements), ISO 9917-1:2007 (powder/liquid acid-base cements), ISO 9917-2:2010 (resin-modified cements), and ISO 4049:2009 (polymer-based cements) standards (Box 13-1). Those requirements, along with other important characteristics are described below.

Biocompatibility

Luting agents are often placed in contact with large areas of exposed dentin. Also, remaining dentin thickness can be insufficient to protect the pulp tissue from external stimuli. The majority of the luting agents show cytotoxicity in vitro, to different degrees. Histological studies also show an early inflammatory reaction to cements placed close to connective tissue. Such responses are usually associated to the initial low pH acid-base cements and self-etch resin cements or monomers present in resin-modified glass ionomers and resin cements.

Interfacial Sealing and Anticariogenic Activity

The perfect sealing of the tooth/restoration interface is important to prevent bacteria penetration that may lead to secondary caries and also, when dentin is involved, prevent excessive fluid movement in the dentinal tubules that may cause hypersensitivity. Sealing is related to the ability of the cement to penetrate in the irregularities of both substrates and establish an intimate contact with them. Ideally, luting cements should not shrink upon setting, or voids may

---

BOX 13.1

ISO Standards for dental cements

ISO 3107:2004 (zinc oxide–eugenol and noneugenol cements)

ISO 9917-1:2007 (powder:liquid acid-base cements)

ISO 9917-2:2010 (resin-modified cements)

ISO 4049:2009 (polymer-based cements)

develop at the interface. Adhesion also contributes for a good interfacial sealing. Fluoride-containing cements are supposed to inhibit bacterial activity, however, the clinical significance of fluoride release from luting cements is yet to be confirmed.

Adhesion

Lack of retention is a common cause of failure of indirect restorations. The use of adhesive materials may reduce the risk of displacement. In some instances (e.g., porcelain crowns), bonding may reduce the risk of restoration fracture. Adhesion may also help improve interfacial sealing. Adhesion may occur by chemical or physical bonding, micromechanical interlocking, or friction. Some acid-base cements and self-adhesive resin cements bond to dental tissues by chelation involving metal ions and carboxylic or phosphate groups. Resin cements require the use of adhesive systems to establish a strong bond to dentin and enamel.

Mechanical Properties

Mechanically, luting cements are described in terms of strength (usually in compression or in flexure), elastic modulus, fatigue resistance, fracture toughness, and wear. Wear is less of a problem when the cement line is not exposed to masticatory forces (e.g., a full crown). Fatigue strength is usually considered more representative of the type of loading cements must endure in the clinic. However, fatigue tests are a lot more time-consuming than static strength tests. Elastic modulus expresses the amount of elastic (recoverable) deformation the cement presents relative to a stress state caused by external loading. Fracture toughness describes the resistance to unstable crack propagation that will cause catastrophic failure of the material.

Permanent luting cements must have high strength (both static and fatigue) and fracture toughness and good wear resistance. Ideal values for elastic modulus are debatable, and values can vary substantially even among permanent cements. Temporary cements, on the other hand, must have a relatively low strength, or removal of temporary restoration can become a difficult task.

Handling Properties and Radiopacity

Ease of use, long working time, and short setting time are desirable characteristics of luting cements. Along with powder and liquid materials, recent products are encapsulated or presented as two-paste, self-dispensing systems, which makes proportioning and mixing faster and less prone to error. A long working time is important to make sure the

cement presents low viscosity while the restoration is seated. Otherwise, adaptation may be compromised. For some materials (e.g., resin cements), removal of excess cement also needs to be done before setting. Radiopacity is important to allow radiographic diagnostic.

Viscosity and Film Thickness

A low film thickness is important to allow for the correct seating of the restoration. Film thickness is usually determined by the cement average particle size and its viscosity. Some cements are pseudoplastic, looking excessively thick at the end of the mixing period, but they flow well under load. Overall, if handled properly and applied within the recommended working time, all currently available materials are able to reach a thickness below that required by the ISO standards. However, some cements may show a sudden increase in viscosity and film thickness in short intervals after the end of the recommended working time.

Solubility

Solubility refers to the resistance to disintegration and dissolution when the cement is immersed in water or other solutions. It affects the marginal integrity of the indirect restoration, which may increase plaque accumulation. Resin-based cements present much lower solubility than acid-base cements.

Esthetics

When used with translucent materials or when restoration margins are exposed, shade and translucency of the cement are important aspects to be considered, because they may affect the final esthetic result of the restoration. It is particularly critic with porcelain laminate veneers. Resin cements are the most esthetic luting materials available. Glass ionomer, resin-modified glass ionomer, compomer, and self-adhesive resin cements also have good esthetics. Zinc polyacrylate, zinc oxide–eugenol, and zinc phosphate are opaque.

ACID-BASE CEMENTS

Zinc Oxide–Eugenol and Noneugenol Cements

The reaction between zinc oxide and eugenol has several applications in dentistry, such as endodontic sealers and root-end filling materials, periodontal coating, inelastic impression materials, cavity base, and temporary restorations. For luting purposes, different formulations of zinc oxide–eugenol (ZOE) cements are available for both temporary cementation and permanent fixation of metallic and metalloceramic crowns and bridges. Due to an inhibitory effect of eugenol on polymerization of methacrylate-based resins and luting composites, temporary cements using nonphenolic components are often preferred over conventional formulations. Their popularity is justified by their ease of use, antibacterial action, and anodyne effect on dental pulp.

Composition

The powder is basically zinc oxide, with up to 8% of other zinc salts (acetate, propionate, or succinate) as accelerators. Rosin (abietic acid) is added to reduce brittleness and increase working time and strength. The liquid contains eugenol (4-allyl-2-methoxy phenol), a weak acid. Acetic acid (up to 2%) is added as accelerator. In two-paste materials used for temporary cementation, one paste contains zinc oxide mixed with mineral or vegetable oils, whereas fillers are incorporated into eugenol to form the other paste. Noneugenol materials use long chain aliphatic acids or aryl-substituted butyric acid to react with zinc oxide particles. Other oils can be added to adjust paste consistency.

An important improvement of ZOE cements was the development of materials in which the liquid is a mixture of 2-ethoxybenzoic acid (EBA) and eugenol, roughly in a 2:1 proportion. Rather than forming a stronger matrix, the addition of EBA allows for the use of very high powder:liquid ratios (6:1) which, *per se*, increases the strength of the set cement. In these materials, alumina (30%) was added to the powder as reinforcing agent. The incorporation of 20% particulated poly(methyl methacrylate) is also used to improve mechanical properties in some products.

Setting Reaction and Structure

The reaction of zinc oxide with eugenol results in the formation of a zinc eugenolate chelate, that is, a complex in which one zinc (Zn) atom binds to two eugenolate molecules. Also, as mentioned above, the dissociation constant of eugenol is small. Therefore, reaction rate is increased with the use of more reactive oxides, along with the presence of accelerators. The acid-base reaction does not take place in an aqueous medium; however, water plays a very important role in the reaction, because it reacts with zinc oxide forming $ZnOH^+$ ions that dissociate in Zn^{2+} and OH^-. The zinc cations then react with the eugenolate, whereas the hydroxyl anions react with the H^+ forming water. Because water is present as reagent and final product, the reaction is autocatalytic. The presence of acetic acid eliminates the need of water to initiate the reaction.

The structure of the set cement is represented by zinc oxide particles bound together by an amorphous zinc eugenolate matrix. EBA also forms a chelate with zinc oxide, and crystalline phases have been identified within the matrix of EBA-eugenol cements.

Manipulation can be found on the book's website http://evolve.elsevier.com/sakaguchi/restorative ⊖

Properties

ZOE cements are considered biocompatible because of their neutral pH, antibacterial action, and anodyne effect on hyperemic pulpal tissue. Their antibacterial activity *in vitro* was shown to be more efficient than those displayed by conventional and resin-modified glass ionomers. That characteristic associated with a good marginal sealing favors the recovery of the pulp. Eugenol released from the salt matrix may contribute to pain relief in preparations with little remaining dentin thickness. However, in high concentrations or when placed directly in contact with connective tissue, it may increase the inflammatory response because of its cytotoxicity.

The low strength displayed by ZOE cements makes them a suitable material for temporary cementation. The ISO 3107 standard (2004) establishes a maximum 24-hour compressive strength of 35 MPa for type 1 materials (i.e., intended for temporary cementation). An important aspect related to the mechanical behavior of ZOE cements is that their properties are very sensitive to temperature. For example, compressive strength at 37° C may represent only 20% of what was found at 23° C. EBA-eugenol cements can be several times stronger than the basic formulation (72 MPa versus 26 MPa, in compression at room temperature). EBA-alumina cements can present 20% higher strength compared to EBA-eugenol materials. Even though these values are above the minimum compressive strength required for type 2 materials (i.e., permanent luting cements) of 35 MPa, both reinforced ZOE cements are the weakest among luting agents used for permanent cementation. The elastic modulus of EBA-eugenol cements (determined at room temperature) is 3 GPa.

ZOE cements present increased plasticity even after set and flow under load. Plastic strain at fracture was shown to be above 15% at 37° C, against a maximum value of 4% presented by other acid-base and resin cements. Creep behavior may explain the good marginal seal achieved with these materials, even considering their setting shrinkage. Linear shrinkage values of wet samples after 24 hours was shown to be 0.31% for the basic ZOE formulation, 0.38% for EBA-eugenol, and 0.12% for EBA-eugenol/alumina cements.

Film thickness measured according to the ISO standard ranges between 16 and 28 μm for

EBA/alumina materials; therefore, it is close to the maximum value allowed. Simulated crowns cemented with a basic formulation and an EBA-eugenol cement showed similar film thicknesses at the occlusal surface (20-25 μm), whereas for the EBA-alumina cement, film thickness was higher (57 μm).

The zinc eugenolate matrix chelate is very unstable in water. Its hydrolysis forms eugenol and zinc hydroxide, releasing the zinc oxide particles exposed in the process. *In vitro* studies showed that zinc 2-ethoxybenzoate matrix formd in EBA-eugenol cements is even more prone to hydrolysis than the zinc eugenolate. In vivo, material loss after 6 months was 3 to 7 times higher for an EBA-alumina compared to other acid-base cements. Clinically, fixed prostheses cemented with EBA-alumina cement showed a success rate of 92% after 2.5 years, whereas for zinc polycarboxylate, it was 95%. Zinc phosphate, for many decades the "gold standard" for permanent luting agents, showed a success rate of 98%.

The inhibitory effect of methoxyphenols such as eugenol on the polymerization of methacrylate resins is of clinical importance. Eugenol is considered a *free-radical scavenger*, due to the presence of the allyl group in its structure acting as a degradative chain-transfer agent (i.e., when activated, it preferably undergoes primary radical termination, rather than propagation). Temporary cements containing eugenol may negatively affect the polymerization of methylmethacrylate used in provisional restorations. If the final restoration will be bonded to the prepared tooth, the polymerization of both the adhesive system and the resin cement may be inhibited, increasing the risk of debonding, or even fracture in case of low-strength ceramic or indirect composite restorations. In fact, in ZOE cement/composite interfaces, composite mechanical properties were reduced up to a 100 μm away from the interface, which may be relevant if the resin cement is applied to a eugenol-contaminated surface. However, several *in vitro* investigations have shown that bond strength to dentin is not adversely affected if the surface is thoroughly cleaned prior to adhesive application.

Glass Ionomer

Glass ionomer (or glass polyalkeonate) cement is arguably one of the most popular materials for permanent cementation used in the clinic, along with resin cements. The chemistry that is the basis for these cements is similar to that in glass ionomer restorative, lining, and preventive materials (see Chapter 9), although there are some important differences in working and setting behavior to fit the needs of luting agents. Besides good physical properties, glass ionomers adhere to the tooth structure and metals and, most importantly, release significant amounts of fluoride, which increase the resistance of enamel and dentin to acid dissolution and act as a bacteriostatic agent. Fluoride release makes this material the first choice for cementation of orthodontic bands. It is indicated for cementation of metallic and metal-ceramic restorations, as well as high-strength ceramic crowns and fixed prostheses. Its setting reaction is sensitive to moisture conditions, and for this reason, it is extremely important to protect the cement against gain and loss of water during the first 24 hours.

Composition

Details of chemical composition and setting reaction are provided in Chapter 9. The powder is a calcium fluoroaluminosilicate glass with maximum particle size of 15 μm. Other glasses can be formulated in which calcium is replaced by strontium or lanthanum to increase radiopacity. The basic character of the glass is defined by its alumina:silica ratio and, in order to react with acids, it must exceed 1:2 by mass. Large amounts of fluoride are incorporated in the glass by adding calcium and sodium fluoride to the other oxides. Fluoride is an important component, because it lowers the melting point and enhances the translucency of the powder and improves the consistency of the mixing paste and the strength of the set material. The presence of electropositive ions, such as Ca^{2+} and Na^+, is important to balance the electrical charges in the basic aluminosilicate lattice. Zinc oxide and barium glasses can be added to the powder to increase radiopacity.

The liquid contains homopolymers of acrylic acid or copolymers of acrylic, itaconic, maleic, and tricarboxylic acids. Overall, high molecular weights and increased acid concentrations improve physical properties of the set cement, but they also increase the viscosity of the liquid. Therefore, commercial materials usually employ polyacids with average molecular weight of 10,000 g/mol and concentrations around 45% by mass. Dextrotartaric, or (+)-tartaric, acid (around 5% by mass) is an important component of the liquid, because it accelerates the setting without shortening working time. Its presence increases cement strength and allows for the use of glasses with higher fluoride content and, therefore, higher translucency.

To avoid the increase in viscosity of the liquid after prolonged storage, some products contain the polyacid freeze-dried and added to the powder. In this case, the powder is mixed with distilled water or a tartaric acid solution. Such presentation adds the advantage of allowing the use of polyacids with higher molecular weight and in higher concentrations, which increases the strength of the set material.

Setting Reaction and Structure

When the powder is brought in contact with the acid solution, H^+ from the acid attacks the glass, releasing metal ions (Al^{3+}, Ca^{2+}, Na^+, and F^-) and silicic acid (general formula: $[SiO_x(OH)_{4-2x}]_n$). Refer to page 182 Chapter 9. The silicic acid condenses on the ion-depleted outer layer of the particle forming a layer of silica gel. Calcium ions are preferentially released from the glass. As the concentration of ions in the solution increases, the pH raises and metal ions begin to condense among the poly(acrylic acid) chains precipitating the polyacrylate salts, initially in a sol state (initial set) and later turning into a gel. The precipitation of aluminum salts initiates after a few hours into the reaction because it is released from the glass as a strong complex with fluoride. The reaction continues until all the ions are bound to the polyacrylate. From a clinical standpoint, the fact that ions remain in solution for extended periods of time before reacting with the polyanions, even after the initial set, is critical. If ions are washed out from the cement, the structure of the polysalt matrix is irreversibly compromised. Also, calcium polyacrylate is more vulnerable to dissolution in water than the aluminum polyacrylate formed at later stages. On the other hand, water plays a very important role in the reaction and in the set cement, because it remains tightly bound to the cement structure, hydrating the silica gel layer and involving the cation-polyacrylate bonds. Therefore, a high relative humidity (approximately 80%) is the ideal condition for the setting reaction to take place.

The (+)-tartaric acid is stronger than poly(acrylic acid) and therefore reacts first with the glass and can form complexes with metal cations at lower pH. Its presence extends working time by delaying the formation of calcium polyacrylate, and upon gelation it accelerates setting by increasing the deposition rate of aluminum polyacrylate.

The set cement is constituted by a hydrogel of calcium, aluminum, and fluoroaluminum polyacrylates involving the unreacted glass particles sheathed by a weakly bonded siliceous hydrogel layer. About 20% to 30% of the glass is dissolved in the reaction. Smaller glass particles may be entirely dissolved and replaced by siliceous hydrogel particles containing fluorite crystallites. The stability of the matrix is given by an association of chain entanglement, weak ionic cross-linking, and hydrogen bonding.

Manipulation can be found on the book's website http://evolve.elsevier.com/sakaguchi/restorative ☺

Properties

Glass ionomer cements are considered mild to the pulp compared to their predecessors, which used phosphoric acid solutions. However, inflammatory response is more intense than that associated with ZOE cements. In fact, the biocompatibility of glass ionomers is controversial, and in vitro results seem to vary according to the commercial brand tested. In general, there is some consensus regarding the fact that freshly mixed cements may present different degrees of cytotoxicity and cause a mild transient inflammatory response when placed in contact with pulpal connective tissue, but such response is greatly attenuated if at least 1-mm thickness of dentin is present. Besides a low remaining dentin thickness, the risk of postoperative sensitivity increases if a faulty technique is used. Thin mixtures seem to increase the risk of sensitivity. Rather than pulpal irritation, it is possible that postoperative pain may be related to the hydrostatic pressure exerted by the cement through the dentin tubules.

Glass ionomer cements release significant amounts of fluoride, both in the short and long term, which was shown to have an important anticariogenic effect. Fluoride release increases the resistance of enamel to acid dissolution, by inhibiting bacterial growth and interfering with the metabolism of the dental plaque. The use of glass ionomer for orthodontic bonding reduced the risk of white spots formation almost by half compared to a resin cement. However, when patients were exposed to fluoride-containing toothpaste, no differences in enamel or dentin demineralization under accumulated plaque were observed in the short term between an ionomeric and a resin cement. It must be emphasized that the surface area of the luting cement exposed to the oral environment is small. Therefore, the amount of fluoride released to the adjacent structures, as well as the fluoride recharging ability of the cement layer may be less clinically relevant compared to direct glass ionomer restorations.

Bonding to tooth structures is one of the main characteristics of glass ionomers. It helps to enhance the marginal sealing of the restoration compared to nonadhesive cements, but is not high enough to significantly increase retention. The proposed adhesion mechanism is twofold: it occurs by the displacement of phosphate and calcium ions from the hydroxyapatite by carboxylate ions pendant from the polyacid chains bond and the incorporation of these carboxylate groups into the hydroxyapatite structure and also by micromechanical interlocking achieved by a shallow hybridization of the partially demineralized dentin. Dentin surface treatment with 10% to 20% polyacrylic acid for 5 to 20 seconds (shorter times for higher concentrations) significantly increases bond strength by removing the smear layer, partially demineralizing the surface creating microporosities for micromechanical interlocking, and enhancing the chemical interaction of poly(alkenoic acid) with the hydroxyapatite. A solution containing 3% to 10%

citric acid is also effective because Fe^{3+} ions deposited on the dentin surface increase the interaction with the cement. Bond strength of glass ionomer to dentin and enamel varies according to commercial product tested, but when loaded in shear it is around 2 to 5 MPa. Glass ionomer cements bond well to stainless steel, noble, and nonnoble alloys and titanium, but not to high-strength core ceramics.

Its mechanical properties are superior to other acid-base cements and increases significantly over long periods. Compressive strength is between 100 and 150 MPa; therefore, it is far beyond the minimum of 70 MPa specified in the ISO 9917 standard. These cements are much weaker in tension because of their brittle nature, with diametral tensile strengths of about 6 MPa. Elastic modulus is around 15 GPa. Film thickness is below the maximum allowed by the ISO standard (25 μm) and should not prevent the correct seating of the restoration, if the cement is properly handled.

Erosion tests in vitro using citric acid showed that the fully set glass ionomers are more resistant than nonadhesive acid-base luting cements and erode in levels similar to those shown by enamel and dentin. Such behavior may be related to the silica gel layer that envelopes the glass particles.

Resin-Modified Glass Ionomer

Resin-modified (or hybrid) glass ionomers set by both an acid-base and a polymerization reaction. The technology was originally developed for direct restoratives, but as with resin cements, the chemistry was adapted to formulate materials for luting cements. Although details of chemistry and setting reactions of resin-modified glass ionomer systems are provided in Chapter 9, this section gives a brief overview pertinent to luting cements. This class of cements does not show the early sensitivity to moisture conditions presented by conventional glass ionomers because of the presence of a polymeric phase, which prevents the loss of water and metal ions from the immature polysalt matrix. Available as a powder-liquid, paste-paste, or capsules, self-cured resin-modified glass ionomer luting cements are indicated for permanent cementation of ceramic-metal crowns and fixed prostheses; metal inlays, onlays, and crowns; prefabricated or cast posts; high-strength core ceramics; and luting of orthodontic appliances. A light-cured version indicated for bracket bonding was also developed.

Composition

The chemistry of resin-modified glass ionomers is more complex than that of conventional glass ionomers (see Chapter 9). In powder-liquid systems, the powder contains fluoroaluminosilicate glass particles similar in composition to those found in conventional glass ionomers. Catalysts for the self-cure (redox) polymerization are added to the powder. The liquid may contain poly(acrylic acids) modified with pendant methacrylate groups replacing a small part of the carboxylic radicals, HEMA (2-hydroxyethyl methacrylate), water, and tartaric acid. HEMA replaces part of the water and is a small molecule (molecular weight: 130 g/mol) soluble in water due to the presence of a hydroxyl group in its structure. Another liquid formulation contains similar concentrations (around 25%-30% each) of a copolymer of poly(acrylic acid), HEMA, and water, and smaller amounts of low-viscosity dimethacrylate resins (such as urethane or triethyleneglycol dimethacrylates). Initiators for the light-cured polymerization, if present, are found in the liquid.

Formulations of paste-paste materials are brand-specific. Basically, one of the pastes contains the glass particles, HEMA, and a dispersing agent. Water and the reducing agent of the self-cure activation may be present, or a urethane dimethacrylate. The other paste contains the modified poly(acrylic acid), water, the oxidizing agent of the activation system, and fillers and may present HEMA or a high-viscosity dimethacrylate monomer, such as Bis-GMA (biphenol A glycidyl methacrylate).

Setting Reaction and Structure

The setting reaction of resin-modified glass ionomer cement comprises two different mechanisms. The initial set is the result of either a light-cured or self-cured polymerization reaction of the methacrylate groups, present as pendant groups in the poly(acrylic acid) chain, in the HEMA molecule, or in the dimethacrylate monomers. Refer to reactions in Chapter 9. The acid-base reaction, described in the previous section, is slower than in conventional glass ionomers because of the lower water content. The HEMA polymer and the polysalt are linked by hydrogen bonds. However, phase separation between the two matrices formed may occur. The use of a modified poly(acrylic acid) prevents phase separation, because the carbon double bond in the HEMA structure may polymerize with the pendant methacrylate from the polyacid chain. As a result, the cement matrix is formed by both ionic and covalent crosslinks. For further discussion, refer to Chapter 9.

Manipulation can be found on the book's website http://evolve.elsevier.com/sakaguchi/restorative ⊖

Properties

Resin-modified glass ionomers are considered less biocompatible than conventional glass ionomers because of the presence of HEMA. Besides its already mentioned allergenic effect, it is a potential source for adverse reactions in the pulp. The largest amounts of HEMA are released in the first 24 hours, but release continues for several days. When resin-modified glass ionomer was placed in direct contact with human pulpal connective tissue, inflammatory responses from mild to severe and a large necrotic area were observed after almost 1 year. It is volatile, so there is risk of inhalation and eye irritation. The release of free HEMA from the cement is higher in undercured materials. Therefore, a correct mixing technique must be used to optimize the polymerization. In light-cured materials, the recommended exposure must be followed.

In vitro fluoride release by conventional and resin-modified luting glass ionomers was found to be similar over a 28-day period, ranging from 99 to 198 ppm. Mineral loss and lesion depth around orthodontic brackets *in vitro* were significantly lower with resin-modified glass ionomers, compared to one resin cement and one luting compomer. Fluoride release is higher after 24 hours, stabilizing after 2 weeks.

Resin-modified glass ionomer cements show shear bond strength to conditioned dentin (10% citric acid, 2% ferric chloride for 20 seconds) or enamel (10% polyacrylic acid solution for 20 seconds) in the range of 8 to 12 MPa. The bonding mechanisms are the same described for conventional glass ionomers. The lower bond strength to enamel compared to resin cements may actually facilitate orthodontic bracket debonding. They bond to metal alloys and high-strength ceramics, with initial shear bond strengths of 2 to 5 MPa. Bond strength to metal alloy is significantly increased with the use of metal primers. Because of the presence of methacrylate groups, these cements bond well to resin composites. Retention of metal-ceramic crowns to prepared teeth may vary significantly between the two-paste and the powder:liquid versions of the same product, and it is usually higher in the latter.

In terms of mechanical properties, resin-modified glass ionomer cements show compressive strength similar to conventional glass ionomers, between 90 and 140 MPa, and lower elastic modulus (3-6 GPa). Flexural strength may vary between 15 and 30 MPa. Film thickness determined at room temperature 2 minutes after the start of mixing may vary between 9 to 25 μm. However, film thickness may increase substantially if the restoration is not placed within the recommended working time.

The presence of HEMA increases the water sorption of resin-modified glass ionomers, compared to conventional glass ionomers and resin cements. In fact, some manufacturers do not recommend its use for luting low-strength ceramic crowns because of the risk of fracture caused by swelling of the cement. Water uptake after 7 days measured according to the

ISO 4049 may be 3 to 9 times higher compared to resin cements. Solubility in water is also higher compared to resin cements, about 2 to 4 times. In lactic acid (pH = 4), the solubility of some resin-modified glass ionomers is about 10 times higher than resin cements.

RESIN-BASED CEMENTS

Resin Cements

Overview

Resin cements are low-viscosity composite materials with filler distribution and initiator content adjusted to allow for a low film thickness and suitable working and setting times. They have a wide range of applications, from inlays to fixed bridges, prefabricated posts, and orthodontic appliances. They are mandatory materials for luting low-strength ceramic and laboratory-processed composite restorations, but can also be used with cast restorations, particularly in cases where extra retention is needed. The ISO specification 4049 (2009) classifies resin cements according to curing mode as class 1 (self-cured), class 2 (light-cured) or class 3 (dual-cured). Most of the commercial products are dual-cured, combining chemical and light-activation mechanisms. These materials show a comfortable working time and cure on command characteristic of light-cured composites, and also the security of high degrees of conversion even in areas not reached by the light. Class 1 and class 3 materials are typically hand- or auto-mixed two-paste systems (base and catalyst). Self-cured and dual-cured materials can be opaque or translucent, and those indicated for cementation of ceramic restorations are usually provided in several shades. Light-cured materials are indicated for bonding of laminated ceramic veneers (esthetic cements) or orthodontic brackets. Some esthetic resin cements used for cementation of veneers include glycerin-based, water-soluble "try-in" pastes to help with shade selection.

Composition

Most resin cements share a very similar composition to that of restorative composites, which are described in Chapter 9. The organic matrix contains dimethacrylate monomers and oligomers. High-molecular-weight molecules such as Bis-GMA (bisphenol-A glycidyl dimethacrylate, Mw = 512 g/mol), UDMA (urethane dimethacrylate, Mw = 480 g/mol), and Bis-EMA (ethoxylated Bis-GMA, Mw = 540 g/mol) are combined with smaller molecules usually derived from ethylene glycol dimethacryles (DEGDMA, Mw = 242 g/mol, and TEGDMA, Mw = 286 g/mol) to achieve a high degree of conversion with a relatively low volumetric shrinkage. The filler fraction may vary between 30% and 66% by volume and contains silanated radiopaque glasses such as barium, strontium, or zirconia, along with silica particles. Average filler size may vary between 0.5 μm to 8.0 μm. Microfilled cements are also available, with an average filler size of 40 nm. Pigments and opacifiers are also present in both pastes.

Some adhesive resin cements contain proprietary monomers. One example combines 10-methacryloyloxydecyl dihydrogen phosphate (MDP), a polymerizable phosphoric acid ester, with Bis-GMA. Another product contains 4-methacryloxyethyl-trimellitic anhydride (4-META) and methylmethacrylate in the liquid, poly(methyl methacrylate) in the powder, and tri-n-butylborane (TBB) as catalyst.

Camphorquinone and a tertiary amine are present in one of the pastes to initiate the light-activated reaction. Benzoyl peroxide, the self-cure activator, is present in the catalyst paste. The amine functions as proton donor and is considered an accelerator of free-radical production. Aromatic amines (such as ethyl 4-dimethylaminobenzoate, EDMAB) are considered more efficient than aliphatic amines (such as 2-(dimethylamino)ethyl methacrylate, DMAEMA). The presence of amine in the composite matrix poses some clinically relevant concerns. First, amines are known to degrade over time, altering the shade of the cement. Second, they become inactive when in contact with acidic adhesive systems, and when cement polymerization takes place in the absence of light activation, the deleterious effect on degree of conversion may increase the risk of restoration debonding. It is important to point out that the relative amounts of self-cure and light-cure initiators vary a lot among commercial brands. Consequently, some materials are more dependent on light activation to achieve a high degree of conversion. Likewise, some commercial materials cure more promptly in the absence of light than others.

Setting Reaction and Structure

Resin cements set by free-radical polymerization resulting in the formation of a densely cross-linked structure involving the filler particles. Free radicals are generated by light activation, in which camphorquinone in the excited state combines with two amine molecules to generate two free-radicals. In the absence of light, free-radicals are formed by redox reaction of the amine-peroxide system. A crosslink is formed when a propagating chain encounters an unreacted carbon double bond in a different polymer chain. Polymerization proceeds until the mobility of the reactive species becomes restricted by the increasing viscosity of the material and free-radicals cannot propagate further, becoming entrapped in the polymer. Final degree of conversion is around 70% and depends on matrix formulation, initial viscosity, and curing mode. Conversion is usually higher in cases where the cement is dual-cured, compared to self-cured.

Manipulation can be found on the book's website http://evolve.elsevier.com/sakaguchi/restorative ⊖

Properties

Monomers released from resin cements are known to produce cytotoxic effects on connective tissue cells. Dual-cure resin cements show higher cytotoxicity at early setting stages when tested in self-cure mode, compared to specimens exposed to light-curing. After 7 days of incubation, Bis-GMA–based dual-cured cements are less cytotoxic than zinc polyacrylate, resin-modified glass ionomer, and a resin cement containing MDP monomer.

Mechanical properties of resin cements are defined by their filler content and degree of conversion reached by the organic matrix. As a rule of thumb, higher filler levels and higher conversion correspond to higher mechanical properties. Degree of conversion of dual-cure cements are between 50% and 73% in self-cure mode and 67% and 85% when light-cured. Compressive strength of dual- and light-cured resin composite cements have been reported from 180 to 300 MPa, therefore much superior to acid-base cements. Flexural strength is between 80 to 100 MPa, higher than the minimum value required by the ISO 4049 standard (50 MPa). Elastic modulus may vary significantly among commercial brands, between 4 and 10 GPa, values comparable to other cements. For dual-cure cements, mechanical properties are slightly higher when the cement is light-cured.

Film thicknesses measured according to ISO standards are between 13 and 20 μm, therefore within the maximum of 50 μm required by the ISO 4049. Water sorption and solubility of resin cements is much lower than that of resin-modified glass ionomer cements. However, the cement line may become apparent after a prolonged period of clinical use because of discoloration. Shrinkage of resin cements varies between 2% and 5%.

Immediate shear bond strength of resin cements to dentin varies between 12 and 18 MPa. MDP can bond to tooth structures, ceramics, and cast alloys by the reaction between its phosphate groups and calcium or with metal oxides. The integrity of the bonded interface is challenged by polymerization stress development. Polymerization stresses arise because of resin cement polymerization shrinkage, associated with the development of elastic behavior. In general, dual-cure cements develop higher polymerization stress values when light-cured because the curing reaction is faster than the self-cure reaction, allowing less time for viscous flow to accommodate the shrinkage before the resin composite reaches the vitrification stage. After the resin cement reaches the degree of conversion corresponding to the vitrification point of the organic matrix, all the shrinkage will contribute for stress build-up. When stresses at the interface surpass the bond strength of the adhesive layer to dentin or enamel, a contraction gap may form.

Compomers (polyacid-modified resin composites) can be found on the book's website http://evolve.elsevier.com/sakaguchi/restorative ⊖

Self-Adhesive Resin Cements

Self-adhesive resin cements were developed to provide clinicians with a luting agent with a very simple application procedure, combining the advantages of glass ionomers (adhesion, fluoride release) with mechanical properties comparable to those of resin cements. Presented as two-paste or powder:liquid, these materials are indicated for cementation of cast alloy single restorations and bridges, ceramic-metal crowns and bridges, ceramic (except veneers), and indirect composite restorations. Good results are also obtained with luting of prefabricated posts and high-strength ceramics.

Composition

Formulations are proprietary and vary among manufacturers. Overall, two-paste materials contain multifunctional monomers with phosphoric acid groups, dimethacrylate resins, and initiators for both light-cured and self-cured reactions in one of the pastes. The other paste contains fluoroaluminosilicate, silanated barium glasses, or both, and silanated silica particles, initiators, and methacrylate monomers. The filler fraction is around 70% by mass (50% by volume).

Setting Reaction and Structure

The main curing mechanism is via free-radical polymerization, either self-activated or dual-cured. An initial low pH is necessary for the adhesion mechanism (described below). At later stages, acidity is neutralized in some cements by the reaction between phosphoric acid groups and the alkaline glass. The structure of the set material is mainly a cross-linked polymer, covalently bonded to filler particles by the silane layer. Some ionic bridging between carboxylic groups and ions released by the glass may also be present.

Manipulation can be found on the book's website http://evolve.elsevier.com/sakaguchi/restorative ⊖

Properties

In terms of biocompatibility, self-adhesive resin cements present higher cytotoxicity than resin cements and acid-base cements. Cytotoxicity is reduced when cements are used in dual-cure mode. Their mechanical properties vary among commercial materials but, in general, are lower than those of conventional resin cements. Flexural strength is in the 50 to 100 MPa range and compressive strength is between 200 and 240 MPa. Values in the lower range are usually associated with the cement tested in self-cure mode, whereas higher values are obtained with light-activation. Film thickness is between 15 and 20 μm. Bonding mechanism to the tooth structures are supposed to occur by micromechanical interlocking and chemical interaction between the acidic groups and the hydroxyapatite. Initial shear bond strength to enamel varies from 3 to 15 MPa, intermediate between resin cements and glass ionomers. On dentin, some products have bond strengths comparable to resin cements. They show good bond strength values to metal alloys and high-strength ceramics. The presence of unreacted acid groups increases water sorption, in comparison to conventional resin cements. Their fluoride content is low (around 10%) and its beneficial effects have not been clinically proven.

Resin Cements for Provisional Restorations

These provisional cements are paste-paste systems, which can be dual- or light-cured. They are useful for cementation of interim restorations in the esthetic zone of the mouth, because they are tooth-colored and fairly translucent. They are easy to clean, and some release fluoride. Resin cementation of provisional restorations is useful when the final cement will also be resin because there is no eugenol present to potentially impair polymerization of the final cement. Composite cements used for cementation of provisional restorations have a substantially lower compressive strength than composite cements used for permanent cementation (25 to 70 MPa and 180 to 265 MPa, respectively).

SELECTED PROBLEMS

PROBLEM 1

The enamel portion of a tooth was etched with phosphoric acid for 15 seconds and rinsed. Upon observation, it did not appear frosty. What might explain the inadequate etch and what is a possible method to obtain a better etch?

Solution

The tooth may contain a higher than normal level of fluoride and thus may be resistant to normal etching. Apply the phosphoric acid for a longer period (up to 120 seconds) to obtain a frosty enamel appearance.

PROBLEM 2

During removal of an impression of a first molar with a composite core build-up, the core material debonded. What might explain the failed bond and what is a possible solution to obtain an adequate bond of the composite core material to the tooth?

Solution a

Self-cured composite core materials are popular because they are esthetic and easy to use. However, some self-cured composite cores are incompatible with certain light-cured bonding agents. Be sure to pick compatible composite core materials and bonding agents for this application.

Solution b

Choose a dual-cured bonding agent or use a light-cured composite core material.

PROBLEM 3

After etching, a dentist inadvertently overdried the tooth. Explain the problem and offer a solution.

Solution

Most modern bonding agents bond best to a moist tooth. If dentin is overdried, it is best to rehydrate it by applying a moist cotton pellet for 15 seconds before applying the primer of the bonding agent.

PROBLEM 4

A gold alloy casting seated properly before cementation but failed to seat when cemented with a glass ionomer cement. What factors might have caused this difficulty, and how can it be corrected?

Solution

An excessive film thickness of glass ionomer cement may result from (1) too high a powder/liquid ratio, (2) too long a time between completion of mixing and cementation, or (3) cement being placed on the tooth before being placed on the casting.

PROBLEM 5

To obtain a root-cement-post and core unit that is bonded, what type of cement would be best to use and what are some pitfalls to avoid?

Solution

Dual- or self-cured resin cement with a compatible adhesive system is the best option for post cementation. Light-cured resin cements may not completely polymerize at the apical end of the root. Many systems contain core build-up materials that are compatible with the cement. One type of adhesive cement forms strong bonds to alloy, ceramic, and tooth structure; however, it sets in anaerobic conditions. Therefore, this type of cement should never be placed inside the root canal, but only on the post before seating.

PROBLEM 6

A pressable, leucite-based ceramic crown was cemented with resin-modified glass ionomer cement. Subsequently, the crown fractured and had to be replaced. What could have been done to prevent this failure?

Solution

Any leucite-based ceramic is etchable and also not as strong as alumina- or zirconia-based materials. Therefore, this restoration should have been etched with hydrofluoric acid gel, silanated, and then bonded with a resin cement. The bonding process imparts strength to the entire restoration-tooth complex. Other all-ceramic materials such as zirconia, or alumina-based restorations are not etchable, but are much stronger, and therefore can be cemented with water-based cements.

Bibliography

Abo-Hamar SE, et al: Effect of temporary cements on the bond strength of ceramic luted to dentin, *Dent Mater* 21(9):794–803, 2005.

Wilson AD, Nicholson J: *Acid-base cements: their biomedical and industrial applications*, New York, 1993, Cambridge University Press, p 398.

Berry EA 3rd, Powers JM: Bond strength of glass ionomers to coronal and radicular dentin, *Oper Dent* 19(4): 122–126, 1994.

Bertolotti RL: Adhesion to porcelain and metal, *Dent Clin North Am* 51(2):433–451, 2007:ix-x.

Boeckh C, et al: Antibacterial activity of restorative dental biomaterials in vitro, *Caries Res* 36(2):101–107, 2002.

Braga RR, Ferracane JL, Condon JR: Polymerization contraction stress in dual-cure cements and its effect on interfacial integrity of bonded inlays, *J Dent* 30(7-8): 333–340, 2002.

Braga RR, et al: Adhesion to tooth structure: a critical review of "macro" test methods. *Dent Mater* 26(2):e38–49, 2010.

Brauer GM: New developments in zinc oxide-eugenol cement, *Ann Dent* 26(2):44–50, 1967.

Cardoso PE, Braga RR, Carrilho MR: Evaluation of microtensile, shear and tensile tests determining the bond strength of three adhesive systems, *Dent Mater* 14(6): 394–398, 1998.

Chin MY, et al: Fluoride release and cariostatic potential of orthodontic adhesives with and without daily fluoride rinsing, *Am J Orthod Dentofacial Orthop* 136(4):547–553, 2009.

Civjan S, Brauer GM: Physical Properties of Cements, Based on Zinc Oxide, Hydrogenated Rosin, O-Ethoxybenzoic Acid, and Eugenol, *J Dent Res* 43:281–299, 1964.

Davidson CL, Mjör IA: Advances in glass-ionomer cements 1999, Carol Stream.

dos Santos JG, et al: Shear bond strength of metal-ceramic repair systems, *J Prosthet Dent* 96(3):165–173, 2006.

Eisenburger M, Addy M, Rossbach A: Acidic solubility of luting cements, *J Dent* 31(2):137–142, 2003.

Farah JW, Powers JM, editors: Self-etching bonding agents, *Dent Advis* 27(9):1, 2010.

Farah JW, Powers JM, editors: Adhesive resin cements, *Dent Advis* 22(8):1, 2005.

Farah JW, Powers JM, editors: Bonding agents-2008, *Dent Advis* 25(5):1, 2008.

Farah JW, Powers JM, editors: Self-adhesive resin cements and esthetic resin cements, *Dent Advis* 26(2):1, 2009.

Farah JW, Powers JM, editors: Traditional crown and bridge cements, *Dent Advis* 23(2):1, 2006.

Fonseca RG, et al: Effect of metal primers on bond strength of resin cements to base metals, *J Prosthet Dent* 101(4):262–268, 2009.

Frankenberger R, Perdigão J, Rosa BT, Lopes M: "No-bottle" vs "multi-bottle" dentin adhesives–a microtensile bond strength and morphology study, *Dent Mater* 17(5):373–380, 2001.

Fujisawa S, Kadoma Y: Effect of phenolic compounds on the polymerization of methyl methacrylate, *Dent Mater* 8(5):324–326, 1992.

Furuchi M, et al: Effect of metal priming agents on bond strength of resin-modified glass ionomers joined to gold alloy, *Dent Mater J* 26(5):728–732, 2007.

Garcia-Godoy F, Donly KJ: Dentin/enamel adhesives in pediatric dentistry, *Pediatr Dent* 24(5):462–464, 2002.

Goracci C, Sadek FT, Monticelli F, Cardoso PE, Ferrari M: Influence of substrate, shape, and thickness on microtensile specimens' structural integrity and their measured bond strengths, *Dent Mater* 20(7):643–654, 2004.

He LH, Purton DG, Swain MV: A suitable base material for composite resin restorations: zinc oxide eugenol, *J Dent* 38(4): 290–295.

Hembree JH Jr, George TA, Hembree ME: Film thickness of cements beneath complete crowns, *J Prosthet Dent* 39(5):533–535, 1978.

Hibino Y, et al: Correlation between the strength of glass ionomer cements and their bond strength to bovine teeth, *Dent Mater J* 23(4):656–660, 2004.

Hibino Y, et al: Relationship between the strength of glass ionomers and their adhesive strength to metals, *Dent Mater* 18(7):552–557, 2002.

Ilie N, Hickel R: Can CQ be completely replaced by alternative initiators in dental adhesives? *Dent Mater J* 27(2):221–228, 2008.

Irie M, et al: Physical properties of dual-cured luting-agents correlated to early no interfacial-gap incidence with composite inlay restorations, *Dent Mater* 26(6): 608–615.

Irie M, Suzuki K, Watts DC: Marginal and flexural integrity of three classes of luting cement, with early finishing and water storage, *Dent Mater* 20(1):3–11, 2004.

Jemt T, Stalblad PA, Oilo G: Adhesion of polycarboxylate-based dental cements to enamel: an in vivo study, *J Dent Res* 65(6):885–887, 1986.

Jivraj SA, Kim TH, Donovan TE: Selection of luting agents, part 1, *J Calif Dent Assoc* 34(2):149–160, 2006.

Johnson GH, et al: Retention of metal-ceramic crowns with contemporary dental cements, *J Am Dent Assoc* 140(9):1125–1136, 2009.

Jongsma LA, Kleverlaan CJ, Feilzer AJ: Influence of surface pretreatment of fiber posts on cement delamination, *Dent Mater* 26(9):901–907, 2010.

Kim TH, Jivraj SA, Donovan TE: Selection of luting agents: part 2, *J Calif Dent Assoc* 34(2):161–166, 2006.

Kious AR, Roberts HW, Brackett WW: Film thicknesses of recently introduced luting cements, *J Prosthet Dent* 101(3):189–192, 2009.

Knobloch LA, et al: Solubility and sorption of resin-based luting cements, *Oper Dent* 25(5):434–440, 2000.

Li Z, White S: Mechanical properties of dental luting cements, *J Prosthet Dent* 81(5):597–609, 1999.

Magni E, et al: Evaluation of the mechanical properties of dental adhesives and glass-ionomer cements, *Clin Oral Investig* 14(1):79–87, 2010.

Mair L, Padipatvuthikul P: Variables related to materials and preparing for bond strength testing irrespective of the test protocol, *Dent Mater* 26(2):e17–23, 2010.

Marcusson A, Norevall LI, Persson M: White spot reduction when using glass ionomer cement for bonding in orthodontics: a longitudinal and comparative study, *Eur J Orthod* 19(3):233–242, 1997.

Marshall SJ, et al: A review of adhesion science, *Dent Mater* 26(2):e11–e16, 2010.

Mausner IK, Goldstein GR, Georgescu M: Effect of two dentinal desensitizing agents on retention of complete cast coping using four cements, *J Prosthet Dent* 75(2): 129–134, 1996.

Mesu FP: Mechanical mixing of zinc oxide-eugenol cements, *J Prosthet Dent* 47(5):522–527, 1982.

Mojon P, et al: Early bond strength of luting cements to a precious alloy, *J Dent Res* 71(9):1633–1639, 1992.

Moura JS, et al: Effect of luting cement on dental biofilm composition and secondary caries around metallic restorations in situ, *Oper Dent* 29(5):509–514, 2004.

Nakamura T, et al: Mechanical properties of new self-adhesive resin-based cement, *J Prosthodont Res* 54(2):59–64.

Negm MM, Beech DR, Grant AA: An evaluation of mechanical and adhesive properties of polycarboxylate and glass ionomer cements, *J Oral Rehabil* 9(2):161–167, 1982.

Nicholson JW, Czarnecka B: The biocompatibility of resin-modified glass-ionomer cements for dentistry, *Dent Mater* 24(12):1702–1708, 2008.

Nicholson JW, Czarnecka B: Review paper: Role of aluminum in glass-ionomer dental cements and its biological effects, *J Biomater Appl* 24(4):293–308, 2009.

Oilo G, Espevik S: Stress/strain behavior of some dental luting cements, *Acta Odontol Scand* 36(1):45–49, 1978.

Osborne JW, et al: A method for assessing the clinical solubility and disintegration of luting cements, *J Prosthet Dent* 40(4):413–417, 1978.

Ozcan M, et al: Bond strength durability of a resin composite on a reinforced ceramic using various repair systems, *Dent Mater* 25(12):1477–1483, 2009.

Perdigao J: New developments in dental adhesion, *Dent Clin North Am* 51(2):333–357, 2007:viii.

Peutzfeldt A: Dual-cure resin cements: in vitro wear and effect of quantity of remaining double bonds, filler volume, and light curing, *Acta Odontol Scand* 53(1):29–34, 1995.

Peutzfeldt A, Asmussen E: Influence of eugenol-containing temporary cement on bonding of self-etching adhesives to dentin, *J Adhes Dent* 8(1):31–34, 2006.

Piwowarczyk A, Lauer HC: Mechanical properties of luting cements after water storage, *Oper Dent* 28(5):535–542, 2003.

Piwowarczyk A, Lauer HC, Sorensen JA: In vitro shear bond strength of cementing agents to fixed prosthodontic restorative materials, *J Prosthet Dent* 92(3):265–273, 2004.

Piwowarczyk A, Lauer HC, Sorensen JA: The shear bond strength between luting cements and zirconia ceramics after two pre-treatments, *Oper Dent* 30(3):382–388, 2005.

Powis DR, Prosser HJ, Wilson AD: Long-term monitoring of microleakage of dental cements by radiochemical diffusion, *J Prosthet Dent* 59(6):651–657, 1988.

Radovic I, et al: Self-adhesive resin cements: a literature review, *J Adhes Dent* 10(4):251–258, 2008.

Rinastiti M, Ozcan M, Siswomihardjo W, Busscher HJ: Effects of surface conditioning on repair bond strengths of non-aged and aged microhybrid, nanohybrid, and nanofilled composite resins, *Clin Oral Investig*, 2010 May 25:[Epub ahead of print].

Robertello FJ, et al: Fluoride release of glass ionomer-based luting cements in vitro, *J Prosthet Dent* 82(2):172–176, 1999.

Schmid-Schwap M, et al: Cytotoxicity of four categories of dental cements, *Dent Mater* 25(3):360–368, 2009.

Schulman A, Vaidyanathan TK: Dental cements for luting and lining, *N Y J Dent* 47(5):142–146, 1977.

Setcos JC, Staninec M, Wilson NH: Bonding of amalgam restorations: existing knowledge and future prospects, *Oper Dent* 25(2):121–129, 2000.

Shaw AJ, Carrick T, McCabe JF: Fluoride release from glass-ionomer and compomer restorative materials: 6-month data, *J Dent* 26(4):355–359, 1998.

Sidhu SK, Schmalz G: The biocompatibility of glass-ionomer cement materials. A status report for the American Journal of Dentistry, *Am J Dent* 14(6):387–396, 2001.

Smith D: The setting of zinc oxide/eugenol mixtures, *British Dental Journal* 105(9):313–321, 1958.

Smith D: A new dental cement, *British Dental Journal* 5:381–384, 1968.

Spinell T, Schedle A, Watts DC: Polymerization shrinkage kinetics of dimethacrylate resin-cements, *Dent Mater* 25(8):1058–1066, 2009.

Summers A, et al: Comparison of bond strength between a conventional resin adhesive and a resin-modified glass ionomer adhesive: an in vitro and in vivo study, *Am J Orthod Dentofacial Orthop* 126(2):200–206, 2004:quiz 254-255.

Swartz ML, Phillips RW, Clark HE: Long-term F release from glass ionomer cements, *J Dent Res* 63(2):158–160, 1984.

Van Meerbeek B, et al: Buonocore memorial lecture. Adhesion to enamel and dentin: current status and future challenges, *Oper Dent* 28(3):215–235, 2003.

Vrochari AD, et al: Water sorption and solubility of four self-etching, self-adhesive resin luting agents, *J Adhes Dent* 12(1):39–43.

White SN, Kipnis V: Effect of adhesive luting agents on the marginal seating of cast restorations, *J Prosthet Dent* 69(1):28–31, 1993.

White SN, Yu Z: Compressive and diametral tensile strengths of current adhesive luting agents, *J Prosthet Dent* 69(6):568–572, 1993.

Wiegand A, Buchalla W, Attin T: Review on fluoride-releasing restorative materials—fluoride release and uptake characteristics, antibacterial activity and influence on caries formation, *Dent Mater* 23(3):343–362, 2007.

Wilson AD, McLean JW: *Glass-ionomer cement*, Chicago, 1988, Quintessence Books.

Wilson AD, Prosser HJ, Powis DM: Mechanism of adhesion of polyelectrolyte cements to hydroxyapatite, *J Dent Res* 62(5):590–592, 1983.

Digital Imaging and Processing for Restorations

DENTAL CAD/CAM SYSTEMS

CAD/CAM, the abbreviation for computer-aided design/computer-aided manufacturing, describes a process in which digital images or models of objects are created and used for the design and fabrication of prototypes or final products using computer numerical control (CNC) or other fabrication methods such as stereolithography. This process has been used for decades in a variety of industries and has become a popular method in restorative dentistry for creating impressions, cast and dies, and provisional and final restorations. Reports of 10-year follow-up studies for one system have shown good outcomes that are improving with each technological enhancement.

Dental CAD/CAM systems consist of three components:

1. A scanner or digitizing instrument that transforms physical geometry into digital data.
2. Software that processes the scanned data and creates images of the digitized object. Some systems then enable restorations to be designed for the digitized object.
3. Fabrication technology that transforms the digital data of the restoration into a physical product. Different systems place the fabrication technology in the dental office, dental laboratory, or centralized facility.

The two types of CAD/CAM systems for dental offices are acquisition (digital impression) only and scan and mill. Acquisition only systems create digital impressions by capturing images of the preparation and then sending the digital file to a center where a model is made upon which a laboratory technician can fabricate the final restoration. A scan and mill system adds an in-office restoration fabrication device to the digital impression instrument, enabling a restoration to be designed, fabricated, and delivered in one appointment. For the acquisition only system, multiple appointments are required as in conventional indirect restorative care, and a provisional restoration is placed in the interim while the restoration is being fabricated by a laboratory technician. Scan and mill systems offer the convenience of one appointment preparation, impression, fabrication, and delivery, but includes a waiting period while the restoration is milled and the additional cost of the milling machine.

Dental CAD/CAM systems have the following benefits:

- Provide improved precision and consistency
- Allow the clinician to visualize the preparation on a computer display from many perspectives
- Allow the clinician to design the restoration on a computer while visualizing the opposing dentition
- Provide a clean and streamlined impression method without the complexity of the many materials required for conventional impressions with an elastomeric material
- Offer instant display and feedback for making corrections immediately
- Reduce the environmental impact of disposing the materials required for conventional impressions

There are several dental CAD/CAM systems currently on the market (Table 14-1). Two of these systems (CEREC AC, Figure 14-1, A, and E4D Dentist, Figure 14-1, B) offer the option of in-office design and milling but also allow design and milling by dental technicians. Two other systems (iTero, Figure 14-2, A, and Lava Chairside Oral Scanner C.O.S., Figure 14-2, B) produce digital impressions that require design and milling at a dental laboratory or milling center. All of these systems can produce models from their digital files.

DIGITAL IMPRESSIONS

After the tooth preparation is complete and the tissues are retracted to visualize the tooth margins, the tooth is dried and readied for scanning. Some

TABLE 14.1   Digital Impression Systems

Product	Manufacturer	Light Source	Number of Images Required	In-office Milling	Laboratory Milling
3M ESPE Lava Chairside Oral Scanner C.O.S.	3M ESPE (St. Paul, MN)	LED	Continuous video	No	Yes
CEREC AC	Sirona Dental Systems (Charlotte, NC)	Bluecam LED	1-3	Yes	Yes
E4D Dentist	D4D Technologies (Richardson, TX)	Laser	9+	Yes	Yes
iTero	Cadent, Inc. (Carlstadt, NJ)	Laser	21	No	Yes

LED, *Light-emitting diode.*

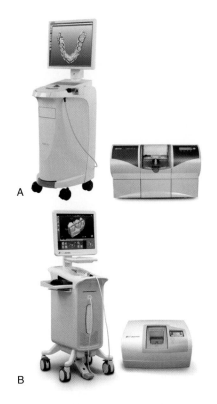

FIGURE 14.1 **In-office CAD/CAM systems. A,** CEREC AC. **B,** E4D Dentist. (*A, Courtesy of Sirona Dental Systems LLC, Charlotte, NC; B, Courtesy of D4D Technologies, Richardson, TX.*)

scanning systems require the use of an oxide powder on the tooth to remove optical highlights from the surface of the preparation and to enhance the scan quality. Scanners use either a series of static images or a stream of video images to capture the geometry of the tooth preparation.

CEREC AC with the CEREC Bluecam has a blue light-emitting diode (LED) and camera system, and uses active triangulation to create images of the tooth surface. Static images of the tooth are stitched together to create a single 3-D model. The E4D Dentist system uses a high-speed swept laser beam combined with a camera to obtain a series of 3-D scans of the tooth using the principle of laser triangulation. Laser utilization allows scanning of a variety of different surface types and colors without the need for a contrast agent (powder). These scans are registered together to form a single 3-D model. The iTero uses parallel confocal imaging to create 100,000 point maps at 300 focal depths spaced 50 micrometers apart. A series of 15 to 30 scanned images record the preparation, opposing teeth, and the occlusal relationship. The LAVA C.O.S. scanner is based on the principle of active optical wavefront sampling, in which 3-D information is collected by a single lens imaging system. Three sensors collect video data simultaneously from different perspectives. Twenty 3-D data sets are captured per second. For a complete digital volume model, about 2400 3-D data sets or 24 million data points per arch are reconstructed.

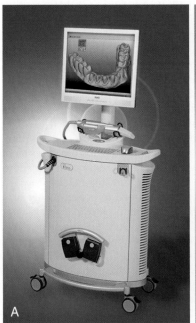
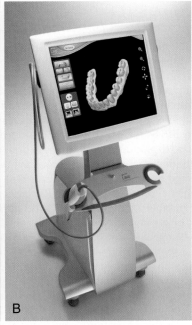
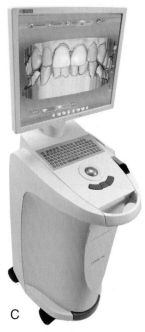

FIGURE 14.2 **Digital impression systems. A,** iTero. **B,** Lava Chairside Oral Scanner C.O.S. **C,** CEREC AC. (*A, Courtesy of Cadent, Inc., Carlstadt, NJ; B, Courtesy of 3M ESPE, St. Paul, MN; C, Courtesy of Sirona, Charlotte, NC.*)

TABLE 14.2   Digital Impression Systems—Choice of Materials (2010)

Product	Company	PFM/Gold	Lithium Disilicate	Leucite-reinforced	Zirconia
iTero	Cadent, Inc.	Yes	Yes	Yes	Yes
E4D Dentist	D4D Technologies	Yes (via E4D Sky)	Yes	Yes	Yes (via E4D Sky)
CEREC AC	Sirona Dental Systems	Yes (via CEREC Connect)	Yes	Yes	Yes (via CEREC Connect)
3M ESPE Lava Chairside Oral Scanner C.O.S.	3M ESPE	Yes	Yes	Yes	Yes

Courtesy of John M. Powers, Ann Arbor, MI.

DESIGN SOFTWARE

Each system includes proprietary software for the visualization of the scanned data and design of restorations. A wide variety of restorations can be designed, including inlays, onlays, full crowns, and fixed dental prostheses. The digital cast and dies can be visualized from any perspective, with or without the opposing dentition. Restorations are designed interactively by the clinician and computer, adapting the contours to harmonize with the adjacent and opposing teeth. A virtual "clay" is used to mold the restoration to the correct emergence profile, interproximal contact, and occlusal scheme. The opposing dentition can be moved through excursive paths to further develop a functional occlusal profile.

PROCESSING DEVICES

Milling centers and dental laboratories produce restorations directly from the digital impression and restoration design data. Restorations can be milled from a variety of materials such as composites, feldspathic porcelain, leucite-reinforced ceramic, lithium disilicate ceramic, and zirconia (Table 14-2). Wax patterns and acrylic provisional restorations can also be milled. The digitally produced models can be used to produce restorations by traditional methods in the dental laboratory.

Milling devices are distinguished by the number of milling axes. The quality of the final product does not necessarily depend on the number of milling axes, but it does affect the level of geometric complexity that can be produced. Three-axis devices are capable of movement in three spatial directions. They are not capable of milling axis divergences and convergences. Three-axis devices can turn the material block used for milling by 180 degrees during processing. Four-axis devices add the ability to rotate the material block infinitely. This enables the fabrication of a fixed prosthesis with a large vertical height difference. Five-axis devices add the ability to rotate the milling spindle so complex geometries can be milled in sections. This enables geometries such as converging abutment teeth to be accommodated.

Metals, resins, composites, and ceramics can be milled by the processing devices. Commercially pure titanium, titanium alloys, and cobalt chrome alloys are metals commonly used in the devices. Resins can be milled to create lost wax frames for casting and also for long-term provisional prostheses. Composite blanks that are prefabricated to mimic enamel and dentin in their translucency and color can be milled to create final anterior restorations. Zirconia, described in Chapter 11, is a high performance ceramic with excellent mechanical characteristics. It is used in milling devices for crowns, fixed partial prostheses, and implant abutments.

CLINICAL OUTCOMES

The performance of restorations produced in CAD/CAM systems have improved dramatically in the last decade. An older perception of poor marginal integrity associated with CAD/CAM restorations is no longer true. Enhancements in image capture, design software, and milling technology along with improvements in materials have all contributed to superior clinical outcomes. Patient selection and attention to margin design and tissue retraction are important factors, as they should be for all restorative procedures.

In recent studies of zirconia-based restorations, digital impressions resulted in better quality of contacts, better fit, and better occlusion than elastomeric impressions (Table 14-3). Digital impressions typically result in 33% shorter seating/adjustment time and fewer incidents of remakes when compared to elastomeric impressions. In a 10-year study of 308 ceramic restorations placed in 74 patients between 1991 and 1994, the restoration survival rate was 94.7% after 5 years and 85.7% after 10 years, which is comparable to the survival rates of cast gold restorations. A systematic review of four studies that reported on implant-supported CAD/CAM fabricated restorations found

TABLE 14.3 Comparison of Restorations Made by Digital Impression vs. Elastomeric Impressions

Parameter	Digital Impression (% perfect)	Elastomeric Impression (% perfect)
Quality of contacts	62	46
Fit	92	71
Occlusion	74	48

Modified from Farah JW, Brown L: Dent. Advis. Res. Rpt. 22, 1-3, 2009.

a cumulative 5-year survival rate of all-ceramic single crowns of 100% (95% CI: 92.4% to 100%). A systematic review of studies that reported on single-tooth restorations fabricated with CAD/CAM technology from 1985 to 2007 revealed a failure rate of 1.75% per year, calculated per 100 restoration years from a total of 1957 restorations and a mean exposure time of 7.9 years. The review estimated a total 5-year survival rate of 91.6% (95% CI: 88.2% to 94.1%). The long-term survival rates for CAD/CAM single-tooth restorations were found to be similar to restorations fabricated with conventional methods.

SELECTED PROBLEMS

PROBLEM 1

What types of materials can be milled with CAD/CAM systems?

Solution

Restorations can be milled from a variety of materials such as composites, feldspathic porcelain, leucite-reinforced ceramic, lithium disilicate ceramic, and zirconia.

PROBLEM 2

Why is it necessary to dust the preparation with titanium oxide powder for some systems?

Solution

CAD/CAM systems use video or static imaging methods that provide the best images when the preparation is void of specular reflection. The powder provides surfaces that are uniform in color and reflectance.

PROBLEM 3

Is the long-term survival rate of CAD/CAM fabricated restorations similar to those fabricated using conventional methods?

Solution

Yes. Systematic reviews found 5-year survival rates between 92% and 95%, which compare favorably with restorations fabricated by conventional methods.

Bibliography

Anderson S: E4D Dentist, E4D Studio and E4D Labworks along the digital skyway, *Dent Advis Clin Case Rpt* 17: 1–3, 2010.

Beuer F, Schweiger J, Edelhoff D: Digital dentistry: an overview of recent development for CAD/CAM generated restorations, *Br Dent J* 204(9):505–511, 2008.

Farah JW, Brown L: Integrating the 3M ESPE Lava Chairside Oral Scanner C.O.S. into daily clinical practice, *Dent Advis Clin Case Rpt* 12:1–4, 2009.

Farah JW, Brown L: Integrating iTero into a busy dental practice, *Dent Advis Clin Case Rpt* 16:1–3, 2009.

Farah JW, Brown L: Comparison of the fit of crowns: 3M ESPE Lava Chairside Oral Scanner C.O.S. vs. traditional impressions, *Dent Advis Res Rpt* 22:1–3, 2009.

Farah JW, Powers JM: CAD/CAM update, *Dent Advis* 26(7):1, 2009.

Farah JW, Powers JM: Digital impressions, *Dent Advis* 27(6):1, 2010.

Fasbinder DJ: Digital dentistry: Innovation for restorative treatment, *Digital Age Dentistry, Compendium of Continuing Education in Dentistry* 31(Spec Iss 4):2–11, 2010.

Giannetopoulos S, van Noort R, Tsitrou E: Evaluation of the marginal integrity of ceramic copings with different marginal angles using two different CAD/CAM systems, *J Dent* 38(12):980–986, 2010.

Harder S, Kern M: Survival and complications of computer aided-designing and computer-aided manufacturing vs. conventionally fabricated implant-supported reconstructions: a systematic review, *Clin Oral Implants Res* 4: 48–54, 2009.

Schroder BK, Brown C: Use of selective open architecture in digital restoration fabrication, In *Digital Age Dentistry, Compendium of Continuing Education in Dentistry* 31(Spec Iss 4):15–22, 2010.

Wittneben J-G, Wright RF, Weber H-P, Gallucci GO: A systematic review of the clinical performance of CAD/CAM single-tooth restorations, *Int J Prosthodont* 22: 466–471, 2009.

Zimmer G, Gohlich O, Ruttemann S, Lang H, Raab WH, Barthel CR: Long-term survival of Cerec restorations: a 10-year study, *Oper Dent* 33(5):484–487, 2008.

Dental and Orofacial Implants

The practice of restorative dentistry seeks to replace the form and function of missing tooth structure. It was therefore expected that dentistry would follow orthopedic medicine in the use of implants to anchor prosthetic devices and as expected, that has happened. In 2010, the global implant market was $3.2 billion. Sales in 2015 is expected to reach nearly $4.2 billion at a compounded annual growth rate of 6%. In 2010, Europe exhibited a 42% market share. By 2015, the Asia-Pacific region will have the highest annual growth rate.

Dental implants are fixtures that serve as replacements for the root of a missing natural tooth. Implants may be placed in the mandible or maxilla. When properly designed and placed, dental implants bond with bone over time and serve as an anchor for dental prostheses. Dental implants are used to replace a single missing tooth or many teeth, or to support a complete removable denture.

Worldwide, modern single-tooth implants have a success rate of nearly 95% survival at 15 years. Implants are permanent devices, surgically anchored in the oral cavity, that often provide significant advantages over other fixed or removable prosthodontic options. Implants are often more conservative than traditional fixed partial dentures because they conserve tooth structure by eliminating the need for reduction of adjacent abutment teeth and they support the maintenance of healthy bone in the region.

CLASSIFICATION

Historically, dental implants have been classified according to their design. This design was in turn based on the way in which they are surgically implanted. The three types of implants commonly used for the past 40 years are the subperiosteal implant, the transosteal implant, and the endosseous implant (Table 15-1).

Endosseous Implant

Endosseous implants are by far the most common type of implant placed today. Implants are placed directly into the mandible or maxilla (Figure 15-1).

A pilot hole is drilled into the alveolar or basal bone beneath (in cases in which the alveolar bone has been partially or completely resorbed), and the implant body is inserted into this site. The top of the implant is positioned so that it either protrudes slightly through the cortical plate or is flush with the surface of the bone. Typically a superstructure containing a prosthetic tooth or teeth connects to the implant body through an abutment that is screwed into the body directly through the mucosa.

OSSEOINTEGRATION AND BIOINTEGRATION

A major issue for implant design is the development of materials that are physically and biologically compatible with alveolar bone. Ideally, bone should integrate with the material, substance, or device and remodel the bone structure around it, rather than responding to the material as a foreign substance by encapsulating it with fibrous tissue.

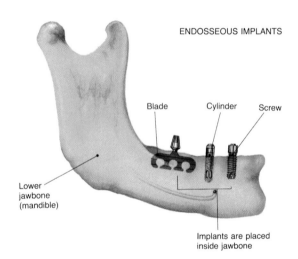

FIGURE 15.1 **Endosteal implant design.** Shown here are three different endosseous implant designs. Notice that all of the designs are implanted directly within the bone. Although the blade design has fallen out of use, the cylinder and screw-shaped versions continue to be the most widely placed implant designs in use today.

TABLE 15.1   Implant Design Classification Scheme

Implant Design	Contact with Bone	Composition	Location Used
Subperiosteal	Directly on bone surface under the gingival tissues; no bone penetration	Co-Cr-Mo (Vitallium)	Maxilla and mandible
Transosteal	Completely through the bone, penetrating the cortical wall twice	Titanium or Ti-alloy	Mandible only
Endosteal	Within the bone, penetrating the cortical wall once	Titanium or Ti-alloy	Maxilla and mandible

Co-Cr-Mo, *Cobalt-chromium-molybdenum; Ti, titanium.*

Under optimum circumstances, bone differentiation occurs directly adjacent to the material (osseointegration). Ideally, this osseointegration provides a stable bone-implant connection that can support a dental prosthesis and transfer applied loads without concentrating stresses at the interface between bone and the implant.

Osseointegration is now formally defined as the close approximation of bone to an implant material (Figure 15-2). To achieve osseointegration, the bone must be viable, the space between the bone and implant must be less than 10 nm and contain no fibrous tissue, and the bone-implant interface must be able to survive loading by a dental prosthesis. In current practice, osseointegration is an absolute requirement for the successful implant-supported dental prosthesis. To achieve osseointegration between an implant and bone, a number of factors must be correct. The bone must be prepared in a way that does not cause necrosis or inflammation. The implant must be allowed to heal for a time without a load. Finally, the proper material must be implanted, because not all materials will promote osseointegration.

In recent years, various surface configurations have been proposed as means of improving the cohesiveness of the implant/tissue interface, maximizing load transfer, minimizing relative motion between the implant and tissue, minimizing fibrous integration and loosening, and lengthening the service life of the construct. Because of the necessity of developing a stable interface before loading, effort has been placed on developing materials and methods to accelerate tissue apposition to the implant surface. Surface-roughened implants and ceramic coatings have been implemented into clinical practice. Other, more experimental techniques include electrical stimulation, bone grafting, and the use of growth factors and other tissue engineering approaches described in Chapter 16.

The application of bioactive ceramics as implant materials was traditionally limited to their use as bone bonding and augmentation materials. There has been interest in coating titanium alloys with bioactive materials to promote an implant bone connection. Bioactive ceramic materials are more than just biocompatible. The use of the term *bioactive* implies that they have the ability to elicit a favorable tissue response when implanted in vivo. These ceramics form a direct chemical bond with natural tissues and are most often designed to bioresorb or biodegrade, having high solubility. Commonly implanted dental ceramics include the calcium phosphates with various calcium-to-phosphorus ratios (e.g., hydroxyapatite and tricalcium phosphate), bioactive glasses (mixtures of SiO_2, CaO, P_2O_5, and sometimes Na_2O, and MgO), and glass ceramics.

Important examples of bioactive glasses and glass ceramics include Bioglass (a glass containing a mixture of silica, phosphate, calcia, and soda); Ceravital (which has a different alkali oxide concentration compared to Bioglass); Biogran (which has a different physical conformation compared to Bioglass); and glass ceramic A-W (a glass

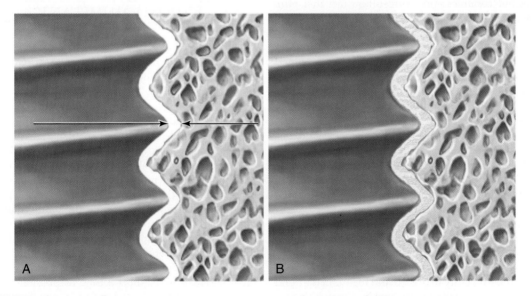

FIGURE 15.2 **Osseointegration and biointegration. A,** In osseointegration, the implant material *(left)* and the bone *(right)* closely approximate one another. This approximation must be closer than 10 nm *(arrows)*. In the intervening space, there can be no fibrous tissue. **B,** In biointegration, the implant and bone are fused and continuous with one another. Osseointegration commonly occurs with titanium alloys, whereas biointegration occurs with ceramics and ceramic-coated metallic implants.

ceramic–containing crystalline oxyapatite and flu-orapatite $(Ca_{10}[PO_4]_6[O,F_2])$ and β-wollastonite (SiO_2CaO) in a $MgO-CaO-SiO_2$ glassy matrix). Additionally, many other glass and glass-ceramic compositions, based on recently developed sol-gel synthesis methods, are being developed. Calcium phosphate ceramics vary in composition, depending on processing-induced physical and chemical changes. Among this group are the apatite ceramics, and of particular interest is hydroxyapatite (HA). This is the synthetic version of the inorganic phase found in tooth and bone and is the bioactive ceramic material that has been most extensively investigated.

The impetus for using synthetic HA as a biomaterial stems from the perceived advantage of using a material similar to the mineral phase in natural tissues for replacing these materials. Because of this similarity, better tissue bonding is expected. Additional perceived advantages of HA and other bioactive ceramics include low thermal and electrical conductivity, elastic properties similar to those of bone, control of in vivo degradation rates through control of material properties, and the possibility of the ceramic functioning as a barrier to metallic corrosion products when it is coated onto a metal substrate.

However, temperature-induced phase transformations while processing HA provoke considerable changes in its in vitro dissolution behavior, and the altered structure changes the biological reaction to the material. Given the multitude of chemical compositions and structures resulting from processing bioactive ceramics and the resultant fact that pure HA is rarely used, the broader term *calcium phosphate ceramics (CPCs)* has been proposed in lieu of the more specific term *hydroxyapatite*. Each individual calcium phosphate ceramic is then defined by its own unique set of chemical and physical properties.

Although calcium phosphate ceramics are too brittle and too stiff to serve as stand-alone dental implants for prosthetic tooth replacement, there has been continuing interest in using a thin (50 to 75 µm) layer of ceramic materials to coat the surface of metallic implants. This provides the beneficial osseointegration characteristics of the ceramic combined with the high strength of the metallic alloy. Most manufacturers provide implants coated with calcium phosphate ceramic for use in sites where poor bone quality exists. A major limitation in using this concept in all clinical situations, however, has revolved around the inability to predict and maintain the bond strength of the coating to the metal. When the bioactive ceramic material resorbs in vivo, an unpredictable change occurs in the implant-bone interface, and implant micromotion and loosening may occur.

This makes the long-term stability of these implants uncertain.

If successful, the ceramic coating becomes completely fused with the surrounding bone. In this case, the interface is called *biointegration* rather than osseointegration, and there is no intervening space between the bone and the implant (see Figure 15-2). A number of ceramic coatings have been used in this manner.

Typically, these coatings have been applied to the surface of an implant via a plasma-spray deposition process. This results in a complex mixture of HA, tricalcium phosphate, and tetracalcium phosphate in the coating, rather than a recapitulation of the starting powder mixture. Physical properties of importance to the functionality of calcium phosphate ceramics include powder particle size, particle shape, pore size, pore shape, pore-size distribution, specific surface area, phases present, crystal structure, crystal size, grain size, density, coating thickness, hardness, and surface roughness.

The long-term integrity of the ceramic coating in vivo is not known, but evidence indicates that these coatings will resorb over time. Additionally, results of ex vivo push-out tests indicate that the ceramic-metal bond fails before the ceramic-tissue bond and is the weak link in the system. Thus the weak ceramic-metal bond and the integrity of that interface over a lengthy service life of functional loading is reason for concern.

FACTORS AFFECTING THE ENDOSTEAL IMPLANT

Geometry

Two primary objectives influence a patient's decision to pursue dental implant treatment: aesthetics and function. To fulfill these objectives over an extended period, a dental implant must be capable of withstanding the occlusal stresses generated in the oral environment and in turn transfer this load to the supporting tissues. Not only must loads be transferred, they should also be of an appropriate direction and magnitude so tissue viability is maintained. In this respect, the implant principally acts to minimize and distribute the biomechanical forces. The forces are characterized by their magnitude, duration, and type. The ability to transfer force largely depends on attaining interfacial fixation. The interface between the implant and bone must stabilize in as short a time as possible postoperatively, and once stable, must remain stable throughout its service life. Designing an "optimal" implant that meets all the foregoing objectives requires the integration of material, physical, chemical, mechanical, biological, and economic factors.

Magnitude of the Force

The amount of load applied during normal chewing varies greatly, depending on location and state of the patient's dentition. Bite force values reported in the literature range from about 40 to 1250 N. The magnitude of force is greatest in the molar region because this area acts like the hinge of a lever (Figure 15-3). The incisor region, in comparison, experiences about 10% of the magnitude seen in the posterior segment. This difference in load borne by the teeth and supporting bone dictates differences in mechanical requirements between anterior and posterior implants. Because stress depends not only on the applied load, but also on the area over which this load is distributed, the loss of some teeth by a patient will greatly increase the stresses applied to the remaining teeth and implants in partially edentulous patients.

A prime requirement for any dental implant is adequate supporting bone height, width, and density. It is well established that bone grows in response to strain, and the presence of an increasing magnitude of stress applied to the bone will result in an increasing magnitude of resorption or loss of bone. However, in the absence of a critical level of strain for normal bone maintenance, the bone will also resorb. Therefore, if the patient has been edentulous for a prolonged time, the underlying bone will have resorbed and become less dense. It is common to place implants preferentially in the anterior mandible, because this region has the greatest trabecular bone density when compared with the premolar or molar regions in both dentate and edentulous patients. When planning implant treatment, careful consideration must be given to the load distribution.

A great majority of the materials considered to be biocompatible are not suitable for use as implants, because their ultimate strength is not high enough to withstand the forces to which they are subjected during normal function. But, in order to survive and continue to function effectively, it is not only the ultimate strength, but also the modulus of elasticity (or stiffness) of the material that must be considered. Unless the bone experiences at least 50 microstrain on a routine basis, it will begin to resorb. Most ceramic materials are extremely stiff, for example, polycrystalline aluminum oxide has a modulus of elasticity ≈372 GPa. This stiffness is too high to transfer an adequate amount of an applied force to the bone. Instead, the stiffer implant material will carry a disproportionate amount of the load, causing stress shielding of the bone. In contrast, titanium has a modulus of elasticity ≈100 GPa, still too high to be ideal, but much closer to that of bone (≈20 GPa). It will permit normal physiological loading of the bone.

Duration of the Force

When considering repetitive loading such as occurs during mastication, it is more appropriate to consider the endurance limit of a material rather than its ultimate strength. The endurance limit is the highest amount of stress to which a material may be repeatedly subjected without failing. This limit is typically only about half of the ultimate strength for the material.

The tooth root-form implant is designed to be loaded parallel to the long axis and is vulnerable to fatigue failure from cyclic bending loads. These bending loads often result from premature contact, bruxism, inappropriate occlusal schemes, and the use of angled abutments. Off-axis loading should be avoided in design of the implant superstructure.

Type of Force

An implant experiences three types of loads in function: tensile forces, compressive forces, and shear forces. As discussed, a well-designed implant transfers and distributes these forces to the supporting bone. Bone is composed of both inorganic and organic constituents, and the inorganic components render it strongest when loaded in compression. Bone is about 30% weaker when placed in tension, and nearly 70% weaker when subjected to shear forces. Therefore, occlusion is a crucial consideration in designing the implant loading.

Smooth-sided cylindrical implant designs place the interface between the implant and the bone in nearly pure shear, the weakest possible loading scenario. These implant designs rely either on microscopic texturing of the implant body to offer some

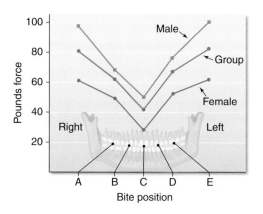

FIGURE 15-3 **Mean adult bite force at different positions in the jaw.** *(From Rugh SD, Solberg WK: Behav. Res. Meth. Instrum. 4, 125, 1972.)*

mechanical interlocking and provide retention, or else they rely on a coating. If the coating on these fails or resorbs, bone loss usually results from the lack of load transfer.

In contrast, screw-shaped implants have threads to engage the bone in compression and transfer the applied load. The thread designs have been extensively researched to provide a minimum of shear forces and maximal compression to the bone. This allows for the most favorable bone response. A number of recent thread designs have been introduced that use rounded thread tips (to reduce shear forces at the tip), changes in the thread angle (to maximize compression), two or more thread profiles on the same implant (which will cut at different locations in the osteotomy, thereby increasing the contact area), and/or a reduced thread height accompanied by an increased thread pitch (spreading the implant loading over a greater contact area while simultaneously increasing the strength of the implant body).

The concept of osseointegration around cylindrical or screw-shaped implants represents a situation of bone ongrowth. An alternative method of implant fixation is based on bone tissue ingrowth into roughened or three-dimensional porous surface layers. Such designs incorporating sintered beads or a sintered wire mesh, are typical of orthopedic implants. Recently, implants with porous metal bodies have been developed and marketed. These new designs incorporate macroscale porosity or porous cellular structures, resembling cancellous bone. This results in a modulus of elasticity close to that of bone, thereby reducing the resulting stress shielding. Such retention systems have been shown to have higher bone/metal shear strength than other types of fixation. Increased interfacial shear strength results in a better stress transfer from the implant to the surrounding bone, a more uniform stress distribution between the implant and bone, and lower stresses in the implant. And, in principle, the result of a stronger interfacial bond is a decreased propensity for implant loosening. The theoretical progression of macroscale surface effects from the lowest implant/tissue shear strength to the highest is as follows: smooth, textured, screw threaded, plasma sprayed, and porous coated, porous body design.

Implant Diameter

An increase in implant length or diameter increases the total surface area of the implant. As a consequence, the area for distribution of the occlusal forces is increased and the stress on the bone is decreased. The bending fracture resistance (and hence rigidity) of the implant increases greatly as the implant width increases and is related to the implant radius raised to the fourth power. This dramatic increase can be deleterious if the diameter chosen causes stress shielding by reducing bone strain to subphysiological levels.

Implant Length

As with increases in the width, increases in implant length also increase the surface area and reduce the bone stress. However, a careful consideration of the bone quality is advised. In the highly dense type of bone usually found in the anterior mandible, overheating of the bone while drilling is a major cause of future failure. Preparation of an extra-long implant site tends to increase heating in this type of bone. Any immediate stability advantages provided by this long implant are transitory, because once the implant osseointegrates, the apical region of the implant receives minimal stress transfer. Most of the stresses are still concentrated around the upper cortical plate through which the implant emerges. Conversely, in regions of poor bone quality, typically found in the posterior mandible and maxilla, anatomical considerations dictate the length of implant placed.

SURFACES AND BIOCOMPATIBILITY

In analyzing an implant/tissue system, three aspects are important: (1) the individual constituents, namely the implant materials and tissues; (2) the effect of the implant and its breakdown products on the local and systemic tissues; and (3) the interfacial zone between the implant and tissue. Regarding the ultrastructure of the implant-tissue interface, it is important to understand that, although this zone is relatively thin (on the order of 0.1 nm), the constituents of the zone (heterogeneous metallic oxide, proteinaceous layer, and connective tissue) have a substantial effect on the maintenance of interfacial integrity. Furthermore, interfacial integrity depends on material, mechanical, chemical, surface, biological, and local environmental factors, all of which change as functions of time in vivo. Thus implant success is a function of biomaterial and biomechanical factors, as well as of surgical techniques, tissue healing, and a patient's overall medical and dental status.

Ion Release

Implant materials may corrode or wear, leading to the generation of particulate debris, which may in turn elicit both local and systemic biological responses. Metals are more susceptible to electrochemical degradation than are ceramics. Therefore, a fundamental criterion when choosing a metallic implant material is that it must *not* elicit significant adverse biological response. Titanium alloys are well tolerated by the body because of their passive oxide layers. The main elemental ingredients, as well as the minor alloying constituents, are endured by the body in trace amounts. However, larger amounts of any metal cannot be tolerated. Therefore, minimizing mechanical and chemical breakdown of implant materials is a primary objective.

Titanium and other implant metals are in their passive state under typical physiological conditions, and breakdown of passivity should not occur. Both commercially pure titanium (CP Ti) and the titanium alloy Ti-6Al-4V possess excellent corrosion resistance for a full range of oxide states and pH levels. It is the extremely coherent, conformal oxide layer and the fact that titanium repassivates almost instantaneously through surface controlled–oxidation kinetics that renders titanium so corrosion resistant. The low dissolution rate and near chemical inertness of titanium dissolution products allow bone to thrive and therefore osseointegrate with titanium. However, even in its passive condition, titanium is not inert. Titanium ion release does occur as a result of the chemical dissolution of titanium oxide.

Surfaces

Analysis of the implant surface is necessary to ensure a twofold requirement. First, implant materials cannot adversely affect local tissues, organ systems, or organ functions. Second, the in vivo environment cannot degrade the implant and compromise its long-term function. The interface zone between an implant and the surrounding tissue is therefore the most important entity in defining the biological response to the implant and the response of the implant to the body.

The success of any implant depends on its bulk and surface properties, the site of implantation, tissue trauma during surgery, and motion at the implant-tissue interface. Surface analysis in implantology therefore aids in material characterization, determining structural and composition changes occurring during processing, identifying biologically induced surface reactions, and analyzing environmental effects on the interfaces.

The surface of a material is always different in chemical composition, form, and structure from the bulk material, because the atoms at the surface are fundamentally different from those in the bulk of the implant metal. The surface of a metal can be considered as an abrupt cessation of the orderly stacking of atoms below. As such, the coordination number of these atoms differs and hence their physical and chemical properties are different from atoms deeper

in the bulk, arising from their molecular arrangement, surface reactions, and potential contamination with other species. These differences may lead to changes in the interaction of the implant with the biological system.

In this regard, interface chemistry is primarily determined by the properties of the metal oxide and not as much by the metal itself. Little or no similarity is found between the properties of the metal and the properties of the oxide, but the adsorption and desorption phenomena can still be influenced by the properties of the underlying metal. Therefore, characterization of surface composition, binding state, form, and function are important in the analysis of implant surfaces and implant-tissue interfaces.

Surface Alterations

In efforts to improve the in vivo performance of dental implants, considerable research is being conducted to investigate the effects of macro-, micro-, and nanoscale surface features on osseointegration. Although many of these research reports are contradictory and few absolutes have been identified, some guiding principles are slowly emerging. The first of these is that cells in vitro (and possibly in vivo) undergo contact guidance on the implant surface. In other words, cells grow preferentially in and along nanometer- to micrometer-sized groove and ridge patterns on the surface of an implant. These minute grooves influence cell behavior by causing the cells to align themselves in the direction of the groove and migrate guided by the surface grooves (Figure 15-4). Furthermore, modification of the implant surface to incorporate micro- and nano scale surface features on top of macrotexturing increases the bone-implant contact area and the biomechanical

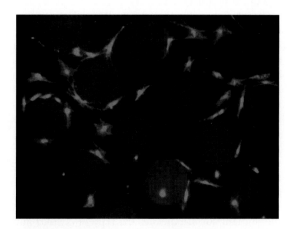

FIGURE 15-4 **Light microscope image of cells grown on a patterned surface.** Notice the contact guidance of the cells provided by the surface texture.

interaction between implant and anchoring bone, especially in the immediate term, after implantation. Cell shape, proliferation rate, and differentiation rate also depend on the texture of the implant surface to a great extent. However, conclusive evidence that this nano- to microscale texture plays a significant role in implant anchorage, in vivo, is as yet lacking.

A second principle is that varying the macroscale surface texture of an implant material significantly affects the interface between the implant and bone in vivo. In general, rough-surfaced implants exhibit greater shear bond strengths than corresponding smooth-surfaced implants. Upon microscopic examination, rough implants exhibit direct bone apposition, whereas smooth implants exhibit various degrees of fibrous tissue encapsulation. Because this direct bone apposition is the method by which dental implants are retained in the jaw, they appear to be significantly affected by macroscale surface texture. Not all surface roughness, however, has the same desirable effects. The exact dimensions or degree of roughness that is optimal remain ambiguous at this time.

As a result of these observations, during the last 10 to 15 years, implant surfaces have changed dramatically. Previously, machined surfaces were the norm. Now, surfaces that are prepared by grit-blasting, followed by either acid etching or coating to enhance the topography and/or remove embedded grit particles, dominate the marketplace. The resulting microscale retentive features not only roughen the implant surface, creating a greater implant-bone contact area but also play a role in activation of key biochemical sequences that ultimately accelerate the wound healing process and encourage osteogenesis.

It is quite clear that the chemistry of the implant surface will also play a significant role in the anchorage of the implant within the bone. This is an area of intense commercial research. Recently, a surface modification technique that incorporates grit blasting, followed by acid etching with a solution that results in fluoride ions on the implant surface, has been brought to the market. This surface preparation procedure results in a surface with varied chemical formulae within the surface oxide layer. This fluoride-containing surface has been shown to enhance gene expression and lead to enhanced osteogenesis. Additional surface chemical treatments being investigated include surface hydroxylation to enhance the hydrophilicity of the surface and electrochemical anodization to grow thick porous oxide layers with varied chemistries. The type of metallic oxide at the implant surface dictates the type of cellular and protein binding onto that surface. Surface oxides are continually altered by the inward diffusion of oxygen, and by hydroxide formation and the outward diffusion of metallic ions. Thus a single oxide stoichiometry rarely exists.

Surface Coatings

The use of an additional surface coating treatment warrants additional discussion. Calcium phosphate–based coatings have traditionally been the most heavily investigated. These materials are commonly applied to the implant surface as a plasma-spray coating. In this high temperature process, a 25 to 50 μm-thick layer of material is deposited onto the roughened implant surface and allowed to cool. These coatings rely on relatively weak mechanical interlocking between the coating and the roughened surface to maintain adhesion to the metallic surface. Furthermore, the rapid cooling of the molten ceramic sprayed onto the surface produces uncontrollable crystallinity changes within the material and results in large-scale cracking of the coating. Although research studies have noted enhanced bioactivity with these types of coatings, their use has been limited in the dental profession because the coating ultimately provides additional interfaces that may undergo stress-induced failure that leads to uncertainty as to their service life, as discussed previously.

Another coating approach under investigation involves the attachment of biological mediators to the implant surface. In particular, the immobilization of short peptide sequences onto the implant surface has been demonstrated to influence cell response in vitro. Cell integrins, which bind to specific short peptide sequences, are responsible for these cell responses. In particular, the tripeptide sequence L-arginine, glycine, and L-aspartic acid (RGD) plays an important role in cell adhesion. This sequence is present in many extracellular matrix proteins, including fibrin, collagen, vitronectin, fibronectin, and osteopontin, and helps to mediate cell adhesion to surfaces. The covalent bonding of recombinant forms of these composed of, via silane chemistry, onto an implant surface may stimulate mesenchymal cell attachment and provoke osteoblast proliferation and differentiation at the site. Additional peptide sequences under investigation include the following: YIGSR, IKVAV, and KRSR (to improve cell adhesion) and FHRRIKA (to increase osteoblast mineralization).

In addition to small peptide sequences, the use of entire recombinant proteins on the implant surface has been investigated. The use of immobilized cytokine growth factors such as bone morphogenetic protein (BMP), transforming growth factor-β (TGF-β), fibroblast growth factor (FGF), vascular endothelial growth factor (VEGF), and platelet-derived growth factor (PDGF) has been shown to positively increase the regeneration of tissues around an implant. However, homogeneous coating of the implant surfaces and the release of these proteins into the surrounding tissues are rather unpredictable and uncontrolled with respect to both duration and dosage. Although further research is needed to illuminate these unresolved issues, this treatment holds promise as a future therapy.

IMPLANT MATERIALS AND PROCESSING

In general, two basic classes of materials (ceramics and metals) are used as implants, either alone or in hybrid fashion. Metallic implant materials are largely titanium based—either CP Ti or Ti-6Al-4V. However, it is essential to note that synergistic relationships between processing, composition, structure, and properties of the bulk metals and their surface oxides effectively leave more than two metals. Casting, forging, and machining, to form near-net-shaped end products, alters the bulk microstructure, surface chemistry, and properties. Similarly, densification of ceramics and deposition of ceramic and metal coatings by hot isostatic pressing or sintering can change bulk and surface composition, structure, and properties. Thus the many material processing sequences necessary to yield the end-stage dental implant have a strong influence on the properties and functionality of the implant, primarily through temperature and pressure effects.

Metallic dental implants are almost exclusively titanium-based alloys, although cobalt-based alloys have been used historically and experimentally in dentistry. The attributes of titanium, namely, corrosion resistance and high strength, are discussed in Chapter 10.

The initial rationale for using ceramics in dentistry was based on the relative biological inertness of ceramics as compared with that of metals. Ceramics are fully oxidized materials and therefore chemically stable. Thus ceramics are less likely to elicit an adverse biological response than are metals, which oxidize only at their surface. As discussed previously, a greater emphasis has been placed recently on bioactive and bioresorbable ceramics, materials that not only elicit normal tissue formation, but that may also form an intimate bond with bone tissue and even be replaced by tissue over time.

CHALLENGES AND THE FUTURE

Although there is no consensus regarding methods of evaluating dental implants and what criteria are most important, clinical evaluations have generally shown that dental implants are successful in about 95% of the cases, 5 years after implantation. Despite advances in synthesis and processing of materials, surgical technique, and clinical protocols, clinical failures occur at rates of approximately 2% to 5% per year. Causes of failure and current problems with dental implants include (1) early loosening from a lack of initial osseointegration; (2) late loosening, or loss of osseointegration; (3) bone resorption; (4) infection; (5) fracture of the implant or abutment; and (6) delamination of the coating from the bulk implant in the case of coated implants. The most common failure mechanism is alveolar crest resorption due to overloading. This inevitably leads to progressive periodontal lesions, decreased areas of supporting tissues, and ultimately to implant loosening. Aseptic failures are most often the cumulative result of more than one of the aforementioned factors.

Changes in implant materials and design will be accomplished by groups composed of dental researchers and the implant manufacturers themselves. They will continue to perform careful, multi-institutional clinical trials and prospective studies of compatibility, stress shielding, and bone loading among other factors. These three areas in particular present a major motivation for change in implant materials. Although very biocompatible, the current alloys suffer from a large elastic modulus mismatch with the supporting bone. Research work is under way to create composite materials that are biologically compatible and have the same modulus of elasticity as bone. Similar modulii will result in a stress distribution that more closely mimics that seen physiologically. Additionally, the work being performed to investigate implant texture effects is sure to reveal additional fundamental principles that will incrementally improve implant designs.

However, in spite of these new research directions, the future of implant dentistry lies in the hands of the restorative dentist. After an implant has been placed and healed, it is the restorative dentist who is responsible for designing and delivering the restoration or prosthesis to the patient. Patient satisfaction of the function and esthetics of the implant-supported prosthesis defines the success, or failure, of an implant case. Implants are in the mainstream of routine dental care in many countries. Their clinical success justifies the offering of implants along with more traditional therapies of fixed and removable partial prostheses for restoring edentulous spaces.

SELECTED PROBLEMS

PROBLEM 1

Name and define the three classifications of dental implants.

Solution

The three classifications are as follows:
1. The subperiosteal implant—a design whereby a metal implant framework rests directly on top of the bone, underlying the periosteum, and provides attachment posts, which extend through the gingival tissue for prosthesis anchorage.
2. The transosteal implant—a design used only in the anterior mandible in which posts extend completely through the mandible and gingiva to provide prosthesis anchorage.
3. The endosteal implant—a cylinder or screw-shaped design whereby the implant is surgically placed directly within the mandible or maxilla and provides prosthesis anchorage via a threaded socket within its body.

PROBLEM 2

A new type of all-metal implant is placed and allowed to heal uneventfully for 12 weeks. Two weeks after restoration, it begins to be mobile and fails. What are the probable causes?

Solution

If an implant moves within the preparation site, it has failed to properly osseointegrate. One crucial aspect in enabling osseointegration is the preparation of the bone. The site should be drilled slowly and prepared with copious irrigation to avoid heating or traumatizing the bone. The site should also be inspected for adequate quantity and quality of the bone tissue prior to placement. Another aspect affecting osseointegration is the material from which the implant was fabricated. Not all materials will promote osseointegration. Titanium or Ti-6Al-4V alloy are the current materials of choice for dental implants. Finally, after loading begins, micromotion between the bone and implant will prevent osseointegration, because the formation of a fibrous encapsulation will result.

PROBLEM 3

Describe the difference between osseointegration and biointegration.

Solution

Osseointegration is the formation of a strong intimate contact between an implant surface and the surrounding bone tissue. The interface that results is capable of withstanding the normal forces generated during mastication. The presence of an intervening ceramic coating on an implant will prevent such a surface contact from forming. At a minimum, two interfaces are created at the inner and outer surfaces of the coating. However, if the ceramic coating is bioactive, it may become chemically fused to the surrounding bone on its exterior surface, while maintaining a tight physical attachment to the metallic implant surface on the interior coating surface. In this case, the interface with the bone is termed *biointegration*, because the bone-implant contact has an intervening layer with two strong interfaces.

PROBLEM 4

Describe the dental implant design that has the best success rate and broadest clinical application.

Solution

Implants are usually classified according to the way in which they are positioned in the patient's jaw. The most successful endosteal implant designs use a cylindrical or screw-shaped implant that is positioned almost completely within the bone site. The coronal end of the implant body permits direct connection of a superstructure through the mucosa. This superstructure is attached to an abutment, which is in turn attached via a screw directly into an internal threaded socket within the implant body.

PROBLEM 5

After a posterior implant and restoration has been in function for a period of time, dark staining of the mucosa around the restoration is seen. What are the probable causes?

Solution

Even in a passive state, ions are constantly released from metal surfaces in the mouth. The staining of the tissue could be the result of titanium ion release from the implant. Alternatively, this could be due to corrosion and ion release from metals in the superstructure restoration.

PROBLEM 6

What role does a bioactive ceramic coating serve on the surface of a metallic implant?

Solution

Bioactive ceramic materials are unique among the biomaterials in that they induce direct chemical bonding to living tissues when implanted in vivo. This response may provide enhanced biocompatibility to a metallic implant. These materials are usually composed of calcium- and phosphorus-containing phases, and they render the surface electrically nonconductive. Also, the dissolution/degradation of the coating provides the major ionic constituents of bone mineral (calcium [Ca] and phosphorus [P]) freely available at the implant site. This is thought to encourage faster osseointegration. Finally, the roughened surface provides contact guidance to migrating cells.

Bibliography

Albrektsson T, Branemark PI, Hansson HA, et al: Osseointegrated titanium implants. Requirements for ensuring a long-lasting, direct bone-to-implant anchorage in man, *Acta. Orthop. Scand* 52:155, 1981.

Ameen AP, Short RD, Johns R, et al: The surface analysis of implant materials. 1. The surface composition of a titanium dental implant material, *Clin Oral Implants Res* 4:144, 1993.

Aparicio C, Gil FJ, Fonseca C, et al: Corrosion behaviour of commercially pure titanium shot blasted with different materials and sizes of shot particles for dental implant applications, *Biomaterials* 24:263, 2003.

Arvidson K, Fartash B, Moberg LE, et al: in vitro and in vivo experimental studies on single crystal sapphire dental implants, *Clin Oral Implants Res* 2:47, 1991.

Baschong W, Suetterlin R, Hefti A, et al: Confocal laser scanning microscopy and scanning electron microscopy of tissue Ti-implant interfaces, *Micron* 32:33, 2001.

Berglundh T, Abrahamsson I, Lang NP, et al: De novo alveolar bone formation adjacent to endosseous implants, *Clin Oral Implants Res* 14:251, 2003.

Block MS, Kent JN: Sinus augmentation for dental implants: the use of autogenous bone, *J Oral Maxillofac Surg* 55:1281, 1997.

Boggan RS, Strong JT, Misch CE, et al: Influence of hex geometry and prosthetic table width on static and fatigue strength of dental implants, *J Prosthet Dent* 82:436, 1999.

Botticelli D, Berglundh T, Lindhe J: The influence of a biomaterial on the closure of a marginal hard tissue defect adjacent to implants. An experimental study in the dog, *Clin Oral Implants Res* 15:285, 2004.

Branemark PI, Adell R, Breine U, et al: Intra-osseous anchorage of dental prostheses. I. Experimental studies, *Scand J Plast Reconstr Surg* 3:81, 1969.

Branemark PI, Albrektsson T: Titanium implants permanently penetrating human skin, *Scand J Plast Reconstr Surg* 16:17, 1982.

Bucci-Sabattini V, Cassinelli C, Coelho PG, et al: Effect of titanium implant surface nanoroughness and calcium phosphate low impregnation on bone cell activity in vitro, *Oral Surg Oral Med Oral Pathol Oral Radiol Endod.* 109(2):217–224, 2010.

Catledge SA, Fries MD, Vohra YK, et al: Nanostructured ceramics for biomedical implants, *J Nanosci Nanotechnol* 2:293, 2002.

Cook SD, Dalton JE: Biocompatibility and biofunctionality of implanted materials, *Alpha Omegan* 85:41, 1992.

Cook SD, Klawitter JJ, Weinstein AM: A model for the implant-bone interface characteristics of porous dental implants, *J Dent Res* 61:1006, 1982.

Cook SD, Weinstein AM, Klawitter JJ, et al: Quantitative histologic evaluation of LTI carbon, carbon-coated aluminum oxide and uncoated aluminum oxide dental implants, *J Biomed Mater Res* 17:519, 1983.

Cooper LF, Masuda T, Yliheikkila PK, et al: Generalizations regarding the process and phenomenon of osseointegration. Part II. in vitro studies, *Int J Oral Maxillofac Implants* 13:163, 1998.

de Lavos-Valereto IC, Deboni MC, Azambuja N Jr, et al: Evaluation of the titanium Ti-6Al-7Nb alloy with and without plasma-sprayed hydroxyapatite coating on growth and viability of cultured osteoblast-like cells, *J Periodontol* 73:900, 2002.

De Maeztu MA, Alava JI, Gay-Escoda C: Ion implantation: surface treatment for improving the bone integration of titanium and Ti6Al4V dental implants, *Clin Oral Implants Res* 14:57, 2003.

Denissen HW, Klein CP, Visch LL, et al: Behavior of calcium phosphate coatings with different chemistries in bone, *Int J Prosthodont* 9:142, 1996.

Dubruille JH, Viguier E, Le Naour G, et al: Evaluation of combinations of titanium, zirconia, and alumina implants with 2 bone fillers in the dog, *Int J Oral Maxillofac Implants* 14:271, 1999.

Elias CN, Meirelles L: Improving osseointegration of dental implants, *Expert Rev Med Devices.* 7(2):241–256, 2010.

Galgut PN, Waite IM, Brookshaw JD, et al: A 4-year controlled clinical study into the use of a ceramic hydroxylapatite implant material for the treatment of periodontal bone defects, *J Clin Periodontol* 19:570, 1992.

Galgut PN, Waite IM, Tinkler SM: Histological investigation of the tissue response to hydroxyapatite used as an implant material in periodontal treatment, *Clin Mater* 6:105, 1990.

Gatti AM, Zaffe D, Poli GP, et al: The evaluation of the interface between bone and a bioceramic dental implant, *J Biomed Mater Res* 21:1005, 1987.

Giannoni P, Muraglia A, Giordano C, et al: Osteogenic differentiation of human mesenchymal stromal cells on surface-modified titanium alloys for orthopedic and dental implants, *Int J Artif Organs* 32(11):811–820, 2009.

Gineste L, Gineste M, Ranz X, et al: Degradation of hydroxylapatite, fluorapatite, and fluorhydroxyapatite coatings of dental implants in dogs, *J Biomed Mater Res* 48:224, 1998.

Glantz PO: The choice of alloplastic materials for oral implants: does it really matter, *Int J Prosthodont* 11:402, 1998.

Guy SC, McQuade MJ, Scheidt MJ, et al: in vitro attachment of human gingival fibroblasts to endosseous implant materials, *J Periodontol* 64:542, 1993.

Haas R, Donath K, Fodinger M, et al: Bovine hydroxyapatite for maxillary sinus grafting: comparative histomorphometric findings in sheep, *Clin Oral Implants Res* 9:107, 1998.

Hall EE, Meffert RM, Hermann JS, et al: Comparison of bioactive glass to demineralized freeze-dried bone allograft in the treatment of intrabony defects around implants in the canine mandible, *J Periodontol* 70:526, 1999.

Haman JD, Scripa RN, Rigsbee JM, et al: Production of thin calcium phosphate coatings from glass source materials, *J Mater Sci Mater Med* 13:175, 2002.

Hatano N, Shimizu Y, Ooya K: A clinical long-term radiographic evaluation of graft height changes after maxillary sinus floor augmentation with a 2:1 autogenous bone/xenograft mixture and simultaneous placement of dental implants, *Clin Oral Implants Res* 15:339, 2004.

Hedia HS, Mahmoud NA: Design optimization of functionally graded dental implant, *Biomed Mater Eng* 14:133, 2004.

Hobkirk JA: Endosseous implants: the host-implant surface, *Ann Acad Med Singapore* 15:403, 1986.

Hodosh M, Shklar G: A polymethacrylate-silica composite material for dental implants, *J Biomed Mater Res* 11:893, 1977.

Holden CM, Bernard GW: Ultrastructural in vitro characterization of a porous hydroxyapatite/bone cell interface, *J Oral Implantol* 16:86, 1990.

Hucke EE, Fuys RA, Craig RG: Glassy carbon: a potential dental implant material, *J Biomed Mater Res* 7:263, 1973.

Hurson S: Threaded implant design criteria, *Int J Dent Symp* 2:38, 1994.

Jarcho M: Retrospective analysis of hydroxyapatite development for oral implant applications, *Dent Clin North Am* 36:19, 1992.

Jokstad A, Braegger U, Brunski JB, et al: Quality of dental implants, *Int Dent J* 53:409, 2003.

Kamel I: A porous and potentially tough dental implant material, *J Dent Res* 55:1143, 1976.

Karoussis IK, Bragger U, Salvi GE, et al: Effect of implant design on survival and success rates of titanium oral implants: a 10-year prospective cohort study of the ITI Dental Implant System, *Clin Oral Implants Res* 15:8, 2004.

Kasemo B, Gold J: Implant surfaces and interface processes, *Adv Dent Res* 13:8, 1999.

Kay JF: Calcium phosphate coatings for dental implants. Current status and future potential, *Dent Clin North Am* 36:1, 1992.

Kikuchi S, Takebe J: Characterization of the surface deposition on anodized-hydrothermally treated commercially pure titanium after immersion in simulated body fluid, *J Prosthodont Res* 54(2):70–77, 2010.

Klinger A, Tadir A, Halabi A, et al: The effect of surface processing of titanium implants on the behavior of human osteoblast-like Saos-2 cells. *Clin Implant Dent Relat Res* 13:64, 2011.

Kohal RJ, Bachle M, Emmerich D, et al: Hard tissue reaction to dual acid-etched titanium implants: influence of plaque accumulation. A histological study in humans, *Clin Oral Implants Res* 14:381, 2003.

Kohal RJ, Weng D, Bachle M, et al: Loaded custom-made zirconia and titanium implants show similar osseointegration: an animal experiment, *J Periodontol* 75:1262, 2004.

Kohn DH: Overview of factors important in implant design, *J Oral Implantol* 18:204, 1992.

Kononen M, Hormia M, Kivilahti J, et al: Effect of surface processing on the attachment, orientation, and proliferation of human gingival fibroblasts on titanium, *J Biomed Mater Res* 26:1325, 1992.

Krennmair G, Seemann R, Schmidinger S, et al: Clinical outcome of root-shaped dental implants of various diameters: 5-year results, *Int J Oral Maxillofac Implants* 25:357, 2010.

Lacefield WR: Current status of ceramic coatings for dental implants, *Implant Dent* 7:315, 1998.

Lemons JE: Dental implant biomaterials, *J Am Dent Assoc* 121:716, 1990.

Linder L, Albrektsson T, Branemark PI, et al: Electron microscopic analysis of the bone-titanium interface, *Acta Orthop Scand* 54:45, 1983.

Liu J, Jin T, Chang S, Czajka-Jakubowska A, et al: The effect of novel fluorapatite surfaces on osteoblast-like cell adhesion, growth, and mineralization, *Tissue Eng. Part A* 16(9):2977–2986, 2010.

Lutz R, Srour S, Nonhoff J, et al: Biofunctionalization of titanium implants with a biomimetic active peptide (P-15) promotes early osseointegration, *Clin. Oral. Implants Res.* 21(7):726–734, 2010.

Marketsandmarkets.com: Global dental implants market (2010-2015), http://www.marketsandmarkets.com/Market-Reports/Dental-Implants-Market-241.html: accessed August 28, 2011.

Massaro C, Rotolo P, De Riccardis F, et al: Comparative investigation of the surface properties of commercial titanium dental implants. Part I: chemical composition, *J Mater Sci Mater Med* 13:535, 2002.

Meyer U, Wiesmann HP, Fillies T, et al: Early tissue reaction at the interface of immediately loaded dental implants, *Int J Oral Maxillofac Implants* 18:489, 2003.

Morris HF, Ochi S: Hydroxyapatite-coated implants: a case for their use, *J Oral Maxillofac Surg* 56:1303, 1998.

Mueller WD, Gross U, Fritz T, et al: Evaluation of the interface between bone and titanium surfaces being blasted by aluminium oxide or bioceramic particles, *Clin Oral Implants Res* 14:349, 2003.

Muller-Mai C, Schmitz HJ, Strunz V, et al: Tissues at the surface of the new composite material titanium/glass-ceramic for replacement of bone and teeth, *J Biomed Mater Res* 23:1149, 1989.

Najjar TA, Lerdrit W, Parsons JR: Enhanced osseointegration of hydroxylapatite implant material, *Oral Surg Oral Med Oral Pathol* 71:9, 1991.

O'Neal RB, Sauk JJ, Somerman MJ: Biological requirements for material integration, *J Oral Implantol* 18:243, 1992.

Paterson HA, Zamanian K: The global dental implant market to experience strong growth despite the economic downturn, *Implant Practice* 2:xx, 2009.

Pelaez-Vargas A, Gallego-Perez D, Ferrell N, et al: Early Spreading and Propagation of Human Bone Marrow Stem Cells on Isotropic and Anisotropic Topographies of Silica Thin Films Produced via Microstamping, *Microsc Microanal* 22:1–7, 2010.

Piattelli A, Scarano A, Piattelli M, et al: Histologic aspects of the bone and soft tissues surrounding three titanium non-submerged plasma-sprayed implants retrieved at autopsy: a case report, *J Periodontol* 68:694, 1997.

Piattelli M, Scarano A, Paolantonio M, et al: Bone response to machined and resorbable blast material titanium implants: an experimental study in rabbits, *J Oral Implantol* 28:2, 2002.

Piddock V: Production of bioceramic surfaces with controlled porosity, *Int J Prosthodont* 4:58, 1991.

Puleo DA, Nanci A: Understanding and controlling the bone-implant interface, *Biomaterials* 20:2311, 1999.

Quaranta A, Iezzi G, Scarano A, et al: A histomorphometric study of nanothickness and plasma-sprayed calcium-phosphorous-coated implant surfaces in rabbit bone, *J. Periodontol* 81(4):556–561, 2010.

Rahal MD, Branemark PI, Osmond DG: Response of bone marrow to titanium implants: osseointegration and the establishment of a bone marrow-titanium interface in mice, *Int J Oral Maxillofac Implants* 8:573, 1993.

Roberts WE: Bone dynamics of osseointegration, ankylosis, and tooth movement, *J Indiana Dent Assoc* 78:24, 1999.

Rugh SD, Solberg WK: The measurement of human oral forces, *Behav Res Meth Instrum* 4:125, 1972.

Ruhling A, Hellweg A, Kocher T, et al: Removal of HA and TPS implant coatings and fibroblast attachment on exposed surfaces, *Clin Oral Implants Res* 12:301, 2001.

Rupprecht S, Bloch A, Rosiwal S, et al: Examination of the bone-metal interface of titanium implants coated by the microwave plasma chemical vapor deposition method, *Int J Oral Maxillofac Implants* 17:778, 2002.

Scarano A, Pecora G, Piattelli M, et al: Osseointegration in a sinus augmented with bovine porous bone mineral: histological results in an implant retrieved 4 years after insertion, *A case report, J Periodontol* 75:1161, 2004.

Schlegel AK, Donath K: BIO-OSS—a resorbable bone substitute, *J Long Term Eff Med Implants* 8:201, 1998.

Schwarz MS: Mechanical complications of dental implants, *Clin Oral Implants Res* 11:156, 2000.

Smith DC: Dental implants: materials and design considerations, *Int J Prosthodont* 6:106, 1993.

Stanford CM, Brand RA: Toward an understanding of implant occlusion and strain adaptive bone modeling and remodeling, *J Prosthet Dent* 81:553, 1999.

Steflik DE, Corpe RS, Young TR, et al: The biologic tissue responses to uncoated and coated implanted biomaterials, *Adv Dent Res* 13:27, 1999.

Steflik DE, McKinney RV Jr, Koth DL, et al: The biomaterial-tissue interface: a morphological study utilizing conventional and alternative ultrastructural modalities, *Scan Electron Microsc* 2:547, 1984.

Steinemann SG: Titanium—the material of choice, *Periodontol 2000* 17:7, 1998.

Sullivan DY, Sherwood RL, Mai TN: Preliminary results of a multicenter study evaluating a chemically enhanced surface for machined commercially pure titanium implants, *J Prosthet Dent* 78:379, 1997.

Sun L, Berndt CC, Gross KA, et al: Material fundamentals and clinical performance of plasma-sprayed hydroxyapatite coatings: a review, *J Biomed Mater Res* 58:570, 2001.

Svanborg LM, Andersson M, Wennerberg A: Surface characterization of commercial oral implants on the nanometer level, *J Biomed Mater Res B Appl Biomater* 92(2):462–469, 2010.

Tamura Y, Yokoyama A, Watari F, et al: Surface properties and biocompatibility of nitrided titanium for abrasion resistant implant materials, *Dent Mater J* 21:355, 2002.

Taylor TD, Laney WR: *Dental implants: Are they for me?* ed 2, Carol Stream, IL, 1993, Quintessence Publishing Co.

Triplett RG, Frohberg U, Sykaras N, et al: Implant materials, design, and surface topographies: their influence on osseointegration of dental implants, *J Long Term Eff Med Implants* 13:485, 2003.

Ungvári K, Pelsöczi IK, Kormos B, et al: Effects on titanium implant surfaces of chemical agents used for the treatment of peri-implantitis, *J Biomed Mater Res B Appl Biomater* 94(1):222–229, 2010.

Variola F, Brunski JB, Orsini G, et al: Nanoscale surface modifications of medically relevant metals: state-of-the art and perspectives, *Nanoscale* 3(2):335–353, 2011, 2010, Oct 26.

Vercaigne S, Wolke JG, Naert I, et al: Bone healing capacity of titanium plasma-sprayed and hydroxylapatite-coated oral implants, *Clin Oral Implants Res* 9:261, 1998.

Vlacic-Zischke J, Hamlet SM, Friis T, et al: The influence of surface microroughness and hydrophilicity of titanium on the up-regulation of TGFβ/BMP signaling in osteoblasts, *Biomaterials* 32(3):665–671, 2011, 2010.

Wagner WC: A brief introduction to advanced surface modification technologies, *J Oral Implantol* 18:231, 1992.

Wataha JC: Materials for endosseous dental implants, *J Oral Rehabil* 23:79, 1996.

Weinlaender M: Bone growth around dental implants, *Dent Clin North Am* 35:585, 1991.

Wennerberg A, Albrektsson T: On implant surfaces: a review of current knowledge and opinions, *Int J Oral Maxillofac Implants* 25(1):63–74, 2010.

Tissue Engineering

Tissue engineering is a term coined at a meeting sponsored by the National Institutes of Health in 1987. This discipline is a rapidly developing multi-disciplinary branch of science that combines many of the basic principles of biology, medicine, and engineering. The primary goal of tissue engineering is the restoration, maintenance, or enhancement of tissue and organ function.

In addition to having therapeutic applications, in which a particular organ is custom grown to replace a failing or missing body part, tissue engineering has diagnostic applications in which tissues are fabricated in vitro and used for in vitro biocompatibility testing of compounds. Examples include application in drug metabolism and uptake, toxicity, or pathogenicity. Tissue engineering research, therefore, translates fundamental knowledge in physics, chemistry, and biology into materials, devices, and strategies. It also integrates biomaterials, cell biology, and stem cell research; engineering characteristics of three-dimensional structures and mass transport issues; biomechanical characteristics of native and replacement tissues, biomolecules and growth factors; and bioinformatics to support gene/protein expression and analysis.

Tissue engineering as a discipline grew out of the pressing need for replacement tissues and organs. During 2010, in the United States alone, over 28,600 solid organs (heart, lung, intestine, kidney, pancreas, and liver) were transplanted. More than three quarters of those organs came from deceased donors. Meanwhile, during this same period, 56,437 new potential recipients were added to the waiting list and nearly 7000 patients died while waiting for a transplant (Box 16-1). Clearly, the demand for organs greatly exceeds the supply. Enthusiasm for tissue engineering comes from the promise of making transplants easier and more common. In dentistry, the disciplines of periodontology and oral and maxillofacial surgery often use bone tissue transplant materials to repair defects.

Today, there are four primary classes of tissue/organ transplants: autograft, allograft, xenograft, and alloplast (Box 16-2).

AUTOGRAFT

An autograft is a tissue or organ that is transferred from one location to another within a single individual (Figure 16-1). It is common to transplant tissues such as hair, blood, and even limited amounts of skin and bone. These tissues regenerate to some extent, repairing the void left after their removal. This method of transplantation avoids immunologic complications and is considered the "gold standard" for success.

BOX 16.1

Summary of Transplant Data, United States

Candidate waiting list as of August 19, 2011[†]

All*	111,733
All—added in 2010	56,437
Kidney	89,442
Pancreas	1,363
Kidney/pancreas	2,137
Liver	16,151
Intestine	255
Heart	3,185
Lung	1,747
Heart/lung	69
Removed from list due to death, 2010	6,946

Transplants performed in 2010[†]

Total	28,662
Deceased donor	22,103
Living donor	6,559

Median waiting times for kidney transplant[‡]

Type O Blood 1999-2000	1763 days (4.8 years)
Type O Blood 2001-2002	1833 days (5.0 years)
Type O Blood 2003-2004	1852 days (5.1 years)

*All candidates will be less than the sum due to candidates waiting for multiple organs.
†Based on Organ Procurement and Transplant Network (OPTN) data as of 08/19/2011.
‡Based on OPTN data (2004—latest data available).

ALLOGRAFT

Allografts are tissues or organs that are transplanted from one individual to another within the same species (Figure 16-2). Routinely, tissues and organs are removed from deceased individuals (as well as living donors) and transferred to a different individual. Blood, bone, skin, corneas, ligaments, and tendons are collected in banks and frozen, to be used in future surgical procedures.

XENOGRAFT

The Center for Biologics Evaluation and Research (CBER) is the Food and Drug Administration (FDA) branch that oversees and regulates human tissue transplants. They define xenotransplants as "transplantation, implantation, or infusion into a human recipient of either (a) live cells, tissues, or organs from a nonhuman animal source or (b) human body fluids, cells, tissues, or organs that have had ex vivo contact with live nonhuman animal cells, tissues, or organs." This therapeutic regimen has been used experimentally to treat neurodegenerative disorders, liver failure, and diabetes, when compatible human materials are not widely available.

Xenografts are now common in dentistry. Two examples are BioOss (a product derived from cow bone) and BioCoral (a corraline product) that are used to augment defects in the maxilla and mandible (Figure 16-3).

ALLOPLASTS

Alloplasts are the newest type of grafting procedure materials. These grafts are fabricated completely from synthetic materials, making them quite different from the other three types of grafts, because no living component is used. Alloplasts, such as dental implants, are becoming increasingly common in dentistry. Dental implants fabricated from metals and ceramics are considered routine restorative treatment in many countries. These materials integrate with bone and help restore function for the patient, with excellent long-term success.

Bone grafting alloplasts are also common (Figure 16-4). Autograft bone placed in the reconstruction of craniofacial structures can be augmented with ceramic and bioactive glasses. These alloplasts are available in nearly unlimited quantity with no adverse immunological reaction. An important benefit is that they do not pose the risk of transmitting disease from one individual to another.

BOX 16.2

Sources of Tissue for Grafting

Autograft: The patient's own tissue
Allograft: Human source other than the patient
   (could be cadaveric)

Xenograft: Tissue from a different species
Alloplast: Synthetic origin

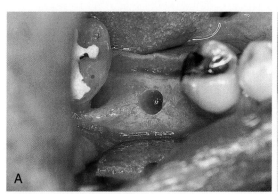 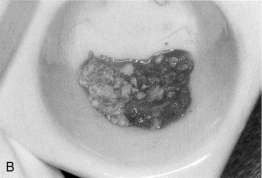

FIGURE 16.1 **Autograft bone (B) is harvested (A) from the patient into whom it will be reimplanted.** *(From Newman MG, Takei HH, Klokkevold PR, et al: Carranza's clinical periodontology, 11ᵗʰ ed. Saunders, St. Louis, 2012.)*

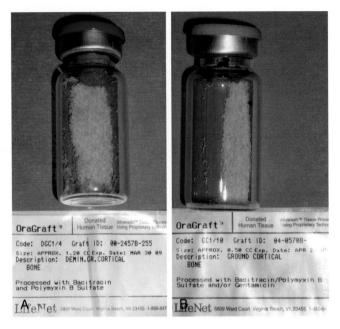

FIGURE 16.2 **Freeze-dried bone allograft is harvested from humans and sold in sterilized vials in both a demineralized form (A) as well as a fully mineralized form (B).** *(Courtesy of Mitchell JC, OHSU School of Dentistry, Portland, OR).*

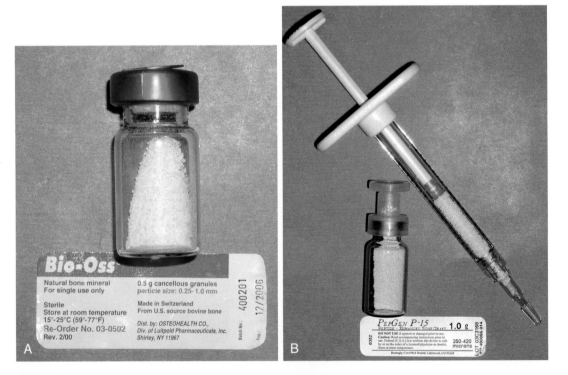

FIGURE 16.3 **Bone matrices.** BioOss, **A**, is a porous bone mineral matrix xenograft prepared from bovine sources; Pepgen P-15, **B**, combines an organic component—a synthetically manufactured amino acid sequence (P-15) designed to elicit cell bonding, with an inorganic calcium-phosphate matrix that acts as a carrier for the amino acid sequence and a scaffold for bone growth. *(Courtesy of Mitchell JC, OHSU School of Dentistry, Portland, OR).*

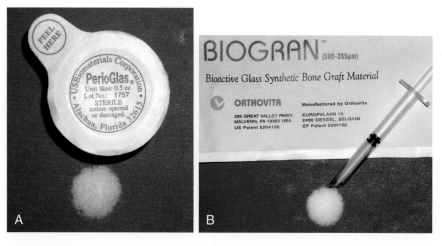

FIGURE 16.4 **Bioactive glasses have received increased attention as a result of their surface bioactivity.** Shown here are PerioGlas, **A,** and Biogran, **B**. *(Courtesy of Mitchell JC, OHSU School of Dentistry, Portland, OR).*

BOX 16.3

Strategies for Tissue Engineering

Injection of cells: Undifferentiated cells (usually not from the patient) are injected directly into the vicinity of injury.

Guided tissue regeneration: Undesired cells are excluded from repopulating a defect or injury site by placing a physical barrier to prevent their migration. Desirable cells are able to enter the site from the surrounding tissue.

Cell induction: Growth and differentiation factors are injected (or implanted with a time-release substrate) within the injury or defect site. Circulating cells are induced to differentiate and populate the site with a desirable phenotype.

Alternatively, gene vectors are injected and cause the growth/differentiation factors to be produced endogenously.

Cells in a scaffold matrix: Preformed scaffolds are seeded with cells from a patient. This construct is grown in vitro to expand the number of cells and to allow the cells to begin to produce a matrix. After a suitable growth interval, the construct is implanted back into the patient. As the cells grow and develop into tissues, the scaffold slowly resorbs, leaving no trace of its former presence.

STRATEGIES FOR TISSUE ENGINEERING

Tissue engineering began with the concept of using biomaterials and cells to assist the body in healing itself. As the discipline matured, its goal shifted to developing logical strategies for optimizing new tissue formation through the judicious selection of conditions that will enhance the performance of tissue progenitors in a graft site, ultimately encouraging the production of a desired tissue or organ. Several strategies are now available for developing new organs and tissues (Box 16-3).

Injection of Cells

With the cell injection method, disaggregated cells at an undifferentiated stage of development are injected into the recipient. Considerable research had been conducted into the use of this method to combat systemic diseases such as Alzheimer's and Parkinson's disease, as well as juvenile-onset diabetes and multiple sclerosis. It also holds potential for treating damaged nerve and muscle sites. Commonly referred to as *stem cells*, the injected cells are more appropriately termed *undifferentiated* or *progenitor cells* (see later discussion under Stem Cells). These cells are capable of forming new tissue with one or more phenotypes. As a therapeutic regimen, the cells

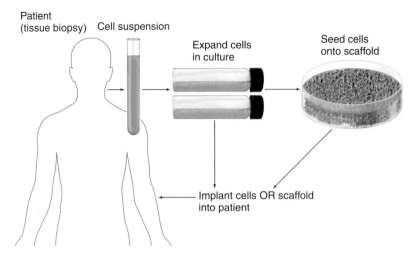

Patient
(tissue biopsy)   Cell suspension

Expand cells
in culture

Seed cells
onto scaffold

Implant cells OR scaffold
into patient

FIGURE 16.5 **Cell injection therapy.** May involve the use of scaffold into which the cells are expanded, or they may be directly injected into their target site without a substrate.

are injected into the vicinity of the site in which they are intended to propagate, and they migrate to the area of injury and begin to replicate and replace the lost tissue, or produce a desired compound such as insulin (Figure 16-5). This strategy has already been successful in regenerating small areas of cartilage in temporomandibular joints.

Guided Tissue Regeneration

Guided tissue regeneration (GTR) is a surgical procedure for regenerating tissue by enhancing the opportunity for one cell type to populate an area while providing contact guidance to the developing cells. The desired cell types can then populate an area without competition because unwanted cell types are excluded. In the laboratory, the method has been successful in creating a biodegradable polymer conduit through which nerve cell regeneration and reconnection can occur. GTR is commonly used in periodontal treatment to regenerate lost periodontal tissues such as the bone, periodontal ligament, and connective tissue attachment that support the teeth. The procedure involves placement of a membrane under the mucosa and over the residual bone (Figure 16-6). The barrier helps to exclude the faster-growing epithelium and gingival connective tissues during the postsurgical healing phase, allowing the slower-growing periodontal ligament and bone cells to migrate into the protected areas.

Cell Induction

In the last decade there has been explosive growth in understanding the role of cytokines, developmental proteins, and growth factors in molecular biology. Many of these growth factors are available

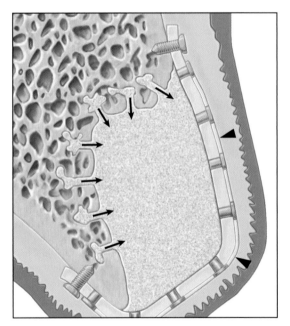

FIGURE 16.6 **Guided bone regeneration (GBR).** GBR is being used to isolate the site being regenerated from the overlying tissues by means of a titanium-reinforced membrane barrier *(arrowheads)*. The newly forming bone may be augmented by the addition of particulate grafting material. The barrier is securely attached to the margins of the defect to prevent displacement during healing. Notice that decortication of the underlying bone bed allows invasion of the site by osteogenic precursor cells from the blood stream and surrounding bone.

as recombinant human lyophilized proteins. There have been tremendous advances in administering various mixtures of these growth factors directly to tissues to force them down a particular differentiation lineage. Often these growth and differentiation factors can be simply injected into the site. This technique, as a tissue-engineering regimen, targets local connective tissue progenitors already present in the region where new tissues are desired and induces those cells to generate the desired tissue. Some of the injected proteins may serve as mitogens in recruiting cells to migrate into the area, where other growth factors cause them to differentiate. Alternatively, they can be delivered by a substrate that releases them over time.

Gene therapy can be used with cell induction methods. In this application, a gene sequence that encodes for production of a particular growth factor or therapeutic compound is inserted wholly into the genome of the recipient cell. Insertion is achieved by a carrier, called a *vector*, to deliver the therapeutic gene to the patient's target cells. The most common vector is a genetically altered virus that has been modified to carry human DNA. Because viruses have evolved a way of encapsulating and delivering their genes to human cells, they can be manipulated to insert these therapeutic genes into the recipient cells. So, vectors are injected into a site along with an initial bolus of the therapeutic compound, and the vectors then upload their genes into resident cells. After incorporating this DNA into their genome, the newly transfected cells begin to replicate the desired growth factor endogenously. This method promotes continuous protein production at the site long after the initially injected growth factors diffuse from their target tissues or degrade enzymatically.

Cells Within Scaffold Matrices

Three-dimensional porous scaffolds can be used with cells to provide many of the advantages of the methods described above. These preformed scaffolds are usually made of bioresorbable materials. The scaffolds promote new tissue formation by providing a surface and void volume that encourages attachment, migration, proliferation, and the desired differentiation of connective tissue progenitors throughout the region where new tissue is required. Typically, the scaffold is seeded with progenitor cells that are allowed to attach and proliferate in vitro. The cell constructs are often grown in a nutrient media supplemented with growth factors necessary for cell and tissue development. During the growth phase, a static or dynamic mechanical load may be applied to the construct, to align the cells in response to the load. The aligned cells tend to produce a highly organized extracellular matrix that results in improved tissue structure and function. After a suitable time in vitro, the entire construct is then implanted in vivo, where the tissue must continue to develop while forming a connection with the existing vascular system. The scaffold gradually degrades until it is completely replaced by new tissues. As the scaffold degrades, the developing tissues gradually experience higher fractions of the loads on the tissue and begin to function as native tissues.

The scaffold can therefore serve a dual function, as both a rigid substrate for cell growth as well as a delivery vehicle for the release of therapeutic regulatory compounds in vivo. Release of bioactive molecules that are attached to the scaffold surface or encapsulated within the scaffold matrix can change the function of connective tissue progenitor cells (activation, proliferation, migration, differentiation, or survival) to create new or enhanced tissues (Figure 16-7). There are several critical variables in design and function of the scaffold design. Variables include the composition of the scaffold, its three-dimensional architecture, surface chemistry, mechanical properties, and the physical, chemical, and biological environment in the area surrounding the scaffold during its functional lifetime, which is often determined by its degradation characteristics.

All cells require access to metabolic molecules (oxygen, glucose, and amino acids) and removal of cellular waste products (carbon dioxide, nitrogen compounds, and salts). There also must be a balance between consumption and delivery of these molecules if cells are to survive. Design of the scaffold must accommodate these issues. Eventually a rich blood supply will perform these tasks, but such a circulatory system takes time to mature.

Patients who receive allogenous tissue and organ transplants are often treated with immunosuppressive drugs for their lifetime to prevent rejection of the grafted tissue. These drugs can have severe side effects. The ideal source of cells for tissue engineering therapies is the patient. Autograft tissue eliminates the potential for adverse immunological reaction. However, autograft tissues usually require an additional surgical site and the associated expense, discomfort, and healing time.

STEM CELLS

Stem cells are used in tissue engineering therapies that are not terminally differentiated and are able to migrate within the body and to self-replicate. Additionally, they are able to produce progeny cells with multiple phenotypes. There are different types of stem cells within the body: pleuripotent cells can become any of the over 200 types of cells in the body, whereas multipotent cells are limited to forming only specific tissues.

Until very recently, most stem cell researchers worked with only two types of cells: embryonic stem cells (which are pleuripotent); and somatic or "adult" stem cells (usually considered to be

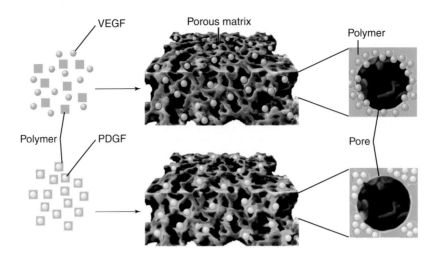

FIGURE 16.7 **Scaffold systems.** These systems may serve as delivery substrates for various therapeutic compounds, in addition to providing the cells with a suitable surface on which to grow. Multiple factors may even be delivered with different release profiles by varying the method in which they are incorporated into the substrate. In this example, vascular endothelial growth factor (VEGF) is incorporated largely near the surface of the scaffold, and is subject to rapid release in vivo. In contrast, the preencapsulated platelet-derived growth factor (PDGF) is more uniformly incorporated throughout the scaffold and is subject to release regulated by the degradation of the matrix polymer. *(Modified from Richardson T, Peters M, Ennett A, et al: Nature Biotech. 19, 1029, 2001.)*

multipotent progenitor cells). Besides their origin, there are important differences between these stem cell types. For example, adult mesenchymal (or stromal) stem cells have been shown to be only capable of transdifferentiation into neural tissue, cartilage, bone, and fat. So, these "adult" cells were thought to be limited to developing into one of only a limited number of cell types. Mesenchymal cells are found in small numbers in bone marrow and also found circulating in the blood stream. Isolating these cells from mature tissues is difficult, and routine methods to multiply them in vitro have not yet been perfected. Embryonic stem cells, on the other hand, can be grown relatively easily in culture. Because a large number of cells are needed for successful stem cell replacement therapy, the choice of cell type is important.

Despite being easier to culture, embryonic stem cells are prone to immunogenic rejection. This is a significant drawback. On the other hand, adult stem cells, and tissues derived from them, are less likely to induce rejection because the origin of the cells is the patient. In that case, the patient's own cells could be multiplied in culture, induced to differentiate into the specific cell type needed, and then reimplanted.

Recently, two additional stem cell types have been found. One previously unknown type has been isolated from the pulp of normally lost deciduous teeth. These cells have been termed *SHED* (Stem cells from Human Exfoliated Deciduous teeth). SHED cells appear to have greater proliferative capabilities than adult stem cells and also maintain the ability to produce the same range of progeny as mesenchymal stem cells (Figure 16-8).

Even more recently, culture conditions and viral vectors have been found in which a limited number of differentiated adult cells can be "reprogrammed" to take on an embryonic stem cell–like state. These new types of stem cells are called *induced pluripotent stem cells (iPSCs)*. They are capable of generating cells that have the characteristics of all three germ layers and can differentiate into many different tissue types. Because these cells and tissues are patient-derived, immunogenic rejection is unlikely. To reduce the potential of cancer development from viral vectors during reprogramming, nonviral delivery methods are being researched. These stem cell types have the greatest promise for future success with stem cell therapies.

Research into stem cell differentiation has led to significant discoveries, but the ultimate cause of differentiation remains unclear. Left in a cell culture plate alone, several tissue types will result from a single group of mesenchymal stem cells. However, with suitably timed administration of the appropriate growth factors, a single cell type emerges and begins to organize into a tissue. The fate of a cell is also controlled by changes in the migration, proliferation, differentiation, or survival of their progeny. Transplanted stem cells may even fuse with existing cells in a body and assume the characteristics of that tissue. Tactile stimulus or other factors to upregulate or downregulate genes to initiate these changes are being studied.

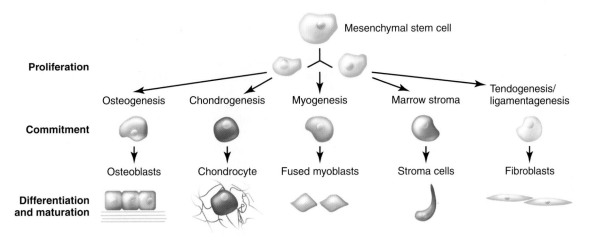

FIGURE 16.8 **Differentiation pathways of mesenchymal cells.** A circulating mesenchymal cell may become one of any of the cell types shown here. The pathway down which it travels is influenced by both local and systemic factors.

BIOMATERIALS AND SCAFFOLDS

Three types of biomaterials have been studied as scaffolds and carrier systems: (1) natural (or biological) materials, (2) ceramic or glass materials, and (3) polymeric materials. Each type has advantages and disadvantages in particular locations and tissues to be regenerated. All scaffolds must be nontoxic and nonimmunogenic, biodegradable, sterilizable, able to withstand mechanical loads, sufficiently porous to permit migration and growth of cells into their interior, and be supportive of a new fractal circulatory system to promote the exchange of metabolic constituents.

Biological Materials

Natural materials such as collagen, lyophilized bone (both allogenous and xenogenous), and coral have been used as tissue engineering substrates. Collagen has been extensively tested as a scaffold for bone regeneration. One of the first materials used for bone tissue engineering was the insoluble collagenous matrix obtained after extraction of the bone matrix with various chemical agents. This collagenous matrix, with freeze-dried bone, formed new endochondral bone when used with growth factors in vivo. Coral, based on calcium carbonate, is strikingly similar to the structure of alveolar bone. When coral is treated with phosphoric acids, the resulting calcium phosphate is very strong and biocompatible. Many patients prefer nonbiological implantable substrates because of the high potential for viral, prion, and disease transmission from these biological materials.

Ceramic and Glass Materials

Three decades of research have shown that certain types of glasses, glass-ceramics, and pure ceramics can bond tightly with living bone tissue. Hydroxyapatite (HA), the major inorganic (ceramic) constituent of bone, was one of the first alloplastic materials used as a bone augmentation scaffold. Ceramic and glass-ceramic materials are generally biocompatible and perform adequately when biomechanical loads are applied. Their use as scaffolds is limited because of their long degradation times in vivo and lack of native porosity.

Some of these limitations might be overcome in the near future with recent advances in sol-gel synthesis methods for nanoporous and nanoparticulate glasses. These newer materials are more bioactive and resorbable than materials fabricated by "melt-derived" processes. In general, the sol-gel process converts a colloidal liquid, *sol*, into a solid *gel* of particles with entrapped pore liquids. The starting precursors are usually metal organic compounds, or alkoxides $M(OR)_n$— in which M is a metal network former and R is an alkyl group. These liquid precursors are mixed and hydrolyzed. This forms silanol groups that condense to create an interconnected network of siloxane bonds, with water and alcohols as byproducts. Precise control of the synthesis and drying steps results in a final glassy solid with a very large degree of interconnected mesoporosity (pore diameters in the range of 2-50 nm) and high specific surface area. This nanoporous glass is an outstanding matrix for entrapping and adsorbing cytokines and drugs, for example. As the glassy matrix resorbs, these compounds are released in an activated form.

Additionally, these bioactive glasses chemically bond to both hard and soft tissues, and they stimulate the formation of new bone in vivo. Bioactive glasses exchange ions with surrounding fluids within seconds of immersion into the body or media. In brief, the processes on the glass surface are characterized by this rapid ion exchange, followed by dissolution of the glass network and reprecipitation and growth of a silica gel layer on the surface, which in turn precipitates a calcium-deficient carbonate apatite (hydroxyl carbonate apatite, HCA) layer onto its surface. This layer reorganizes and quickly results in the formation of a crystalline HCA layer on the glass surface. As these layers are forming and growing outward from the surface, extracellular proteins become entrapped in the growing layers and invoke subsequent cellular reactions including cell attachment and colonization, proliferation, and differentiation into relevant progenitor cells (Figure 16-9).

The interaction of bioactive glasses with living tissue, in particular forming strong chemical bonds

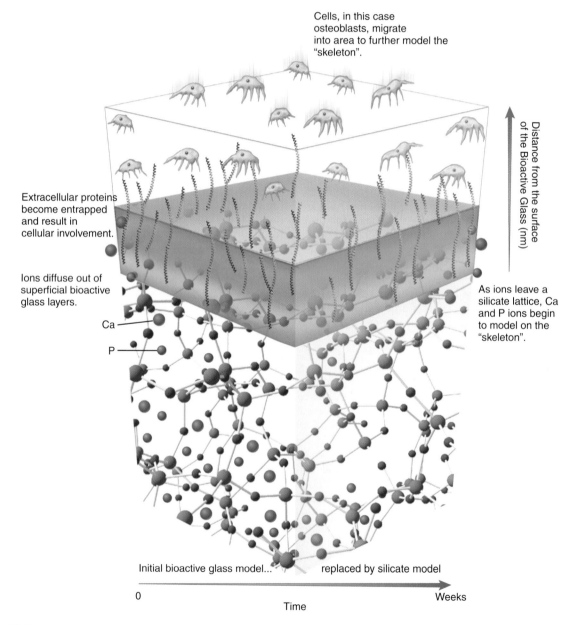

Cells, in this case osteoblasts, migrate into area to further model the "skeleton".

Distance from the surface of the Bioactive Glass (nm)

Extracellular proteins become entrapped and result in cellular involvement.

Ions diffuse out of superficial bioactive glass layers.

As ions leave a silicate lattice, Ca and P ions begin to model on the "skeleton".

Ca

P

Initial bioactive glass model... replaced by silicate model

0   Weeks

Time

FIGURE 16.9 **The in-vivo reactions that occur when a bioactive glass is implanted.** *Ca,* Calcium (green); *P,* phosphorus (purple).

to a tissue, is called *bioreactivity* or *bioactivity*. It is now believed that a biologically induced active apatite surface layer must form at the interface between the material and the bone to create a material bond with bone. In addition, the ionic species released from the reacting glasses up-regulate at least seven families of genes found in mesenchymal cells and osteoblasts.

Polymeric Materials

Polymers are by far the most common materials used for tissue-engineering scaffolds. Polylactic acid and polyglycolic acid (and co-polymers of these two) as well as polycaprolactone are common examples. These polymers are metabolized in vivo, and their acidic degradation products are easily removed from the body. They can easily be cast into a mesh or other desired shape or can simply be extruded as fibers, which are used to loosely pack an anatomically designed mold. The same material from which the scaffold is designed can be used to encapsulate growth factors to provide a timed release of the protein as the capsule degrades. Polymers release acidic and toxic products when they degrade; that creates inflammation around the implantation site. Their survival time in the body is difficult to control, and they become stiff as they degrade.

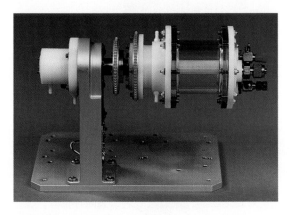

FIGURE 16.10 **Image of National Aeronautics and Space Administration (NASA) bioreactor.** *(Courtesy of NASA/Johnson Space Center, Houston, TX.)*

CELL CULTURE METHODS

Cells can be grown as a monolayer (or sheet) on a polystyrene growth plate treated to optimize cell attachment and proliferation. Culturing cells on three-dimensional scaffolds for later implantation is more difficult. Scaffolds thicker than 1 mm often produce a shell of viable cells and new extracellular matrix surrounding a necrotic core. Some type of perfusion bioreactor system (Figure 16-10) must be used to more closely mimic the mass transport in vivo environment. Alternatively, the tissues can be fabricated in a well-vascularized region, in vivo. This allows a circulatory system to develop along with the cells.

Optimal culture conditions for tissue-engineering scaffolds require high seeding efficiency to minimize growth time and a homogeneous cell distribution in the scaffolds to ensure a uniform, organized tissue. Mechanical loads can improve tissue

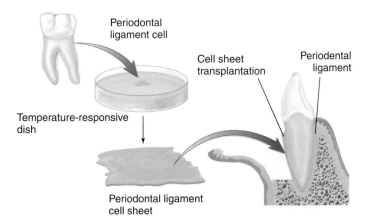

FIGURE 16.11 **One method of periodontal ligament engineering under development.** Periodontal cells are extracted from a patient's tooth and grown on temperature responsive culture plates in vitro. Upon lowering the temperature on these cultures, the confluent layer of cells spontaneously lifts off of the plate as a sheet of cells with intact cell junctions. These sheets are then implanted with various treatments to attempt regeneration of the periodontal tissues. *(Modified from Yamato M, Okano T: Mater. Today. 7, 42, 2004.)*

organization if they are applied to the developing cells as the cells begin to embed themselves within their extracellular matrix. Physiological loads are continually applied to natural tissues during development and use, so some loads applied in vitro begin to prepare the cells and tissues for implantation. Early loading aligns the cells into a stronger, more organized matrix, which in turn creates improved tissue function.

TISSUE-ENGINEERED DENTAL TISSUES

A great amount of research has been done to develop methods for regenerating tooth structure and its supporting tissues. The FDA has already approved two tissue-engineered living skin products and these are commercially available. It is probable that tissue-engineered bone and cartilage will soon follow.

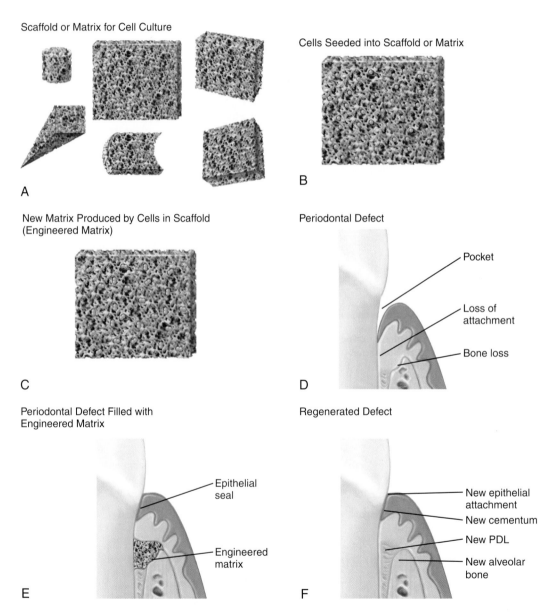

FIGURE 16.12 **A more classical approach to periodontal tissue regeneration being developed. A,** The support scaffold is developed and shaped to the desired geometry. **B,** In this method, cells are again harvested from the patient's periodontal ligament (*PDL*) and seeded into a scaffold, where they are expanded in vitro. **C,** The cells are allowed to grow for a time to allow synthesis of an appropriate matrix for implantation. **D,** A periodontal defect is shown. **E,** The tissue-engineered matrix is implanted into the defect site, leading to a regenerative response. **F,** In this method the fully regenerated periodontal defect is expected to be indistinguishable from other sites in the patient's mouth. (*Modified from Bartold PM, McCulloch CA, Narayanan AS, et al: Periodontology. 24, 253, 2000.*)

Two approaches are being used to fabricate periodontal ligament (PDL). The first harvests existing PDL cells from the patient. The cells are grown and expanded in vitro (Figure 16-11). They are then cultured as a monolayer without any substrate. Once the layer is continuous, with tight intercellular junctions, the sheet of cells is released from the culture plate and placed in situ on the tooth surface to repair the periodontal defect.

The second approach is a cell and scaffold method in which cells are again harvested from the PDL of the patient. The cells are then seeded onto a three-dimensional polymer matrix. This is grown in vitro and eventually implanted back into the patient's periodontal defect (Figure 16-12).

Another oral tissue being targeted by considerable research is a tissue-engineered salivary gland. The technique uses human parotid cells grown in vitro to develop an orally implantable, functioning, fluid-secreting tissue.

Finally, several research groups announced in 2004 that they had succeeded in growing primitive teeth using tissue-engineering methods. They created a tooth-shaped porous scaffold of bioresorbable polymer and seeded it with individual cells taken from a tooth bud. This cell-seeded construct was implanted into the omentum of a rat to provide the fluid and nutrient transfer during growth and development. A mixture of cell types from the tooth bud migrated to the appropriate region during growth, and differentiated to form pulp tissue, dentin, and enamel in the correct anatomical relationships and ratios. Although these initial experiments have only produced teeth that were about 2 mm wide, they have shown that the concept will work to create entire teeth de novo.

SELECTED PROBLEMS

PROBLEM 1

A completely edentulous patient desires to have dental implants placed but does not have sufficient bone height and width to support the implants. What are the types of grafting material currently available to augment the deficient bone? Discuss the merits and limitations of each for this patient.

Solution

Currently, one can use autograft, allograft, xenograft, or alloplast. An autograft is the preferred source because generally ample numbers of cells are present and there is no risk of immunological rejection. However, the limited supply of bone to harvest, especially in an edentulous patient, coupled with additional costs and the risks and discomforts of a second surgical site limit the attractiveness of this source. An allograft has the advantages of normal bone morphology and generally good surgical outcome. However, the risk of disease or viral transmission has caused this option to be unacceptable to many patients. The xenograft has advantages similar to the allograft. However, with the demonstrated possibility of cross-species viral transmission, this technique has also fallen under patient scrutiny. The final option, alloplast grafting, has the advantage of unlimited supply. It does not, however, provide any biological activity and may not provide a suitable geometry for cell growth and resorption.

PROBLEM 2

List and discuss the classes of biomaterials used as tissue-engineering scaffolds.

Solution

The materials are classified as biological materials, ceramic and glass materials, and polymeric materials. Biological materials have two distinct advantages over synthetic materials: (1) they have a geometry already evolved to allow circulation of nutrients to all cells with their structure; and (2) they may contain native cells and proteins, which may be beneficial to the regeneration of the tissue. This latter advantage is also a liability. Considering the possibility that these scaffolds might transmit an undesirable or deadly virus or disease to the implantation site, a nonbiologically derived substrate is desirable. The ceramic and glass materials may be bioactive and form chemical bonds directly with living tissues. They also provide moderate mechanical advantages in compressive load-bearing situations over the other two scaffold classes. However, they generally have limited porosity and are not easily degraded and resorbed in vivo. The final class is the polymers. These materials are relatively easy to fabricate into a desired shape, can be designed to degrade with some degree of predictability, and may serve as a delivery substrate for therapeutic compounds encapsulated within their matrix. However, they are not useful in load-bearing situations and generally cause inflammation during degradation. As such, no one scaffold material type is suitable for all applications.

PROBLEM 3

The use of stem cells is a topic of great controversy in the popular press. Which tissue-engineering strategies make use of implanting these cells and why are these particular cells desired?

Solution

The cell injection method and the method of growing cells within a scaffold matrix both use this type of cell. Stem cells are important because they are capable of migrating within the body, undergo self-replication, and are not terminally differentiated. Stem cells are not committed to becoming any one particular type of cell, so they and their progeny may form any tissue type needed in the body.

Bibliography

Abukawa H, Terai H, Hannouche D, et al: Formation of a mandibular condyle in vitro by tissue engineering, *J Oral Maxillofac Surg* 61:94, 2003.

Aframian DJ, David R, Ben-Bassat H, et al: Characterization of murine autologous salivary gland graft cells: a model for use with an artificial salivary gland, *Tissue Eng* 10:914, 2004.

Agrawal CM, Ray RB: Biodegradable polymeric scaffolds for musculoskeletal tissue engineering, *J Biomed Mater Res* 55:141, 2001.

Almany L, Seliktar D: Biosynthetic hydrogel scaffolds made from fibrinogen and polyethylene glycol for 3D cell cultures, *Biomaterials* 26:2467, 2005.

Al-Salihi KA, Samsudin AR: Bone marrow mesenchymal stem cells differentiation and proliferation on the surface of coral implant, *Med J Malaysia* 59:45, 2004.

Alsberg E, Hill EE, Mooney DJ: Craniofacial tissue engineering, *Crit Rev Oral Biol Med* 12:64, 2001.

Altman GH, Diaz F, Jakuba C, et al: Silk-based biomaterials, *Biomaterials* 24:401, 2003.

Angelini L, Eleuteri E, Coppola M: Surgery in Italy, *Arch Surg* 136:1318, 2001.

Anusaksathien O, Giannobile WV: Growth factor delivery to re-engineer periodontal tissues, *Curr Pharm Biotechnol* 3:129, 2002.

Auger FA, Berthod F, Moulin V, et al: Tissue-engineered skin substitutes: from in vitro constructs to in vivo applications, *Biotechnol Appl Biochem* 39:263, 2004.

Badylak SF: Xenogeneic extracellular matrix as a scaffold for tissue reconstruction, *Transpl Immunol* 12:367, 2004.

Bartold PM, McCulloch CA, Narayanan AS, et al: Tissue engineering: a new paradigm for periodontal regeneration based on molecular and cell biology, *Periodontology* 24:253, 2000.

Baum BJ, Mooney DJ: The impact of tissue engineering on dentistry, *J Am Dent Assoc* 131:309, 2000.

Baum BJ: Prospects for re-engineering salivary glands, *Adv Dent Res* 14:84, 2000.

Beele H: Artificial skin: past, present and future, *Int J Artif Organs* 25:163, 2002.

Bhishagratna KL: *An English translation of the Sushruta Samhita*, Varanasi, India, 1963, Chowkhamba Sanskrit Series Office, Varanasi, pp 352-356.

Blum JS, Barry MA, Mikos AG: Bone regeneration through transplantation of genetically modified cells, *Clin Plast Surg* 30:611, 2003.

Bohl KS, Shon J, Rutherford B, et al: Role of synthetic extracellular matrix in development of engineered dental pulp, *J Biomater Sci Polym Ed* 9:749, 1998.

Bonassar LJ, Vacanti CA: Tissue engineering: the first decade and beyond, *J Cell Biochem Suppl* 30:297, 1998.

Buckley MJ, Agarwal S, Gassner R: Tissue engineering and dentistry, *Clin Plast Surg* 26:657, 1999.

Chai Y, Slavkin HC: Prospects for tooth regeneration in the 21st century: a perspective, *Microsc Res Tech* 60:469, 2003.

Chen FM, Jin Y: Periodontal tissue engineering and regeneration: current approaches and expanding opportunities, *Tissue Eng Part B Rev* 16(2):219–255, 2010.

Cordeiro MM, Dong Z, Kaneko T, et al: Dental pulp tissue engineering with stem cells from exfoliated deciduous teeth, *J Endod* 34:962–969, 2008.

Dard M, Sewing A, Meyer J, et al: Tools for tissue engineering of mineralized oral structures, *Clin Oral Investig* 4:126, 2000.

Demarco FF, Casagrande L, Zhang Z, et al: Effects of morphogen and scaffold porogen on the differentiation of dental pulp stem cells, *J Endod* 36(11):1805–1811, 2010.

Deporter D: Surgical site development in the partially edentulous patient. In Zarb G, Lekholm U, Albrektsson T, et al: *2002. Aging, osteoporosis and dental implants*, Carol Stream, IL, 2002, Quintessence Publishing Co.

Di Silvio L, Gurav N, Sambrook R: The fundamentals of tissue engineering: new scaffolds, *Med J Malaysia* 59:89, 2004.

Du C, Moradian-Oldak J: Tooth regeneration: challenges and opportunities for biomedical material research, *Biomed Mater* 1(1):R10–R17, 2006.

Duailibi MT, Duailibi SE, Young CS, et al: Bioengineered teeth from cultured rat tooth bud cells, *J Dent Res* 83:523, 2004.

Duan X, Tu Q, Zhang J, et al: Application of induced pluripotent stem (iPS) cells in periodontal tissue regeneration, *J Cell Physiol* 226(1):150–157, 2011.

Earthman JC, Sheets CG, Paquette JM, et al: Tissue engineering in dentistry, *Clin Plast Surg* 30:621, 2003.

Giannobile WV: What does the future hold for periodontal tissue engineering? *Int J Periodontics Restorative Dent* 22:6, 2002.

Goldberg M, Smith AJ: Cells and extracellular matrices of dentin and pulp: A biological basis for repair and tissue engineering, *Crit Rev Oral Biol Med* 15:13, 2004.

Gosain AK, Persing JA: Biomaterials in the face: benefits and risks, *J Craniofac Surg* 10:404, 1999.

Gunatillake PA, Adhikari R: Biodegradable synthetic polymers for tissue engineering, *Eur Cell Mater* 20:1, 2003.

Hadlock TA, Vacanti JP, Cheney ML: Tissue engineering in facial plastic and reconstructive surgery, *Facial Plast Surg* 14:197, 1998.

Hollister SJ, Maddox RD, Taboas JM: Optimal design and fabrication of scaffolds to mimic tissue properties and satisfy biological constraints, *Biomaterials* 23:4095, 2002.

Hubbell JA: Biomaterials in tissue engineering, *Bio-technology* 13:565, 1995.

Ikeda H, Sumita Y, Ikeda M, et al: 2001. Engineering bone formation from human dental pulp- and periodontal ligament-derived cells, *Ann Biomed Eng* 39(1):26–34, 2011.

Jin Q, Anusaksathien O, Webb SA, et al: Engineering of tooth-supporting structures by delivery of PDGF gene therapy vectors, *Mol Ther* 9:519, 2004.

Jin QM, Zhao M, Webb SA, et al: Cementum engineering with three-dimensional polymer scaffolds, *J Biomed Mater Res A* 67:54, 2003.

Kaigler D, Mooney D: Tissue engineering's impact on dentistry, *J Dent Educ* 65:456, 2001.

Kim YS, Min KS, Jeong DH, et al: Effects of fibroblast growth factor-2 on the expression and regulation of chemokines in human dental pulp cells, *J Endod* 36(11): 1824–1830, 2010.

Krebsbach PH, Robey PG: Dental and skeletal stem cells: potential cellular therapeutics for craniofacial regeneration, *J Dent Educ* 66:766, 2002.

Kuboki Y, Sasaki M, Saito A, et al: Regeneration of periodontal ligament and cementum by BMP-applied tissue engineering, *Eur J Oral Sci* 106:197, 1998.

Lalan S, Pomerantseva I, Vacanti JP: Tissue engineering and its potential impact on surgery, *World J Surg* 25:1458, 2001.

Langer R: Tissue engineering, *Mol Ther* 1:12, 2001.

Lavik E, Langer R: Tissue engineering: current state and perspectives, *Appl Microbiol Biotechnol* 65:1, 2004.

Lee KY, Mooney DJ: Hydrogels for tissue engineering, *Chem Rev* 101:1869, 2001.

LeGeros RZ: Properties of osteoconductive biomaterials: calcium phosphates, *Clin Orthop* 395:81, 2002.

Lenza RF, Jones JR, Vasconcelos WL, et al: in vitro release kinetics of proteins from bioactive foams, *J Biomed Mater Res A* 1:121, 2003.

Letic-Gavrilovic A, Todorovic L, Abe K: Oral tissue engineering of complex tooth structures on biodegradable DLPLG/beta-TCP scaffolds, *Adv Exp Med Biol* 553:267, 2004.

MacNeil RL, Somerman MJ: Development and regeneration of the periodontium: parallels and contrasts, *Periodontol 2000* 19:8–20, 1999.

Malhotra N, Kundabala M, Acharya S: Current strategies and applications of tissue engineering in dentistry–a review Part 2, *Dent Update* 36(10):639–642, 2009:644–646.

Mantesso A, Sharpe P: Dental stem cells for tooth regeneration and repair, *Expert Opin Biol Ther* 9(9):1143–1154, 2009.

Matalova E, Fleischmannova J, Sharpe PT, et al: Tooth agenesis: from molecular genetics to molecular dentistry, *J Dent Res* 87(7):617–623, 2008.

Miura M, Gronthos S, Zhao M, et al: SHED: stem cells from human exfoliated deciduous teeth, *Proc Natl Acad Sci USA* 100:5807, 2003.

Murphy WL, Mooney DJ: Controlled delivery of inductive proteins, plasmid DNA and cells from tissue engineering matrices, *J Periodontal Res* 34:413, 1999.

Murray PE, Garcia-Godoy F: Stem cell responses in tooth regeneration, *Stem Cells Dev* 13:255, 2004.

Nakahara T, Nakamura T, Kobayashi E, et al: In situ tissue engineering of periodontal tissues by seeding with periodontal ligament-derived cells, *Tissue Eng* 10:537, 2004.

Nakashima M, Reddi AH: The application of bone morphogenetic proteins to dental tissue engineering, *Nat Biotechnol* 21:1025, 2003.

Nör JE: Tooth regeneration in operative dentistry, *Oper Dent* 31(6):633–642, 2006.

Ohazama A, Modino SA, Miletich I, et al: Stem-cell-based tissue engineering of murine teeth, *J Dent Res* 83:518, 2004.

Ohgushi H, Miyake J, Tateishi T: Mesenchymal stem cells and bioceramics: strategies to regenerate the skeleton, *Novartis Found Symp* 249:118, 2003.

Pappalardo S, Carlino V, Brutto D, et al: How do biomaterials affect the biological activities and responses of cells? An in vitro study, *Minerva Stomatol* 59(9):445–464, 2010.

Pradeep AR, Karthikeyan BV: Tissue engineering: prospect for regenerating periodontal tissues, *Indian J Dent Res* 14:224, 2003.

Ratner D: Skin grafting from here to there, *Dermatol Clin* 16:75, 1998.

Ratner BD: Replacing and renewing: synthetic materials, biomimetics, and tissue engineering in implant dentistry, *J Dent Educ* 65:1340, 2001.

Richardson T, Peters M, Ennett A, et al: Polymeric system for dual growth factor delivery, *Nature Biotech* 19:1029, 2001.

Ripamonti U, Reddi AH: Tissue engineering, morphogenesis, and regeneration of the periodontal tissues by bone morphogenetic proteins, *Crit Rev Oral Biol Med* 8:154, 1997.

Saber SE: Tissue engineering in endodontics, *J Oral Sci* 51(4):495–507, 2009.

Salgado AJ, Coutinho OP, Reis RL: Bone tissue engineering: state of the art and future trends, *Macromol Biosci* 9:743, 2004.

Saltzman WM, Olbricht WL: Building drug delivery into tissue engineering, *Nat Rev Drug Discov* 1:177, 2002.

Schmelzeisen R, Schimming R, Sittinger M: Soft tissue and hard tissue engineering in oral and maxillofacial surgery, *Ann R Australas Coll Dent Surg* 16:50, 2002.

Seong JM, Kim BC, Park JH, et al: Stem cells in bone tissue engineering, *Biomed Mater* 5(6):062001, 2010.

Shin H, Jo S, Mikos AG: Biomimetic materials for tissue engineering, *Biomaterials* 24:4353, 2003.

Smith AJ, Lesot H: Induction and regulation of crown dentinogenesis—embryonic events as a template for dental tissue repair, *Crit Rev Oral Biol Med* 12:425–437, 2001.

Smith AJ: Tooth tissue engineering and regeneration—a translational vision, *J Dent Res* 83:517, 2004.

Stock UA, Vacanti JP: Tissue engineering: current state and prospects, *Annu Rev Med* 52:443, 2001.

Thesleff I, Tummers M: Stem cells and tissue engineering: prospects for regenerating tissues in dental practice, *Med Princ Pract* 12:43, 2003.

Ueda M, Tohnai I, Nakai H: Tissue engineering research in oral implant surgery, *Artif Organs* 25:164, 2001.

Vacanti JP, Langer R: Tissue engineering: the design and fabrication of living replacement devices for surgical reconstruction and transplantation, *Lancet* 354:SI32, 1999.

Vacanti CA, Vacanti JP: The science of tissue engineering, *Orthop Clin North Am* 31:351, 2000.

Vunjak-Novakovic G: The fundamentals of tissue engineering: scaffolds and bioreactors, *Novartis Found Symp* 249:34, 2003.

Whitaker MJ, Quirk RA, Howdle SM, et al: Growth factor release from tissue engineering scaffolds, *J Pharm Pharmacol* 53:1427, 2001.

Xu HH, Zhao L, Weir MD: Stem Cell-Calcium Phosphate Constructs for Bone Engineering, *J Dent Res* 89(12): 1482–1488, 2010.

Xue Y, Dånmark S, Xing Z, et al: Growth and differentiation of bone marrow stromal cells on biodegradable polymer scaffolds: An in vitro study, *J Biomed Mater Res A* 95(4):1244–1251, 2010.

Yamato M, Okano T: Cell sheet engineering, *Mater Today* 7:42, 2004.

Yannas IV: Synthesis of tissues and organs, *Chembiochem* 5:26, 2004.

Young CS, Terada S, Vacanti JP, et al: Tissue engineering of complex tooth structures on biodegradable polymer scaffolds, *J Dent Res* 81:695, 2002.

Zaky SH, Cancedda R: Engineering craniofacial structures: facing the challenge, *J Dent Res* 88(12):1077–1091, 2009.

Zhao M, Jin Q, Berry JE, et al: Cementoblast delivery for periodontal tissue engineering, *J Periodontol* 75:154, 2004.

Websites

Organ Procurement and Transplantation Network: *http://optn.transplant.hrsa.gov/*

Center for Biologics Evaluation and Research (CBER): *http://www.fda.gov/BiologicsBloodVaccines/TissueTissue Products/default.htm*

Conversion of Units

This appendix presents several tables that will assist the reader in converting units.

TABLE OF WEIGHTS AND MEASURES

LENGTHS

1 millimeter (mm)	= 0.001 meter	= 0.03937 inch
1 centimeter (cm)	= 0.01 meter	= 0.3937 inch
1 meter (m)		= 39.37 inches
1 yard (yd)	= 0.9144 meter	= 36 inches
1 inch (in)	= 2.54 centimeters	= 25.4 millimeters
1 micrometer (μm)	= 0.001 millimeter	= 0.00003937 inch
1 micrometer (μm)	= 10,000 Angstrom units	
1 Angstrom unit (Å)	= 0.1 nanometer	= $3.937 \times 10-9$ inch
1 nanometer (nm)	= 0.001 micrometer	= 10 Angstrom units

WEIGHTS

1 milligram (mg)	= 0.001 gram	= 0.015 grain
1 gram (g)	= 0.0022 pound	= 15.432 grains
1 gram (g)	= 0.035 ounce	
1 kilogram (kg)	= 1000 grams	= 2.2046 pounds
1 ounce (oz)	= 28.35 grams	
1 pound (lb)	= 453.59 grams	= 16 ounces
1 pennyweight (Troy dwt)	= 1.555 grams	= 24 grains
1 grain (gr)	= 0.0648 gram	

FORCES

1 Newton (N)	= 0.2248 pound force	= 0.102 kilogram force = 100,000 dynes
1 dyne (d)	= 0.00102 gram force	

CAPACITY (LIQUID)

1 milliliter (mL)	= 1 cubic centimeter	= 0.0021 pint
1 liter (L)	= 1000 cubic centimeters	= 1.057 quarts
1 quart (qt)	= 0.946 liter	= 32 ounces
1 ounce (oz)	= 29.6 milliliters	
1 cubic foot (cu ft)	= 28.32 liters	

AREA

sq in (in^2)	sq ft (ft^2)	sq mm (mm^2)	sq cm (cm^2)
1	0.00694	645.16	6.4516
144	1	92,903	929.03
0.00155	0.000011	1	0.01
0.155	0.0011	100	1

VOLUME

cu in (in^3)	cu mm (mm^3)	cu cm (cc, cm^3)
1	16,387	16.387
0.0000610	1	0.001
0.0610	1000	1

NOTE: *1 mL (or cc) of distilled water at 4° C weighs 1 g*

CONVERSION TABLES

CONVERSION FACTORS (LINEAR)

	Millimeters (mm)	Centimeters (cm)	Inches (in)
1 Angstrom unit (Å)	0.0000001	0.00000001	0.000000003937
1 nanometer (nm)	0.000001	0.0000001	0.00000003937
1 micrometer (μm)	0.001	0.0001	0.00003937

CONVERSION FACTORS (FORCE PER AREA)

To change kilograms force per square centimeter (kgf/cm^2) to pounds force per square inch (lbf/in^2), multiply by 14.223 (1 kgf/cm^2 = 14.223 lbf/in^2).

To change kilograms force per square centimeter (kgf/cm^2) to megapascals (MPa), multiply by 0.0981 (1 kgf/cm^2 = 0.0981 MPa). NOTE: 1 MN/m^2 = 1 MPa.

To change kilograms force per square millimeters (kgf/mm^2) to gigapascals (GPa), multiply by 0.00981.

To change pounds force per square inch (lbf/in^2) to megapascals (MPa), multiply by 0.00689.

To change meganewtons force per square meter (MN/m^2) to pounds force per square inch (lbf/in^2), multiply by 145 (1 MN/m^2 = 145 lb/m^2).

To change meganewtons per square meter (MN/m^2) to gigapascals (GPa), divide by 1000.

CONVERSION OF THERMOMETER SCALES

Temperature Fahrenheit (° F) = (⅘ Temperature Celsius) + 32°
Temperature Celsius (° C) = ⅚ (Temperature Fahrenheit – 32°)
    or

$$(°C \times 1.8) + 32° = °F$$

$$(°F - 32°) / 1.8 = °C$$

CONVERSION FACTORS (MISCELLANEOUS)

1 foot-pound (ft-lb) = 13,826 gram-centimeters = 1.356 Newton-meters
1 radian = 57.3 degrees
1 watt = 14.3 calories/minute

CONVERSION OF EXPONENTIALS TO DECIMALS

Exponential no.	Decimal no.
1×10^{-5} (or 10^{-5})	0.00001
1×10^{-3}	0.001
1×10^{-1}	0.1
1×10^{0} (or 10^{0})	1
1×10^{1}	10
1×10^{4}	10,000
1×10^{7} (or 10^{7})	10,000,000

COMPARATIVE TABLE OF TROY, AVOIRDUPOIS, AND METRIC WEIGHTS

Grain	Troy dwt	Troy oz	Avoirdupois oz	Avoirdupois lb	Gram g
1	0.042	0.002	0.00228	0.00014	0.065
24	1	0.05	0.0548	0.0034	1.555
480	20	1	1.097	0.0686	31.10
437.5	18.23	0.91	1	0.063	28.35
7000	291.67	14.58	16	1	453.59
15.43	0.64	0.032	0.035	0.0022	1

PREFIXES AND SYMBOLS FOR EXPONENTIAL NUMBERS

Factor	Prefix	Symbol
10^{18}	exa	E
10^{15}	peta	P
10^{12}	tera	T
10^{9}	giga	G
10^{6}	mega	M
10^{3}	kilo	k
10^{2}	hecto	h
10	deca	da
10^{-1}	deci	d
10^{-2}	centi	c
10^{-3}	milli	m
10^{-6}	micro	μ
10^{-9}	nano	n
10^{-12}	pico	p
10^{-15}	femto	f
10^{-18}	atto	a

Index

Page references followed by "f" indicate figure, by "b" indicate box, and by "t" indicate table.